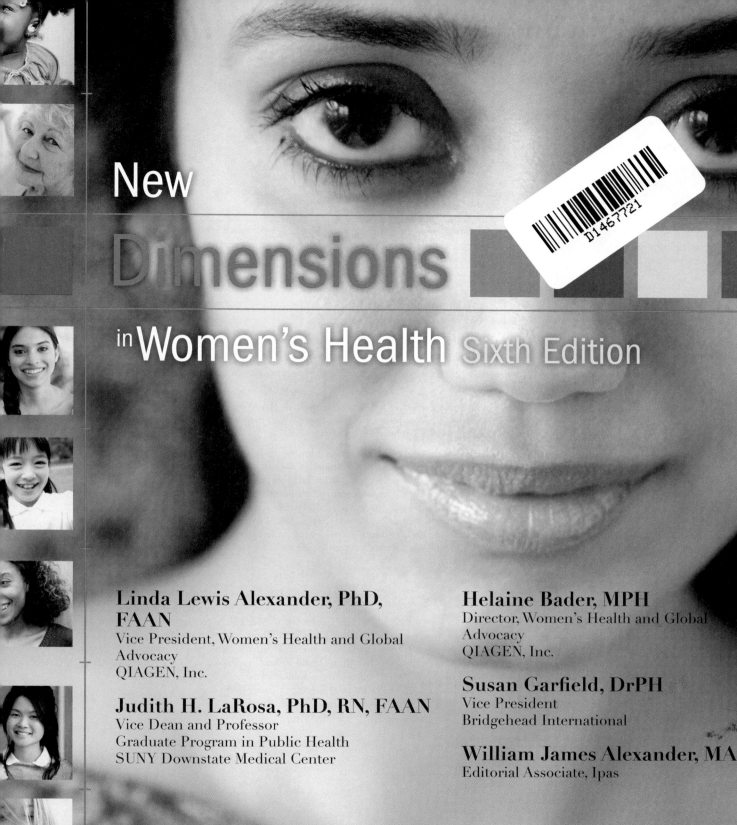

New
Dimensions
in Women's Health Sixth Edition

Linda Lewis Alexander, PhD, FAAN
Vice President, Women's Health and Global Advocacy
QIAGEN, Inc.

Judith H. LaRosa, PhD, RN, FAAN
Vice Dean and Professor
Graduate Program in Public Health
SUNY Downstate Medical Center

Helaine Bader, MPH
Director, Women's Health and Global Advocacy
QIAGEN, Inc.

Susan Garfield, DrPH
Vice President
Bridgehead International

William James Alexander, MA
Editorial Associate, Ipas

JONES & BARTLETT
LEARNING

World Headquarters
Jones & Bartlett Learning
5 Wall Street
Burlington, MA 01803
978-443-5000
info@jblearning.com
www.jblearning.com

Jones & Bartlett Learning books and products are available through most bookstores and online booksellers. To contact Jones & Bartlett Learning directly, call 800-832-0034, fax 978-443-8000, or visit our website, www.jblearning.com.

Substantial discounts on bulk quantities of Jones & Bartlett Learning publications are available to corporations, professional associations, and other qualified organizations. For details and specific discount information, contact the special sales department at Jones & Bartlett Learning via the above contact information or send an email to specialsales@jblearning.com.

New Dimensions in Women's Health, Sixth Edition is an independent publication and has not been authorized, sponsored, or otherwise approved by the owners of the trademarks or service marks referenced in this product.

Some images in this book feature models. These models do not necessarily endorse, represent, or participate in the activities represented in the images.

The screenshots in this product are for educational and instructive purposes only. All trademarks displayed are the trademarks of the parties noted therein. Such use of trademarks is not an endorsement by said parties of Jones & Bartlett Learning, its products, or its services, nor should such use be deemed an endorsement by Jones & Bartlett Learning of said third party's products or services.

The authors, editor, and publisher have made every effort to provide accurate information. However, they are not responsible for errors, omissions, or for any outcomes related to the use of the contents of this book and take no responsibility for the use of the products and procedures described. Treatments and side effects described in this book may not be applicable to all people; likewise, some people may require a dose or experience a side effect that is not described herein. Drugs and medical devices are discussed that may have limited availability controlled by the Food and Drug Administration (FDA) for use only in a research study or clinical trial. Research, clinical practice, and government regulations often change the accepted standard in this field. When consideration is being given to use of any drug in the clinical setting, the health care provider or reader is responsible for determining FDA status of the drug, reading the package insert, and reviewing prescribing information for the most up-to-date recommendations on dose, precautions, and contraindications, and determining the appropriate usage for the product. This is especially important in the case of drugs that are new or seldom used.

Production Credits

Publisher: William Brottmiller
Executive Editor: Cathy L. Esperti
Senior Editorial Assistant: Sean Coombs
Production Editor: Cindie Bryan
Senior Marketing Manager: Andrea DeFronzo
V.P., Manufacturing and Inventory Control: Therese Connell
Composition: Publishers' Design and Production Services, Inc.
Cover Design: Kristin E. Parker
Director of Photo Research and Permissions: Amy Wrynn
Rights & Photo Research Intern: Shaun Steele

Cover Images: (main) © Jupiterimages/Brand X Pictures/Thinkstock; (side images top to bottom) © Image Source/Thinkstock, © Pixland/Thinkstock, © Maria Teijeiro/Photodisc/Thinkstock, © TongRo Image Stock/Thinkstock, © Jupiterimages/Creatas/Getty Images/Thinkstock, © Ingram Publishing/Thinkstock, © Thomas Northcut/Digital Vision/Thinkstock, © Ryan McVay/Photodisc/Getty Images/Thinkstock
Printing and Binding: Courier Companies
Cover Printing: Courier Companies

To order this product, use ISBN: 1-978-1-4496-9813-3

Library of Congress Cataloging-in-Publication Data
New dimensions in women's health / Linda Lewis Alexander . . . [et al.]. — 6th ed.
   p. ; cm.
  Includes bibliographical references and index.
  ISBN 978-1-4496-8375-7 (pbk.) — ISBN 1-4496-8375-4 (pbk.)
  I. Alexander, Linda Lewis.
  [DNLM: 1. Women's Health—United States.   WA 309 AA1]
  613'.04244—dc23
   2012039314

6048

Printed in the United States of America
17   16   15   14   13   10 9 8 7 6 5 4 3

BRIEF CONTENTS

CONTENTS

The sixth edition of *New Dimensions in Women's Health* discusses health issues that affect all women: women of all racial and ethnic groups, of all ages, of different sexual orientations, and with various degrees of physical ability. The text presents unbiased, accurate information free from any specific political agenda while allowing its readers to appreciate the range of perspectives that influence how women in the United States and around the world think about health and make decisions that affect their well-being. *New Dimensions in Women's Health* discusses prevention, health promotion, research, clinical intervention, and public policy as well as how these factors affect the rate of different diseases, disorders, and conditions that afflict women. This book is written for women, recognizing their outstanding contributions as daughters, sisters, mothers, nurses, doctors, scientists, laborers, advocates, and much more.

Organization of the Book

This book is organized into four parts, each of which covers a different dimension of women's health.

Part One, Foundations of Women's Health, takes a population-based approach. It introduces students to the concepts of women's health, public health, health economics, and issues of health across the lifespan. Chapter 1 provides a brief history of the women's health movement and the political climate around women's health. Chapter 2 is focuses on the economics of health, including the payer system in the United States, various insurance plans, healthcare reform, and the impact on the aging population. Chapter 3 introduces the concepts of health promotion and disease prevention and discusses how these efforts benefit women through the different stages of life.

Part Two, Sexual and Reproductive Dimensions of Women's Health, addresses issues regarding sexual health and sexuality, as well as sexual violence as a public health problem. Chapter 4 defines sexual health and discusses the cultural, economic, and biological factors that influence women's sexual health. Chapter 5 discusses contraceptive methods, abortion, and provides information that will help inform a woman's decision around reproduction.

Building on this, Chapter 6 covers pregnancy, childbirth, breastfeeding, and infertility. Chapter 7 is devoted to the clinical, sociological, and epidemiological dimensions and treatment issues of sexually transmitted infections, including HIV/AIDS. In Chapter 8, menopause is explored as a biological and cultural phenomenon, and the benefits, drawbacks, and effects of hormone replacement therapy are discussed.

Part Three, Physical and Lifespan Dimensions of Women's Health, comprises Chapters 9 through 12. Chapter 9 discusses exercise, nutrition, and weight management. Chapter 10 examines how cardiovascular disease and cancer affect women as well as how these diseases progress and can be prevented, treated, and managed. Chapter 11 discusses other chronic diseases important to women's health, including osteoporosis, arthritis, diabetes, autoimmune diseases, and Alzheimer's disease. Chapter 12 offers definitions of mental health and mental illness, explores the reasons why good mental health is essential, and provides information on various mental disorders.

The final section, Interpersonal and Social Dimensions of Women's Health, opens with Chapter 13, which discusses substance use and abuse of both legal and illegal drugs. Chapter 14 provides different perspectives on violence, abuse, and harassment, while Chapter 15 discusses current trends and issues for women in the workforce.

New to This Edition

The sixth edition of *New Dimensions in Women's Health* has been expanded, updated, and revised. It presents the most current, accurate, and relevant women's health information in an organized, easily understood manner. New features to this edition include:

- Major content updates for Chapters 2, 3, 5, 6, and 7
- New material discussing healthcare reform and its implications for individual women and the country as a whole
- Expanded discussions of women's health from a global perspective, with discussions of how women's health

issues in developing countries, Canada and Europe compare to those in the United States

- New and expanded information on testing and prevention for sexually transmitted infections, including the HPV vaccination

- New quotes from women of all ages and backgrounds discussing their feelings and experiences dealing with anorexia, hormone replacement therapy, birth control, and other issues

The most current guidelines, surveillance, and statistics are included in every chapter. Highlights include:

- The 2010 Dietary Guidelines for Americans

- Revised WHO and CDC estimates for the global and national incidence and prevalence of chronic and infectious diseases

- Updated Youth Risk Behavior Survey data on teenage women's eating habits, physical activity levels, alcohol and tobacco use, and other factors

Features of This Text

Each chapter reviews an important aspect of women's general health and examines how epidemiological, historical, psychosocial, cultural, ethnic, legal, political, and economic influences shape that topic. *New Dimensions in Women's Health* also discusses how age, ethnicity and race, sexual orientation, and other factors influence women's needs. In addition, special features distributed throughout each chapter highlight and summarize important concepts and promote healthy lifestyle choices:

- **It's Your Health** highlights key facts that help readers improve their own health, such as disease symptoms, screening recommendations, and benefits of healthy behaviors.

- **Informed Decision Making** provides students with detailed information for making appropriate decisions regarding their health and well-being.

- **Self-Assessments** provide exercises to help students determine their risk of disease and need for modifying behaviors.

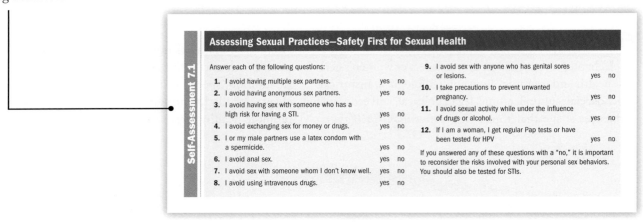

Assessing Sexual Practices—Safety First for Sexual Health

Self-Assessment 7.1

Answer each of the following questions:

1. I avoid having multiple sex partners.   yes   no
2. I avoid having anonymous sex partners.   yes   no
3. I avoid having sex with someone who has a high risk for having a STI.   yes   no
4. I avoid exchanging sex for money or drugs.   yes   no
5. I or my male partners use a latex condom with a spermicide.   yes   no
6. I avoid anal sex.   yes   no
7. I avoid sex with someone whom I don't know well.   yes   no
8. I avoid using intravenous drugs.   yes   no

9. I avoid sex with anyone who has genital sores or lesions.   yes   no
10. I take precautions to prevent unwanted pregnancy.   yes   no
11. I avoid sexual activity while under the influence of drugs or alcohol.   yes   no
12. If I am a woman, I get regular Pap tests or have been tested for HPV   yes   no

If you answered any of these questions with a "no," it is important to reconsider the risks involved with your personal sex behaviors. You should also be tested for STIs.

- **Gender Dimensions** discuss how specific health issues, ranging from breast cancer to obesity, vary between the genders.

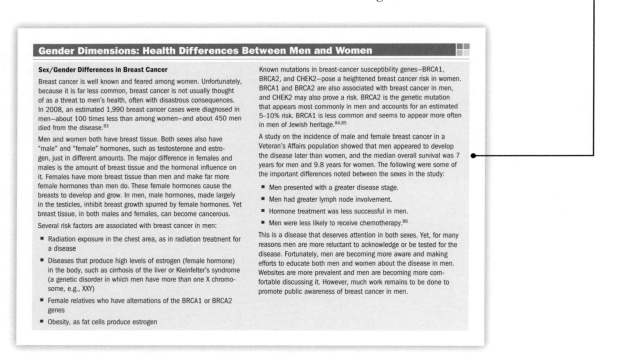

Gender Dimensions: Health Differences Between Men and Women

Sex/Gender Differences in Breast Cancer

Breast cancer is well known and feared among women. Unfortunately, because it is far less common, breast cancer is not usually thought of as a threat to men's health, often with disastrous consequences. In 2008, an estimated 1,990 breast cancer cases were diagnosed in men—about 100 times less than among women—and about 450 men died from the disease.[83]

Men and women both have breast tissue. Both sexes also have "male" and "female" hormones, such as testosterone and estrogen, just in different amounts. The major difference in females and males is the amount of breast tissue and the hormonal influence on it. Females have more breast tissue than men and make far more female hormones than men do. These female hormones cause the breasts to develop and grow. In men, male hormones, made largely in the testicles, inhibit breast growth spurred by female hormones. Yet breast tissue, in both males and females, can become cancerous.

Several risk factors are associated with breast cancer in men:

- Radiation exposure in the chest area, as in radiation treatment for a disease
- Diseases that produce high levels of estrogen (female hormone) in the body, such as cirrhosis of the liver or Kleinfelter's syndrome (a genetic disorder in which men have more than one X chromosome, e.g., XXY)
- Female relatives who have alternations of the BRCA1 or BRCA2 genes
- Obesity, as fat cells produce estrogen

Known mutations in breast-cancer susceptibility genes—BRCA1, BRCA2, and CHEK2—pose a heightened breast cancer risk in women. BRCA1 and BRCA2 are also associated with breast cancer in men, and CHEK2 may also prove a risk. BRCA2 is the genetic mutation that appears most commonly in men and accounts for an estimated 5–10% risk. BRCA1 is less common and seems to appear more often in men of Jewish heritage.[84,85]

A study on the incidence of male and female breast cancer in a Veteran's Affairs population showed that men appeared to develop the disease later than women, and the median overall survival was 7 years for men and 9.8 years for women. The following were some of the important differences noted between the sexes in the study:

- Men presented with a greater disease stage.
- Men had greater lymph node involvement.
- Hormone treatment was less successful in men.
- Men were less likely to receive chemotherapy.[86]

This is a disease that deserves attention in both sexes. Yet, for many reasons men are more reluctant to acknowledge or be tested for the disease. Fortunately, men are becoming more aware and making efforts to educate both men and women about the disease in men. Websites are more prevalent and men are becoming more comfortable discussing it. However, much work remains to be done to promote public awareness of breast cancer in men.

- **Quotes** offer students experiences, opinions, and thoughts from women of all ages, races, and cultures.

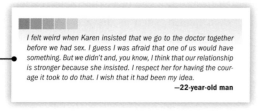

I felt weird when Karen insisted that we go to the doctor together before we had sex. I guess I was afraid that one of us would have something. But we didn't and, you know, I think that our relationship is stronger because she insisted. I respect her for having the courage it took to do that. I wish that it had been my idea.

—22-year-old man

▪ **Profiles of Remarkable Women** highlight individuals who contributed to the health and well-being of all women. These profiles showcase women as champions of health across all ages and life spans.

Profiles of Remarkable Women

Michelle Obama (1964–)

Michelle Obama is a lawyer, community activist, a mother of two, and the husband of the 44th U.S. President, Barack Obama. Since becoming the First Lady of the United States in 2008, she has been a strong advocate for a balanced diet and physical fitness. In 2010, she launched a national initiative, *Let's Move!*, to reduce and prevent childhood obesity and improve the health of American children. *Let's Move* takes a multipronged approach by working to improve access to healthful, affordable foods; increase children's physical activity; provide healthful foods in school;, and educate and empower parents and guardians.

Mrs. Obama was born and raised in Chicago as the second of two children of Marian and Fraser Robinson. She was an excellent student and went on to study sociology in Princeton, and then law at Harvard Law School. She joined Sidley Austin, a Chicago law firm and met her future husband when she was assigned to be his mentor. Mrs. Obama left Sidley Austin in 1991 to work for the government of Chicago and to direct a Chicago nonprofit that encouraged young people to become socially active and participate in public service. Mr. and Mrs. Obama were married in 1992.

From 1996 to 2002, Mrs. Obama worked for the University of Chicago, where she helped build the University's Community Service Center. She later worked for the University of Chicago hospitals and the University of Chicago Medical Center. Mrs. Obama continued to work part-time while she raised their two daughters, Sasha and Malia, and to help with her husband's Senate, and later, Presidential campaigns.

In addition to working to improve children's physical fitness, Mrs. Obama works to help support military families, promote national service, help women balance career goals and family aspirations, and encourage education in the arts.

Topics for Discussion

1. How well do your eating habits compare to those outlined in the *2010 Dietary Guidelines for Americans*? What patterns are healthful, and what patterns could use improvement?

2. How does the modern American lifestyle make getting regular physical activity and a balanced diet difficult? What are some ways to overcome these challenges?

3. Women who are physically active are healthier and therefore at lower risk of chronic disease and early mortality than those who are inactive. Should they have to pay the same insurance rates as those women whose lifestyles place them at greater risk for illness? If so, how should insurance policies be implemented to be fair and accurate?

▪ **Topics for Discussion** at the end of each chapter encourage students to consider their own opinions on a topic and to explore the philosophical dimensions surrounding issues of women's health.

▪ A list of **websites** at the end of each chapter enables students to further explore topics of interest.

Ancillary Material

New Dimensions in Women's Health, Sixth Edition includes learning tools for students and teaching tools for instructors. The companion website (**go.jblearning.com/Alexander6e**) offers flashcards, chapter outlines, crossword puzzles, an interactive glossary, practice quizzes, self-assessments, and Web exercises designed to help students learn to evaluate health information found on the Web.

For instructors teaching this course, an instructor's manual, PowerPoint Lecture Outlines and a TestBank are available as secure downloads.

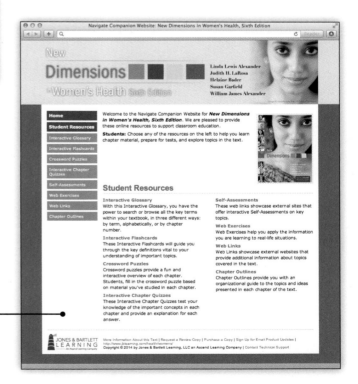

ACKNOWLEDGMENTS

This sixth edition of *New Dimensions in Women's Health* builds on the success of all previous editions. The authors remain indebted to family and friends for their support, guidance, patience, and sacrifices as we dissected and reconstructed the entire text again. Lastly, we'd like to acknowledge and remember the following remarkable women: Elizabeth Bennett, EdD, RN (1926–1998), Gail Addlestone, MD (1969–2007), and Lucille Dorey Lewis (1915–1993).

We also thank the reviewers of the *Sixth Edition* for their valuable suggestions:

Andrea Hope, EdD, Assistant Professor, Monmouth University

Francoise Grossmann, Tulane University

Julie Williams Merten, MSH, MCHES, University of North Florida

Kim A. Sleder, MPH, Long Beach City College

Patricia Kelley RN, MSN, BC, Clinical Instructor, Nursing, North Carolina A&T State University

Linda Lewis Alexander, PhD, FAAN

Linda Alexander recently retired as VP, Women's Health and Global Advocacy at QIAGEN Corporation. Her previous professional positions included VP, Women's Health at Digene Corporation, President/CEO of the American Social Health Association, and VP at United Information Systems. She is also a retired lieutenant colonel, with the U.S. Army Nurse Corps and has held faculty positions at the Uniformed Services University of Health Sciences and the University of Maryland. She currently serves as Chair, Board of Directors, for Women Deliver, an international NGO dedicated to resolving the disparity in health needs among women throughout the world.

Dr. Alexander is nationally known for her leadership in women's health advocacy and has published extensively on women's health issues. Her many honors include appointments to national advisory panels on infectious diseases and women's health; she is also a fellow in the American Academy of Nursing. Dr. Alexander holds a baccalaureate degree in nursing, master's degrees in education/counseling and community health, and a doctoral degree in health education.

Judith H. LaRosa, PhD, RN, FAAN

Dr. Judith LaRosa's career has spanned education, research, clinical practice, and administration. Her present position is Vice Dean and Professor, State University of New York (SUNY) Downstate School of Public Health, where her current research focus is on cultural perceptions of health and disease. She is currently on the editorial board of the *Journal of Community Health* and she serves on the board of the Bedford Stuyvesant Family Health Center—a federally qualified health center.

Before this, Dr. LaRosa served as Professor and Chair, Department of Community Health Sciences, Tulane University School of Public Health and Tropical Medicine, and Director, Tulane Xavier National Center of Excellence in Women's Health. From 1991 to 1994, she served as the first Deputy Director of the Office of Research on Women's Health, National Institutes of Health (NIH). She is a co-author of the legislatively mandated 1994 Guidelines on the Inclusion of Women and Minorities as Subjects in Clinical Research. From 1978 to1991, Dr. LaRosa served at the NIH's National Heart, Lung, and Blood Institute (NHLBI) as the first coordinator of the NHLBI Workplace Initiative in cardiovascular disease risk factor reduction.

Dr. LaRosa has served on the Institute of Medicine's Committee on Understanding the Biology of Sex and gender as well as the Committee on Assessing the Medical Risks of Human Oocyte Donation for Stem Cell Research; the National Institute for Nursing Research Advisory Council; the Armed Forces Epidemiological Board; and the National Science Foundation/Institute of Medicine Committee on Defense Women's Health Research. Dr. LaRosa received her Bachelor of Science degree in nursing and her Master of Nursing Education degree from the University of Pittsburgh and her PhD in health education from the University of Maryland.

Helaine Bader, MPH

A global health advocacy and education consultant with a focus in women's health. She is passionate about helping people understand how to prevent disease, have healthy lives, and become advocates for their own health. Working with nonprofit organizations, corporations, academic institutions, and individuals, she brings groups together to tackle issues through collective action. Previously, Ms. Bader was responsible for corporate relations at a global maternal health organization, where she helped bring the private sector into the conversation around the Millennium Development Goals. In her prior position as Director, Women's Health and Global Advocacy at QIAGEN, Inc., she developed and implemented partnerships and educational initiatives with the NGO community. She also worked on increasing access to cervical cancer screening in low-income countries.

Ms. Bader also worked for GlaxoSmithKline, where she was responsible for media relations and community outreach within the Cardiovascular and Urology Center for Excellence in Drug Discovery. Ms. Bader has more than 20 years of experience in women's health research, health communications, and health education. She has worked on multimedia and Web-based health campaigns in both the public and private sectors and has developed, implemented, and evaluated health education projects for various issues affecting women and children. Ms. Bader received her baccalaureate degree in English with a minor in premedical sciences from the University of Pennsylvania and her master's degree in public health from University of Pittsburgh.

Susan Garfield, DrPH

Susan Garfield is a market access, reimbursement and economics strategist, with an expertise in demand creation and advocacy. For fifteen years, her professional career has focused on innovations in healthcare, the economics of practice change, and the role of reimbursement and policy to the adoption of new technologies. Dr. Garfield's work has included economic modeling, coding analyses and applications, payer coverage campaigns, market strategies for innovative technologies, health policy development, government relations, and creating partnerships between industry and advocacy groups.

Currently, she is Vice President GfK Bridgehead a division of GfK Healthcare. Gfk Bridgehead is a market leading health care consultancy focusing on the market access needs of biotech, medical device, diagnostic, specialty, and pharmaceutical clients. Prior to joining GfK Bridgehead, Dr. Garfield was the Director, Global Reimbursement, Policy and Economic Strategy at QIAGEN Corporation (formally Digene Corporation). In this role, she planned and executed a reimbursement strategy that resulted in near universal coverage for the company's leading cancer diagnostic product. In addition, she directed global economic and pricing analyses for the company's clinical diagnostic portfolio.

Dr. Garfield received her Bachelors of Art in English and Women's Studies from the University of Pennsylvania, a Master's of Science in Population and Development from the London School of Economics, and a Master's of Science in Health Policy and Management from Harvard University, School of Public Health, and her Doctorate of Public Health from Boston University.

William Alexander, MA

William Alexander is a medical and science writer focusing on women's health and global public health. He currently works as a writer for the Duke University School of Medicine, where he writes online, interactive lessons on health and wellness.

Before joining Duke University, Mr. Alexander worked at TCL Institute, a private medical education company. He also worked at Ipas, an international nonprofit organization dealing with women's reproductive health, and MEASURE Evaluation, a global organization that helps USAID-funded countries improve their systems to confront disease, population issues, and poverty. He has also written for the North Carolina Department of Health and Human Services, Escapist Magazine, the Embassy of Kazakhstan, the American Social Health Association and other organizations.

Mr. Alexander received his baccalaureate degree in English from St. Mary's College of Maryland and his master's degree in medical and science journalism from UNC-Chapel Hill.

Part One

Foundations of Women's Health

1

Chapter One

Introduction to Women's Health

Chapter Objectives

On completion of this chapter, the student should be able to discuss:

1. Major ways of thinking about and defining women's health.

2. How the women's health movement has grown and changed over the past 200 years.

3. The government's role in protecting and promoting the health of the public.

4. The responsibilities of the National Institutes of Health and the Office of Research on Women's Health.

5. The federal government's role in funding and conducting research on women's health.

6. The importance of investing in biomedical research and the inclusion of women and minorities in research studies.

7. The concept of gender-based research and basic health differences between women and men.

8. Reproductive rights, the global gag rule, and the effects that restricting abortion has on global health.

9. How lack of access to health care, lack of health insurance, cultural insensitivity, and other obstacles affect the health of women.

10. The need to train health professionals about women's health and cultural sensitivity.

11. Global efforts to support women's health and gender equity.

womenshealth.jbpub.com

Women's Health Online is a great source for supplementary women's health information for both students and instructors. Visit

http://womenshealth.jbpub.com

to find a variety of useful tools for learning, thinking, and teaching.

Introduction

Women's health is a fascinatingly complex area of study. Thousands, even millions, of factors affect the ways women develop, get sick, get well, interact with others, reproduce, age, and receive health care. Some books on women's health attempt to provide a deep but narrow level of detail by focusing on a few of these factors. This book, however, attempts to explore, or at least introduce, the significant facets of women's health from many different angles. The following paragraphs describe areas of concern and ways of thinking about women's health and well-being that are included in the following 15 chapters.

Women's health includes the study of the whole body. Women's health examines biological characteristics unique to women, the most obvious being the reproductive organs, but also differences in body structure, childhood development, hormones, and brain chemistry. Yet women's health is also concerned with factors that affect both genders, including the common cold, heart disease, depression, and the benefits of regular physical exercise. Women's health includes the study of disease, but it also examines factors that affect a woman's physical and mental well-being.

Women's health can study populations or an individual woman. Women's health benefits from examining patterns of health and disease in populations—for example, whether women who are exposed to secondhand cigarette smoke have a greater risk for developing lung cancer than women who are not. But women's health also includes the study of how diseases affect individuals, such as ways a woman can reduce her personal risk of getting cancer; what the signs, effects, and treatments of cancer are for an individual woman who has it; how that woman's unique body acts and reacts to disease; and how a woman copes after being diagnosed.

The entire spectrum of research and social sciences can provide insight into women's health. A full understanding of women's sexual and reproductive health requires biological, cultural, historical, psychological, and political perspectives. The physical components of the reproductive system influence a woman's sexual response, but so do cultural mores and traditions that dictate when and how women are supposed to enjoy and think about their sexuality. Women's health includes reproductive health, defined as the well-being of a person's reproductive system, including their ability to decide if and when to have children.[1] Studying reproductive health requires examining the laws, practices, and cultural beliefs that influence when and where women learn about childbirth, family planning,

and birth control, and their legal options for ending a pregnancy. Because women's unequal treatment affects their well-being and lives in many ways, **feminism**—the idea that women should have the same political, economic, and social rights and opportunities as men—is also an important part of women's health. Not all women become mothers, but because all mothers are women, women's health also includes studying pregnancy, fetal development, and mother–infant interactions.

Finally, society and culture also influence women's health. Women's place in society affects if and how often rape, sexual harassment, and other forms of sexual violence occur. Sociocultural factors also influence where and when women can enter the workforce, as well as what sort of workplace they encounter. Women's health includes women's ability to get and benefit from health care. The study of access to health care has increased dramatically over the past 20 years. Access to health care not only includes whether women can physically get to a doctor or healthcare provider, but also whether they trust that provider, whether they have insurance or some other way to pay for health care, and whether they know if and when something is wrong. Access to health care and healthcare decision making is especially important for women's health, because women are more likely than men to make decisions regarding health care for their relatives and families.

Historical Dimensions: The Women's Health Movement

The past 200 years have seen enormous improvements in women's health, political and economic rights, and place in society. The following section provides a brief history of the women's health movement and advances in women's health in the United States.

Reductions in morbidity and mortality—or injuries and deaths resulting from pregnancy and childbirth—are one of the most important human achievements over the past 200 years. Until the late 1800s, rates of maternal death in the United States and Europe ranged from 25/1000 to 85/1000.[2] This means women had a 2.5% to 8.5% chance of dying every time they gave birth. Without access to family planning, the large family sizes that were often the norm made childbirth a major cause of death for women.

Today, the maternal mortality rate in the United States is about 13/1000, (1.3%), less than half of what they were in the 19th century. Maternal mortality rates are even lower throughout most of Western Europe. Rates of infant mortality have fallen even more dramatically.

In the late 1800s, anywhere between 10% and 25% of infants died either during or shortly after childbirth in Europe and the United States.[3] Today, just 0.7% of U.S. infants die during or shortly after childbirth. The medical advances that allowed these changes include the knowledge of germ theory, which helped reduce infections during childbirth; improved birthing assistance techniques from doctors and midwives; access to basic medical care during childbirth; and access to family planning services.

Women's political and economic rights have also grown enormously since the 1800s. In the early 19th century, women had no rights to vote and were legally restricted to a small number of professions, most of them low paying and menial in nature. Women could not legally attend college, and rarely had the opportunity to complete a high school education. Methods of birth control such as condoms and diaphragms existed, but they were illegal and difficult to obtain. The legal system also limited how and when women could own property, the circumstances under which they could marry and get divorced, and many other areas of women's legal life. While there are still opportunities for improving women's health and for ending existing sources of discrimination, women today can be grateful for the advances made by previous generations of women (and men) to advance women's health.

1830s and 1840s: The Health Movement

Many historians believe the women's health movement began in the 1830s and 1840s, when small groups of women began advocating taking an active role in preventing disease and staying healthy, rather than relying on formally trained physicians for treatment. This first wave of advocacy focused on eating a proper diet, the elimination of the **corset**, and periodic sexual abstinence in marriage to control family size. For the first time, a few middle-class women who became interested in their own health sought entry into the medical profession. Elizabeth Blackwell, for example, entered medical school in 1847 and prompted the opening of several medical schools for women. In 1848, the first women's rights convention was held in Seneca Falls, New York; the convention marked the official beginning of the women's rights movement.

1861–1865: The Civil War

The Civil War prompted many women to volunteer as doctors and nurses; some women even disguised themselves as men to tend to wounded soldiers on the battlefield. Dorothea Dix and Clara Barton led a national effort to organize a nursing corps to care for the war's wounded and sick.

Women's participation in the war led to the opening of the first training schools for nurses in 1873; by 1890, 35 such schools existed. Although this trend represented advancement for women, the relationship between male doctors and female nurses mirrored the domestic sexual division of labor, with males as the authority figures and females as the subordinates.

Mid- to Late-1800s: The Women's Medical Movement

After the Civil War, educational and employment opportunities, though still severely limited, increased for women. The women's medical movement emerged from the growing numbers of women attending medical schools, their struggles to achieve equal status within the profession, and the popularity of challenging historical notions regarding women's fragility.

■ During the Popular Health Movement, women were encouraged to eliminate the corset. Corsets were worn as an undergarment or outergarment to support and shape the waistline, hips, and breasts.

© Index Stock/age fotostock

■ Elizabeth Blackwell was responsible for the opening of several medical schools for women in the mid-1800s.

© National Library of Medicine

My grandmother was a physician at a time when all of her peers were men. I have always admired her but now that I have reached the same age as she was when she started her practice, I have a better understanding of the challenges she must have faced at my age in her time.

—24-year-old woman

1890s–1920s: The Progressive Era

The women's medical movement gave way to the Progressive Era, which advanced the roles of women and women's rights as well as women's health. In 1920, the 19th Amendment to the U.S. Constitution, which guaranteed women the right to vote, was ratified. A few years later, the National Women's Party, formed in 1917, proposed the Equal Rights Amendment, which to this day remains unratified (see **It's Your Health**).

During this time, Margaret Sanger and other activists pushed to legalize birth control. In 1916, Sanger opened the nation's first birth control clinic in Brooklyn and was arrested shortly afterward for violating a federal ban on contraception. Sanger was found guilty and sentenced to 30 days' labor; however, in an appeal, a judge legalized contraception—but only to married couples with a doctor's prescription. Other progressives worked to promote healthy motherhood through prenatal care and child health services. The Sheppard–Towner Act of 1921 greatly increased the availability of prenatal and child health care, especially in rural areas where care was scarce. This legislation provided federal funding for programs that opened clinics for women and children, educated women about pregnancy and childbirth, and trained midwives and physicians about childbirth. The Act lasted until 1929, when a conservative Congress refused to continue its funding.

It's Your Health

Equal Rights Amendment

The Equal Rights Amendment was written in 1921 by **suffragist** Alice Paul. Although it passed both houses of Congress in 1972, it was not ratified by enough state legislatures to be added to the Constitution.

Section 1. Equality of Rights under the law shall not be denied or abridged by the United States or any state on account of sex.

Section 2. The Congress shall have the power to enforce, by appropriate legislation, the provisions of this article.

Section 3. This amendment shall take effect two years after the date of ratification.

■ The number of women employed in the United States increased by 50% during World War II. Many of these women were forced to leave their jobs when the war ended.

1930s–1950s: World War II and Postwar Years

The United States dramatically increased its production during World War II while millions of male workers were leaving to join the military. Women made a vital contribution to this effort. Twelve million women were working when the United States entered the war; by the time the war ended, 18 million women were employed.[3] Women began receiving more pay and worked in a greater variety of positions, though they were rarely, if ever, employed in skilled labor or managerial positions. When the war ended, women were pressured to leave their jobs and return to being homemakers.

Although many women were using birth control by the 1950s, popular culture still reinforced the idea that sexuality was simply a means for married couples to produce children. The Kinsey reports on human sexuality, issued in 1953, started to dispel this idea by revealing that, for many men and women, marriage was not a prerequisite for sex.

1960s–1970s: The Grassroots Movement

During the 1960s and 1970s, grassroots organizations challenged medical authority in the delivery of health care to

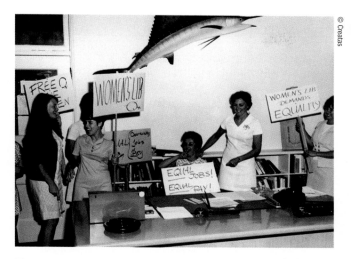

■ During the 1960s and 1970s, women challenged the authorities on many issues regarding gender equality.

women. These groups believed that the overwhelmingly male medical community excluded women from making decisions about their own health care, and they addressed issues such as unnecessary hysterectomies and cesarean sections, postpartum depression, abortion, and childbirth reform from a feminist perspective. The self-help manual *Our Bodies, Ourselves* epitomized this effort. This health book and guide to women's bodies, originally published in 1970, was written and self-published by 12 feminist activists. Today the book has been expanded greatly, is in its 13th edition, and has sold millions of copies worldwide.

Legal reforms during this time gave greater rights to women. The Food and Drug Administration (FDA) approved the birth control pill in 1960. In 1964, Congress passed the Civil Rights Act, including Title VII, which protected women against employment discrimination. In 1972, Congress passed the Equal Rights Amendment, though this amendment fell short of the 38 states needed to ratify it and add it to the Constitution. Also in 1972, legislation known as Title IX forced schools to provide equal funding for men and women in athletic programs.

For decades, the women's health movement had been composed mostly of middle-class white women. During the 1960s and 1970s, this movement began to be more

Before I came to college, I thought that you had to be pretty radical and a little "anti-man" to be a feminist. Now I understand that feminists simply want women to have the same chances to make a name for themselves, have their voices heard, and live a good life as men do. I guess I've always been a feminist, but I just didn't know it.
—19-year-old student

I have an inherited condition that affects most of the women in my family. I don't know what we would have done without the support of an advocacy organization that is focused on our condition.
—21-year-old woman

inclusive. Organizations such as the National Black Women's Health Project (now called the Black Women's Health Imperative), the National Latina Women's Health Organization, the National Asian Women's Health Organization, and the Native American Women's Health Education and Resource Center were developed to focus on issues and diseases that disproportionately affect women of color.

1980s: Changing Public Policy

In the 1980s, the U.S. Public Health Service's Task Force on Women's Health Issues formed to assess the status of women's health. The Task Force issued recommendations to increase gender equity in **biomedical research** and establish guidelines for the inclusion of women in federally sponsored studies. In 1990, the National Institutes of Health (NIH) strengthened its guidelines and established the Office of Research on Women's Health (ORWH). The ORWH ensures women's participation in clinical trials, strengthens research on diseases affecting women, and promotes the career advancement of women in science. The Women's Health Equity Act also was passed, allocating

■ The past five years have seen the first major female candidate for president of the United States (Hillary Clinton), the first female vice presidential candidate for the Republican party (Sarah Palin), the first African-American woman as secretary of state (Condoleeza Rice), and the first female speaker of the House of Representatives (Nancy Pelosi).

It's Your Health

Feminism

Feminism is the idea that women should have the same political, economic, and social rights and opportunities as men. Feminism has achieved great advances for women over the past 100 years. Feminism has evolved to help different generations of women, and it will continue to evolve as women face new challenges and opportunities.

The first wave of feminism began in the late-19th and early-20th centuries, when suffragists and abolitionists worked to secure basic rights for women such as the rights to vote, own property, and inherit property.

The second wave of feminism occurred in the 1960s and 1970s. It fought against specific injustices, such as the lack of reproductive freedom, the lack of equal pay for equal work, and women's inability to receive equal access to jobs and education. The second wave of feminism attempted to highlight ways that society legally and professionally subjugated women, and thus turned women's personal struggles into political action.

The third wave of feminism began in the late 1980s and early 1990s. This new movement addressed domestic violence, access to safe and legal abortions, and sexual harassment, as well as ensuring equal status of women in educational, work, athletic, and social environments. The first two waves of feminism had largely come from a white, middle-class perspective. In this third movement, activists attempted to broaden the scope of feminism to include perspectives of women of color and different social classes. The third feminist wave also looked at all aspects of society, art, and science through a feminist lens. This perspective provided insights into where inequality persists and how women often contribute to supporting the status quo instead of actively fighting for change. The third wave has also focused on practical ways to help women achieve equality, such as by promoting

flexible work scheduling, demanding the availability of child care, and making time off available for maternity leave and caring for sick family members.

Today, many young women are living the dreams of the women who started the feminist movement. Millions of women pursue careers and family, are equal partners in their relationships, and support feminist political agendas. Although the current generation of women may appreciate advances that feminism has made possible, they do not always feel the same personal connection with the feminist movement that women from earlier generations felt (and feel).

Women in the United States enjoy more power and opportunities than they ever have before. Women's wages have risen, and women now constitute a majority of college and university students. The past decade has seen the first African American woman as secretary of state, the first female speaker of the House of Representatives, the first major female candidate for president of the United States, and the first female vice-presidential candidate for the Republican party. However, women continue to face discrimination at home, in public, and at the workplace because of their gender; and progress on issues from rape and sexual assault to access to reproductive health care has stalled in many ways over the past 20 years.

Today, feminism is exploring many aspects of women's lives. Modern feminism acknowledges that gender differences exist even while working to eliminate gender-based favoritism and bias. Feminism also acknowledges that women may not all want to focus on their careers or even have careers (though they continue to be grateful for the opportunity). Feminists come from both genders, and different political and cultural backgrounds, ages, ethnicities, and sexual orientations; in short, they are as diverse a group as women themselves.

---

money to fund health research on particular areas of concern to women, including contraception, infertility, breast cancer, ovarian cancer, HIV/AIDS, and osteoporosis.

1990s: Women's Health at the Forefront

The 1990s brought together government, healthcare institutions, academia, and advocacy organizations to analyze and promote women's health and well-being. New women's health offices in federal agencies and in regional public health service offices opened throughout the country. Existing centers broadened their scope beyond reproductive issues to take a more comprehensive look at health and disease among women.

In the 1993 NIH Revitalization Act, Congress required that women and minorities be included as subjects in all human subject research funded by NIH. This decision was a bold and innovative step. The inclusion of women in research has broadened the scientific knowledge base necessary for developing sex-specific diagnostic techniques,

preventive measures, and effective treatments for diseases and conditions affecting women throughout their life span.

The Family and Medical Leave Act, also introduced in 1993, gives employees unpaid medical leave for themselves or for the care of a family member or a newborn or adopted infant. In 1994, the Violence Against Women Act mandated a unified judicial response to sexual crimes committed against women.

The 21st Century

The new millennium has brought many contributions to improving the health of the public—for example, the identification of the **human genome**, improvements in HIV/AIDS medications, public health programs targeting behavior-related health problems, the inclusion of children in **clinical trials**, and the passage of the Patient Protection and Affordable Care Act to extend health insurance to millions of women, men, and children. Nevertheless, women still face many difficulties in the healthcare arena. There has been a rollback of many of the advances made in the 1990s. Funding for reproductive health initiatives fell both domestically and internationally for the first decade of the 21st century. In 2012, a record number of women were elected to Congress, with 20 women serving in the Senate and more than 80 women serving in the House of Representatives. However, women remain underrepresented in national, local, and state governments. Millions of Americans lack health insurance or are underinsured; women are living longer but not necessarily with better quality of life; and women across the United States and the world continue to be victims of individual and societal violence and discrimination.

Political Dimensions of Women's Health

Government plays an important role in protecting and promoting women's health, and is involved in six main areas relating to women's health:

1. Policymaking
2. Financing
3. Protecting the health of the public
4. Collecting and disseminating information about health and healthcare delivery systems
5. Capacity building for population health
6. Managing of health services

The government directly and indirectly influences many of the areas affecting women's health. The federal government ensures that the food supply is safe, provides highway funding for states that adopt a legal drinking age, and regulates businesses that provide medications to the public.

During the 1990s, the government established many organizations and agencies devoted to women's health. The Department of Health and Human Services' Office on Women's Health (DHHS-OWH) serves as the coordinating agency for women's health initiatives throughout the agencies and offices of the U.S. DHHS, including the National Institutes of Health, Food and Drug Administration, Centers for Disease Control and Prevention (CDC), and other agencies and departments. The Office on Women's Health finds and addresses inequities in research, healthcare services, and education that have placed the health of women at risk.

The Office of Research on Women's Health (ORWH) within NIH is the government's focal point for women's biomedical research.

- It advises the NIH director and staff on women's health research.
- It strengthens and enhances research related to diseases, disorders, and conditions affecting women.
- It ensures that NIH research addresses issues regarding women's health.
- It develops opportunities for and supports recruitment, retention, reentry, and advancement of women in biomedical careers.
- It ensures that biomedical and behavioral research studies supported by NIH represent women and women's health issues.
- It supports research on women's health issues.

The ORWH has been critical in national and international efforts to make women's health research part of the scientific and educational infrastructure. The ORWH works with scientists, practitioners, legislators, and lay advocates to identify research priorities and set a comprehensive research agenda. The ORWH also encourages research that examines the biological differences between the sexes—that is, gender-based biology—to more fully understand each and thereby enhance knowledge and practice.

The Healthy People initiative joined U.S. DHHS with other federal agencies, nonprofit organizations, and members of various medical industries to educate women and provide them with the knowledge needed to live long and healthy lives. Every 10 years, this initiative creates goals and objectives to guide health promotion and disease prevention efforts on a national scale. By identifying diseases that affect women the most, scientists can set future directions and goals for research. The current iteration of this initiative, Healthy People 2020, will track and analyze almost 600 public health objectives that are important to women.

U.S. DHHS also works to provide family planning services, prevent sexually transmitted infections, and reduce unintended pregnancies. The Title X program provides funding to millions of people for reproductive health and family planning services. Funding has also increased for research and programs aimed at improving the health of older women. The Administration on Aging has launched a resource center to educate older women about issues such as income security, housing, and caregiving. The Administration on Aging has also increased support for community nutrition services to combat nutrition-related illnesses in the elderly.

The reasons for excluding women from clinical investigations are less obvious than one might expect. In spite of a significant body of opinion to the contrary, the reasons have very little to do with male chauvinism or the gender of the investigating scientist—until the 1990s, female scientists were every bit as likely as men to exclude females from clinical protocols. Even at the most sophisticated academic medical centers, senior investigators taught young scientists that data obtained from male subjects could be extrapolated to women without modification. They assumed that women were essentially small men—identical in all respects except for their reproductive physiology. It is astonishing that in a scientific system that prides itself on its critical sense and accepts no hypothesis as true until it has been rigorously tested, we have tolerated such a leap of faith for so long.[7]

—**Marianne Legato,** founder and director of the
Partnership for Gender-Specific Medicine

Investment in Biomedical Research

The federal government plays a critical role in funding biomedical research. The National Institutes of Health is the main federal agency responsible for distributing money to private and public institutions and organizations for conducting medical and health research. Along with the CDC and other agencies, it advances basic research to discover new and better methods of treatment and prevention of numerous health conditions. Funding also comes from the private sector, philanthropic organizations, universities, and voluntary health agencies.

Pharmaceutical companies and private corporations also invest millions of dollars each year to research and develop new drugs, vaccines, and technologies. Investment in biomedical research and new technologies has led to increased **life expectancy**, improved health throughout the life span, and, in many cases, decreased cost of illness.

However, newer medicines, technologies, and equipment are not the only way to improve health. About one-half of the deaths in the United States are directly or indirectly caused by people's behavior choices.[5] Research can also find better ways to educate people about basic health measures, such as preventing disease; eating a healthful, balanced diet; exercising; and avoiding tobacco and other drugs, offering the potential to improve the health of millions of Americans. Promoting healthful behaviors and preventing disease are usually cheaper, more effective methods than intervening after a disease or harmful event occurs. Unfortunately, these types of programs typically receive little funding compared to pharmaceutical drugs or technologies promising the next "miracle cure" (or, for shareholders, the next revenue source).

Research on women's health has seen unprecedented growth over the past 35 years, especially with the push to include women in clinical trials. By demanding that women are included in health research, women as well as men become the studied models for the conditions that affect them and the drugs used to treat these conditions. This trend has led to the integration of women-specific data into clinical practice and the formulation of new questions in regard to women and specific diseases.

Another approach to improving women's health relies on gender-based research—studies that examine the similarities and differences between men and women to learn more about the causes of disease and responses to medication in these populations. Gender-based studies identify and investigate the biological and physiological differences between men and women. Males and females can manifest different symptoms of a disease, experience the course of a disease differently, or respond in distinct ways to pharmaceuticals. Identifying and studying gender-based differences offers remarkable potential for understanding disease epidemiology and health outcomes in both men and women. The **Gender Dimensions** box discusses several areas of women's health research that have benefited from increased funding and attention. These topics are discussed in greater detail in later chapters of this book.

Fat and body water content, steroidal sex hormone levels, and **genetic phenotype** all affect drug metabolism through pharmacokinetics (concentration of the drug) and pharmacodynamics (ability to metabolize the drug).[7] Medical literature has documented significant differences in the ways that men and women process aspirin, acetaminophen (Tylenol), lidocaine, and other commonly prescribed medications.[8] Differences such as age, hormonal status, race and ethnicity, and socioeconomic status can also affect how women metabolize drugs. The extent to which these differences prevail among the range of drugs used to prevent and treat disease is still not fully known or understood.

Food and Drug Administration guidelines urge drug investigators to account for gender differences in drug metabolism throughout the development process and to include women of childbearing age in both Phase I and Phase II clinical trials (**Table 1.1**). The FDA once excluded women of childbearing potential from clinical trials, but has revised its guidelines to call for gender-specific analyses of safety and effectiveness in new drugs. The FDA also changed its policy of excluding women of childbearing potential from early drug studies. These measures have helped the FDA acquire better information on drug effects in women.[9]

Gender Dimensions: Health Differences Between Men and Women

Differences between men and women are not just limited to the reproductive organs. Women and men react differently to certain medications, have distinct reactions and vulnerabilities to disease, and may show disease in different ways.

The following 10 examples show some of the ways that diseases affect men and women differently.

Heart Disease. Heart disease kills 500,000 U.S. women each year—more than 50,000 more women than men. Heart disease also strikes women, on average, 10 years later than men. Compared to men, women are also more likely to have a second heart attack within a year of the first one. Symptoms of a heart attack tend to be less obvious and easier to overlook in women than in men.

Depression. Depression is two to three times more likely to affect women than men, in part because women's brains make less of the neurotransmitter serotonin, which regulates emotions.

Drug Reactions. Many common drugs, like antihistamines and antibiotics, cause different reactions and side effects in women than in men.

Autoimmune Diseases. Three out of four people suffering from autoimmune diseases, such as multiple sclerosis, rheumatoid arthritis, and lupus, are women.

Osteoporosis. Women have a higher rate of bone loss than men. Four out of five people suffering from osteoporosis are women.

Smoking. Smoking causes more cardiovascular damage in women than in men. Women have stronger withdrawal symptoms of smoking and are less likely to be able to successfully quit smoking.

Sexually Transmitted Infections. If exposed to a sexually transmitted infection, women are twice as likely as men to become infected.

Anesthesia. Women, on average, wake up from anesthesia after 7 minutes, whereas men, on average, wake up after 11 minutes.

Alcohol. Women produce less of the gastric enzyme that breaks down ethanol (alcohol) in the stomach. Therefore, even after allowing for size differences, women will have a higher blood alcohol content after drinking.

Pain. Some pain medications, such as kappa-opiates, are far more effective in relieving pain in women than in men.

Source: Society for Women's Health Research. http://www.women-shealthresearch.org.

Table 1.1   Phases of a Clinical Trial

- **Phase I:** A new drug tested in a small group (20–80) of healthy volunteers to evaluate its safety, determine a safe dosage range, and identify side effects.
- **Phase II:** The study drug is given to a larger group (100–300) of people to further evaluate its safety and effectiveness.
- **Phase III:** The study drug is given to large groups (1,000–3,000 subjects) in clinics and hospitals to confirm its effectiveness, monitor side effects, and compare it with other treatments.
- **Phase IV:** The study done after the drug is marketed to continue collecting information regarding the drug's effects in various populations.

Gender-based research has posed challenges as well as opportunities for pharmaceutical manufacturers. If research shows that a drug is effective for only one gender, the potential market for that drug could be limited, which would diminish the company's profits. However, targeting drugs for women or other specific populations can also allow researchers and pharmaceutical companies to create much more effective products.

Even with advances toward inclusion of women and minority groups in research studies, one major barrier to women's participation in biomedical research still exists. Many women are unable to take part in clinical trials because of they lack health insurance. Some states have passed legislation requiring health plans to pay for routine medical care that a person may receive as a participant in a clinical trial. In 2000, **Medicare** began covering **beneficiaries'** patient care costs in clinical trials. Clinical trials still are considered experimental by some insurance companies, however, and therefore are not covered under all standard health policies.

Including women in clinical studies may pose challenges, but leaving them out courts disaster through ignorance. Using women, particularly women of childbearing age, presents challenges to the investigation as the researchers must consider the effect of hormonal cycling on the hypothesis being tested. Furthermore, the potential for pregnancy and possible **teratogenic** effects in the fetus must be considered. These factors weigh heavily in designing and conducting any study.

Reproductive Rights

The history and politics surrounding women's decisions to control when and if to have children are long and complex. (See Chapter 5 for more information.) For nearly 100 years, abortion was illegal in the United States. On January 22, 1973, the landmark Supreme Court decision *Roe v. Wade* legalized abortion. However, since then, the

■ The potential for pregnancy and possible teratogenic effects in the fetus must be considered in clinical trials.

© Terry Walsh/ShutterStock, Inc.

battle has shifted to the state level, with many states with socially conservative governments imposing restrictions that limit where, when, and under what conditions women may receive abortions.

Roe v. Wade has also not prevented the federal government from imposing abortion restrictions in countries that

---

It's Your Health

Research Studies

Epidemiologists (scientists who study trends of disease and health in populations) conduct many types of studies. Each type of study has its own advantages and disadvantages. Most of these studies are either descriptive or analytic in nature.

Descriptive studies attempt to describe or examine a disease in a population or populations, as well as how that disease or phenomenon relates to variables such as race, age, or gender. Descriptive studies can find correlations between the disease and variables, but cannot say if one causes the other. A descriptive cross-sectional survey might find that people who work in factories (variable) are more likely than other people to develop cancer (disease), but it could not say that working in a factory causes disease—there could be some other common factor involved, such as an environmental contaminant that affects people living near the factory. Descriptive studies include population studies, case-report studies, and cross-sectional studies.

Analytic studies compare people who are exposed to a certain variable to people who are not exposed to see if that variable influences their chances of developing a disease. Unlike descriptive studies, analytic studies can find a cause-and-effect ratio, though they are generally more difficult to perform. Studies that have followed otherwise equal groups of smokers and non-smokers over time and found that smokers were more likely to develop lung cancer were responsible for linking the variable of smoking to the disease of lung cancer. Analytic studies include case-control studies, cohort studies, intervention studies, and clinical trials.

---

receive U.S funding. In 1984, President Reagan imposed the Mexico City policy, or "global gag rule." This rule has been particularly contentious, having been eliminated by President Bill Clinton in 1993, reimposed by President George W. Bush in 2001, and removed once more by President Barack Obama in 2009. This policy withheld U.S. assistance from foreign family planning agencies if they provided the following services, even if U.S. funds were not used for these services:

■ Performing abortions in cases of pregnancy that are not life-threatening to the woman or the result of rape or incest

■ Providing counseling and referral for abortions

■ Lobbying to legalize abortion or increase its availability in the country in which the nongovernmental organization (NGO) is operating[10]

The global gag rule's restrictions have had serious effects on women's health in many developing countries. Under this rule, developing countries faced a dilemma: If they agreed to the rule and accepted U.S. family planning assistance, they risked seeing death and injuries from unsafe abortions increase because women who cannot obtain safe and legal abortions may visit unqualified practitioners in secret to end their pregnancies. But if these countries rejected U.S. assistance, they lost funding for all areas of family planning, including reducing unplanned pregnancy, preventing HIV, and reducing maternal and infant deaths. This increase in unplanned pregnancies and reduction in the number of safe medical services for pregnant women may have encouraged more women in these countries to seek abortions.

Access to Healthcare Providers, Services, and Health Information

Advances in public health and medicine have improved the prevention, diagnosis, and treatment of disease. Many people are living longer and healthier lives as a result. Over the years, women have learned to seek out medical information on their own, thereby becoming informed consumers of medicine.

Unfortunately, healthcare promotion and disease prevention are not simple. Many factors prevent women from receiving adequate health care, including:

■ Poverty or insufficient income to pay for care

■ Lack of health insurance

■ Lack of access to healthcare facilities

- Inability to understand medical personnel because of language barriers or illiteracy
- Unfair treatment by medical personnel because of race, ethnicity, or sexual orientation
- Inability to pay for the costs of medications needed for treatment
- Declined coverage for healthcare costs that are deemed unnecessary or experimental
- Fear of doctors and avoidance of seeking health care altogether

Lack of adequate access to healthcare services and information is a serious issue in the United States, with a lack of health insurance being one of the most formidable barriers. In 2010, 19 million women between the ages of 19 and 64 had no health insurance; another 17 million were underinsured, meaning their health insurance had limitations that prevented them from receiving necessary services.[11] The Patient Protection and Affordable Care Act, passed in 2010, will eventually help insure many of these women. However, all of the provisions will take until between 2014 and 2020 to take effect; in addition, state and national opposition to the Act may cause additional delays or prevent many citizens from receiving insurance coverage entirely. Health insurance for underinsured Americans may not cover serious illnesses or extended hospital stays, or it may require holders to pay large copayments or deductibles for health services. When costs for health care are great, lack of insurance or underinsurance can either prevent people from affording health care or force them to devote most of their resources to pay for care. Often, as unemployment rates rise, the number of people covered by insurance steadily declines. **Premiums** for private health insurance are extremely expensive and, therefore, many people opt to take a chance and remain uninsured when an employer does not sponsor them. (For more information on this issue, see Chapter 2.)

A lack of cultural and gender sensitivity, as well as a lack of knowledge about specific health concerns of women, also seriously affects women's health. The health needs of women are different from those of men. Additionally, health needs vary from woman to woman, depending on many factors, including her age, ethnicity/race, and sexual orientation. Several steps are being taken to make healthcare providers aware of these specific needs. The ORWH has developed coursework for medical students to make them more sensitive toward and aware of women's health issues. Dental, nursing, and pharmacy programs, as well as **osteopathic** and **allopathic schools**, also are developing

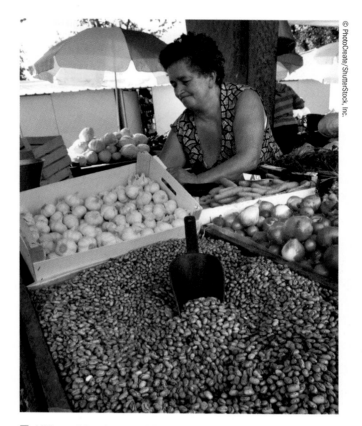

■ Millions of Americans work but do not have access to health care.

similar coursework. Healthcare providers who receive this training are better equipped to care for the diverse population of women in the United States.

Global Perspective on Women's Health

Around the world, women continue to be less likely than men to receive adequate health care, to have opportunities for economic advancement, and to have political representation. Women who live in the developing world (most countries outside of Western Europe, the United States, Canada, and Japan) are also much more likely than women in industrialized countries to die or be injured from a variety of illnesses, injuries, and diseases. Global threats to women's health include poverty, underweight and malnutrition, HIV/AIDS, violence, and **maternal morbidity and mortality** (disability, disease, or death related to pregnancy or childbirth). Women are burdened by disease and by violations of their human rights that directly affect their health. These problems include domestic violence, **female genital mutilation**, **honor killings**, **trafficking**, and barriers to reproductive health services.

■ Around the world, women are working to improve their lives and make their voices heard.

Access to clean water, nutritious food, and medical care, as well as protection from violence and poor working conditions, are basic, inexpensive factors that could greatly improve global health; unfortunately, hundreds of millions of women lack these basic human rights. Social inequalities, such as lack of education, money, and decision-making freedom, pose a greater threat to women than to men; women consequently have a disproportionately higher burden of disease and poverty. In addition, women are often the primary caregivers for their children and families.

The United Nations (U.N) has worked to advance the status of women and achieve equity in the treatment, opportunities, and status of both genders for the past 35 years. In 1979, the U.N. adopted the Convention on the Elimination of All forms of Discrimination (CEDAW), also referred to as the international bill of rights for women.

Profiles of Remarkable Women

Susan F. Wood, PhD (1959–)

Dr. Susan F. Wood has dedicated her career to advancing women's health, both by using scientific evidence to make better decisions about health policy and by taking a principled stand against political interference in the scientific process.

Wood studied biology and psychology and graduated with a Bachelor's of Science degree from Southwestern at Memphis in 1980; she earned a PhD in Biology at Boston University in 1989, and received research fellowship training in neuroscience from Johns Hopkins School of Medicine in 1990. Wood has studied the biochemistry of smells, researched how medications affect women during pregnancy, and advocated for women participating in clinical trial research.

Wood joined the FDA in 2000. She later became the assistant commissioner for women's health, the top agency official for women's health issues. In 2005, Wood resigned from the FDA to protest the agency's continued delays on ruling about the emergency birth control pill known as Plan B. (See Chapter 5 for more information.) Wood believed that decisions to delay the contraceptive were politically motivated.

The FDA's independent, scientific expert advisory committees had recommended that Plan B be approved in 2003, but leadership in the FDA, appointed by President George W. Bush, refused to approve the contraceptive. Before Wood resigned, the FDA regulatory staff, an advisory committee, and the head of the FDA drug center had all found Plan B to be safe and effective and had recommended that the drug be approved for over-the-counter use. Lester M. Crawford, the head of the FDA during this time, overruled these recommendations and said the decision would be "indefinitely delayed." Wood and many other scientists believed that Crawford's decision amounted to political interference from the Bush administration over a scientific decision.

"I can no longer serve as staff when scientific and clinical evidence, fully evaluated and recommended for approval by the professional staff here, has been overruled," she wrote in an email explaining her decision.[1]

Wood's decision brought immediate national attention to the FDA approval process. In August 2006, less than a year later, the FDA made Plan B available without a prescription to women 18 years of age or older. Wood is currently a research professor in George Washington University's School of Public Health.

[1]FDA Quits over Delay on Plan B, *Washington Post*, September 1, 2005.

CEDAW legally binds 165 U.N. member states to take steps to promote women's equity and to report on the steps they have taken. However, even if a country legally recognized women's rights, women in that country were not always able to exercise them. Many factors contribute to this discrepancy. Sexist attitudes often persist in popular culture and among those with political and economic power. In addition, educational opportunities for women may be limited, there are often insufficient childcare support systems for women, and men may be indifferent or even hostile toward improving women's place in society.[12]

In 1995, the U.N. identified 12 critical obstacles to women's advancement (**Table 1.2**). Five years later, at the "Women 2000: Gender Equality, Development and Peace for the 21st Century" conference, held in New York, the U.N. evaluated the achievements of different governments and new action plans. In the same year, the U.N.

Table 1.2 U.N. Conference in Beijing: Twelve Critical Areas of Concern for Women's Health
• Women and poverty
• Education and training of women
• Women and health
• Violence against women
• Women and armed conflict
• Women and the economy
• Women in power and decision making
• Institutional mechanisms for the advancement of women
• Human rights of women
• Women and the media
• Women and the environment
• The girl child

Source: United Nations WomenWatch. (2000). *The four global women's conferences, 1975–1995: Historical perspective.* United Nations Department of Public Information: DPI/2035/M.

Profiles of Remarkable Women

Gloria Steinem (1934–)

Gloria Steinem, a well-known feminist leader, activist, and journalist, is the daughter of a newspaperwoman and the granddaughter of the noted suffragette, Pauline Steinem. Steinem studied in India for two years, an experience that made her aware of the extent of human suffering in the world. Steinem returned from India strongly motivated to fight social injustice and decided to begin her career as a journalist.

In 1960, Steinem moved to New York and began working as a freelance writer for popular magazines. One of her first major assignments in investigative journalism was a two-part series for *Show* magazine on the working conditions of Playboy bunnies. Steinem worked as a Playboy bunny for three weeks to prepare for the article. The articles she wrote exposed the poor working conditions and meager wages of the Playboy bunnies and the discrimination and sexual harassment that occurred at New York's Playboy Club.

In 1968, Steinem joined the staff of *New York* magazine as a contributing editor and political columnist. During these years Steinem moved into politics, covering everything from the assassination of Martin Luther King, Jr. to demonstrations of United Farm Workers led by Cesar Chavez. She also worked for various Democratic candidates. Steinem's shift to the women's liberation movement and feminism began when she started attending abortion hearings. She found herself deeply moved by the stories she heard and realized that society oppressed women in many ways.

By the late 1960s, Steinem had positioned herself as a leader of the women's liberation movement through her research, writing, and activism. In 1971, she joined Bella Abzug, Shirley Chisholm, and Betty Friedan to form the National Women's Political Caucus, encouraging women's participation in the 1972 election.

Steinem became friendly with Dorothy Pitman Hughes, an African American childcare pioneer. Steinem and Hughes spoke together publicly throughout the United States to promote women's rights, civil rights, and children's rights. In 1971 they formed the Women's Action Alliance to develop women's educational programs. Although the alliance folded in 1997, its offshoot WISE (Women Initiating Self-Empowerment) continues.

In 1972, Steinem gained funding for the first mass-circulation feminist magazine, *Ms.* The preview issue sold out, and within five years *Ms.* had a circulation of 500,000. As editor of the magazine, Steinem became an influential spokesperson for women's rights issues while continuing her active political life. In 1975, she helped plan the women's agenda for the Democratic National Convention, and she continued to exert pressure on liberal politicians on behalf of women's concerns. In 1977, Steinem participated in the National Conference of Women in Houston, Texas. The conference—the first of its kind—drew attention to feminist issues and women's rights leaders.

As a writer and an activist, Gloria Steinem continues to be a leader in the women's rights movement. Steinem's books include *Outrageous Acts and Everyday Rebellions* (1983), *Marilyn: Norma Jean* (1986), *Revolution from Within: A Book of Self-Esteem* (1992), *Moving Beyond Words* (1994), and *Doing Sixty and Seventy* (2006).

developed eight Millennium Development Goals (MDGs). The MDGs set global goals toward lowering global poverty, improving health, reaching environmental sustainability, and other issues to be reached by 2015. Two of the eight MDGs—improving maternal health and reaching gender equality—directly deal with women's health, while several others, such as ending poverty and hunger and providing universal education, are issues that affect women more than men. The U.N. estimates progress toward the MDGs through measures such as the ratio of boys to girls in school; the ratio of literate women to literate men; the percentage of women with waged employment; the proportion of seats in parliament held by women; and the percentage of births attended by a skilled health professional.

Despite gains around the world in women's lifespans, quality of health, and political opportunities, women still face discrimination, violence, and marginalization around the world, and women account for the majority of the world's poor.[13] The United Nations has created a set of common objectives aimed at building equity and fair treatment for everyone, and has started progress toward meeting these goals. Women and men around the world will need to work together to make this goal a reality.

■■■■
Informed Decision Making: Take Action

There are many ways to advocate for women's health. Women's health organizations encourage donating, getting involved by sending letters to legislators and helping to organize events, and educating oneself on women's health issues. Visiting the Internet can be a good first step in learning about organizations and deciding where to focus personal interest and commitment. The websites section of this chapter lists several organizations that offer ways to become involved in promoting women's health.

■■■■
Summary

Women's health is a wide area of study that examines the biology of the female body, human development throughout the lifespan, the health of individuals and entire populations, factors that contribute to mental and physical health, women's place in society, and other factors. Over the past 200 years, many organizations and individuals have worked to improve women's health, rights, and status. Women's health is now recognized as a national priority,

and tremendous progress has been achieved in expanding the scope and depth of women's health research. Continued success in the women's health movement depends on political commitment; sufficient funds; educated and interested scientific and lay communities; advocacy by professionals, patients, and the public; and involvement of women, men, and communities in working for equality and recognizing gender differences. These factors have driven the explosion in women's health research and are responsible for advances in developed countries and throughout the world. Findings from biological, behavioral, and social sciences all provide insights and important data that can improve women's health and well-being.

■■■■
Topics for Discussion

1. What are some of the different ways of envisioning women's health? What do you think are the most important aspects of women's health?

2. How has the definition of feminism changed over the past 100 years? What elements have remained the same? Do you consider yourself a feminist? Can a person have socially conservative views about women's health and rights and still be a feminist?

3. What are some of the major differences in how men and women react to medications?

4. Why is it important for women to be included in clinical trials? What is gender-based research, and what areas of health could benefit from further gender-based research?

5. Discuss the ways the government is involved in the following areas in relation to health:
   - Policymaking
   - Financing
   - Protecting the health of the public
   - Conducting research
   - Influencing how and where people receive health care

■■■■
Key Terms

Allopathic school: A school that teaches a system of medical practice making use of all measures proved of value in treatment of disease (i.e., convention medicine exclusive of homeopathic practices).

Beneficiary: In terms of insurance, an individual who is eligible to receive benefits under an insurance policy.

Biomedical research: Studies relating to the activities and applications of science to clinical medicine.

Clinical trial: A research study designed to answer specific questions about new vaccines, new therapies, or new ways of using known treatments. Clinical trials are used to determine whether drugs or treatments are both safe and effective.

Corset: A close-fitting undergarment or outer garment worn to support and shape the waistline, hips, and breasts.

Female genital mutilation (FGM): Any of the three types of genital mutilation: removal of the prepuce and/or the tip of the clitoris; removal of the entire clitoris (both prepuce and glans) and the adjacent labia; or removal of the clitoris, the adjacent labia (majora and minora), and the joining of the scraped sides of the vulva across the vagina. Often referred to as female circumcision or female genital cutting.

Feminism: The policy, practice, or advocacy of political, economic, and social equality for women. It is the principle that women should have rights equal to those of me.

Genetic phenotype: The observable traits or characteristics of an organism—for example, hair color, weight, or the presence or absence of a disease.

Honor killings: The killing of a woman who has a (sexual) contact with a man outside the frame of marriage, even when she has been a victim of rape. It is intended to maintain and protect the honor of the family. Offenders often are younger than age 18 and are sometimes treated as heroes in their communities. Such killings have been reported in Pakistan, Jordan, Yemen, Lebanon, Egypt, the Gaza Strip, and the West Bank.

Human genome: The DNA contained in an organism or a cell, which includes both the chromosomes within the nucleus and the DNA in mitochondria.

Life expectancy: The number of years a person born at a given point in time is expected to live from birth.

Maternal morbidity and mortality: Death or illness while pregnant or within a defined time period of the termination of pregnancy, irrespective of the duration and the site of the pregnancy, from any cause related to or aggravated by the pregnancy or its management but not from accidental or incidental causes.

Medicare: A health insurance program providing benefits to approximately 30 million elderly (aged 65 or older) and disabled Americans. It is funded by the federal government and administered by the Centers for Medicare and Medicaid Services (CMS).

Osteopathic school: A school that focuses on natural medicine, which aims to restore function to the organism by treating the causes of pain and imbalance.

Premium: In terms of health insurance, a regular periodic payment.

Suffragist: An advocate of the right to vote and the ability to exercise that right.

Teratogenic: The characteristic of producing a permanent abnormality in structure or function, causing growth retardation, or causing death when an embryo or fetus is exposed to a certain substance, organism, or physical agent.

Trafficking: In regard to women, the use of force and deception to transfer women into situations of extreme exploitation; the recruitment, transportation, transfer, harboring, or receipt of persons by the threat or use of force or the abuse of power for the purpose of exploitation.

Websites

Black Women's Health Imperative: http://www.blackwomenshealth.org

Centers for Disease Control and Prevention (CDC): http://www.cdc.gov/women/

The Children's Bureau: http://www.acf.hhs.gov/programs/cb/

Equal Rights Amendment (ERA): http://www.equalrightsamendment.org

Feminist Women's Health Center: http://www.fwhc.org

Global Health Council: http://www.globalhealth.org

National Organization for Women (NOW): http://www.now.org

Office of Research on Women's Health (ORWH): http://orwh.od.nih.gov/

Planned Parenthood Federation of America: http://www.plannedparenthood.org

Society for Women's Health Research: http://www.womenshealthresearch.org

U.S. Food and Drug Administration (FDA): http://www.fda.gov

Women's Issues in Congress: http://www.womenspolicy.org

■■■■

References

1. World Health Organization. (2012). *Reproductive health*. Available at: http://www.who.int/topics/reproductive_health/en/

2. Chamberlain, G. (2006). British maternal mortality in the 19th and early 20th centuries. *Journal of the Royal Society of Medicine* 99(11):559–563.

3. Corsini, C., & Viazzo, P. (1993). *The decline of infant mortality in Europe, 1800–1950: Four national case studies*. UNICEF Innocenti Research Centre. Available at: http://ideas.repec.org/p/ucf/hisper/hisper93-3.html#biblio

4. Sorensen, A. (2004). *Rosie the riveter: Women working during World War II*. National Parks Service. Available at: http://www.nps.gov/pwro/collection/website/rosie.htm

5. Steen, J. (2007). *The primacy of public health*. American Public Health Association: Community Health Planning and Policy Development. Available at: http://www.apha.org/membergroups/newsletters/sectionnewsletters/comm/spring07/primacyph.htm

6. Legato, M. J. (1998). Belling the cat: Clinical investigation in vulnerable populations (a good idea, but who's going to volunteer?). *Journal of Gender-Specific Medicine* 1(1): 18–22.

7. Owens, N. J., & Hume, A. L. (1994). Pharmacotherapy in women: Do clinically important gender-related issues exist? *Rhode Island Medicine* 77: 412–416.

8. Merkatz, R. B., Temple, R., Subel, S., et al. (1993). Women in clinical trials of new drugs: A change in the FDA. *New England Journal of Medicine* 329: 292–296.

9. U.S. Food and Drug Administration [FDA]. (2012). *About the Office of Women's Health*. Available at: http://www.fda.gov/womens/programs.html

10. Center for Reproductive Rights. (2009). *Myths and realities: Debunking USAID's analysis of the Global Gag Rule*. Available at: http://reproductiverights.org/en/document/myths-and-realities-debunking-usaid%E2%80%99s-analysis-of-the-global-gag-rule

11. Robertson, R., Squires, D., Garber. T., et al. (2012). *Realizing health reform's potential*. Washington, DC: The Commonwealth Fund. Available at: http://www.commonwealthfund.org/~/media/Files/Publications/Issue%20Brief/2012/Jul/1606_Robertson_oceans_apart_reform_brief.pdf

12. Murthy, P., & Smith, C. (2010). *Women's global health and human rights*. Sudbury, MA. Jones and Bartlett.

13. World Health Organization [WHO]. (2009). *Women and health: Today's evidence, tomorrow's agenda*. Available at: http://www.who.int/gender/documents/9789241563857/en/index.html

Chapter Two

The Economics of Women's Health

Chapter Objectives

On completion of this chapter, the student should be able to discuss:

1. The third-party payer system.

2. The fee-for-service model versus managed care.

3. Factors to consider when choosing an insurance plan.

4. Types of public health insurance, including Medicare and Medicaid.

5. The substantial risks associated with being uninsured.

6. Ways that women as healthcare consumers affect demand within the healthcare system.

7. Healthcare reform and the arguments for and against a universal health system.

8. The financial burden of aging and how it disproportionately affects women.

9. Long-term care and its associated costs.

10. The impact of the 2008 recession on health care.

womenshealth.jbpub.com

Women's Health Online is a great source for supplementary women's health information for both students and instructors. Visit

http://womenshealth.jbpub.com

to find a variety of useful tools for learning, thinking, and teaching.

Introduction

Medical knowledge is not the only factor affecting women's health. Money also influences almost every aspect of health care, from when and where people go to get medical care, to the behaviors that they perform, to who pays for health care. Around the world, various systems of health insurance have evolved. Health insurance is a policy that pays for medical care (or part of medical care) when a person gets sick and injured. Most industrialized countries have a system of universal health insurance, or insurance provided by the government, financed through taxes, and offered to every individual. In the United States, a unique hodgepodge system exists, with some Americans receiving insurance through their jobs, some Americans receiving insurance through a variety of government agencies, some individuals purchasing private insurance, and many Americans going uninsured. As a result, patients, the government, hospitals and the healthcare system, employers, and the public all pay for health care.

The details surrounding health insurance—including whether health insurance should be mandatory, how much it should cost, and who it should cover—has been one of the most controversial and most discussed political topics in the United States for decades. Most people with private insurance share the cost of medical care with insurers via premiums, deductibles, copays, and coinsurance in addition to the negotiated fee schedule some providers have with insurers. People without insurance who receive care must pay for it "out-of-pocket," or with their own funds. The government provides some free health care via public health clinics and other venues.

Different participants in the healthcare system all shape the direction of health care. Major healthcare stakeholders include providers (such as physicians, nurses, and social workers), patients, hospitals, health insurers, policymakers, health education firms, and medical manufacturers such as pharmaceutical, medical device, and diagnostic companies. Each has a different perspective on healthcare delivery and funding.

Increasingly, health care has become a consumer- or patient-oriented industry. Manufacturers, pharmaceutical companies, hospitals, and private doctors' offices develop goods and services to court consumers and drive demand for specific services. Patients are more willing to shop around for different providers, an increasing demand for wide access to services, and a growing eagerness to pursue litigation in cases of perceived substandard care.

Understanding the effects of women's growing economic power on women's health and the persistent limitations that marginalized women face in accessing quality women's health care is critical. Other important issues include the economics of aging and the effects of an aging population on women's health, public policy that influences the economics of health care, and the roles that women as caregivers have in the delivery of health care.

Paying for Health Care

Since World War II, the money Americans spend on health care has continued to grow, both in terms of dollars spent and as a percentage of the gross domestic product (GDP), the total value of all goods and services produced in the United States in one year. This growth has accelerated over the past 30 years, slowing only after the national economy contracted after the economic recession in 2008. In 1950, Americans spent 4.6% of the GDP on health care; this number increased to 9.2% in 1980, 12.5% in 1990, 13.8% in 2000, and 17.9% in 2010.[1,2] This rapid growth has led politicians, employers, healthcare providers, individual tax payers, and others to call for healthcare reform to curb the growth in expenditures, protect individuals from healthcare-related costs, and protect access to services. Before understanding how healthcare reform policies were developed and the debates surrounding their merit, an understanding of current funding structures is needed.

In the United States, health care functions much like a traditional market setting. Individuals and patients purchase medical care as needed, much like they do other goods and services. However, unlike other markets (such as real estate or retail sales) all individuals need health care at one stage or another of their lives, often at unpredictable times or levels. People do not have control over their need for health care in the same way that they do when deciding whether to purchase a television. If a woman has heart disease and needs to go to a cardiologist, she has very little choice except to purchase the services needed or go without care. In addition, a patient must trust her physician to tell her which goods and services she needs instead of making that decision on her own. From an economic perspective, the necessity of health care and an individual's inability to have full information to make purchasing choices make health care a unique market.

In the United States, the healthcare system is based on a **third-party payer system**, in which most individuals do not pay directly for the delivery of care (**Figure 2.1**).

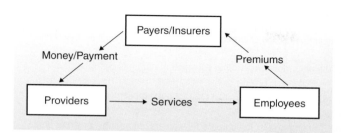

Figure 2.1

The third-party payer system.

■ Before World War II, few Americans had health insurance.

Instead, many have health insurance, which, in return for a monthly or yearly payment called a premium plus a per-doctor's encounter fee called a copayment and/or deductible, provides coverage for health-related goods and services. Before third-party payers became a mainstay of the U.S. system, patients would pay out-of-pocket for health care, either to their doctor or to hospitals. Medical care was purchased and delivered like most other commodities. If an individual became sick or was injured on the job, the financial repercussions of paying for medical care could be extreme. Private health insurance was introduced in the early 1930s as a method to lower the economic risk associated with hospital care costs. Health insurance was developed and based on an **indemnity** or **fee-for-service** system. Through this system, insurers reimbursed hospitals based on a list of charges for services rendered. Individuals paid insurers a flat fee regardless of whether they had encounters with the healthcare system. As the third-party payer system matured, it grew to include fee-for-service payments to physicians and other outpatient providers of health care (**Table 2.1**).

Table 2.1   Paying for Health Care Timeline

1900s	■ American Medical Association (AMA) becomes a powerful national force.
	■ In 1901, AMA reorganizes as the national organization of state and local associations. Membership increases from about 8,000 physicians in 1900 to 70,000 in 1910—half the physicians in the country. This period is the beginning of "organized medicine."
	■ Doctors are no longer expected to provide free services to all hospital patients.
	■ The United States lags behind European countries in offering health insurance.
	■ Railroads are the leading industry to develop extensive employee medical programs.
1910s	■ U.S. hospitals become modern scientific institutions, valuing antiseptics and cleanliness and using medications for the relief of pain.
	■ American Association for Labor Legislation (AALL) organizes first national conference on "social insurance."
	■ Progressive reformers argue for health insurance and seem to be gaining support.
	■ Opposition from physicians and other interest groups, plus the entry of the United States into the war in 1917, undermine the reform effort.
1920s	■ Consistent with the general mood of political complacency, there is no strong effort to change health insurance.
	■ Reformers now emphasize the cost of medical care instead of wages lost to sickness. The relatively higher cost of medical care is a new and dramatic development, especially for the middle class.
	■ The cultural influence of the medical profession grows—physicians' incomes are higher and prestige is established.
	■ General Motors signs a contract with Metropolitan Life to insure 180,000 workers.
	■ Penicillin is discovered. However, it will be 20 years before this antibiotic is used to combat infection and disease.

(continues)

Table 2.1   Paying for Health Care Timeline *(continued)*

1930s	■ The Depression changes priorities, with greater emphasis being placed on unemployment insurance and "old age" benefits. ■ The Social Security Act is passed, omitting health insurance. ■ There is a push for health insurance within the Roosevelt Administration, but internal government conflicts over priorities undermine this effort. ■ Against the advice of insurance professionals, Blue Cross begins offering private coverage for hospital care in dozens of states.
1940s	■ Prepaid group health care begins; it is seen as radical. ■ During World War II, wage and price controls are placed on U.S. employers. To compete for workers, companies begin to offer health benefits, giving rise to the employer-based system in place today. ■ President Roosevelt asks Congress for an "economic bill of rights," including the right to adequate medical care. ■ President Truman offers a national health program plan, proposing a single system that would include all of U.S. society. ■ Truman's plan is denounced by the AMA and is called a Communist plot by a House subcommittee.
1950s	■ At the start of the decade, national healthcare expenditures are 4.5% of the gross national product. ■ Attention turns to the Korean War and away from health reform. ■ Federal responsibility for the sick poor is firmly established. ■ Many legislative proposals are made to offer hospital insurance, but none succeeds. ■ Many more medications are available to treat a range of diseases, including infections, glaucoma, and arthritis. New vaccines become available that prevent dreaded childhood diseases, including polio. The first successful organ transplant is performed.
1960s	■ In the 1950s, the price of hospital care doubled. In the early 1960s, those outside the workplace, and especially the elderly, have difficulty affording insurance. ■ More than 700 insurance companies sell health insurance. ■ Concern about a "doctor shortage" and the need for more "health manpower" leads to federal measures to expand education in the health professions. ■ Major medical insurance endorses high-cost medicine. ■ President Lyndon Johnson signs Medicare and Medicaid into law. ■ "Compulsory health insurance" advocates are no longer optimistic. ■ The number of doctors reporting themselves to be full-time specialists grows from 55% in 1960 to 69% by 1969.
1970s	■ President Richard Nixon renames prepaid group healthcare plans as health maintenance organizations (HMOs), with legislation providing federal endorsement, certification, and assistance. ■ Healthcare costs escalate rapidly, partly due to unexpectedly high Medicare expenditures, rapid inflation in the economy, expansion of hospital expenses and profits, and changes in medical care, including greater use of technology, medications, and conservative approaches to treatment. U.S. medicine is now seen as in crisis. ■ President Nixon's plan for national health insurance is rejected by liberals and labor unions, but his "War on Cancer" centralizes research at NIH. ■ The number of women entering the medical profession rises dramatically. In 1970, 9% of medical students are women; by the end of the decade, the proportion exceeds 25%.
1980s	■ Corporations begin to integrate the hospital system (previously a decentralized structure), enter many other healthcare-related businesses, and consolidate control. Overall, there is a shift toward privatization and corporatization of health care. ■ Under President Reagan, Medicare shifts to payment by diagnosis (DRG) instead of by treatment. Private plans quickly follow suit. ■ Insurance companies voice complaints that the traditional fee-for-service method of payment to doctors is being exploited. ■ "Capitation" payments to doctors become more common.
1990s	■ Healthcare costs rise at double the rate of inflation. ■ Expansion of managed care helps to moderate increases in healthcare costs. ■ Federal healthcare reform legislation fails again to pass in the U.S. Congress. ■ By the end of the decade, 44 million Americans, 16% of the nation, have no health insurance at all. ■ The Human Genome Project to identify all of the more than 100,000 genes in human DNA gets under way. ■ By June 1990, 139,765 people in the United States have HIV/AIDS, with a 60% mortality rate.
2000s	■ Healthcare costs continue to rise. ■ Medicare is viewed by some as unsustainable under the present structure and must be "rescued." ■ Changing demographics of the workplace lead many to believe the employer-based system of insurance cannot last. ■ The Human Genome Project is completed 2 years ahead of schedule, in 2003. ■ Direct-to-consumer advertising for pharmaceuticals and medical devices increases. ■ Medicare expands to include a prescription drug benefit in 2006. ■ Employers continue to cut health insurance benefits in an attempt to address persistent increases in costs. ■ Medical savings accounts become common.

Table 2.1	**Paying for Health Care Timeline** *(continued)*
	▪ President George W. Bush unsuccessfully tries to privatize Social Security. ▪ Congress passes a major expansion to State Children's Health Insurance Program (SCHIP), which will provide insurance for an additional 4 million low-income children, in 2009.
2010s	▪ The Patient Protection and Affordable Care Act (PPACA) is passed in 2010; among other features, the Supreme Court upholds the vast majority of the Act in 2012. The PPACA includes a patient's bill of rights, increases cost-free preventive services, and reduces brand-name drug prices for people with Medicare. Additional provisions of the PPACA include: ▪ Providing small business health insurance tax credits ▪ Relief for four million seniors who hit the Medicare prescription drug "donut hole." ▪ Cutting down on healthcare fraud. ▪ Providing access to insurance for uninsured Americans with preexisting conditions. ▪ Extending coverage for young adults (up to age 26).

Sources: Reprinted with permission from *Healthcare crisis: Who's at risk?* Healthcare Timeline, PBS. Produced by Issues TV, 2000; Data from What's Changing and When. US Department of Health and Human Services. Available at http://www.healthcare.gov/law/timeline/index.html#event1-pane.

In 2010, about two-thirds (64%) of Americans were covered by private health insurance, either provided by their employer or purchased individually.[3] Many private health insurance plans are now structured within a managed care plan. **Managed care** was introduced as a method to control costs by changing how the delivery of care is coordinated and how health care is reimbursed. In contrast to a fee-for-service model, managed care requires patients to go to specific providers and have access to care only when certain criteria are met. In some cases, physicians are receive a predetermined lump sum for all care delivered as opposed to a fee for each service rendered.

Managed care has been perceived both as a form of reform (by keeping costs down and providing broad access to services) and as a barrier to care (by placing limits on access to care). Managed care is blamed for decreased access to care by shortening physician office visits, increasing copayments, and placing more restrictions on which doctors patients can see. Managed care is continually evolving to meet the changing needs and demands of patients, employers, and providers.

The limitations on access that lead patients and physicians to vilify managed care resulted in slowing the rate at which health-related expenditures grew in the United States in the 1990s (see **Figure 2.2**). Managed care limited expenditure growth by asking for stringent proof of medical necessity before services are paid for. For example, health insurers often require physicians to get prior authorizations from the payer before certain care is rendered—thereby restricting access to certain prescriptions, procedures, or referrals to only those patients they see as appropriate or medically indicated.

Another method for cost-containment has been to allow members to get care only from a specific network of physicians who have contracted with insurance companies to offer lower-cost care, or to make patients pay higher copayments if they see doctors who are not members of the designated network. By controlling the supply of healthcare resources, managed care organizations have been able to provide patients with a wider range of services, such as pharmaceuticals and rehabilitation services, at than many fee-for-service models. Some health insurers also own the physician and hospital networks where participants are served. These are called Integrated Delivery Networks (IDNs) or Integrated Health Networks (IHNs). Large IDNs and IHNs include Kaiser Permanente, Geisinger Health System, and Intermountain Health.

It's Your Health

Employment-based health benefit programs have existed in the United States for more than 100 years. In the 1870s, for example, railroad, mining, and other industries began to provide the services of company doctors to workers. In 1910, Montgomery Ward entered into one of the earliest group insurance contracts. Before World War II, few Americans had health insurance, and most policies covered only hospital room, board, and ancillary services. During World War II, the number of persons with employment-based health insurance coverage started to increase for several reasons. When wages were frozen by the National War Labor Board and a shortage of workers occurred, employers sought ways to get around the wage controls to attract scarce workers. Health insurance was an attractive means to recruit and retain workers during a labor shortage for two reasons: unions supported employment-based health insurance, and workers' health benefits were not subject to income tax or Social Security payroll taxes, as were cash wages. Under the current tax code, health insurance premiums paid by employers are deductible for employers as a business expense, and are excluded, without limit, from workers' taxable income.[1]

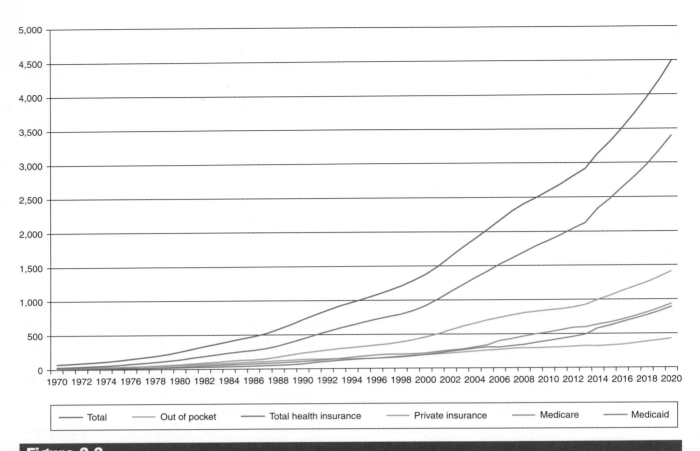

Figure 2.2

National Health Expenditures: 1970–2020 (projected).

Source: Data from Centers for Medicare & Medicare Services, Office of the Actuary. National Health Expenditures data. Released January 2011.

It's Your Health

Drive-Through Deliveries

In the 1990s, HMOs and other managed care plans shortened average maternity stays for normal births. Such programs were dubbed "drive-through deliveries." Because women were being discharged from hospitals only 24 to 48 hours after giving birth, many lawmakers, alarmed that the practice would endanger newborns, adopted laws to require insurance coverage for at least 48 hours of care after delivery.

In a study conducted at Harvard Medical School, researchers found that newborns needed the same number of later emergency room visits and hospital readmissions regardless of whether they had longer initial stays or shorter ones. In essence, the shorter stays were not adding risk to the newborns, even though the "common sense" of many women and legislators suggested that it would. The study looked at 20,366 normal deliveries in the 1990s. During the period studied, newborn visits to emergency rooms kept steady at an average of about 1% every 3 months. Hospital readmissions hovered around 1.5%. The same pattern held for a more vulnerable group of young, lower-income mothers with less education.

Larry Akey, a spokesman for the Health Insurance Association of America, said that short-stay programs were designed "not entirely as cost-saving measures, but an opportunity for the mother to get home" faster. The debate continues among women's advocacy groups, health insurers, and hospitals.

The Breast Cancer Patient Protection Act, first introduced in January 1997 by Congresswoman Rosa DeLauro of Connecticut as H.R. 135, proposed a similar 48-hour hospitalization postmastectomy. The bill languished in committee, never being brought to the floor for vote, so Rep. DeLauro reintroduced it five more times, never being voted on by both houses of Congress. In March 2009, the bill was reintroduced again (H.R. 1691) with Senator Olympia Snowe of Maine introducing the same bill in the Senate, where it currently resides in committee (S.688).

Sources: Data from DeLauro, R. *Breast Cancer Patient Protection Act of 2009*. The Library of Congress. March 24, 2009. Available at http://thomas.loc.gov/cgi-bin/bdquery/z?d111:h.r.01691:; Data from Snowe, O. *Breast Cancer Patient Protection Act of 2009*. The Library of Congress. March 24, 2009. Available at http://thomas.loc.gov/cgi-bin/bdquery/z?d111:s.00688:

Table 2.2   Managed Care Plans

Health Maintenance Organization (HMO): An HMO is a managed care plan that offers a full range of services for a fixed, prepaid fee rather than charging patients for each service provided. Patients normally pay a small copayment for care. With some plans and for some services, patients also have to satisfy a deductible. Usually, patients don't have to file claims.

HMO plans typically fall into one of two categories:

- Staff Model: A staff model HMO has salaried physicians who provide services only to plan members. They offer care at a hospital, clinic, or health center in the community.

- Independent Practice Association (IPA): An IPA maintains contracts with a number of physicians and/or physician group practices. These physicians see patients in their own offices.

Point-of-Service (POS) Plan: POS plans function much like IPAs. Patients select a primary care physician who coordinates all care within the participating provider network, including specialist referrals.

Preferred Provider Organization (PPO): A PPO plan functions much like a POS plan, but it eliminates the primary care physician. As with the POS plan, patients can use a healthcare provider outside of the preferred provider network for an additional cost. Patients can usually see any participating provider—whether a primary care physician or a specialist—without a referral, at no additional cost. PPO plans often cost slightly more than HMOs.

High Deductible Health Plan (HDHP) with a Health Savings Account (HSA) or a Health Reimbursement Arrangement (HRA): An HDAR/HSA or HRA provides traditional medical coverage and a tax-free way to build savings for future medical expenses. It gives patients flexibility and discretion over how healthcare benefits are used. The HDHP features higher annual deductibles than other plans (usually $1,000 to $2,000) and usually has some upper limit on out-of-pocket liability. However, HDHPs make consumers share the financial burden of healthcare utilization. Most plans' coverage does not kick in until a large deductible is met, though many plans will pay for routine preventive care before the deductible is met.

Managed care plans differ based on how much they control the services patients receive. Types of managed care plans include preferred provider organizations (PPOs), health maintenance organizations (HMOs), and point-of-service (POS) plans. **Table 2.2** describes the various types of managed care plans. Almost all health insurers today offer some form of managed care products or include elements of managed care products such as physician networks or tiered copayments into their existing product lines. The least expensive option typically has the highest deductible and greatest degree of management (such as limitations on providers and requirements for prior authorization for expensive procedures).

Insurance companies decide which types of services they will cover (see **Figure 2.3**). As patient demand evolves, some health insurance companies are beginning to cover

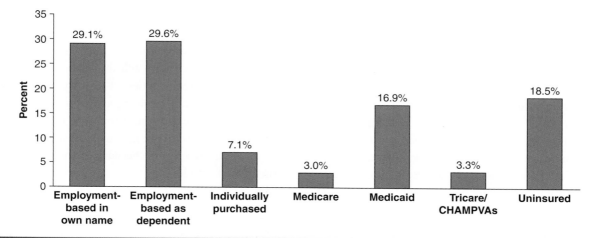

Figure 2.3

Health Insurance Coverage of Nonelderly Americans by Source of Coverage, 2010.

Source: Data from Employee Benefit Research Institute estimates of the Current Population Survey, March 1995–2011 Supplements.

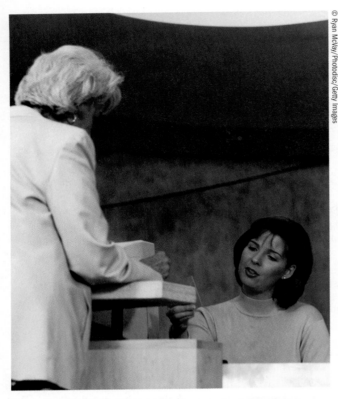

© Ryan McVay/Photodisc/Getty Images

■ A co-pay is money that a patient must pay to receive health-care services; co-pays are either a fixed amount of money or a percentage of the overall charge for a given service.

complementary, alternative therapies and preventive care services, such as massage, acupuncture, and chiropractic care.[4]

Choosing an Insurance Plan

When people choose between different insurance options, their choices are often influenced by which services are covered or what percentage of the total cost the insurer will pay. If a woman thinks that she is unlikely to use many services, as a 24-year-old woman without any existing medical conditions might, she may opt for a less expensive insurance program like an HMO, making the compromise to have more restricted coverage at a lower cost rather than pay more for broader coverage. Regardless of the insurance program selected, an individual is at considerable financial risk if her insurance does not cover or only partially covers the services she uses. The inability to pay for health care beyond insurance premiums leads many people to avoid going to the doctor when necessary or to cut short therapy if it becomes too expensive.

As a method to manage rising costs, employers and health insurance companies are increasingly requiring

patients to pay out-of-pocket for a portion of their health care. A **copayment** (or **copay**) is the amount of money a patient is responsible for paying to receive healthcare services. Copays can be either a fixed amount of money, like a $10 or $20 copay for a routine office visit, or a percentage of the overall charge for a given service (referred to as coinsurance). Insurance plans may often pay 80% or 90% of a patient's bill, with the patient responsible for the remaining amount.

With prescription drugs, many payers use a tiered copay system, which requires different payment levels for different types of medications. Most tiered copays reward patients for purchasing lower-cost generic drugs by requiring no or very low copays for these drugs and higher copays for more expensive brand-name drugs. **Generic drugs** are the chemical equivalents of brand-name drugs, but are far less expensive; they become available when the patent protecting the manufacturer's exclusive ability to market the drug expires, enabling greater competition in the marketplace. Within a tiered copay system, for example, a woman may pay $5 for a generic antibiotic, $25 for a preferred brand-name drug, and $50 or more for the premium-cost brand-name drug. In addition to copays, some health insurance plans require patients to try the lower cost generics and document treatment failure before agreeing to cover the higher-cost branded products.

Women pay more than men under many health insurance policies. Insurance policies often force women to pay sizeable copays for birth control pills or for hormone therapy, with many prescriptions falling into the highest copay tier. As a result, a woman may have to pay $20 to $40 per month to control her fertility and manage her transition into menopause. Health insurers have lists of drugs for which they provide reimbursement (i.e., **formularies**), which describe to patients and doctors which drugs are covered, into which tier each drug falls, and how much each drug will cost the patient. Out-of-pocket costs often prevent women from receiving appropriate care and from properly taking medication. A report by the Kaiser Family Foundation found that one in five (21%) nonelderly women did not fill a prescription because of the cost, compared with 13% of men.[5]

Types of Health Insurance

Employer-sponsored health insurance, as well as health insurance purchased by individuals, is considered **private health insurance**. Employers purchase and subsidize most private health insurance in the United States. When an

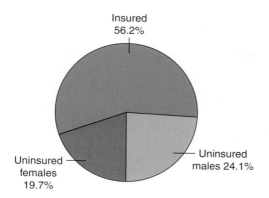

Figure 2.4

Percentage of total uninsured by gender.

Source: Data from Employee Benefit Research Institute estimates from the March Current Population Survey, 2011 Supplement.

■ Due to the aging population and the fact that women live longer than men, an increasing majority of Medicare beneficiaries are women.

individual has a full-time job, health insurance is often an integral benefit. Employer-sponsored health insurance can often be extended to cover the family of the insured individual. The government is also a major provider of health insurance, with 31% of Americans receiving some form of government-sponsored health insurance (also known as **public health insurance**).[6] The federal government is the largest health insurer in the United States through its Medicare, Medicaid, Veterans Administration, Department of Defense, and Bureau of Indian Affairs insurance programs (see **Figure 2.4**). Medicare is the result of a bill enacted by Congress in 1965 to provide health insurance at a reasonable cost to Americans aged 65 and older. Medicare is provided in three parts:

- Part A is provided to all enrollees and covers inpatient hospitalization.
- Part B is optional and covers outpatient services.
- Part D was instituted in 2006 and is optional, covering a portion of prescription drug costs.

Since 1965, Medicare has grown to cover disabled individuals and patients with end-stage renal disease. Most recently, it has expanded to include a portion of prescription drug coverage. Medicare's prescription drug coverage has already had substantial effects on who pays for prescription drugs in the United States (see **Figure 2.5**). In the 2010 census, Medicare was the largest single insurer in the United States, covering more than 44.3 million people, 56% of whom are women. Due to the aging of the population

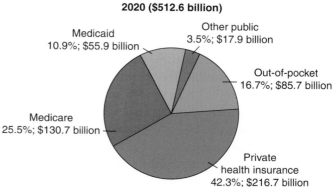

Figure 2.5

Prescription drug spending, by payer, 2009 and 2020 (projected).

Source: Data from National Health Expenditures (NHE) released January 2011. Centers for Medicare and Medicaid, Office of the Actuary, National Health Statistics Group.

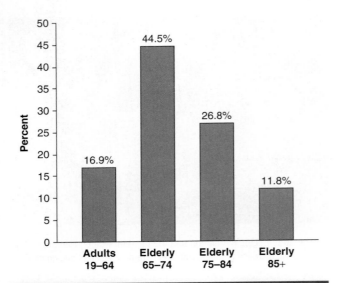

Figure 2.6

Medicare Population by Age

Source: Data from Centers for Medicare & Medicaid services, Office of Information Services: Data from the 100-percent Denominator File; data development by the Center for Strategic Planning.

and the fact that women live longer than men, a majority of the eldest Medicare beneficiaries are women (**Figure 2.6**). The aging of the U.S. population and the 2008 economic recession (with its corresponding decrease in taxes received due to declining incomes) threatens the solvency of the Medicare system; healthcare reform implemented through the Patient Protection and Affordable Care Act may reduce some Medicare costs, but these costs will likely continue to rise.[7]

Medicaid is a program jointly administered by federal and state governments that provides health insurance to low-income Americans. Whereas Medicare is a federally controlled health system, Medicaid is largely run at the state level. In some states, such as California and Tennessee, Medicaid has a state-specific name, such as MediCal or TennCare, respectively. The vast majority of Medicaid recipients are low-income women and their children; the children are covered through State Children's Health Insurance Programs (SCHIPs). Medicaid and the benefits it provides are fundamental part of providing health care to economically disadvantaged women and children in the United States. In 2009, legislation expanded SCHIP to provide coverage to an additional four million low-income children. Funded by an increased federal cigarette tax, the new SCHIP now insures 11 million low-income children.

In the 2010 census, Medicaid covered 48.6 million people, or nearly 16% of insured population.[3] Individuals qualify based on income status, level of disability or need for long-term care, or by being a dependent of a Medicaid recipient. All hospitals and most physicians accept Medicaid as a form of payment, but some private physicians refuse Medicaid patients due to the lower reimbursement rates the system provides compared to private insurance. All states cover the following basic services for Medicaid recipients:

- Inpatient and outpatient medical care
- Laboratory and X-ray services
- Chronic care facilities for persons older than 21 years
- Home health care for those eligible for nursing facility services
- Services provided by a physician or nurse practitioner
- Necessary transportation

States may cover some additional services, such as prescription drugs, case management, dental care, prosthetic devices, medical transportation, intermediate care facilities, optometry, and tuberculosis-related services. Federal law requires the delivery of services that are "medically necessary." However, states exercise substantial independence in determining the amount and duration of services covered by establishing criteria for medical necessity and utilization control.

In addition to Medicare and Medicaid, the federal government provides health insurance to veterans through the Veterans Administration (VA), active service military personnel through the Department of Defense (DOD), government workers through the government's own health insurance program (Federal Employees Health Benefits Program), and Native Americans through the Indian Health Services. These programs are all separately administered and have different organizational structures. For example, the VA is a payer for health care and a network of providers. Veterans covered within this system are eligible for care at VA hospitals and clinics. This approach is similar to how the DOD provides health insurance and healthcare services to active-duty military personnel.

Uninsured Americans

In addition to those people with private insurance and those with public insurance, 49.9 million Americans were uninsured for all of 2010—more than the populations of Texas, Florida, and Connecticut combined (**Figure 2.7**). A larger number of Americans are uninsured for a portion of the year (such as seasonal workers who only have health insurance for the portion of the year for which they are employed). One study found that close to one in three

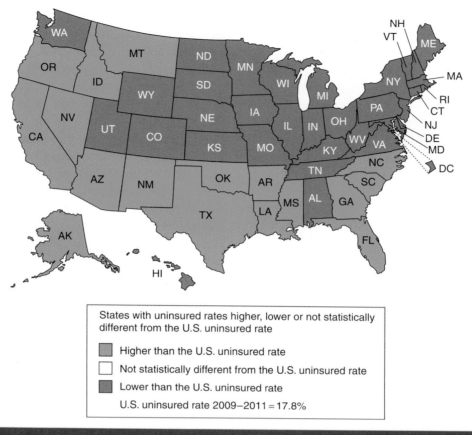

States with uninsured rates higher, lower or not statistically different from the U.S. uninsured rate

■ Higher than the U.S. uninsured rate

□ Not statistically different from the U.S. uninsured rate

■ Lower than the U.S. uninsured rate

U.S. uninsured rate 2009–2011 = 17.8%

Figure 2.7

Uninsured rates by state, using three-year average: 2009–2011.

Source: Data from Employee Benefit Research Institute estimates of the 2009–2011 Current Population Survey, March Supplement.

Americans were uninsured for all or part of the period studied. Two-thirds of these partially uninsured Americans were uninsured for 6 months or longer.[8]

The uninsured are men, women, and children, though today, men are less likely to have health insurance than women. Uninsured individuals are more likely to be sick or injured, have a more difficult time accessing care, and to die prematurely than people with insurance. Nearly one in five families has at least one uninsured member. Most uninsured individuals are younger than age 30. In fact, 9.8% of children under 18 are uninsured, and 15.4% of children in poverty (and therefore by definition eligible for Medicaid).[7] These numbers are expected to fall under the Patient Protection and Affordable Care Act, which will both offer insurance to a greater number of Americans and financially penalize individuals who choose to go without health insurance.

People without health insurance are at significant financial risk if they get sick or have an accident requiring emergency medical care. Because the uninsured must pay for medical services such as doctors' office visits or prescription drugs themselves, they often avoid preventive care or proper followup care because of cost concerns. In addition, the uninsured pay more for medical care because they are not eligible for the discounted pricing structures that health insurance companies negotiate with hospitals and doctors. As a result, the cost of care often strains family finances, jeopardizing families' physical, emotional, and economic health.[9] Long-term implications from being uninsured may include lack of preventative care, worsening of health status due to lack of appropriate care, and not being accurately monitored by a physician, leading to suboptimal care.

African Americans and Hispanic Americans are less likely to have insurance than White or Asian Americans (see **Figure 2.8**). People with small to moderate incomes are the least likely to be insured: Only 7.1% of people in the $75,000-plus income bracket are uninsured, compared to 35.7% of people with family income below $10,000.[9]

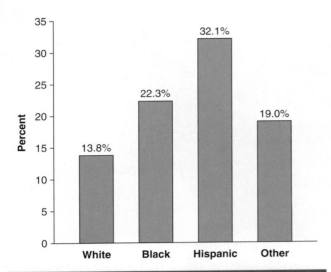

Figure 2.8

Percentage within race category uninsured among the nonelderly population by race, 2010.

Source: Data from Employee Benefit Research Institute estimates from the March Current Population Survey, March 2011 Supplement.

Lack of health insurance affects access to health services and contributes to poorer health, higher hospitalization rates, and more advanced disease states by the time health services are finally received. The 2009 expansion of Medicaid and the State Children's Health Insurance Program has reduced the number of uninsured children, though more than 1 in 10 children still lack health coverage. Nearly 20% of uninsured Americans—8.7 million individuals—are children. The likelihood that a child is uninsured fell from 13.9% in 1998 to 10.5% in 2004 to 9.8% in 2010 (**Figure 2.9**).[7] SCHIP expansions are responsible for reducing this number, but these changes will likely take years for their full effects to be felt. Health insurance is particularly important for children. Uninsured children are more likely than insured children to lack a usual source of health care, to go without needed care, and to become sick, injured, or unhealthy.[10]

Unemployment has increased significantly because of a weakening economy and rising healthcare costs for employers; as a result, many individuals who were formerly covered by their employers have suddenly lost their health insurance. A decline in coverage through employer-based health plans, rising out-of-pocket costs associated with these plans, and skyrocketing costs for insurance premiums are seen as major drivers of this trend.

Healthcare Reform

In most industrialized countries, such as Canada and the United Kingdom, the government provides health insurance to all citizens through a system of **universal health insurance**. Universal healthcare systems attempt to make sure that all citizens have access to basic levels of medical care. Individuals are often allowed to purchase supplementary insurance to pay for items not covered under the national health systems. Proponents of universal health insurance systems argue that health care is a right, not a privilege, and should therefore be available to all citizens.

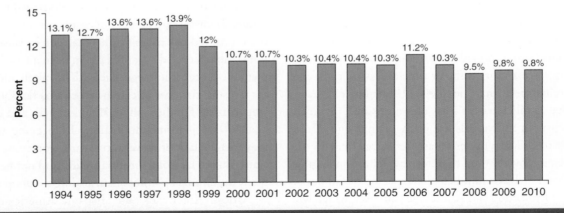

Figure 2.9

Percentage of children under age 18 without health insurance, 1994–2010.

Source: Adapted from Employee Benefit Research Institute estimates from the March Current Population Survey, March 1995–2011 Supplements.

Note: Data from 1994–1998 are not directly comparable with data from 1999–2010 because of a change in the way coverage were counted.

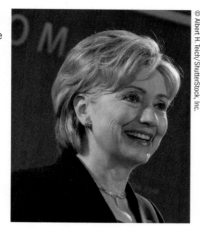

■ Healthcare reform is a major political topic in the United States.

was to expand coverage to uninsured Americans, provide coverage to previously uninsurable individuals like those with preexisting conditions, and make insurance more affordable for small businesses and individuals. Litigation brought the PPACA before the Supreme Court in 2012; a 5–4 majority ruled the vast majority of the PPACA as constitutional, allowing it to stay in effect.

Some of the changes became effective immediately, such as tax credits to small businesses to provide health benefits to workers and matching grants to states to expand their Medicaid programs to more individuals and families. Others, such as increasing Medicaid payments to primary care doctors and establishing affordable insurance exchanges will be instituted between 2014 and 2020. One of the bill's main tenets requires individuals to have health insurance and for states to expand coverage to uninsured low-income individuals provided by Medicaid programs. An estimated 40 million people, many of which are women and families, will gain insurance as a result of the bill. The PPACA will also require health insurers to accept patients with preexisting conditions. Before the bill's passage, a

Their opponents counter that universal health care is an overly costly approach and prefer that the private sector manages and funds health care through a free-market approach. In the early 1990s, President Bill Clinton led a major drive to establish universal health insurance in the United States. Although those efforts ultimately failed, healthcare reform has remained a major political topic. (See **It's Your Health** for more information.) In 2010, President Barack Obama signed into law the Patient Protection and Affordable Care Act (PPACA). The law's main goal

It's Your Health

Universal Health Care

Lack of health insurance harms individuals, their families, and the community-at-large. Because of the high costs of health care, uninsured individuals and their families have difficulties getting quality health care when they are sick. They tend to delay treatments until their illnesses become serious, and they are less likely to seek routine preventive health services that can avert or detect major illnesses early on. As a result, they tend to die sooner than people with health insurance.

The lack of health insurance aggravates the financial burden placed on the community as a whole. Because the uninsured tend to delay necessary treatment, they are often sicker and therefore more expensive to treat when they finally seek care. Uninsured people frequently turn to the nearest hospital emergency room, which is an expensive and inefficient way to get care. Furthermore, the primary providers of care to the uninsured—such as public hospitals, teaching hospitals, academic health centers, and nonprofit community hospitals—incur heavy losses from high rates of uncompensated care. In turn, these providers are forced to cut back on their services to all patients or even close their facilities.

Source: Reproduced from *Universal Health Care.* American Public Health Association. Available at http://www.apha.org/advocacy/reports/facts/advocacyfacthealthcare.htm; Related APHA Policy: *Public Health's Critical Role in Health Reform in the United States.* 2009, 200911. Available at http://www.apha.org/advocacy/policy/policysearch/default.htm?id=1386

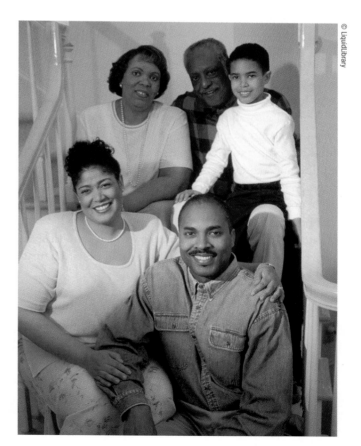

■ Many women are "sandwiched" with requirements for elder care and child care.

Gender Dimensions: Health Differences Between Men and Women

The population of the United States is getting older as disease prevention, health promotion, and innovative treatments prevent or delay disease and prolong life. In 2012, the average life expectancy for all Americans was 78 years of age: 76 years for white men and 70 years for black men, and 81 years for white women and 77 years for black women. On average, women now live 6 years longer than men. In 2000, there were only 70 men per 100 women over age 65; there were only 41 men per 100 women age 85 or older (see **Figure 2.10**). Note, however, that these figures are an aggregate of all U.S. women. When examined by race and ethnicity, life expectancy varies among both women and men.

As a result, most of the burden of aging rests on women, and increasingly women are aging into their oldest years without the support or help of spouses.[8] The aging trends have enormous economic ramifications. As women age, they become more likely to suffer from chronic diseases such as heart disease, cancer, and arthritis. These illnesses create significant morbidity as well as costs to affected individuals.[9] Currently, Medicare provides health insurance for all Americans over the age of 65, ensuring that all older Americans have at least some access to health care. Because Medicare covers only 80% of costs, however, a significant financial burden is often imposed on older patients when seeking care.[10]

The economic realities faced by elderly women also affect women's health. As women age, they are likely to need increased access to prescription drugs, perhaps specialty medical assistance, durable

medical equipment (such as walkers and orthopedic beds), and other expensive goods and services.

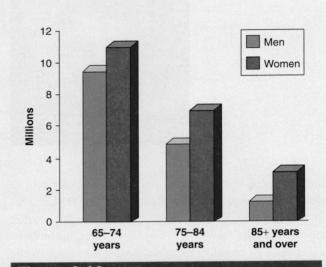

Figure 2.10
Population 65 years and over by age and gender, 2010.

Source: Data from U.S. Census Bureau, 2010 Census Summary File 1.

new insurer could deny coverage to women who had cervical cancer, diabetes, or other conditions based on her health history.

The bill also allows the government to explore novel ways to encourage more cost-effective care. This includes funding comparative effective research that considers the clinical and economic benefits of new technologies compared to the standard of care. This type of research is helpful in understanding the real world impact of new products and helping payers to fund technologies likely to have the greatest impact. An example in the women's health space includes research on the most effective diagnosis and treatment for osteoporosis in aging women.

Healthcare reform also began federal funding of Accountable Care Organizations (ACOs). ACOs are provider groups like hospitals or physicians' group practices who take complete responsibility for the care of a patient rather than just providing isolated services. ACOs receive a fixed fee for the broader provision of care and are rewarded if patients' health improves. The theory is that by shifting the financial risk to providers—if providers are no longer paid for each medical encounter but are instead paid for overall care and quality—that care will be more appropriate and effective. Some ACOs are implementing

pilot programs for the care of chronic diseases like diabetes, while others are delivering more comprehensive care. These ACOs are attempting to provide a more cohesive and rational delivery of preventive services, disease management, and acute care. ACOs' influence on the costs and quality of care will take several years to evaluate.

The research and development of new technologies will influence both the types of medical care available as well as how it is delivered. Major advances in women's health will arise from research into genetic engineering, stem cell research, microscopic surgical techniques, and personalized medicine. Paying for these advancements and making them accessible to the majority of people will remain a policy challenge.

Preventive Care and a Focus on Women's Health

Preventative care is medical or health care designed to prevent or reduce the effects of disease or injury. Preventative care can improve quality of life and often save money by eliminating the need for expensive procedures. A positive outcome of this trend has been widespread support for many preventive services, such as mammograms, cervical cancer screening, and smoking cessation programs. The old saying that "an ounce of prevention is worth a pound of cure" has been proven true in most studies. (See Chapter 3 for more on primary, secondary, and tertiary prevention.) Investing in preventive services and education leads to members with fewer major medical problems, such as heart disease, and the ability to diagnose diseases, such as breast cancer, at an earlier stage.

Preventive services and health education are the cornerstones of effective women's health care. As awareness and support of these and other women-specific health issues has grown, many payers have established whole departments dedicated to women's health. These departments educate patients and physicians about best practices and new treatments for women; they also analyze the benefits of new technologies. Women's health departments within payer organizations have prioritized women's health issues by supporting prenatal check-ups and strict monitoring regimens for pregnant women, promoting women's cardiac health, and ensuring universal coverage of gynecological exams. Under the PPACA, women will not have to pay copays for core preventive care like mammograms, vaccinations, and cervical cancer screening.

Women as Healthcare Consumers

Women make most of the decisions regarding health care, both for themselves and their families: one large survey found that women make 90% of their families' health-related decisions.[11] As a group, women have seen their economic power and ability to affect the overall demand within the healthcare system increase substantially. Women in the workforce collectively earn more than $1 trillion annually.[12] According to a study by the Commonwealth Institute, more than 68% of women, compared to 55% of men, say they manage the bills in their household. Women's growing economic power has made them increasingly important in the eyes of pharmaceutical, medical device, and diagnostics manufacturers. More research and development dollars are being poured into discovering both necessary and voluntary treatments for women. In addition, women are taking a more active role in their own health care, by learning more about their health status, taking part in preventive health care, and articulating their needs to providers, payers, manufacturers, and legislatures. Together, these factors have raised awareness of women's health issues and made women's health a priority within the healthcare industry.

Despite advances over the past 40 years, however, health care is lacking for many women, especially for women who need it the most—women living under or just above the poverty line. Whether due to being unemployed or underemployed, not having adequate childcare support, lacking education, being in poor health, lacking access to resources, or just not having adequate support, these women often lack the decision-making freedom of women with additional resources. Today, lower-income women are disproportionately more likely than other women to be in poor health. Thus, women with the least resources often carry the largest burden of healthcare costs, disability, and responsibility in caring for others. Women with health problems may have difficulties obtaining care because of coverage restrictions, high costs, and logistical barriers, such as transportation. For many women, coverage and access to care are unstable. Health coverage, involvement with health plans, and relationships with doctors are often short lived, resulting in spotty and fragmented care. A survey by the Kaiser Family Foundation found that almost one-quarter (24%) of nonelderly women, compared with 16% of nonelderly men, delayed or went without care in the past year because they could not afford it.[5]

Long-Term Care and Women as Caregivers

Women are more likely than men to be responsible for taking care of friends and relatives who need care, and to make decisions about long-term care or assisted living communities that care for elderly or disabled persons. Additionally, because women on average live longer than men, the vast majority of residents in these facilities are women.

© Photodisc/Getty Images

■ Most older women in nursing homes spend down their life savings to pay for services until Medicaid begins to cover the remaining costs of care.

Long-term facilities provide ongoing care for people who need lengthy or even lifelong assistance with daily living due to an illness, injury, or severe cognitive impairment (such as Alzheimer's disease). Care can be provided either in a nursing home, in an assisted living facility, or at the patient's home. The national average annual cost for care in a nursing home exceeds $75,190 for a private and $52,000 for a semiprivate room.[13] Costs of long-term care and long-term care insurance are expected to continue to increase dramatically, with a semiprivate room costing $190,600 by 2030.[14] Paying for long-term care is an open-ended proposition, as some people may live in an assisted care facility and then move on to a nursing home and live for 20+ years or more in a facility; actuarial calculations on the costs have driven insurance prices up and, in 2010, forced the largest long-term care insurer (MetLife) from accepting new policies. Two insurance options are available to cover these expenses:

- Private long-term care insurance programs are very expensive and are predominantly purchased by wealthier Americans.

- Medicaid covers Americans in long-term care facilities once they have exhausted all other resources. Most older women in nursing homes spend their life savings to pay for services until Medicaid begins to cover the remaining costs of care.

With the U.S. population aging and the average lifespan increasing, informal caregiving by family members in the home has become a vital part of the healthcare delivery system. One national study estimates the value of unpaid caregiving at approximately $450 billion per year, twice as much as is spent on home care and nursing home services.[13] Women provide most of this care, even though most working-age women now participate in the labor force. As a result of shouldering the stress and burden for elder caregiving, women caregivers tend to suffer more adverse health events than noncaregivers.[14] According to the Commonwealth Fund, one-fourth (25%) of women caring for a sick or disabled family member rate their own health as fair or poor, compared with one-sixth (17%) of other women.[15] More than half (54%) of women caregivers have one or more chronic health conditions, compared with two-fifths (41%) of other women. In addition, one-half (51%) of all caregivers exhibit high depressive symptoms and sleeplessness.[16]

■■■■

Informed Decision Making

Choosing health insurance is often a baffling undertaking. Many options may mean little to the individual other than being associated with different monthly premiums. Most people receive their health insurance through their employers, so they usually have either a single option or a small menu of plans to choose from.

When choosing a health insurance plan, it is important to consider the following:

- **Deductibles:** Deductibles are set amounts that individuals must pay out-of-pocket before the benefit kicks in. For example, if a woman has a $500 deductible on her insurance plan, she must pay for the first $500 worth of healthcare services she receives before the insurance plan begins to pick up the cost. Usually, the less expensive the plan, the higher the deductible. Deductibles are common in all types of insurance programs.

- **Benefits:** The different benefits insurance provides vary from plan to plan. Look closely at the list of covered services. For example, does the insurance plan cover prescription drugs? Does it cover open access to relevant specialists or provide medical equipment needed for specific health problems?

- **Network:** Consider the implications of a restrictive network to the costs of care and access to care. Does the insurance plan restrict access to a specific network of physicians? Is your preferred doctor a member of that network? If not, what are the costs for going to a doctor

■ Choice of health insurance plans is often a baffling undertaking; there are many important factors to consider other than simply the monthly premium.

© Thinkstock/Creatas

out of the network? Are the major local hospitals part of the health plan's network?

- **Coinsurance:** Many plans require patients to pay a set percentage of charges, often 10–20%. While coinsurance can keep premiums affordable, patient costs can be very high if hospitalization or long-term care is required. Consumers should inquire whether their insurance plan has a maximum amount that a patient is required to pay if a hospitalization or other high-cost event occurs.

- **Emergency Services:** Often health insurance programs have restrictive criteria for use of emergency services. What is the process for receiving emergency services? Is prior authorization needed before going to the emergency room?

- **Copayments:** Copayments are fixed amounts of money a patient must pay to receive health-related goods or services. Copays usually have to be paid out-of-pocket, either at the doctor's office, at the pharmacy, or at the hospital.

By considering these factors when choosing health insurance, a woman is more likely to get a package that is right for her and her family.

■■■■
Summary

Health care is one of the top expenses in modern American life. In the United States, both public and private health insurance exists to help individuals afford health care. However, millions of Americans are currently uninsured or underinsured. The Patient Protection and Affordable Care Act, enacted in 2010, will reduce but not eliminate the number of people without insurance. Lacking health insurance has many negative effects on health: People without insurance are less likely than people with insurance to be able to afford regular medical care and are more likely to be sick, injured, or unhealthy. Different health insurance plans affect the amount individuals have to pay for healthcare goods, such as prescription drugs, and services, such as physician office visits.

Among the elderly population, issues of access to and payment for healthcare goods and services continue to be a major problem. Although most are covered by Medicare and Medicaid, the elderly, who are predominantly women, face a unique set of economic challenges in managing their health.

Profiles of Remarkable Women

Katherine Swartz (1950–)

Katherine Swartz is a Professor of Health Policy and Economics at the Harvard School of Public Health. She is a demonstrated leader in health policy research, with a focus on the issue of the uninsured. She has been involved in research concerning health insurance issues since she graduated from college and went to work at what was then the U.S. Department of Health, Education, and Welfare (now the Department of Health and Human Services). For the last 20 years, Prof. Swartz's research interests have focused on the population without health insurance and efforts to increase access to healthcare coverage. Her research contributed to policymakers' understanding that people without health insurance are not all alike—many different types of people lack insurance. Prof. Swartz also was the first researcher to show that people differ in terms of the length of time they may go without health insurance. In fact, many spells without health insurance last less than 6 months, but a significant percentage of uninsured spells last more than 2 years. The dynamic nature of health insurance coverage means that over the course of a year, many more people are at risk for the financial costs of medical care than the number estimated to be uninsured when a survey is conducted.

Prof. Swartz's interest in how health insurance might be made more affordable and more accessible to the uninsured has led her to analyze the markets for health insurance, particularly for individuals who may not be covered through work in a group insurance plan. This research has focused on insurance companies' fear of being left with the sickest and therefore most expensive people in these markets. Findings from her research have emphasized the need for government policy to reduce such fears so as to allow the nongroup insurance markets to expand health insurance coverage. One such policy that Prof. Swartz has proposed is that the government act as the reinsurer and take responsibility for the extremely high-cost people each year in the nongroup markets. Her most recent book, *Reinsuring health: Why more middle-class people are uninsured and what government can do*, was published in 2006.

■■■■
Topics for Discussion

1. How can a person's health insurance status affect his or her health status?

2. Should everyone have access to health insurance, even if he or she can't afford it?

3. Is access to health care a right or a privilege?

4. How will the expansion of coverage enabled by healthcare reform impact women?

5. What are some common health-related items that often are not covered by health insurance?

6. What role do employers have in the delivery of health care?

7. What are potential implications of Medicare becoming more like a managed care program and less of a fee-for-service program?

8. How can health insurance status be affected by women's different stages of life?

9. What are some central issues related to the elderly population's healthcare needs?

■■■■
Key Terms

Copayment/copay: A type of cost sharing whereby the enrollee or covered person pays a specified flat amount per unit of service or unit of time, and the healthcare insurer pays the remainder of the cost.

Fee-for-service: A traditional method of healthcare payment in which physicians and other providers receive payment that does not exceed their billed charges for each unit of service rendered.

Formularies: Lists of drug products that a payer has identified as part of a given health insurance product's covered benefits.

Generic drug: The chemical equivalent of a brand-name drug that is available once the brand-name drug goes off patent. Generic drugs are typically less expensive than their brand-name counterparts.

Indemnity: A form of health insurance in which a person prepays a premium in exchange for a specific amount of monetary coverage in the event of illnesses or accidents. If an illness or accident occurs, the enrollee or the care provider submits a claim to the insurance organization.

The insurance organization then reimburses the party for all or, in most cases, a percentage of the incurred costs.

Long-term facilities: Facilities in which custodial care is provided over a prolonged or indefinite period of time, required because of a person's disability or aging. Skilled nursing facilities, or nursing homes, are the most common types of long-term care facilities.

Managed care: A system of healthcare delivery that aims to manage utilization of services and cost of services, while measuring performance. The goal is a system that delivers value by giving people access to quality, cost-effective health care.

Medicaid: A joint federal/state health insurance program for low-income persons who receive public assistance or whose medical expenses "spend down" their income to qualify for the program. This program is administered by each state, and places fairly tight restrictions on payments for physician services and drugs. Also known as Title XIX.

Private health insurance: Health insurance provided by third-party payers to individuals or employer groups either through indemnity or managed care systems.

Public health insurance: Health insurance provided by government sources including Medicare, Medicaid, the Department of Defense (DOD), Veterans Administration (VA), and the Bureau of Indian Affairs.

Third-party payer system: A payment system whereby an insurer (or third party) pays for services rendered to an individual by a provider of care.

Universal health insurance: A system by which the government provides health insurance to all citizens, thereby controlling health insurance at the federal level.

■■■■
Websites

Academy Health: http://www.academyhealth.org

America's Health Insurance Plans: http://www.ahip.org

Center for Medicare and Medicaid Services: http://www.cms.hhs.gov

Kaiser Family Foundation: http://www.kaisernetwork.org

National Center for Quality Assurance: http://www.ncqa.org

The Patient Protection and Affordable Care Act: http://www.healthcare.gov/law/index.html

■■■■

References

1. Fuchs, V. (2012) Major trends in the U.S. health economy since 1950. *New England Journal of Medicine* 366:973–977.

2. Martin A., Lassman D., Washington B., et al. (2012). The National Health Expenditure Accounts Team. Growth in US health spending remained slow in 2010; Health share of gross domestic product was unchanged from 2009. *Health Affairs* 31(1): 208–219.

3. DeNavas-Walt, C., Proctor, B., & Smith, J. (2011). *U.S. Census Bureau, Current Population Reports, P60-239, Income, poverty, and health insurance coverage in the United States: 2010.* U.S. Government Printing Office, Washington, DC. Available at: http://www.census.gov/prod/2011pubs/p60-239.pdf

4. Tait, E., Laditka, S., Laditka. J., et al. (2012). Use of complementary and alternative medicine for physical performance, energy, immune function, and general health among older women and men in the United States. *Journal of Women & Aging* 24(1): 23–43.

5. Kaiser Family Foundation. (2011). *Key findings from the Kaiser Women's Health Survey.* Available at: http://www.kff.org/womenshealth/upload/8164.pdf

6. EBRI Databook on Employee Benefits (4th ed.). (2008). Washington, DC: Employee Benefits Research Institute; and Fronstin, P. *The future of employment-based health benefits: Have employers reached a tipping point?* Washington, DC: National Academies Press.

7. U.S. Department of Health and Human Services. (August 5, 2010). *Trustees announce solvency of Medicare trust fund extended by 12 Years to 2029.* Available at: http://www.hhs.gov/news/press/2010pres/08/20100805d.html

8. Families USA. (2007). *Wrong direction: One out of three Americans are uninsured.* Publication 07-108. Available at: http://www.policyarchive.org/handle/10207/5864

9. Collins, S., Kriss, J., Davis, K., et al. (2006). *Squeezed: Why rising exposure to health care costs threatens the health and financial well-being of American families, prepared by the Commonwealth Fund.* Washington, DC: The Commonwealth Fund.

10. Shaller, D. (2005). *Consumers in health care: The burden of choice, prepared for the California HealthCare Foundation.* Sacramento, CA: California Hospital Association.

11. Fronstin, P., & Collins, S. (2008). *Findings from the 2007 EBRI/Commonwealth Fund consumerism in health survey.*

12. U.S. Bureau of Labor Statistics. (2011). *Women's earnings and employment by industry, 2009.* Available at: http://www.bls.gov/opub/ted/2011/ted_20110216.htm

13. U.S. Department of Health and Human Services. (2012). *The Federal Long Term Care Insurance Program on-line calculator.* Available at: http://www.healthcare.gov/law/timeline/index.html

14. Coughlin, J., (2010). *Estimating the impact of caregiving and employment on well-being. Outcomes & insights in health management.* Available at: http://www.well-beingindex.com/files/20100513_CHR_CareGiving.pdf

15. Ho, A., Collins, S., Davis, K., et al. (August 2005). A look at working-age caregivers' roles, health concerns, and need for support. *The Commonwealth Fund* 854(1): 1–12.

16. Johnson, R. W., & Wiener, J. M. (2006). *A profile of older Americans and their caregivers* (Occasional Paper Number 8). Washington, DC: The Urban Institute.

Chapter Three

Health Promotion and Disease Prevention

Chapter Objectives

On completion of this chapter, the student should be able to discuss:

1. Health promotion and disease prevention at the individual and population levels.

2. Concepts of epidemiology, incidence, prevalence, morbidity, and mortality, and why they are important.

3. Primary, secondary, and tertiary levels of prevention.

4. How race, ethnicity, age, sexual orientation, and other factors influence public health.

5. Barriers to healthcare access experienced by different groups of women.

6. Major health concerns in the developing world, and how these concerns compare to those in developed countries.

7. How life expectancy differs by gender and race.

8. Healthcare concerns and preventive measures for adolescents.

9. Healthcare concerns and preventive measures for young adults.

10. Healthcare concerns and preventive measures for women in midlife.

11. Healthcare concerns and preventive measures for senior women.

12. Taking responsibility for one's own health.

womenshealth.jbpub.com

Women's Health Online is a great source for supplementary women's health information for both students and instructors. Visit

http://womenshealth.jbpub.com

to find a variety of useful tools for learning, thinking, and teaching.

Introduction

Health is more than the absence of disease. Health depends on many positive factors as well, including what people eat, how often they are physically active, how they interact with their environment, and what kinds of relationships they have. Fully one-half of the deaths in the United States are due to people's behavioral choices.[1] Health promotion is the act of encouraging people to improve their health and maintain a healthy lifestyle.

A specific type of health promotion called disease prevention attempts to improve public health by preventing diseases. Heart disease, stroke, cancer, and many other chronic diseases lack simple cures, but diet, physical activity, and other lifestyle choices can often either prevent them from occurring or help manage the conditions after they develop. In addition, many diseases or conditions can be prevented, partially mitigated, or treated more easily if they are found and treated early.

At an individual level, health promotion can consist of efforts to learn about one's own health and to develop and maintain healthful behaviors. At the population level, health promotion often consists of major public health campaigns run by government entities, nongovernmental organizations, universities, and other organizations. These campaigns may seek to change a law, encourage a healthful behavior, educate a group of people, or improve the areas that people live in. A health promotion campaign could be as broad as a national cigarette tax or speed limit, or as narrow as an effort to increase knowledge of birth defects to teenage Latina women living in a specific Chicago neighborhood.

At both the individual and population levels, effective health promotion depends upon knowledge of the target audience. The population of women can be examined in many ways, including by race, ethnicity, age, geography, sexual orientation, body type, and psychological temperament.

Recognizing this diversity, and how it influences causes, diagnoses, progression, and treatment of disease, is important for women's health. These differences create a need for tailoring the delivery of health education and health-care services. The health needs of a White, 54-year-old single actress living in New York City may differ sharply from those of a Black, married, 24-year-old homemaker in rural Alabama, but the needs of both women are equally important.

Political Dimensions

There are many players in the health system, including government agencies, advocacy groups, national health education associations, hospitals, and volunteer groups. The federal health infrastructure starts with the Department of Health and Human Services (DHHS), part of the U.S. cabinet. Led by the Secretary of Health and Human Services, this Department provides basic human services and protects the health of all Americans. As the U.S. government's principal health agency, the DHHS includes more than 300 programs. DHHS works with state, local, and tribal governments, and funds some local services. Eleven DHHS operation divisions—eight agencies in the U.S. Public Health Service and three human service agencies (**Figure 3.1**)—administer the DHHS's programs.

Within the DHHS and underneath the Secretary of Health and Human Services is the Surgeon General, who acts as the country's leading spokesperson about public health. Nicknamed "America's doctor," the Surgeon General advises the President and provides the public with information on how to improve health and lower the chances of disease and injury. The Surgeon General publishes reports and publications on topics such as the smoking, nutrition, mental health, violence, overweight and obesity, suicide, and sexual health. One of these initiatives, Healthy People, aims to identify national health improvement priorities, increase awareness of public health issues, and improve the health of all Americans. The current phase of the initiative, Healthy People 2020, offers a set of national disease prevention and health promotion objectives for the United States. These objectives range from reducing obesity and lowering the number of infections acquired in hospitals and clinics to improving sleep and reducing racial and ethnic disparities in health care.

■ Women are not a homogenous population.

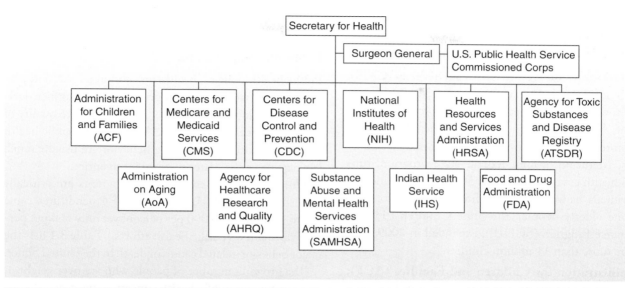

Figure 3.1

The U.S. Department of Health and Human Services (DHHS).

The eight agencies of the U.S. Public Health Service have different mandates:

- **National Institutes of Health (NIH):** The world's premier medical research organization, NIH supports more than 35,000 research projects nationwide studying diseases such as cancer, Alzheimer's disease, diabetes, arthritis, cardiovascular disease, and AIDS.

- **Food and Drug Administration (FDA):** The FDA assures the safety of foods and cosmetics, and the safety and efficacy of pharmaceuticals, biological products, and medical devices.

- **Centers for Disease Control and Prevention (CDC):** Working with states and other partners, CDC provides health surveillance to monitor and prevent disease outbreaks, implement disease prevention strategies, and maintain national health statistics.

- **Agency for Toxic Substances and Disease Registry (ATSDR):** ATSDR helps prevent exposure to hazardous substances from waste sites on the U.S. Environmental Protection Agency's National Priorities List, and it develops toxicological profiles of chemicals found at these sites.

- **Indian Health Service (IHS):** The IHS provides health services to the 1.9 million American Indians and Alaska Natives of 564 federally recognized tribes in 35 states.

- **Health Resources and Services Administration (HRSA):** HRSA provides access to essential health services for people who are poor, uninsured, or live in rural and urban neighborhoods where health care is scarce. Working with state and community organizations, HRSA also helps insure healthy mothers and children, increase the number and diversity of healthcare professionals in underserved communities, and support people fighting human immunodeficiency virus (HIV) infection and acquired immune deficiency syndrome (AIDS) through the Ryan White Care Act.

- **Substance Abuse and Mental Health Services Administration (SAMHSA):** SAMHSA funds and collects information on substance abuse prevention, addiction treatment, and mental health services. This agency provides federal block grants to the states to support and maintain substance abuse and mental health services.

- **Agency for Healthcare Research and Quality (AHRQ):** AHRQ supports research designed to improve the quality of health care, reduce its cost, improve patient safety, address medical errors, and broaden access to essential services. It provides evidence-based information on healthcare outcomes; quality; and cost, use, and access.

The Assistant Secretary for Health oversees these eight health agency divisions of HHS as well as the

Commissioned Corps, a uniformed service of more than 6,000 health professionals who serve at DHHS and other federal agencies.

The DHHS also includes three human service agencies:

- **Centers for Medicare and Medicaid Services (CMS):** CMS administers the Medicare and Medicaid programs, which provide health care to approximately one in four Americans. Medicare provides health insurance for more than 48 million elderly and disabled Americans. Medicaid, a joint federal–state program, provides health coverage for about 50 million low-income individuals, as well as nursing home coverage for low-income elderly people. The State Children's Health Insurance Program (SCHIP), expanded in 2009, now covers more than 11 million children.

- **Administration for Children and Families (ACF):** This agency administers the state–federal welfare program, the national child support enforcement system, and the Head Start program. The ACF oversees some 60 programs that promote the economic and social well-being of families, children, individuals, and communities.

- **Administration on Aging (AoA):** AoA is the Federal agency in charge of the interests and concerns of the elderly and their caregivers. Among other duties, the AoA provides services to the elderly, such as home meal delivery and transportation services, that enable them to remain independent.

Economic Dimensions

Public health policies, health-promotion efforts, and prevention campaigns can help people make healthier decisions and reduce the burden of illness, enhance quality of life, and increase the lifespan. Additionally, public health efforts that focus on changing behavior are usually much less expensive than later medical intervention.

Unfortunately, these types of programs are critically underfunded. In 2005, total medical expenditures came out to more than $7,000 per person, yet only $60 per person was spent on public health efforts.[1] **Table 3.1** lists the major behavior-related causes of death in the United States.

The growing number of people who are overweight or obese is a major public health concern. An estimate of the direct medical costs of treating obesity and overweight in the United States in 2008 found these costs came to more than $147 billion per year.[2] The indirect costs are also great: Obesity may cost U.S. employers more than $45 billion a year in lost productivity and health expenditures.[3] By changing their behaviors, such as modifying diet and increasing exercise, individuals can improve their own health and greatly reduce healthcare costs down the road. But education efforts and policies that promote healthy behaviors are also important to promote health. Requiring that school lunches meet basic nutritional requirements, or helping to fund local farmer's markets so that people can purchase fresh fruits and vegetables, for example, are two ways to encourage healthful decision making.

It's Your Health

Cost Benefits of Prevention Programs

Some examples from the National Center for Chronic Disease Prevention and Health Promotion show the cost benefits of prevention programs:

- One quality-adjusted year of life is saved for the cost of a smoking cessation program ($1,109 to $4,542).

- For each $1 spent on a school HIV, other sexually transmitted infection (STI), and pregnancy prevention program, roughly $2.65 is saved on medical and social costs.

- For every $1 spent on preconception care programs for women with diabetes, $1.86 can be saved by preventing birth defects among their offspring.

- A mammogram every 2 years for women ages 50–69 years costs only about $9,000 per year of life saved.

- For the cost of 100 Papanicolaou (Pap) tests for low-income elderly women, about $5,907 and 3.7 years of life are saved.

Source: United States Department of Health and Human Services, Centers for Disease Control and Prevention, National Center for Chronic Disease Prevention and Health Promotion. Available at http://www.cdc.gov/nccdphp/index.htm.

Table 3.1   Leading Behavior-Related Causes of Death in the United States

Cause	Number of Deaths Per Year	Percentage of Total Deaths
Tobacco	435,000	18.1
Poor diet and inactivity	365,000	15.2
Alcohol consumption	85,000	3.5
Motor vehicle accidents	43,000	1.8
Firearm (gun) accidents	29,000	1.2
Sexual behavior	20,000	0.8
Illegal drug use	17,000	0.7

Source: Steen, J. (2007). *The primacy of public health.*

Total costs associated with diseases are often significantly lower for people who take part in preventive care measures. For example, according to the American Cancer Society, the 5-year survival rate for cancers detected at the earliest invasive stage is 93%; the 5-year survival rate for cancers detected at the latest stages is only 15%. The costs and associated morbidity of treating women with early cellular changes, or minor cervical cancers, is significantly lower than that associated with treating women for invasive disease once cervical cancer has spread. Early detection can reduce both the financial cost and the human costs counted in pain, suffering, and anxiety.

Some health insurers and employers have grown to understand the economic value of health promotion and preventive care, and they recognize their importance by covering these services. Some insurers and employers now offer incentives for joining a health club, or provide partial payment or reimbursement for alternative therapy services such as massage or chiropractic adjustments.

Epidemiology

Health promotion and disease prevention depends on epidemiology, the study of patterns of disease in the population. Although many people think of health and disease as issues relating to individuals, epidemiologists examine the health of communities, specific populations, and entire countries. Epidemiology examines the frequency and types of diseases in groups of people and the factors that influence the distribution of disease. Epidemiologists use the following terms to describe conditions or diseases within a population:

- **Incidence:** new cases of a condition that occur during a specified period of time.

- **Prevalence:** the total number of people affected by a given condition at a point in time or during a period of time.

- **Mortality rate:** the incidence of death in a given population during a particular time period. It is calculated by dividing the number of deaths in a population by the total population.

- **Morbidity rate:** the incidence of illness in a given population during a particular time period. Morbidity rate is calculated in a similar manner to mortality rate.

Incidence and prevalence rates allow epidemiologists to examine how diseases or conditions progress. A condition with a high prevalence and a low incidence (a common

It's Your Health

Important Epidemiological Terms

Measures of Morbidity (illness)

Incidence = number of new cases of a disease during a given period of time/total population at risk

Prevalence = number of existing cases of a disease at a given point in time/total population at risk

Measures of Mortality (death)

Mortality rate = number of deaths in a population in a given period of time/total population

condition with few new cases), for example, might eventually stabilize or drop within a population, whereas a condition with a low prevalence but a high incidence (a rare condition with many new cases) may indicate a new and dangerous outbreak. Morbidity and mortality rates can be calculated across the entire population or within a specific subpopulation, such as age, gender, or race, to show relevant variations across those groups.

Within the field of epidemiology, health education and health promotion are two important public health concepts. Health education consists of efforts to improve people's knowledge and awareness about health. Health education can focus on teaching individuals, communities, or entire populations. Health education can cover any health-related topic, including prenatal care, improving physical fitness, or recognizing signs of stroke. Health promotion focuses on getting people to change their behavior. Health promotion includes health education as well as policies designed to improve the public health. (New York City's recent ban of trans fats in foods in restaurants is one such policy.) Health promotion deals primarily with lifestyle and chronic disease factors, such as smoking, drinking, use of primary care facilities, and sexual activity.

Many diseases and conditions are a result of lifestyle factors, such as poor nutrition or smoking, and are therefore preventable. Health promotion efforts attempt to allow individuals and populations to make informed decisions regarding lifestyle behaviors and disease prevention practices. Prevention is practiced at three different levels—primary, secondary, and tertiary.

- **Primary prevention** involves reducing exposure to a risk factor that may lead to disease or injury. Primary preventive measures include healthful diet, regular physical activity, cessation of smoking, and safe sexual practices.

- **Secondary prevention** refers to early detection and prompt treatment of disease. Secondary prevention includes screening tools such as mammography and Pap tests that detect disease before it spreads, thereby preventing further complications or disease progression. Secondary prevention also includes the use of medications and lifestyle behaviors to control chronic diseases that cannot be prevented.

- **Tertiary prevention**, which takes place once a disease has advanced, involves alleviating pain, providing comfort, halting progression of an illness, and limiting disability that may result from disease. It consists of rehabilitation in situations where a person can work on restoring certain functions, such as those lost after suffering a stroke.

Primary prevention is largely the responsibility of the individual. Secondary prevention requires both the guidance of the healthcare provider and the compliance of the individual. Tertiary prevention remains a goal of both healthcare providers and caregivers.

Women as a Population

The population of the United States is always evolving. As this population changes, its health needs also change. Some of these developments are along racial and ethnic lines, such as the growth of the Hispanic and Asian American sectors of the population, as well as in the increased numbers of people of mixed racial backgrounds. By 2030, one in five American women will be of Hispanic heritage, and one in 14 will be Asian (**Figure 3.2**). Significant diversity exists among women based on age as well. By 2030, one in four American women will be over the age of 65.[4] Because a majority of the elderly population in the United States is female, the needs of the elderly represent a significant women's health issue.

Women's increased educational attainment adds to the diversity of the population. Educated women tend to be more knowledgeable in their decisions about health care. Differing education levels create heterogeneity among women, as women with little or no education and women with advanced education may have different health and health education needs. The increased number of women in the workforce has presented new opportunities and challenges in women's health. Women work in a variety of settings, creating differences in their healthcare needs. For example, women working at home, in factories, in offices, in agriculture, and in retail will encounter different work-related health issues.

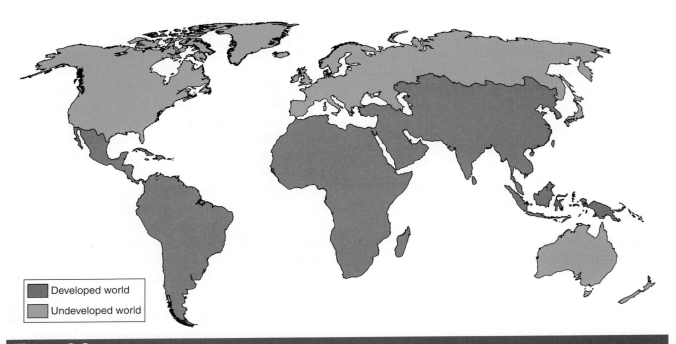

Developed world

Undeveloped world

Figure 3.2

World Map: Developed and Developing Countries

Source: Adapted from British Broadcasting Company, 2012. Development and Health. Available at http://www.bbc.co.uk/scotland/education/int/geog/health/revision/question2_physical.shtml

Another difference in the female population relates to the ways and stages of life in which women become mothers. Many women are delaying marriage and family to focus on careers, and thus are having children at a later age than they were one or two generations ago. This trend creates new issues surrounding childbirth, fertility, and parenting that target women in their thirties, forties, and fifties as opposed to primarily women in their teens and twenties. Other women are having children at younger ages, becoming teenage mothers. Many of these women are either raising their children alone or having their parents take a leadership role in childrearing responsibilities. Some women choose not to have children, instead pursuing careers and other opportunities.

Health needs of women also differ by sexual orientation. Health concerns specific to lesbians are often overlooked, leaving many women without proper guidance and medical attention. When lesbians share health concerns and risks with heterosexual women, misconceptions about the health needs of lesbians by healthcare providers and lesbians themselves may create barriers to receiving adequate care. Both lesbians and healthcare providers often believe that women who have sex with women do not need cervical cancer screening, routine gynecological care, or information about sexually transmitted infections (STIs), including HIV/AIDS. Other barriers to health care may include homophobia among providers and lack of health insurance coverage, because many lesbians are unable to share their partner's benefits or are eligible for less complete benefit coverage than a spouse of the same gender would be.[5]

Incarcerated women face special health-related challenges. Many have unmet medical needs that relate to drug addiction, mental health, and reproductive health. Women in prison often lack access to regular gynecological visits, breast exams, and basic medical care. Many women in prison are survivors of physical and sexual abuse, putting them at increased risk for high-risk pregnancies, HIV/AIDS, hepatitis C, and cervical cancer. Pregnant incarcerated women face challenges to their health and to the health of their developing fetuses.

Women with disabilities face unique challenges to their health. Physical barriers, such as facilities or examination

■ By 2030, one in five American women will be of Hispanic heritage.

equipment that are inaccessible or difficult to access, present major problems for these women in obtaining adequate health care. Communication barriers may pose a problem if a patient has visual, hearing, or verbal disabilities. Women with disabilities, as well as uninformed healthcare professionals, may believe that they are not at risk for sexually transmitted infections or other diseases. Many times, healthcare providers focus on the woman's disability and associated issues, rather than on basic routine healthcare needs.[6] Whether a woman's disability is a mobility, vision, hearing, speech, or cognitive challenge, greater levels of research, support, and compassion are needed to adequately address her health concerns.

Global Health Issues for Women

Standards of living vary greatly around the world. Traditionally, experts have distinguished between developed and developing countries (see **Figure 3.3**). Developed countries (Western Europe, the United States, Russia, Canada, Japan, South Korea, Australia, and New Zealand) have economies, health infrastructure, and standards of living that are significantly higher and more developed than those in developing countries (Latin America and the Caribbean, Eastern Europe, Africa, Latin America, Oceania, and most of Asia and Oceania). In practice these generalizations do not always hold (countries like Mexico, Brazil, and China have seen rapid growth and development, and standards of living may vary widely within a country), but as a broad tool, these terms are useful.

In developing countries, the health needs of women are extensive and often differ from the needs of U.S. women. The World Health Organization (WHO) lists 10 factors

I had a bad experience with a former gynecologist after she found out I was a lesbian. She went from being friendly and chatty to stiff and formal. I felt so uncomfortable I started missing appointments. I'm glad I have a better provider now.

31-year-old woman

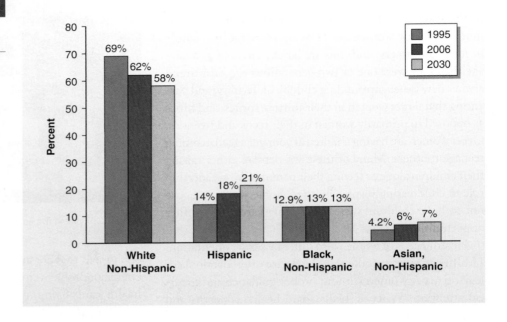

Figure 3.3

Projected U.S. population by race and Hispanic origin, 1995–2030

Source: U.S Census Bureau

that account for more than 40% of the disease burden worldwide[6] (**Figure 3.4**). Major behavioral and environmental risk factors that contribute to death and disease worldwide include the following:

- Underweight
- Unsafe sex
- High blood pressure

- Tobacco consumption
- Alcohol consumption
- Unsafe water, sanitation, and hygiene
- Iron deficiency
- Indoor smoke from solid fuels
- High cholesterol
- Obesity

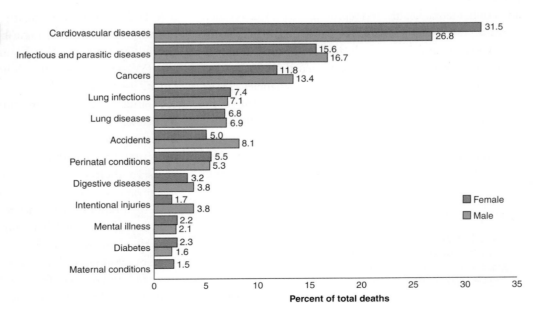

Figure 3.4

Global Causes of Death for Males and Females

Source: Adapted from *World Health Report*. 2004. World Health Organization.

All ages are at risk for **underweight** (living below a healthy weight), but this condition is most common among children younger than 5 years of age. Unsafe sex closely follows underweight as a risk factor and is the major factor in the spread of HIV/AIDS. HIV/AIDS is now the world's fourth leading cause of death. More than 15 million women are living with the disease; two-thirds of these women live in sub-Saharan Africa. Each year, about 2.7 million people are newly infected with HIV, and 1.8 million people will die from AIDS.[7] AIDS is a devastating disease. It primarily infects the adolescent and young adult sectors of the population—people who are parents, caregivers, and primary breadwinners. AIDS is wreaking havoc on already fragile health systems in many of the countries most dramatically affected. Over the past decade, the global community has organized an unprecedented campaign to fight the spread of HIV and to treat people who are affected. This effort has made enormous progress, but much works needs to be done.

Antiretroviral therapy (ART), though not a cure, can greatly increase the quality of life and life expectancy for people living with HIV. Yet, for years, these treatments were prohibitively expensive for most of the people living in the developing world. Recent efforts have mobilized billions of dollars to provide treatment and to prevent transmission of HIV; however, deciding how to most effectively spend these funds remains an important concern. Private companies are working with both **nongovernmental organizations (NGOs)** and governments to address the issue. The World Bank defines NGOs as "private organizations that pursue activities to relieve suffering, promote the interests of the poor, protect the environment, provide basic social services, or undertake community development." In wider usage, the label NGO can be applied to any nonprofit organization that is independent from government, including a large charity, community-based self-help group, research institute, church, professional association, or lobbying group.

Diseases caused or influenced by the local environment, such as cholera and tuberculosis, often occur when people do not have access to clean water or regular trash removal, and lack of regulations providing bacteria-free meat and food sources. People in developed countries often take for granted the infrastructures that make these systems available and reliable in their countries. In contrast, many developing countries have no system in place for sanitation and often use the same polluted water sources for bathing, drinking, and washing clothes. Parasitic infections from contaminated water and food sources are major causes of death and injury in countries throughout the world. Increasing access to preventive care, vaccinations, safe drinking water, and proper sanitation has been a primary focus of global health initiatives. Making this challenge even more difficult is the fact that the developing world faces a chronic shortage of trained healthcare providers, particularly physicians.

Despite the very real differences between the developed world and developing countries, many health risks are the same around the world. Risk factors for mortality such as high blood pressure, tobacco use, physical inactivity, and overweight/obesity were once considered "diseases of excess," or problems that were only of concern in wealthy, developed countries. Over the past 40 years, however, these same risk factors have become the leading risks for death around the world.

Around the globe, women are the primary caregivers for children and elderly family members. Although family composition varies from culture to culture, women consistently shoulder the burden of reproduction and feeding, clothing, and caring for children and elderly relatives. The health risks associated with motherhood in developing countries are many times higher than those experienced by women in more developed countries. Iron deficiency, one of the most prevalent nutrient deficiencies in the world, most severely affects young children and their mothers because of the high iron demands of infant growth and pregnancy. Sources of iron, such as meat, fish, and beans, are not always regularly available to families living in developing countries. Indoor smoke from solid fuels also primarily affects women because they are inside cooking for their families and working in the home far more often than men. In developing countries, about 700 million people—mainly women and children in poor rural areas—inhale harmful smoke from burning wood and other fuels. These and other factors put women at high risk for developing acute respiratory infections, especially pneumonia.[10] According to the World Health Organization:

In some communities, inequality of girl children and women is the transcending risk factor that explains the prevalence not only of maternal mortality and morbidity, but also of higher vulnerability of girls to childhood mortality. Risk factors like malnutrition of girl children resulting in anemia, and early marriage resulting in premature pregnancy, can be traced to the fact that women do not enjoy the status and significance in their communities that men enjoy.... Barriers to improving women's health are often rooted in social, economic, cultural, legal, and related conditions that transcend health considerations. Social factors,

■ Health risks and concerns change as a woman develops from a child to an adolescent, from a young adult to an older adult.

such as lack of literacy and of educational or employment opportunities, deny young women alternatives to early marriage and early childbearing, and economic and other means of access to contraception. Women's vulnerability to sexual and other abuses, in and out of marriage, increases risks of unsafe pregnancy and motherhood.[8]

Stages of Life

Health risks and concerns change as a woman ages. Reaching women with effective health promotion, or even taking care of oneself as one ages, requires some knowledge of these differences. Accidents, for example, are the leading cause of death for women aged 10–34, but drop to the ninth leading cause of death by age 65. As women age, the risks for diseases also change, as do their consequences. Many factors related to age have indirect effects on health: Women in their twenties face very different social pressures, challenges, and opportunities than women in their fifties.

However, some factors remain constant at any age. Good nutrition, regular physical activity, and adequate sleep are essential for health at all stages of life. Healthy living also encompasses avoidance of harmful substances, such as tobacco, drugs, and excessive alcohol. Mental health is equally as important as physical health. Maximizing mental health requires recognizing signs and symptoms of mental health threats, such as depression, drug or alcohol abuse, and physical or mental abuse. In addition, healthy sexuality and responsible sexual behavior are important for a woman's overall health. Healthy sexuality is expressed throughout life by exploring one's sexuality in adolescence, establishing long-term intimate relations in adulthood, and maintaining sexual pleasure in the senior years.

Health risks and concerns change as a woman develops from a child to an adolescent, and then from a young adult to an older adult. The risk of disease often varies throughout life, and, therefore, the methods of prevention differ depending on one's age as well as multiple other factors. **Table 3.2** highlights the major primary preventive measures that should be taken throughout one's life span.

Adolescence

The transition from childhood to adolescence is a time of major change. Adolescence begins with the onset of puberty and continues until the approximate age of 17, when adult physical development is generally realized. During adolescence, a girl becomes a woman and begins to form her identity and sense of independence. Parents should provide guidance and support during this time and help their children make appropriate decisions, but should also encourage adolescents to learn on their own and begin to understand how to take responsibility for oneself and one's actions.

Puberty encompasses changes in nearly every aspect of development, from physical to intellectual maturation. During this period in life, girls begin to differ in appearance from boys. Secondary sexual characteristics appear, such as widening hips, breast development, height and weight gain, and body hair growth. Perspiration and body odor increase, and vaginal discharge creates a new awareness of sexuality for girls. Menstruation, the onset of a woman's reproductive capability, also begins. As these changes occur,

Table 3.2 Primary Preventive Measures Throughout the Life Span
Avoid tobacco and other drugs.
Moderate alcohol intake to one drink per day or less. Avoid alcohol completely if you are pregnant.
Consume a healthful, balanced diet.
Participate in regular physical activity.
Learn appropriate and effective weight-management techniques.
Practice safe behaviors, such as using seat belts, wearing motorcycle and bicycle helmets, not driving under the influence of alcohol, and not riding with someone under the influence of alcohol.
Learn nonviolent measures to achieve conflict resolution.
If engaging in sexual activity, use condoms to reduce the risk of STIs, HIV/AIDS, and pregnancy.
Maintain an overall sense of well-being through stress reduction techniques, relaxation methods, socializing with friends and family, and seeking counseling if needed.
Balance work, school, family, friends, and time for yourself.

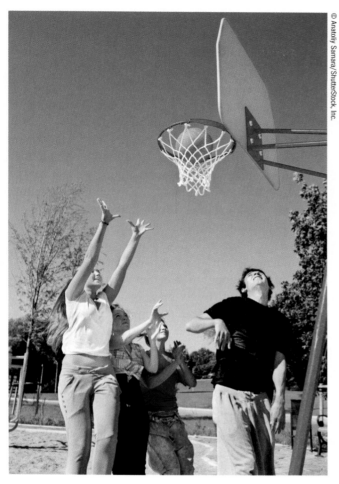

© Anatoliy Samara/ShutterStock, Inc.

■ Adolescence is a time when friends become an important influence in a girl's life.

adolescents begin to separate from their parents and assume greater independence. Teens may display rebelliousness, with friends often influencing decision making. Peer pressure also affects self-esteem and self-perception. Adolescent girls often focus on and define themselves through their relationships with both friends and romantic interests. Their concerns often revolve around popularity, attractiveness, and body weight. They face many challenges as they adjust to their sexual maturation and their increased independence.[10]

Specific Health Concerns for Adolescents

Adolescence is generally a healthy time of life, especially for young women. In the United States, the top four causes of death for females ages 15 to 19 are accidents (unintentional injuries), cancer, assault, and suicide (see **Table 3.3**). Mortality rates for boys in the same age group are more than twice as high as for girls.[11] Behaviors such as not using seat belts, not wearing motorcycle and bicycle helmets, riding with a driver who has been drinking alcohol,

and driving after drinking alcohol are responsible for many of the injuries that result in death. Homicide is the third leading cause of death for adolescents ages 15 to 19 years and the sixth leading cause of death for adolescents ages 10 to 14 years.[10] On average, guns kill 10 to 12 children

Table 3.3 Leading Causes of Death for U.S. Females Aged 10–24

Ages 10–14

Cause	Percentage of Total Deaths
1. Accidents	33.4
2. Malignant neoplasms (cancer)	14.9
3. Assault	5.4
4. Heart disease	5.4
5. Congenital and chromosomal abnormalities	5.3
6. Suicide	4.9
7. Benign and in situ neoplasms	1.6
8. Cerebrovascular disease (stroke)	1.5
9. Chronic respiratory disease	1.3
10. Septicimia (blood infections)	1.3

Ages 15–19

Cause	Percentage of Total Deaths
1. Accidents	51.3
2. Suicide	7.9
3. Assault	7.7
4. Malignant neoplasms (cancer)	6.8
5. Heart disease	3.2
6. Congenital and chromosomal abnormalities	2.3
7. Pregnancy and childbirth	1.0
8. Chronic respiratory diseases	1.0
8. Cerebrovascular disease (stroke)	0.9
10. Influenza and pneumonia	0.8

Ages 20–24

Cause	Percentage of Total Deaths
1. Accidents	40.7
2. Assault	8.5
3. Malignant neoplasms (cancer)	7.6
4. Suicide	7.4
5. Heart disease	4.8
6. Pregnancy and childbirth	2.9
7. Congenital and chromosomal abnormalities	1.9
8. HIV/AIDS	1.4
9. Cerebrovascular disease (stroke)	1.2
10. Diabetes	1.0

Source: Modified from Heron, M. (2010). Deaths: Leading causes for 2006. *National Vital Statistics Reports* 58(14). Hyattsville, MD: National Center for Health Statistics. Available from: http://www.cdc.gov/nchs/data/nvsr/nvsr58/nvsr58_14.pdf

(ages 0–19) in the United States every day. About 25% of these children and teenagers take their own lives, while the other deaths are homicides or unintentional injuries. In contrast, in the developing world, major health issues for young people typically involve infections, diarrheal diseases, and other communicable diseases like tuberculosis.

Although many adolescents display moody behavior and signs of rebelliousness (normal behaviors during the teenage years), this should not be confused with depression, a significant concern during adolescence. As girls reach adolescence, there is a noted increase in the rate of depression and the rate of suicide attempts. At any given time, between 10% and 15% of children and adolescents have some symptoms of depression. After age 15, depression is twice as common in girls and women as in boys and men.[11] Suicide is the second leading cause of death for adolescents ages 15–19 years and the third leading cause of death for younger adolescents.[10] A national survey found that 14% of high school students have seriously considered attempting suicide and 7% of students had attempted suicide. Of the students surveyed, girls were more likely than boys to have considered attempting suicide (17% versus 10%) and more likely to actually attempt suicide (8% versus 5%).[12]

Trying new behaviors during adolescence is essential for healthy development; however, risky behaviors, such as sexual experimentation or drug and alcohol abuse, may have dangerous, life-altering consequences. Sexual relations often occur before adolescents have experience and skills in self-protection and in setting and expressing the kinds of behaviors they feel comfortable with, before they have acquired adequate information about sexually transmitted infections (STIs), and before they have access to health services and supplies (such as condoms). Almost one-half (46%) of U.S. high school students have had sex at least once, and more than one-third (34%) are currently sexually active.[12] This problem is often amplified in developing countries, where girls typically have less access to health care and information. While teen pregnancy rates dropped for much of the 1990s and into the 2000s, each year approximately one million U.S. teenagers become pregnant.[13] Increased condom use, the adoption of the effective injectable and implantable contraceptives, and the leveling off of teen sexual activity are some of the factors believed to be driving this downturn in teen pregnancies. Of the students who were currently sexually active, 61% reported that they had used a condom during their last act of sexual intercourse, leaving four in ten sexually active students at high risk for various STIs, including HIV infection.[12] Approximately three million cases of STIs occur annually among teenagers.[14] HIV infection is the seventh-leading cause of death among persons ages 20 to 24 years in the United States.[10] Chlamydia infection during adolescence is more likely to result in pelvic inflammatory disease and, potentially, lead to infertility.

Globally, more than half of all new HIV infections affect members of the 15–24 age group. According to UNAIDS, "7,000 girls and women become infected with HIV every day. In South Africa, Zambia, and Zimbabwe, young women (ages 15–24) are five to six times more likely to be infected than young men of the same age."[15] In one study in Zambia, more than 12% of the 15- and 16-year-olds seen at antenatal clinics were already infected with HIV. Girls appear to be especially vulnerable to infection.

Adolescents may also engage in substance use, another risky behavior. Alcohol and drug use are detrimental activities on their own (see Chapter 13), but they also lead to other situations that may compromise one's health. The Youth Risk Behavior Survey, an annual national survey of high school students, found that 42% of high school students had drunk alcohol within the past month, and 24% had drunk five or more alcoholic drinks in a row in the past month. Almost one-quarter (22%) of sexually active students had had at least one drink the last time they had intercourse. Just over 10% of students had driven a car or other vehicle while drinking, while almost 3 in 10 (28%) had been in a car while the driver had been drinking.[12] In addition to their direct affects on health, alcohol and drug

It's Your Health

Tattoos

The following advice has been prepared by professional tattooists working with local, state, and national health authorities.

1. Always insist that you see your tattooist remove a new needle and tube set-up from a sealed envelope immediately prior to your tattoo.

2. Be certain that you see your tattooist pour a new ink supply into a new disposable container.

3. Make sure your artist puts on a new pair of disposable gloves before setting up tubes, needles, and ink supplies.

4. Satisfy yourself that the shop furnishings and tattooist are clean and orderly in appearance—much like a *medical facility*.

5. Feel free to question the tattooist about any of his or her sterile procedures and isolation techniques. Take time to observe the tattooist at work and do not hesitate to inquire about his or her *experience* and *qualifications* in the tattoo field.

6. If the tattooist is a qualified professional, he or she will have no problem complying with standards above and beyond these simple guidelines.

7. If the artist or studio does not appear up to these standards or if the person becomes evasive when questioned, seek out a different professional tattooist.

Source: Alliance of Professional Tattooists, www.safe-tattoos.com. Reprinted with permission.

use increase the likelihood that a person will choose casual, high-risk sexual activities.

Cigarette smoking, the cause of one in every five deaths in the United States every year, typically begins during adolescence, before it is legal to smoke and before the mind is fully capable of making rational decisions. Nearly one-half (46%) of surveyed high school students admitted to trying cigarettes and 20% had smoked in the past month. More than one-half (51%) of these students had tried to quit at least once in the past year. [12]

Overweight and obesity have steadily grown to epidemic proportions among adolescents over the past 40 years (**Figure 3.5**). Increased consumption of high-fat, high-sugar foods, as well as reduced physical activity, appear to be the primary culprits behind this increase. However, this does not mean that American children and adolescents today are inherently lazier or less disciplined than they were in previous generations. Instead, epidemiologists believe the environment Americans grow up in has made it more difficult to eat a healthful diet and to engage in regular physical activity. The CDC has identified many environmental factors contributing to child and adolescent obesity and overweight, including:

- Sugary drinks and unhealthful foods on school campuses
- Reduced access to healthful, affordable foods
- Fewer safe, appealing places to play and be active
- Growing numbers of high-calorie foods and sugary drinks
- Less daily, high-quality physical activity in public schools
- Increased portion sizes in restaurants, grocery stores, and vending machines
- Increased advertising of high-calorie, high-fat foods
- Lack of breastfeeding support
- Increased presence and use of television, video games, and electronic media

Obese children are at risk for type 2 diabetes, low self-esteem, and many other adverse health outcomes. In 2009, 12% of high school students were obese, and 16% were

Figure 3.5

Prevalence of overweight among children and adolescents aged 6–19 years.

Source: Data from Ogden, C., Carroll, M., Kit, B., Flegal, K. (2012). Prevalence of Obesity in the United States, 2009-2010. NCHS Data Brief 82. Hyattsville, MD: National Center for Health Statistics.

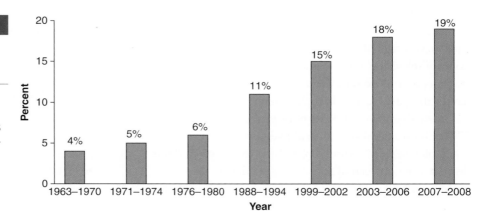

overweight. Nearly half (44%) of high school students were attempting to lose weight. Although male students are more likely than female students to be overweight, female students are twice as likely to attempt to lose weight. Female students are also more likely than male students to try to lose weight using dangerous, unhealthy methods (going more than a day without food; vomiting or taking laxatives; or taking diet pills, powders, or liquids).[12]

Tattoos and piercings have also become popular with adolescents and young adults. These activities hold inherent risks of infection and have been associated with serious complications. Increasingly, people are choosing to have body parts such as the lips, eyebrows, septums, or genitalia pierced, in addition to the more standard ear piercing. These piercings increase risks of infections, scarring, and nerve damage. Individuals can minimize the risks associated with these behaviors by choosing experienced professionals who uphold high safety and cleanliness standards. Some primary care physicians have ear-piercing kits and can perform the service in the safety of a clinical setting. Anyone getting either a piercing or a tattoo should be fully sober, both for safety reasons and to ensure this permanent decision is made with a clear mind.

Preventive Behaviors

Behavioral decisions are by far the greatest influence on adolescent health. Harmful behaviors include smoking, alcohol and drug use, unhealthy dietary behaviors, inadequate physical activity, and risky sexual behaviors. Many of them are contributing factors to major killers among other age groups, such as heart disease, cancer, and injuries.

Regular physical activity and good nutrition are two especially important aspects of health promotion for adolescents. However, comparatively few young Americans are engaging in these behaviors, despite their numerous, well-documented benefits. Just over one-third (37%) of U.S. high school students met the recommended levels of physical activity (were active for a total of 60 minutes or more for at least five days in the past week). A roughly equal percentage of high school students watch 3 or more hours of television a day. Nationwide, 23% of high school students do not exercise for 1 hour or more in any given day in the past week.[12] Female students are significantly less likely than male students to be physically active. Only 22% of high school students eat five servings of fruits and vegetables per day. Almost one-third (30%) of students drink at least one can of soft drinks per day.[12]

Although all of the essential nutrients are important for good health, calcium is especially important for adolescent

girls. Girls need to consume enough calcium to develop good bone health and protect themselves from osteoporosis in their later years. Unfortunately, many adolescent girls become concerned about their widening hips and weight gain, and consequently follow diets that lack sufficient nutrients. The average calcium intake of adolescent

It's Your Health

Safe Piercing

Here are 10 things to look for that will help you choose a safe piercer or piercing studio.

© IS Stock/Valueline/Thinkstock

1. **Cleanliness:** A good studio should have a separate counter, waiting room, piercing room, bathroom, and an enclosed sterilizing room. All of these, as well as studio staff, should be neat and clean.

2. **An autoclave and spore tests:** Studios should have an autoclave (a steam sterilizer) and a spore test to check whether the autoclave is working correctly. Chemical soaks or "dry heat" systems do not provide adequate sterilization.

3. **Single-use needles:** Needles should be opened while you are present, as well as individually packaged, sterile, and single use. Needles should go into an approved sharps container.

4. **Good piercing room practices:** Ideally, watch the piercer prepare for the piercing. Beforehand, the piercer should wash his or her hands and then wear latex gloves, changing gloves if he or she touches anything nonsterile.

5. **No ear-piercing guns:** In many cases, ear-piercing guns can't be adequately sterilized.

6. **Knowledgeable staff:** Ask the staff questions. Do they seem knowledgeable and friendly? How long has the piercer been doing his or her job? Does he or she seem well informed?

7. **An after-care sheet:** Studios should have a sheet that explains how to best take care of your new piercing. Make sure this sheet is up to industry standards.

8. **Listen to your instincts (and friends):** Have your friends had experience with a given studio or piercer? What did they think, and how does their piercing look? Do you feel comfortable with the studio/piercer? If not, go somewhere else.

9. **A license:** States and cities have different requirements for a studio or piercer, usually requiring regular inspections. Call your local health department to find the standards in your area.

10. **APP recognition:** Studios or piercers that have joined the Association of Professional Piercers have agreed to standards of cleanliness and jewelry quality set forth by the organization. APP members should have a membership certificate displayed on premises; make sure this certificate is up to date.

girls is about 800 mg per day, just two-thirds of the Recommended Dietary Allowance for adolescents of 1,200 mg per day.[16] Millions of teenage girls face even greater long-term consequences when they develop eating disorders as a result of poor body image, unhealthy eating habits, and dangerous purging behaviors (discussed further in Chapters 9 and 12).

Heavy sun exposure during early life has been strongly correlated with an increased lifetime incidence of both **melanoma** and **nonmelanoma** skin cancers. Tanned skin remains fashionable, however, and many teenagers and young adults regularly visit beaches or tanning salons. A major study of more than 10,000 young people found that sunscreen use was low (about 35%), but was likely to be higher among girls than boys. Eighty-three percent of survey respondents reported a recent sunburn, and 36% of respondents reported three or more sunburns. About one-tenth of teenagers indicated use of tanning beds. This use was mostly among girls and increased as the girls approached age 18.[17]

Generally, adolescence is a period of good health; however, millions of teens experience the health concerns mentioned here. In addition, behaviors started during adolescence can become habits that continue throughout life. Therefore, adolescence is an excellent time for young men and women, with guidance from their parents and healthcare providers, to make healthful and sensible choices about their own lives and behaviors (**Table 3.4**).

Young Adulthood

As adolescents become adults, they generally become independent of their parents and gain rights that were not afforded to them as children. Yet, the age of adulthood is often confusing considering that one can vote and can

■ Many young women avoid routine health examinations.

Table 3.4	Secondary Preventive Measures for Adolescents

Pap test 3 years after onset of sexual activity or by age 21.

Annual STI screening for sexually active adolescents.

HIV screening for high-risk adolescents with their consent.

Annual preventive services visit to screen for depression, risk of suicide, abuse (emotional, physical, and sexual), eating disorders, learning or school problems, and drug use.

Physical exam recommended at least once between ages 11 and 14, once between 15 and 17, and once between 18 and 21.

Annual screening for high blood pressure, cholesterol (if risk factors are present), and tuberculin test (PPD) if risk factors are present.

Annual screening for anemia if any of the following risk factors are present: heavy menstruation, chronic weight loss, nutritional deficit, or excessive athletic activity.

enlist in the military service at the age of 18, yet cannot legally drink alcohol until age 21. In addition, postsecondary school and the high financial burdens associated with advanced education keep many people at least partially dependent on their parents well into their twenties. Nevertheless, as a woman ages, her increased independence and age bring new health challenges and risks.

For some women, the first stage of young adulthood occurs in college. College can be an extension of adolescence in the sense that many women continue to experiment with new behaviors and explore their sense of self. Some use the freedom of being away from home to engage in behaviors that were not permitted in high school. Young women experience many of the same health threats that affect them as adolescents, including drug and alcohol use, smoking, violence (such as date rape), risky sexual behaviors, poor nutrition, and lack of exercise. Different health challenges face women who graduate from high school and then directly enter the workforce or begin parenting, as well as for women after graduation from college.

Specific Health Concerns for Young Adults

For women between the ages of 15 and 24, accidents, assault, and suicide are the top three causes of death, followed by heart disease and cancer. As women reach their mid-twenties, deaths from heart disease, cancer, and other chronic diseases increase. **Chronic diseases** (as opposed to **acute diseases**) are diseases or conditions that are permanent or semipermanent. They include heart disease and cancer, as well as diabetes, HIV/AIDS, and **autoimmune diseases**. Although chronic diseases are generally thought of as afflictions of the elderly, they are significant causes of

Table 3.5	Leading Causes of Death for U.S. Females Aged 25–44

Ages 25–34		Ages 35–44	
Cause	Percentage of Total Deaths	Cause	Percentage of Total Deaths
1. Accidents	27.3	1. Malignant neoplasms (cancer)	25.7
2. Malignant neoplasms (cancer)	14.8	2. Accidents	16.5
3. Heart disease	7.9	3. Heart disease	12.0
4. Suicide	7.3	4. Suicide	4.9
5. Assault	5.8	5. HIV/AIDS	3.8
6. HIV/AIDS	3.5	6. Cerebrovascular disease (stroke)	3.4
7. Pregnancy and childbirth	2.5	7. Liver disease and cirrhosis	2.9
8. Diabetes	2.3	8. Diabetes	2.6
9. Cerebrovascular disease (stroke)	1.9	8. Assault	2.4
10. Congenital and chromosomal abnormalities	1.4	10. Chronic respiratory disease	1.4

Source: Modified from Heron, M. (2010). Deaths: Leading causes for 2006. *National Vital Statistics Reports* 58(14). Hyattsville, MD: National Center for Health Statistics. Available from: http://www.cdc.gov/nchs/data/nvsr/nvsr58/nvsr58_14.pdf

death for all age groups; additionally, healthful behavior choices and prevention strategies begun early in life can often prevent these diseases from developing later in life or reduce the harm that these diseases cause.

Causes of death for young adult women vary dramatically by race and ethnicity. These variations are especially pronounced during the young adult years. HIV-related diseases are the leading cause of death for Black women ages 25–34, but only the seventh-leading cause for Hispanic women, and the tenth-leading cause for White and Asian American women in that same age group (see **Table 3.5**).[10] White women ages 25–34, meanwhile, are more likely to die from suicide or accidents than other women their same age. Black women are more likely than any other racial or ethnic group to die during these years, followed respectively by White, Hispanic, and Asian women.[10] Cultural, economic, social, and individual factors all contribute to these differences.

In developing countries, young adult women are at high risk from reproductive health–related disease and infectious disease. The top causes of death for young adult women in developing countries in this age group are six infectious diseases:

- Pneumonia
- Tuberculosis
- Diarrheal diseases
- Malaria
- Measles
- HIV/AIDS

Young adulthood can be rewarding as well as stressful. During this time, many women seek or develop long-term intimate relationships. They may start a family and have children. Women may be defining their career path,

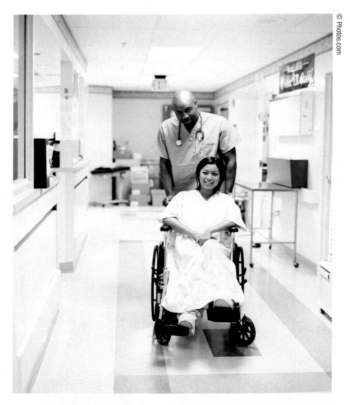

■ Women with disabilities often face condescending attitudes or discrimination when visiting healthcare providers.

advancing within their career, or still searching for the right career. Many women face obstacles along the way, such as a lack of adequate childcare and the juggling of family and work responsibilities. As women with disabilities enter the workforce, they may encounter new challenges, including discrimination from employers and employees, difficulty moving throughout the workplace, and adjustment to new tasks. Some women find it difficult to cope as their friends transition into different stages of life while they feel as if they are standing still. Managing stress and maintaining emotional well-being are important for achieving a healthy perspective.

Although women and men report similar levels of stress, causes of stress and coping mechanisms often differ between women and men. A study of 1,600 Americans found that women are more apt to attribute stress to family and health issues than are men. Most women surveyed (52%) were personally concerned about the effect of stress on their health and 30% (versus 24% of men) said that they found it "very challenging" to manage the stress and tension they confront. Men were more likely than women to report watching more television (42% versus 36%) and drinking alcohol (29% versus 18%) as a way of dealing with the stress in their lives. Women report either increased eating of "comfort foods" or decreased contact with the stressor as common strategies of coping.[18]

Alcohol and drug abuse affect the lives of many young women, including women who have children. An estimated 6 million children younger than 18 years of age have a parent who has used illicit drugs in the past month. Marijuana is the drug parents are most likely to use. Heavy drinking, defined as consumption of five or more drinks at one time on at least three occasions in the past 30 days, was reported by 5.2 million parents (3% of mothers and 14% of fathers).[19]

Young women deal with health-related issues associated with dating and sexual relationships, including sexual violence, STIs, and pregnancy. Consider these statistics:

- Almost 18% of the women in the United States have been the victim of rape or attempted rape at some point during their lives.

- In college, one in four female students is a rape survivor; experts estimate about 60% of the victims in reported rapes know their assailant.

- One-third of the 333 million global cases of STIs that occur every year occur among young people under 25 years of age.

- According to Planned Parenthood International, nearly 4 in 10 pregnancies are unplanned.

■ Physical activity is important for both physical and mental well-being.

- The WHO estimates that between 8 and 30 million unplanned pregnancies result from inconsistent or incorrect use of contraceptive methods, or from method-related failure.

Women who desire children may face fertility problems or other complications regarding pregnancy or childbearing. Infertility can lead to physical and emotional stress, financial burdens, and the anxiety and discomfort that often accompany fertility tests and treatment (see Chapter 6). Lesbians and women with disabilities may face disapproval from healthcare providers as well as friends and family members who feel they should not have children. Lesbians who want to have children may run into opposition or prejudice while they explore options for sperm donors or adoption agencies.

Preventive Behaviors

Because many chronic diseases can be prevented or controlled by behavioral changes, a young woman should continue following a healthful diet, participating in regular physical activity, avoiding smoking and drug abuse, and

Contributors to Improved Life Expectancy for Women

Identification, treatment, eradication, and control of some infectious and parasitic diseases

Better prenatal and antenatal care

More efficient, effective methods for assisting childbirth

Greater awareness, identification, and control of threats to health and ways to promote and maximize health

Improved protection from environmental and workplace toxins and hazards

moderating her alcohol intake. Secondary preventive measures, such as screenings for cancer, Pap and human papillomavirus (HPV) tests, and blood pressure screenings, are essential during this time as well (see **It's Your Health**).

As in all stages of life, positive mental well-being is essential for a young woman's overall health. Finding ways to cope with stress and addressing any mental health issues will help to establish a more balanced sense of well-being. Physical activity, healthy relationships with an intimate partner as well as close friends, and participation in enjoyable activities are all effective ways of reducing stress.

Sexual assault is a concern for women of all ages, but women in their late teens and twenties especially should be aware of this possibility. It is not healthy for women to consider themselves victims or targets for violence at all times, but education about how to avoid compromising situations and how to fight off an attack if it should occur can help women to maintain their independence and peace of mind.

During this period of life, some women have multiple sexual partners or may be sexually involved with someone who has multiple partners. These women are at high risk

■ Many women no longer choose to begin their families in their twenties.

for contracting STIs if they do not protect themselves by using latex condoms or other barrier contraception methods. Most sexually transmitted infections can exist with or without symptoms, and if untreated, cause infertility or other health problems (see Chapter 7).

Many women experience pregnancy for the first time in their twenties and thirties. Roughly one-half of all pregnancies are unplanned, causing anxiety and difficult choices for many women. Whether a woman is in a relationship or dealing with a pregnancy on her own, an unplanned pregnancy can be an enormously stressful experience. Seeking advice and counseling from friends, family, healthcare providers, and knowledgeable reproductive health agencies can help women make the decision that is best for them.

For a woman who is planning to become pregnant, proper nutrition and consumption of essential minerals and vitamins like folic acid are important measures to prevent birth defects. For a woman who is sexually active and does not want to become pregnant, effective birth control and risk reduction for STIs become very important preventive health behaviors. Other lifestyle choices become significant preventive health choices as well, such as wearing sunblock, reducing unnecessary stress, and making sure that routine medical appointments are made. In the case of skin cancers, routine visits to the dermatologist or primary care physician for full body checks are important for all women, but vital for women with fair skin or a family history of skin cancer.

Midlife

Many women in their forties have completed their families and either remain at home or continue working outside of the home. Some have established productive careers, whereas others struggle to find and maintain a job with decent wages, advancement opportunities, and a satisfactory work environment. Women in this stage of life are often busy raising children, caring for elderly parents, and working to keep their relationships healthy. As they reach their fifties and sixties, many must deal with the mortality of their parents as well as their own aging. Some may be fearful of getting older, while others are looking forward to retirement. Some grandparents, often women in their fifties and sixties, are raising their grandchildren. The parents of these children, for various reasons, have left the responsibility of childrearing with the grandparent, creating a different dimension of aging for these women.

Thanks to increasing physical fitness and greater access to effective medical treatment, many women discover midlife to be an ideal time to focus on themselves. They realize some of the benefits of the healthier lifestyles they have adopted over the past 20 years and consequently find their retirement years to be filled with physical activity, travel, healthy sexuality, and relaxation.

Specific Health Concerns for Women During Midlife

Between the ages of 45 and 64, the top five causes of death for women are chronic diseases. Cancer, heart disease, cerebrovascular disease (stroke), chronic obstructive pulmonary disease, and diabetes all benefit from behavioral changes (**Table 3.6**). In developing countries, the leading causes of death for women in this age group are a mix of infectious diseases, diseases of the reproductive system, and chronic diseases. Chronic diseases such as cancer and heart disease are increasingly dominant causes of death for women in this age group in developing countries as well.

■ Significant controversy and confusion remain over the use of hormone replacement therapy and dietary supplements for perimenopause and menopause.

Table 3.6 **Leading Causes of Death for U.S. Females Aged 45 and Older**

Ages 45–54

Cause	Percentage of Total Deaths
1. Malignant neoplasms (cancer)	35.8
2. Heart disease	15.3
3. Accidents	8.4
4. Cerebrovascular disease (stroke)	4.1
5. Liver disease and cirrhosis	3.1
6. Diabetes	3.1
7. Chronic respiratory disease	2.8
8. Suicide	2.6
9. HIV/AIDS	1.6
10. Septicemia (blood infections)	1.5

Ages 55–64

Cause	Percentage of Total Deaths
1. Malignant neoplasms (cancer)	41.0
2. Heart disease	18.1
3. Chronic respiratory disease	5.3
4. Diabetes	4.2
5. Cerebrovascular disease (stroke)	4.1
6. Accidents	3.2
7. Liver disease and cirrhosis	1.9
8. Kidney disease	1.7
8. Septicemia (blood infections)	1.7
10. Influenza and pneumonia	1.1

Ages 65 and older

Cause	Percentage of Total Deaths
1. Heart disease	28.7
2. Malignant neoplasm (cancer)	19.3
3. Cerebrovascular disease (stroke)	7.6
4. Chronic respiratory disease	5.8
5. Alzheimer's disease	5.2
6. Diabetes	2.9
7. Influenza and pneumonia	2.9
8. Kidney disease	2.0
9. Accidents	1.9
10. Septicemia (blood infections)	1.5

Source: Modified from Heron, M. (2010). Deaths: Leading causes for 2006. *National Vital Statistics Reports* 58(14). Hyattsville, MD: National Center for Health Statistics. Available from: http://www.cdc.gov/nchs/data/nvsr/nvsr58/nvsr58_14.pdf

Menopause, the cessation of the menstrual cycle, is a significant transition for women during their midlife years (see Chapter 8). For some women, menopause is a welcome change, eliminating their menstrual cycle and the need

© Thinkstock Images/Comstock/Thinkstock

for contraception. Other women experience bothersome symptoms or more serious health concerns associated with menopause and have difficulty finding an effective therapy. Women entering menopause today are encountering more confusion than in the past due to recent controversy surrounding hormone replacement therapy (HRT). The controversy has limited the medical options for dealing with the distressing side effects of menopause. Women in perimenopause, the period just before menopause, may find themselves experiencing discomfort during sex or lack of libido.

Many women in their forties, fifties, and sixties find themselves sandwiched between the demands of their children and their parents. The recent economic recession, along with continuing high unemployment, has increased the number of students living at home while attending college and the number of adult children who return home after a divorce or loss of job. These "boomerang" children change the dynamics of life for many women in their middle years who assumed their children would grow up, leave home, and live as independent, self-supporting adults. Instead, many women must deal with a child at home again precisely at the time when their caregiver roles increase for their own parents.

Preventive Behaviors

As a woman ages, secondary preventive measures, such as mammograms and colonoscopies, become extremely important to ensure early detection of disease and, consequently, timely treatment. **Table 3.7** lists secondary preventive behaviors for middle-aged women.

As in other stages of life, maintaining mental wellness is a critical part of maintaining health. Women who are caregivers for children, elderly relatives, or both often find themselves suffering from severe stress, depression, and anxiety. Many of these women may see the effects spill over from their home life into their work life. Finding support groups, seeking professional help, and establishing time to take care of oneself are effective means for improving the mental health of many women.

Discussing options with a healthcare provider can help improve sexual functioning and desire, if necessary. Many women may still require contraception for preventing pregnancy or STIs if they are not in a mutually monogamous relationship.

The Senior Years

Over the past 110 years, the average life expectancy in the United States has increased by more than 30 years, from

Table 3.7   Secondary Preventive Measures for Women During Midlife
Annual screening for high blood pressure.
Periodic height and weight measurement to monitor for overweight and obesity.
Clinical breast examinations yearly.
Periodic screening for high cholesterol levels, at least once every 5 years.
Behavioral assessment to detect depression and other problems.
Annual fecal occult blood test plus sigmoidoscopy every 5 years or colonoscopy every 10 years or barium enema every 5–10 years; a digital rectal examination should also be performed at the time of screening—for adults age 40 years or older with a family history of colorectal cancer and all adults age 50 years or older.
Annual mammography for women at high risk beginning at age 35 and for all women after age 50. Some authorities recommend screening mammograms every 1 to 2 years for women 40 to 49 years of age.
Annual Pap test or HPV test; after three or more consecutive normal exams, the Pap test may be performed less frequently in low-risk women at the discretion of the patient and clinician.
Counseling about the benefits and risks of postmenopausal hormone replacement therapy.
Bone density measurements for women at risk of osteoporosis.

48 in 1900 to 78 in 2010.[10] Public health initiatives are responsible for 25 of those years; all the medical advances over the past century have only increased the average life expectancy by about 5 years.[1]

On average, women live several years longer than men. The life expectancy for women in 2010 was 81 years, while the life expectancy for men was 76. Cardiovascular disease typically appears later in women than in men, accounting for part of this difference. In addition, women are less likely to engage in dangerous behaviors such as drinking to excess or not wearing seatbelts or motorcycle helmets.

■ Living a healthy life from childhood on may lead to fulfilling and enjoyable senior years.

Life expectancy also varies by race (**Figure 3.6**). In 2010, life expectancy was 81 years for White, non-Hispanic women, 78 for Black women, and 84 for Hispanic women.[10] Social factors, rather than any biological differences between these groups, appear to be responsible for these differences. These differences shrink as women age. By age 65, the difference in life expectancy between non-Hispanic White and Black women shrinks from more than 3 years to 1.6, and by age 85, life expectancy for the two groups is nearly equal.

Increasing life expectancies have led to a "graying" of the U.S. population. Today, nearly one out of seven people in the United States is 65 or older. By 2030, one in four American women will be older than 65.[20] Furthermore, the fastest growing section of the population is people over age 85. In 2050, an estimated 18 million people over the age of 85 will live in the United States; in this year people in this age group will make up 4.6% of the U.S. population.[20] Because of their longer life expectancies, women constitute a majority of both these populations. The aging of the population presents a unique challenge to society, individuals, and healthcare providers, along with opportunities to allow this growing population to live healthier, more satisfying lives.

Health Concerns During the Senior Years

Women 65 or older face a spectrum of health issues. Some women remain healthy into their eighties and beyond, while other women struggle with continual health issues as they age. From the age of 65 on, chronic diseases are

■ A major health concern related to aging is the side effects of taking multiple drugs.

the leading cause of death for women in the United States (**Table 3.7**).[3] For women ages 65–74, the five leading causes of death are cancer, heart disease, chronic lower respiratory diseases, stroke, and diabetes. For women 75 and older, heart disease becomes the leading cause of death. As women's bodies grow frailer with age, Alzheimer's disease, influenza, and pneumonia become increasingly common killers.

Debilitating conditions such as osteoporosis and arthritis often make it harder for women over 65 to maintain their independence. Fall-related fractures are a major concern for anyone, but they can be extremely detrimental to a woman whose bone health is suffering (see Chapter 11). Arthritis can impede a woman's ability to perform daily activities, such as opening jars, lifting objects, bending to pick up an item that has fallen, or lifting herself from the toilet seat. A woman also may begin having problems with vision or hearing, creating new challenges in performing everyday tasks and maintaining independent living.

Women over the age of 65 often take multiple medications on a regular basis. The combination of these drugs may produce serious side effects. The risk of side effects is especially high for women who have multiple conditions or who take a medication that requires other medications to treat side effects it causes. Healthcare providers are not always aware of harmful drug interactions. Harmful effects of drug interaction may include abnormal heart rate and/or rhythm, depression, dizziness and imbalance, constipation, increased blood pressure, and confusion.

Healthcare providers and other caregivers can also harm elderly people by treating them with a lack of respect. This lack of respect is not necessarily deliberate. It can include a nurse withholding medical information from an elderly woman on the assumption that a woman "won't understand" the information, or a physician who calls her elderly

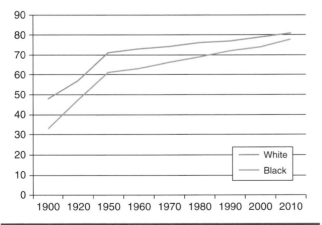

Figure 3.6

Life expectancy for Black women and White women, 1900–2010

Source: Data from Murphy, S., Xu, J., & Kochanek, K. Deaths: Prelinary Data for 2010. *National Vital Statistics Reports* 60(4). January 11, 2012. Hyattsville, MD: National Center for Health Statistics patients names like "dear" or "sweetie" in an effort to be friendly. Research has found that these kinds of habits reduce elderly patients' self-esteem and perceptions of themselves; these reduced perceptions in turn actually lower patients' life expectancies.[21]

The loss of a spouse and close friends may affect a woman's well-being as she ages. The number of women who are widowed doubles after the age of 65. Learning to cope with grief and loss is essential for physical and mental well-being. Maintaining independence and fostering social relationships may help women deal with feelings of grief, sadness, and loneliness. Diagnosable depression, however, is not the same as sadness, grief, or the emotional effects of loss. Depression is a significant health concern for aging women and may result from medication interactions, chronic disease, pain, or loneliness; it should not be viewed as a normal part of aging. The CDC estimates that 7% of Americans age 65 or older suffer from diagnosable depression in any given year.[11]

Women typically bear the responsibility of caring for their parents or loved ones when they need help. Women account for more than 80% of the family caregivers for

Gender Dimensions: Health Differences Between Men and Women

On average, a woman born in the United States can expect to live almost 7 years longer than a man born under the same conditions. Two major contributors to this discrepancy are women's lower rates of death for accidents and suicide. Accidents cause about 6.5% of total deaths for males, but only 3.5% of deaths for females, roughly half that amount. More than 2% of men, but only 0.6% of women, die from suicide.[11] Suicide and accidents dramatically reduce life expectancy because they typically happen while men are relatively young.

A man who dies at age 25 from a work-related accident reduces the average life expectancy for males far more than a woman who dies from a heart attack at age 70.

Compared to men, women are significantly more likely than men to die of stroke (6.7% of women's deaths versus 4.5% of men's deaths) and Alzheimer's disease (4.2% of women's deaths versus 1.8% of men's deaths), in large part because women are likely to reach the ages at which these diseases typically strike.[11]

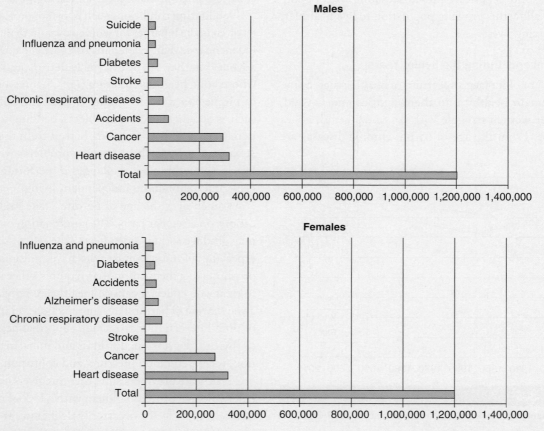

Source: Modified from Heron, M. (2010). Deaths: Leading causes for 2006. *National Vital Statistics Reports* 58(14). Hyattsville, MD: National Center for Health Statistics. 2010. Available from: http://www.cdc.gov/nchs/data/nvsr/nvsr58/nvsr58_14.pdf

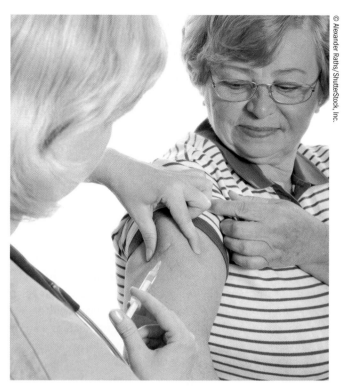

Flu immunizations significantly reduce the chance of an older woman getting influenza or pneumonia.

chronically ill elders, and 73% of these women caregivers are 65 or older.[22] The value of services caregivers provide is estimated to be more than $350 billion per year. Some women may experience cognitive decline and depression as a result of being the primary caregiver for a partner, relative, or friend.[23] Healthcare providers also need to be aware of the possibility of abuse by a relative or caregiver and help provide protection when a woman is unable to or afraid to protect herself (see Chapter 14).

As women age, their skin becomes thinner, loses some of its elastic quality, suffers injury more easily, and heals more slowly. Women who have spent a lot of time in the sun during their lives may develop skin cancers at this stage of their lives. Most skin cancers can be removed safely and easily with a simple procedure if they are found early. If left untreated, however, skin cancers can pose a serious health risk. Proper attention to skin care throughout life can prevent serious consequences as women age.

Sexuality also remains an issue for older women. Although many healthcare providers do not view their patients as sexual beings at this age, many women continue to desire sexual relations and may need advice for maintaining healthy sexuality as they age. An American Association of Retired People (AARP) study found that 61% of women ages 45 and older believe that "a satisfying sexual relationship" is important to their quality of life.[24] Chapter 4 discusses this issue in more depth.

Preventive Behaviors

The senior years can be a time of relaxation and fulfillment for women who are fortunate enough to have achieved financial stability, who have maintained their physical and mental health, and who are surrounded by loving family and friends. Other women may be less fortunate and experience considerable concerns regarding their future. Planning for one's future and maintaining one's health from childhood on may help women to have an easier time in their later years.

As throughout life, good nutrition, exercise, and avoidance of harmful substances can prevent harmful diseases and reduce their consequences in old age. Regular healthcare screening and preventive checkups are essential, as is continual monitoring for drug interactions and signs or symptoms that may signal a health concern. Additionally, women living in their senior years may wish to consider lifestyle changes, such as making safety arrangements to reduce the danger of falling, thus reducing their risks of accidents while maintaining their independence. Getting a flu vaccination and paying close attention to colds and minor illnesses can help keep a woman safe from pneumonia and influenza (**Table 3.8**).

Table 3.8 **Secondary Preventive Measures for Seniors**
Annual screening for high blood pressure.
Cholesterol screening every 3 to 5 years or as recommended by the healthcare provider.
Periodic height and weight measurement to monitor for overweight and obesity.
Clinical breast examinations yearly or as recommended by one's healthcare provider.
Initial assessment of cognitive function and monitoring of changes as part of a routine preventive visit.
Behavioral assessment to detect depression and other problems.
Annual fecal occult blood test plus sigmoidoscopy every 5 years or colonoscopy every 10 years or barium enema every 5 to 10 years; a digital rectal examination should also be performed at the time of screening.
Routine mammography screening as recommended by the healthcare provider.
Periodic evaluation for hearing loss and visual acuity.
Thyroid-stimulating hormone test every 3 to 5 years.
Bone mineral density test as recommended by the healthcare provider; counseling on fall prevention.
Annual influenza and pneumococcal pneumonia vaccines.

Women should also take special care of their skin as they age, using proper moisturizers and barriers to protect against skin breakdown. In addition, women should get bone density screenings to make sure they are not at risk for developing osteoporosis.

■■■■
Informed Decision Making

To take personal responsibility for their own health and wellness, all women should educate themselves about their health status. Integrating primary prevention methods into one's daily life can improve both present and future health (see **Self-Assessment 3.1**). By understanding their own secondary prevention needs, such as the appropriate screening methods for women at certain ages, women can better inform their healthcare providers about their health status and demand the healthcare services that they require and deserve.

The Internet has evolved into a valuable resource for health information. Yet the quality of health information on websites and shared through social networks like Facebook is extremely variable and difficult to assess. Evaluating the information can be a significant challenge, even for experienced users. Being able to identify the validity of the material in a given website is crucial, as it could potentially affect health outcomes for millions of people. Most online material is posted without any form of approval or review for accuracy and reliability, or it is posted by a company having a financial stake in the information being communicated (for example, pharmaceutical firms or physicians offering specific surgical procedures). Individuals must often rely on their own common sense and judgment. Keeping a critical eye and relying on trustworthy sources can help women find reliable information online. In addition, women should understand that open communication with their physicians is their right. Better communication between physicians and patients can improve both the quality of the care women receive and their health promotion knowledge base.

■■■■
Summary

Health promotion is the act of encouraging people to improve their health and maintain a healthy lifestyle. Health promotion may consist of an individual effort, such as a young woman learning how to protect her health, or it may consist of a large public health effort, such as a study to prevent deaths from lung cancer by educating teenagers about the dangers of smoking.

Health prevention may occur at the primary, secondary, or tertiary level. Primary prevention consists of avoiding a disease or injury, secondary prevention consists of early detection and prompt treatment, and tertiary prevention consists of managing a disease once it has advanced.

Global inequities in access to proper health care, including preventive services, medical treatments, family planning, or proper maternal and child health, threaten and reduce women's quality of life. These services are essential to women who seek to lead active, healthy, and happy lives at all stages of life.

Self-Assessment 3.1

Rate Your Preventive Practices

Answer the following questions:

1. Do you eat a healthful diet consisting of the appropriate servings of fruits and vegetables, grains, protein, vitamins, and minerals?

2. Do you participate in moderate-intensity physical activity at least four days a week?

3. Do you get enough sleep so that you do not feel tired throughout the day?

4. Do you avoid using tobacco products and drugs?

5. If you consume alcohol, do you do so in moderation?

6. If you are sexually active, do you use condoms or other barrier contraceptives to protect against STIs?

7. Do you employ methods to reduce stress, find time to socialize with friends and relax, and maintain an overall sense of mental wellness?

8. Do you practice safe behaviors, such as using seat belts, wearing motorcycle and bicycle helmets, not driving under the influence of alcohol, and not riding with someone under the influence of alcohol?

9. Do you use nonviolent methods of conflict resolution?

10. Do you receive routine preventive care from a healthcare provider?

The more questions to which you answered "yes," the better off you are! If you answered "no" to any questions, try to change that behavior to achieve a better state of overall health.

Profiles of Remarkable Women

Margaret Chan (1947–)

© Rick Gershon/iStockphoto.com

Margaret Chan is the Director-General of the World Health Organization (WHO), the United Nations organization that directs global health efforts.

Chan was born in Hong Kong in 1947 and obtained her medical degree from the University of Western Ontario in Canada. She started working in public health in 1978, when she joined the Hong Kong Department of Health.

Chan became Director of Hong Kong's public health system in 1994. There, Chan introduced initiatives to improve recording of and response to disease outbreaks, train public health professionals, and improve relationships between Hong Kong's public health department and local and international groups. She effectively managed outbreaks of avian influenza (bird flu) and of severe acute respiratory syndrome (SARS).

Chan's position leading public health efforts in Hong Kong required difficult decisions on a daily basis. To avoid a possible outbreak of influenza among humans, Chan ordered the slaughter of 1.5 million chickens in Hong Kong.[26] Chan had no way of knowing at the time how many chickens were infected, or if the outbreak would occur. The decision to destroy Hong Kong's poultry population also brought considerable economic consequences. But the consequences of a new influenza outbreak, both for Hong Kong and the world, would have been catastrophic. Today, many public health experts believe that Chan's actions may have prevented a global disease outbreak.

In a 2007 interview, Chan said, "In public health, especially when you're dealing with new and emerging infections, science is always lagging behind time and in the absence of solid evidence. But based on the best available information and evidence, one has to make difficult and often times unpopular decisions. Of course the recommendation ... was a very difficult decision we took, but all in all, that was the right decision."[27]

Chan joined WHO in 2003 and was nominated as Director-General in November 2006. Her first term ran through 2012; her second term will run through 2017.

Profiles of Remarkable Women

Eleanor Hinton Hoytt

Courtesy of Eleanor Hinton Hoytt

Eleanor Hinton Hoytt has served as President and CEO of the Black Women's Health Imperative since 2006. The Imperative is the only organization devoted solely to advancing the health and wellness of America's 19.5 million Black women and girls through advocacy, education, and leadership development. Before she joined the Imperative, Ms. Hinton Hoytt spent 10 years as the president of Hinton Hoytt & Associates. The firm provided strategic counsel to nonprofit organizations, foundations, and government agencies on effective organizational infrastructure, programs, and strategies for working with women of color. Before establishing this consulting firm, Ms. Hinton Hoytt was a director at the National Council of Negro Women, where she expanded their national presence as an active voice in women's health, including reproductive health and HIV/AIDS. She is a member of the Alliance for Nonprofit Management, has served as chair of the board of directors of the Avery Institute for Social Change, and is the founding chair of the board of directors of the Imperative (formerly known as the National Black Women's Health Project). Hinton Hoytt also produced the groundbreaking book *Tomorrow Begins Today: African American Women As We Age* for the National Council of Negro Women. She has received the NAACP's Thurgood Marshall Legacy Award and the Keystone Award for Women's Research Advocacy from the NIH Office on Women's Research. Most recently, she is the co-author of *Health First!: The Black Woman's Wellness Guide*. The *Guide* explores Black women's most critical health challenges today with discussions with experts and the uncensored voices of real women—from adolescence through elderhood. The focus is on prevention and awareness, across generations and circumstances—from candid conversations about reproductive health and HIV/AIDS to frank explorations of Black women's top 10 health risks, including cancer, obesity, and violence.

Many factors, including race, age, and sexual orientation, influence women's health needs. Certain preventive measures, such as a balanced, healthful diet; regular physical activity; positive, healthy relationships; and avoidance of drugs, tobacco and alcohol, are important for any stage of life. Other preventative measures, such as cancer screening tests, are recommended for women at specific ages. All women should take responsibility for their own health and wellness by educating themselves about their health status and risks.

■■■■
Topics for Discussion

1. How can parents, healthcare providers, and health educators encourage adolescents to follow healthy behaviors? How can they convince adolescents that their present behaviors will affect their future health?

2. What are some ways in which you can improve your health? Are there preventive practices from which your parents can benefit that they are not practicing?

3. How do the health needs of women in developing countries differ from those of women in the United States? How are they similar?

4. What are some barriers to health care experienced by lesbians? What are some barriers experienced by physically challenged women?

5. Some health behaviors are detrimental to well-being. Should policies such as restricting smoking or mandating bicycle helmets be mandatory or voluntary? How should these decisions be made?

■■■■
Key Terms

Acute disease: A disease that begins and ends quickly. Examples include pneumonia and localized infection.

Autoimmune disease: A disease caused by autoantibodies or lymphocytes that attack normal components of the body—molecules, cells, or tissues—by the organism producing them. It is more common among women than men.

Chronic disease: A disease that lasts longer than several weeks, often for the length of a person's life; it may be ongoing or progress slowly. Examples include diabetes, heart disease, and lupus.

Incidence: The number of new cases of a disease or condition in a given period of time.

Melanoma: A cancer that originates within the melanocytes.

Morbidity rate: The rate of illness in a given population over a period of time.

Mortality rate: The rate of death in a given population over a period of time.

Nongovernmental organizations (NGOs): According to the World Bank, "private organizations that pursue activities to relieve suffering, promote the interests of the poor, protect the environment, provide basic social services, or undertake community development." This term can be applied to any nonprofit organization that is independent from government, including a large charity, community-based self-help group, research institute, church, professional association, and lobby group.

Nonmelanoma: The most common cancers of the skin (usually basal cell and squamous cell cancers). Nonmelanoma cancers include all skin cancers except malignant melanoma.

Prevalence: The total number of people with a given condition at a point in time.

Primary prevention: Prevention of disease by reducing exposure to a risk factor that may lead to the disease. Primary preventive measures include healthy nutrition, regular physical activity, cessation of smoking, and safe sexual practices.

Puberty: The stage of life between childhood and adulthood during which the reproductive organs mature and secondary sexual characteristics begin to develop. For girls, it is the time of the onset of menstruation, the development of breasts and body hair, and usually some level of growth spurt.

Secondary prevention: Early detection and prompt treatment of disease. Examples of secondary preventive measures include screening tools such as mammography and Pap smears, which may detect disease before it spreads and thereby prevent further complications from the disease.

Tertiary prevention: Prevention measures that take place once a disease has advanced. They may involve alleviating pain, providing comfort, halting progression of an illness, and limiting disability that may result from disease.

Underweight: An individual who is below the acceptable average weight for his or her height or body type.

■■■■
Websites

Administration for Children and Families: http://www.acf.hhs.gov

Administration on Aging: http://www.aoa.gov

Agency for Healthcare Research and Quality: http://www.ahrq.gov

Centers for Disease Control and Prevention: http://www.cdc.gov

Centers for Medicare and Medicaid Services: http://www.cms.hhs.gov

Food and Drug Administration: http://www.fda.gov

Health Resources and Services Administration: http://www.hrsa.gov

Healthy People 2020: http://www.healthypeople.gov

Indian Health Service: http://www.ihs.gov

National Institutes of Health: http://www.nih.gov

Office of the Surgeon General: http://www.surgeongeneral.gov

Substance Abuse and Mental Health Services Administration: http://www.samhsa.gov

U.S. Department of Health and Human Services: http://www.hhs.gov

U.S. Public Health Service Commissioned Corps: http://www.usphs.gov

■■■■
References

1. Steen, J. (2007). *The primacy of public health*. American Public Health Association: Community Health Planning and Policy Development. Available at: http://www.apha.org/membergroups/newsletters/sectionnewsletters/comm/spring07/primacyph.htm

2. Finkelstein, E., Trogdon, J., Cohen, J., et al. (2009). Annual medical spending attributable to obesity: Payer- and service-specific estimates. *Health Affairs* 28(5): w822–w831.

3. Barrington, L., & Rosen, B. (2008). *Weights and measures: What employers should know about obesity*. New York, NY: The Conference Board.

4. National Center for Health Statistics. (2004). *Health, United States 2004 with chartbook on trends in the health of Americans*. Hyattsville, MD: Department of Health and Human Services.

5. Solarz, A. L. (Ed.). (1999). *Lesbian health: Current assessment and directions for the future*. Committee on Lesbian Health Research Priorities. Institute of Medicine. Washington, DC: National Academy Press.

6. World Health Organization. (2004). *The World health report 2004*. Geneva, Switzerland: WHO.

7. Joint U.N. Programme on HIV/AIDS (UNAIDS). (2010). *UNAIDS report on the global epidemic, 2010*. Geneva, Switzerland: UNAIDS.

8. World Health Organization. (2001). *Advancing safe motherhood through human rights*. Geneva, Switzerland: Author.

9. Benderly, B. L., for the Institute of Medicine. (1997). *In her own right: The Institute of Medicine's guide to women's health issues*. Washington, DC: National Academy Press.

10. Murphy, S., Xu, J., & Kochanek, K. (2012). *Deaths: Preliminary data for 2010*. National Vital Statistics Reports 60(4). Hyattsville, MD: National Center for Health Statistics.

11. Centers for Disease Control and Prevention. (2010). Current depression among adults—United States, 2006 and 2008. *Morbidity & Mortality Weekly Report* 59(38): 1229–1235.

12. Eaton, D., Kann, L., Kinchen, S., et al. (2011). *Youth risk behavior surveillance—United States, 2009*. Atlanta, GA: Centers for Disease Control and Prevention.

13. Ventura, S., Abma, J., Mosher, W., et al. (2006). *Recent trends in teenage pregnancy in the United States, 1990–2002*. Health E-stats. Hyattsville, MD: National Center for Health Statistics.

14. Centers for Disease Control and Prevention. (2000). *Tracking the hidden epidemic: Trends in STDs in the United States 2000*. Atlanta, GA: CDC.

15. UNAIDS Global Coalition on Women and AIDS. (2005). *2005 progress report*. Available at: http://data.unaids.org/Publications/IRC-pub07/JC1210-GCWA-ProgressReport-2005_en.pdf

16. Centers for Disease Control and Prevention. (2000). *Promoting lifelong healthy eating: CDC's guidelines for school health programs*. Division of Adolescent and School Health. Atlanta, GA: CDC.

17. Geller, A. C., Colditz, G., Oliveria, S., et al. (2002). Use of sunscreen, sunburning rates, and tanning bed

use among more than 10,000 U.S. children and adolescents. *Pediatrics* 109(6): 1009–1014.

18. The Tension Tracker 2002. Based on 1,805 interviews among a representative sample of Americans 18 years or older. Harris Interactive conducted interviews from April 29, 2002, to May 8, 2002.

19. Centers for Disease Control and Prevention. (2005). *Summary health statistics for U.S. adults: National Health Interview, 2004 Survey.* Atlanta, GA: CDC.

20. Expectation of life at birth, 1960–2004, and projections, 2010 and 2015. National Center for Health Statistics. (August 21, 2007). *National Vital Statistics Reports* 55(19): 246–254.

21. Leland, John. (October 6, 2008). In "Sweetie" and "Dear," a hurt for the elderly. *New York Times.* Available at: http://www.nytimes.com/2008/10/07/us/07aging.html

22. Hooyman, N. R., & Kiyak, H. A. (1996). *Social gerontology* (4th ed.). Boston: Allyn and Bacon.

23. Gross, J. (October 14, 2008). Who cares for the caregivers? *New York Times.* Available at: http://newoldage.blogs.nytimes.com/2008/10/14/who-cares-for-the-caregivers/

24. American Association of Retired People. (2010). *Sex, romance, and relationships: AARP survey of midlife and older adults.* Washington, DC: AARP.

25. Associated Press (November 8, 2006). Margaret Chan rose to prominence in Hong Kong's battle with bird flu. International Herald-Tribune. Available at: http://www.iht.com/articles/ap/2006/11/08/news/UN_GEN_UN_WHO_Chan_Profile.php

26. CNN. (April 16, 2007). Interview with Dr. Margaret Chan. Available at: http://www.cnn.com/2007/WORLD/asiapcf/04/13/talkasia.chan.script/index.html

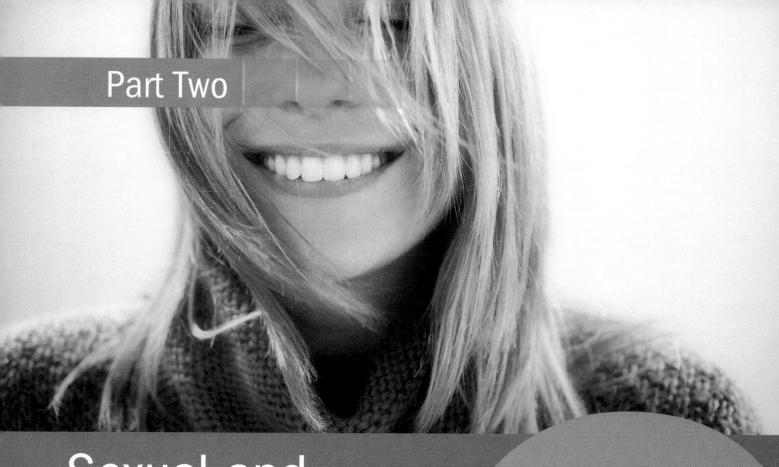

Sexual and Reproductive Dimensions of Women's Health

2

Chapter Four

Sexual Health

Chapter Objectives

On completion of this chapter, the student should be able to discuss:

1. The ways that cultural values, stereotypes, and socialization define or influence sexual behavior.

2. The economic, legal, and political dimensions of sexual health.

3. The importance of research on sexual behavior and major contributors to this body of research.

4. The difference between sex and gender and the concepts of gender identity and gender role.

5. Homosexual, heterosexual, and bisexual orientation and issues surrounding homophobia.

6. The location and function of the major external and internal female genital structures.

7. The three phases of the menstrual cycle.

8. The four basic phases of the female sexual response cycle.

9. Several examples of sexual expression.

10. The importance of the gynecological examination and the procedures involved.

11. Sexual dysfunction in women and its treatment.

12. Expression of sexuality throughout a person's life span.

13. Sexual violence as a public health problem.

14. The significance of communication in intimate relationships and with a woman's healthcare provider.

womenshealth.jbpub.com

Women's Health Online is a great source for supplementary women's health information for both students and instructors. Visit

http://womenshealth.jbpub.com

to find a variety of useful tools for learning, thinking, and teaching.

Introduction

Sexual health refers to the physical, psychological, social, cultural, and emotional facets of sexual human interactions. The World Health Organization (WHO) defines sexual health as:

> A state of physical, emotional, mental and social well-being related to sexuality; it is not merely the absence of disease, dysfunction or infirmity. Sexual health requires a positive and respectful approach to sexuality and sexual relationships, as well as the possibility of having pleasurable and safe sexual experiences, free of coercion, discrimination, and violence. For sexual health to be attained and maintained, the sexual rights of all persons must be respected, protected, and fulfilled.[1]

Both scientific and psychological perspectives are needed to understand sexual health. Sexual health entails the need for responsible sexual behavior to avoid sexually transmitted infections (STIs); unintended pregnancy; and sexual abuse, coercion, or violence. Positive sexuality requires thoughtful and respectful discussion of issues that may be difficult or awkward for some people to talk about. Learning about the physical and emotional aspects of sexuality and respecting the variations in forms of sexual behavior can improve sexual health and responsible sexual behavior.

Cultural and Religious Perspectives on Sexuality

Cultural values often influence sexual behavior and how men and women interact sexually. The structure of various societies affects sexuality in many ways by creating

■ Marriage is a central social underpinning of most societies.

normative sex roles, accepted types of sexual activity, preferences for sexual arousal, and sanctions and prohibitions on sexual behavior. One consistent theme exists, however—that of "marriage" in some form or another. Within all cultures, marriage provides sanctioned sexual privileges and obligations.

Some cultures have strong values warning against premarital sex; people, especially women, participating in sexual activity before marriage bring shame to themselves and their families, and they may be ostracized from their communities. Other cultures insist on modesty and sexual restraint for females, but have a greater acceptance for male sexual behavior. Many cultures stigmatize the open display of certain behaviors, such same-sex relationships, while offering greater acceptance for those behaviors as long as they occur behind closed doors. Other cultural influences extend into contraceptive decision making. Some cultures consider it acceptable for a woman to decide what form of birth control to use, as well as to purchase condoms and ask her partner to use them. In other cultures, men take charge of this decision and consider it disrespectful for a woman to mention the use of contraception to her partner. The tremendous cultural diversity in the United States results in a spectrum of perspectives, values, and messages to women about sexual practices.

Economic Dimensions

Historically, marriage was not simply the union of two people, but a formal arrangement made for financial, political, or social reasons between two families or within society as a whole. While many marriages are now a celebration of the romantic bond between two people, other unions continue to be for reasons other than love. In some cultures,

■ Society influences how boys and girls think, act, and express themselves as they grow up.

lengthy financial transactions taking the form of a bride-price or dowry are still common.

Throughout history, and even today in some parts of the world, the value of a bride often depends on her virginity. A girl who has lost her virginity before marriage, either willingly or unwillingly, can be seen as less valuable to both her family and the groom's family she is entering. In the United States and other Western countries, it has become extremely common for young women to have sex before marriage, though rates for U.S. teens ever having sexual intercourse have decreased over the past 20 years. In 1991, 54% of U.S. high school students surveyed had ever had sexual intercourse, while in 2009, 46% of students had sexual intercourse [2] (**Figure 4.1**).

Sexuality can be viewed within a frame of power and economic dynamics. The less power a woman has, based on either cultural or individual factors, the less able she is to control a given sexual encounter. Significant power imbalances, like those seen between rich and poor, educated and uneducated, and young and old, have been strongly associated with sexual violence and abuse. For example, within the commercial sex industry in Thailand, the highest incidence of sexual violence is documented between Western adult males and native girl sex workers under the age of 12. Social and economic factors that give men power over women can undermine women's abilities to say "no" to unwanted sexual advances or aggression. Educating men and women about healthful, mature relationships and about how women can empower themselves in relationships have helped reduce sexual violence and give women greater power in contraceptive decision making.

One direct relationship between sexuality and economics occurs between a commercial sex worker, or prostitute, and a sex consumer. In this relationship, sexual acts, with prices attached to them, are delineated between sex workers and their clients. Some intellectuals have argued that prostitution creates the ultimate power inversion, whereby women take control of sexuality and reap the financial rewards of performing sexual acts. The reality for most sex workers is quite different. The vast majority of sex workers are working under some level of indentured servitude, with a male pimp typically taking a portion of their earnings in exchange for protection and limiting competition. Pimps are individuals who act as brokers and supposed protectors for sex workers. They often require their sex workers to perform sexual acts on them for free, and they use physical abuse and threats to maintain power in the relationship.

Legal Dimensions

Laws criminalizing sexual intimacy once existed in all 50 states. These laws were enacted to impose norms on the lives of the nation's citizens and, sometimes, to prevent sexual activity not intended for procreation. Cohabitation, or unmarried sexual partners sharing a living space, and fornication, defined as sexual intercourse between unmarried partners, were also illegal in most states. Although these laws still exist in a handful of states, they are rarely

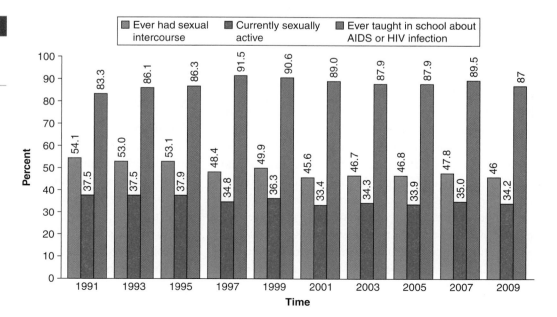

Figure 4.1

Trends in Sexual Behaviors among U.S. Youth, 1991–2009

Source: Data from Centers for Disease Control and Prevention. (2010). Youth Risk Behavior Surveillance–United States 2009. Surveillance Summaries, June 4, 2010. MMWR 2010;59 (No. SS-5).

enforced. Cohabitation is common today. By age 30, about one-half of U.S. women have cohabitated outside marriage.[3] Sodomy laws, laws that define certain sexual acts as sex crimes, no longer exist in the United States, since in 2003, the Supreme Court struck down state laws that ban sodomy, calling them an unconstitutional violation of privacy. Many sodomy laws had explicit rules, but courts typically interpreted the term to include any sexual act that does not lead to procreation, such as oral sex, anal sex, and bestiality; in practice such laws were rarely enforced against heterosexual couples.

Same-sex partners face discrimination when it comes to legalizing their partnership. Same-sex marriages are currently legal in only a few countries around the world. The Netherlands was the first country to legalize same-sex marriage in 2001. Other countries that have since legalized same sex marriage include Belgium, Spain, Canada, South Africa, Norway, Sweden, Portugal, Iceland, and Argentina. It is expected that Nepal, which only decriminalized homosexuality in 2007, also will legalize same-sex marriage in its new constitution. In the United States, eight states (Massachusetts, Connecticut, Iowa, Vermont, New Hampshire, New York, Washington, and Maryland) and the District of Columbia have passed laws allowing same-sex marriages. California also legalized same-sex marriage in 2008; however, an amendment to the California constitution and various subsequent court orders kept the marriages from becoming legal. Thirty-eight states have adopted state laws or constitutional prohibitions of same-sex marriage. Many of these states adopted "defense of marriage" language that defines marriage as a legal union between a man and a woman. Some states allow civil unions, which offer some, but not all, of the rights of a civil marriage.

Political Dimensions

Controversy about school-based sex education programs has been intense since these programs have existed. The federal government had endorsed abstinence-only until marriage (AOUM) as the primary approach to sex education starting with President Bill Clinton and continuing with President George W. Bush. Federally funded AOUM programs promoted abstinence from sexual activity and limited discussion of condoms and contraception, despite evidence that comprehensive sexuality education effectively promotes sexual health and that parents support these programs in public schools.[4] No research has shown that AOUM education programs are effective at preventing teen pregnancies or sexually transmitted infections

(STIs), and the programs typically contained misleading and inaccurate information.[5,6] Proponents of AOUM programs have argued that comprehensive sex education might lead to an increase in teens having sex; however, research shows that comprehensive sexual education programs either delay or have no effect on initiation of sexual activity. Studies have also shown that teaching about contraception was not associated with increased risk of adolescent sexual activity or STIs; in fact, adolescents who received comprehensive sex education had a lower risk of pregnancy than adolescents who received abstinence-only or no sex education.[7]

President Barack Obama eliminated federal funding for most abstinence-only education programs in his 2010 budget, with the following programs for teens receiving funding:[8]

- In December 2009, Congress replaced the Abstinence Education program with a teen pregnancy prevention program to support evidence-based interventions.

- In March 2010, through healthcare reform, Congress created a 5-year Personal Responsibility Education Program to educate adolescents on both abstinence and contraception. The program also teaches about healthy relationships, parent–child communication, and decision making.

- Congress also renewed the Title V abstinence-only program run by the Administration on Children, Youth, and Families. The $50 million program provides states with funding for abstinence-only until marriage programs.

Currently, 20 states and the District of Columbia require both sex and HIV education, 37 states require that sex education include abstinence, and 18 states and the District of Columbia require that information on contraception is included.[9]

Sex Research

Despite its importance, there has been less systematic, scientific research on the sexual behavior of Americans than on most other health and social topics of importance. The AIDS epidemic has improved the accuracy and increased the availability of information on sexual behavior, but the collection of scientific information on sexual matters continues to face strong political opposition.

Researchers attempting to understand sexual behavior face many of the same problems that handicap all research into human social behavior. Human subjects cannot be placed in a laboratory setting where variables that influence outcome measures can be controlled. Human behavior is complex, and studies, particularly on human behavior, are prone to contamination and bias. As a personal, private behavior, sex is such is more limited than other areas of behavioral research. Clearly, many problematic issues arise with any attempt to understand the prevalence and nature of contemporary sexual behavior.

Even with these limitations, there are ways to measure or analyze sexual activity and study sexual behavior, such as case studies, direct observation, experimental laboratory research, and surveys. Studies can address sexual research directly, for example, by determining the prevalence of sexual activities such as oral sex or homosexual couplings. Indirect assessments, such as adolescent pregnancy rates or sexually transmitted disease rates, provide insight into the consequences of sexual behavior.

Definitions create another technical difficulty in research. For years, researchers used the term "premarital sex" to describe penile–vaginal intercourse that takes place before a couple is married. However, as a measure of sexual activity outside of marriage, this definition is misleading because it excludes many noncoital heterosexual and homosexual activities. Heavy petting can include extensive types of sexual contact, often resulting in orgasm. The traditional definition of "virginity" as not having had sexual intercourse, therefore, may not reflect a lack of sexual activity. The term "premarital" has connotations that may be inappropriate to some individuals, especially to couples in same-sex relationships or relationships in cultures that offer commitments equal to marriage. Not all couples that engage in sexual activity have intentions toward long-term commitment with that partner. Any review of sex studies must consider the inherent limitations of such research.

© AbleStock

■ Definitions of "virginity" are subjective and may include (or exclude) a number of sexual behaviors.

Well-Known Studies

Several important studies on sexual behavior have provided valuable information and insight into sexual practices, behaviors, and attitudes.

- In 1948 and 1953, Alfred Kinsey conducted the most comprehensive taxonomic surveys of human sexual behavior to date.[10, 11] The 1948 study researched sexual behavior in men, and the 1953 study researched sexual behavior in women. Both studies attempted to present objective data on sexual behavior. The researchers interviewed thousands of people of various socioeconomic statuses, educational levels, marital statuses, and sex education experiences. The results showed how factors such as age, religious adherence, and gender influenced the incidence, frequency, and patterns of sexual behavior.

- In 1966, through direct observation techniques, Masters and Johnson observed and recorded more than 10,000 completed sexual response cycles.[12] Before their work, no significant empirical data had been gathered about male and female sexual arousal. Masters and Johnson are considered pioneers in sexual research for determining the four phases of the sexual response cycle: excitement, plateau, orgasm, and resolution.

- In 1976, the Hite Report, a questionnaire survey on female sexuality, also provided extensive narrative answers to several important questions about the sexual practices of American women.[13] The Report, which brought to light the fact that the majority of women can reach orgasm through self-stimulation but not during sexual intercourse, helped fuel the sexual revolution of the 1970s.

- The *Redbook* Survey (1977) was a questionnaire sent to more than 100,000 U.S. women that examined sexual behavior and attitudes.[14] This survey documented women's sexual fulfillment in respect to their marital status, age at sexual initiation, and sexual fidelity.

- Blumstein and Schwartz (1983) elicited excellent information about sexual and nonsexual components of relationships from a large national sample. Their book, *American Couples: Money, Work, Sex*, explored couples as cohabitating, married, or same-sex, comparing the dynamics of decision making between partners on the major issues faced by couples.[15]

- In 1992, the National Health and Social Life Survey interviewed more than 3,400 adults. The survey asked about sexual behavior over the lifetime, including childhood and adolescence, as well as sexually transmitted infections, sexual dysfunctions, and sexual attitudes and opinions. This landmark survey had significant implications for public health and provided further insight into the sexual behavior of American adults.[16]

- In 2001, the Surgeon General released the *Call to Action to Promote Sexual Health and Responsible Sexual Behavior*. The *Call to Action* contained strategies and information for promoting sexual health and responsible sexual behavior.[17] The *Call to Action* was the first time that the promotion of responsible sexual behavior and the improvement of sexual health were addressed as significant public health challenges (see **It's Your Health**).

- In 2003, Bancroft and colleagues conducted The National Survey of Women in Heterosexual Relationships.[18] Nearly 1,000 women ages 20 to 65 were surveyed, assessing the prevalence and predictors of sexual distress among women; it found that the best predictors of sexual distress were a woman's emotional well-being and her emotional relationship with her sexual partner, as opposed to physical aspects of the sexual response cycle.

It's Your Health

Call to Action to Promote Sexual Health and Responsible Sexual Behavior

Individual responsibility includes the following duties:

- Understanding and awareness of one's sexuality and sexual development
- Respect for oneself and one's partner
- Avoidance of physical and emotional harm to oneself or one's partner
- Ensuring that pregnancy occurs only when welcomed
- Recognition and tolerance of the diversity of sexual values within any community

Community responsibility includes assurance that its members have the following characteristics:

- Access to developmentally and culturally appropriate sexuality education as well as sexual and reproductive health care and counseling
- The latitude to make appropriate sexual and reproductive choices
- Respect for diversity
- Freedom from stigmatization and violence on the basis of gender, race, ethnicity, religion, or sexual orientation

Source: *The Surgeon General's Call to Action to Promote Sexual Health and Responsible Sexual Behavior.* (2001). U.S. Department of Health and Human Services.

- In a 2004 *ABC News Primetime Live* poll, more than 1,500 adults were randomly queried in a telephone survey about sexual activities, fantasies, and attitudes. The vast majority of respondents said they were monogamous and that they were happy about it.[19]

- The 2010 National Survey of Sexual Health and Behavior (NSSHB) is one of the most comprehensive and nationally representative studies on sexual and sexual-health behaviors. It includes the sexual experiences and condom-use behaviors of more than 5,800 adolescents and adults ages 14 to 94.[20]

Although some of the above studies have been criticized for overrepresenting or underrepresenting certain population segments, these studies have provided valuable information and insight into sexual behavior and attitudes. With any study of sexual behavior, however, it is important to consider the quality of the study method and the sampling techniques employed.

Sex and Gender

The terms gender and sex refer to partially overlapping, yet distinct, concepts. Gender refers to the economic, social, and cultural attributes and opportunities associated with being male or female, whereas the term sex refers to an individual's biological status as male or female. Issues surrounding sex and gender differences in health have been evolving for the past several decades.

Gender Identity

Gender identity refers to an individual's personal, subjective sense of being male or female. Biological sex, along with many other variables, clearly influence gender identity; a person's gender identity is not necessarily consistent with his or her biological sex.

The genetic material in a fertilized egg is organized within structures known as chromosomes. Chromosomes give rise to the process of sexual differentiation, whereby an individual develops distinct physical male or female characteristics. The physical femaleness or maleness is not just a result of this chromosome mix, however, but rather the result of processes that occur at various levels of sexual differentiation. In early prenatal development, male and female external genitalia are undifferentiated and will remain so unless a specific gene on the Y chromosome involved in sex determination is present and is activated. This gene is necessary for the development of the testes, so it is involved in initiating the male sexing process. Through a series of complex interactions involving gonadal sex hormones, both the internal and the external sex structures differentiate into male or female genitalia. Because the external genitals, gonads, and some of the internal structures of males and females originate from the same embryonic tissues, it is not surprising that they have homologous, or corresponding, parts (**Figure 4.2**).

Scientists have found important structural and functional differences in the brains of males and females. Sex differentiation in human brains occurs largely during prenatal development. Sex differences in the brain and sex hormones contribute to differences in processes such as thinking, remembering, language use, and ability to perceive spatial relationships. Other gender differences such as sensory perception and emotional responses may also affect sexual behavior. Clearly, environmental factors and psychosocial factors can also affect these differences. It is premature to suggest which factors play the most important role in determining these female–male differences.

Gender Roles

Gender role refers to the public expression of one's gender identity, as well as cultural expectations of male and female behaviors. Gender-role expectations are culturally defined and vary from society to society; they can also change as a culture develops.

Social-learning theory suggests that the identification with either feminine or masculine roles or a combination (androgyny) results primarily from the social and cultural models and influences to which the individual is exposed from birth. Parents typically dress boys and girls differently. Children grow up with toys specifically designed for their gender and receive reinforcement for gender-expected behaviors. At some point, most children develop a firm sense of being a girl or a boy, as well as a strong desire to adopt behaviors that are considered by society to be appropriate for their sex. Parents, peer groups, schools, textbooks, and the media frequently help develop and reinforce traditional gender-role assumptions and behaviors. Gender-role conditioning affects all facets of an individual's life, perhaps most importantly in influencing sexuality.

Gender-role expectations and their resulting stereotypes have clearly influenced the women's ability to succeed in traditional male arenas such as sports and professional careers. Stereotyping also influences the sexual health and behavior of women, who naturally find conflict with expectations that they be passive, submissive, dependent,

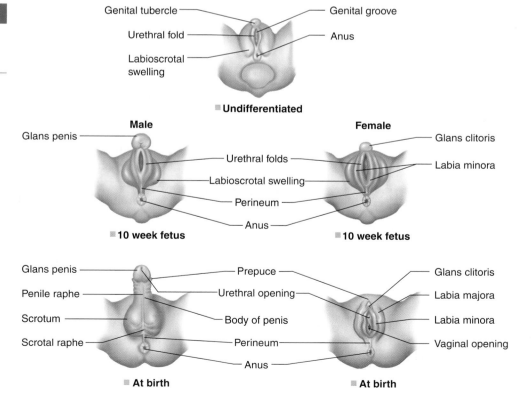

Figure 4.2

External genital differentiation—male and female.

Genital tubercle
Genital groove
Urethral fold
Anus
Labioscrotal swelling
Undifferentiated

Male
Female
Glans penis
Glans clitoris
Urethral folds
Labia minora
Labioscrotal swelling
Perineum
Anus
10 week fetus
10 week fetus

Glans penis
Prepuce
Glans clitoris
Penile raphe
Urethral opening
Labia majora
Scrotum
Body of penis
Labia minora
Scrotal raphe
Perineum
Vaginal opening
Anus
At birth
At birth

> *I used to feel confused about what was feminine or what was masculine. I finally decided that it didn't matter. How I talk and dress, and what I do in the bedroom, are my business. That really does not make me less of a woman.*
>
> **18-year-old student**

emotional, and subordinate. Stereotypical expectations of men and women clearly influence gender-role expectations. These expectations hinder both men and women in becoming mature individuals and in establishing fulfilling relationships. Despite the constraints associated with rigid, stereotypical gender roles, many men and women behave in a manner that is remarkably consistent with the norms that these roles establish (see **It's Your Health**).

Androgyny refers to having characteristics of both sexes, but appearing gender neutral (or not specifically male or female). Androgyny has physiological, behavioral, and psychological aspects. Physiological androgyny describes an individual whose appearance suggests gender ambiguity; behavioral androgyny refers to the manner in which people presents themselves, such as a male who displays traditionally feminine behaviors; and psychological androgyny describes an individual whose gender identity may differ from their sex. Androgynous individuals of both sexes are more likely to engage in behavior typically ascribed to the other sex than are gender-typed individuals.

Transgender

A transsexual is a person whose gender identity is opposite to her or his biological sex. Like other people, transgender people can be straight, gay, lesbian, or bisexual. A transsexual should not be confused with cross-dressing, the act of putting on clothes of the opposite sex (often for the

It's Your Health

Sexual Stereotypes of Women and Men

Women are undersexed, and men are oversexed.

Women are inexperienced, and men are experts.

Women are recipients, and men are initiators.

Women are controllers, and men are movers.

Women are nurturing and supportive, and men are strong and unemotional.

Women are sensitive, and men are insensitive.

Women are dependent, and men are independent.

Women are passive, and men are aggressive.

purposes of sexual excitement). The American Psychiatric Association classifies transsexualism as a gender identity disorder (GID), a mental disorder characterized by strong and persistent cross-gender identification; however, significant controversy exists regarding this classification of transsexualism. For many transsexuals, their gender identities do not cause distress or disability and therefore they do not identify themselves as having a mental disorder. However, some proponents of classifying transsexualism as a mental disorder argue that it is essential to retain a diagnosis to ensure access to affordable resources and health care, such as counseling, hormone therapy, medical procedures, and social support services.

Gender dysphoria is a psychological term used to describe negative or conflicting feelings about one's sex or gender roles. Almost all transgender people suffer from some degree of gender dysphoria. **Transitioning** is the process in which transsexuals work to change their appearance and societal identity so as to match their gender identity. To acknowledge their transition, transsexuals self-identify as male to female (MTF) or female to male (FTM). Changes are often medical, via surgery and hormones, as well as legal, through name and sex changes on legal documents and forms of identification.

No clear understanding of the nature and causes of transsexualism has yet emerged. Possible explanations include both biological and social-learning hypotheses. Data support the view that transsexualism may reflect a form of brain hermaphroditism, meaning that structures in the brain are sexually differentiated in a manner opposite to the transsexual's genetic and genital sex.[22] As described by one transgender group, these findings propose "a medical model of transsexuality as an 'obscured' congenital intersex condition in which the genitalia are spared but the brain is not."[23]

Intersexuality refers to the sexual physiology of an individual. A person who is born intersexed is born with sex chromosomes, external genitalia, or internal reproductive organs that are not considered "standard" as male or female. This condition can be manifested as a girl without ovaries, a boy without testes, or a child with genitalia that may appear as neither a vagina nor a penis.

Health care is a major challenge for transgender and intersex individuals. Research describing their healthcare needs is in its infancy, and much remains to be done to design effective medical and mental health programs and interventions.[24] For intersex individuals, recent activism has drawn attention to harmful childhood surgeries performed to "assign" a sex to an infant.

© Jack Dagley Photography/ShutterStock, Inc

■ Cultural expectations of gender roles and behaviors evolve over time.

Sexual Orientation

Sexual orientation refers to a person's erotic, romantic, and affectional attraction to other people. **Homosexual** orientation is attraction to same-sex partners, and **heterosexual** orientation is attraction to other-sex partners. A **bisexual** person is attracted to both sexes.

Although these concepts imply a clear distinction between the terms, the actual delineation is not always so precise. Kinsey described a seven-point continuum that ranged from exclusive contact with and attraction to the other sex to varying degrees of heterosexual and homosexual orientation.[10,11] Although Kinsey's methodology and conclusions have been criticized, the continuum of orientation provides a model for understanding differences in sexual orientation. The presumption that most people are heterosexual and the idea that heterosexuality and homosexuality represent sharply distinct behaviors are inconsistent with the complex, often unpredictable arena of human behavior.

A homosexual is a person whose primary erotic, psychological, emotional, and social interest is in a member of the same sex. Gay is another word often used to describe homosexual men or women as well as social and political issues related to homosexual orientation.

I am a lesbian. I am still "in the closet." I would like to be more open about my identity, but I am afraid. I still hear jokes and comments about lesbians from friends and family, like how someone "acts like a lesbian," or how shoes or an outfit looks "like something a lesbian would wear." I know they would say they don't mean any harm, but it scares me—and pisses me off.

27-year-old woman

Homosexual women are often referred to as lesbians. There is no profile that fits all lesbian women. They may be of any ethnicity, single, married, divorced, rich, poor, teenagers, middle-aged, or seniors. Many self-identified lesbians exhibit a variety of sexual practices, including heterosexual and bisexual activity. The extent to which a lesbian decides to be secretive or open about her sexual orientation has a significant effect on her lifestyle. There are various degrees of being "in the closet" and several steps in the process of "coming out." These steps are usually incremental and include self-acknowledgment, self-acceptance, and disclosure. These steps are particularly difficult because of homophobia.

Homophobia, an irrational fear or hatred of homosexuality, leads to many problems, including discrimination in medical care.[25] Misconceptions about health needs are also present with healthcare providers and patients. For example, many healthcare providers, as well as women who self-identify as lesbians, believe that lesbians are not at risk for sexually transmitted infections, gynecological infections, or cancers, and therefore do not require contraception education, regular cervical cancer screening, or pelvic exams. Some healthcare providers do not address the issue of sexual orientation and assume that any sexually active woman of reproductive age should practice methods of birth control to prevent pregnancy. After encountering physicians who either ignore the facts or respond negatively, many lesbians hesitate to disclose their sexual orientation or even to visit a healthcare provider regularly. Better awareness and training among healthcare providers would allow lesbians to receive better preventive services, health care, and health education.[26]

© bilderlounge/Yashoda/Alamy Images

■ There is no profile of a lesbian woman. Women of all ages, classes, races, and body types are lesbians.

Biological Basis of Sexual Health

Female Sexual Anatomy and Physiology

External Structures

Unfortunately, many women not only harbor misconceptions about their bodies, but also are unfamiliar with their own genitalia. Gaining knowledge and understanding of how her body functions and performs is an important aspect of a woman's sexual health and well-being. One way to begin understanding female sexual anatomy is to examine the vaginal area with a mirror.

All women have the same genital structures, but there are individual variances in terms of colors, shapes, and textures (**Figure 4.3**). The **vulva** encompasses all the female external genital structures, including the pubic hair, folds of skin, and urinary and vaginal openings. The **mons veneris**, or "mound of Venus," is the area covering the pubic bone. It consists of pads of fatty tissue between the bone and the skin. Nerve endings in this area are responsible for the pleasure sensations from touch and pressure. At puberty, the mons becomes covered with pubic hair that varies in color, texture, and thickness.

The **labia majora** consist of outer lips that extend downward from the mons and extend toward each side of the vulva. The color of the labia majora is usually darker than the color of the thighs. The nerve endings and underlying fatty tissue are similar to those in the mons. The **labia minora**, or inner lips, are located within the outer lips and often protrude between them.

The **clitoris** consists of an external shaft and glans and parts known as internal crura; its function is sexual arousal. The shaft and glans of the clitoris are located just below the mons area, where the inner lips converge. They are covered by the clitoral hood, or prepuce. Initially, it may be easier for a woman to locate her clitoris by touch rather than by sight or location because of its sensitive nerve endings and small size. The external part of the clitoris, although tiny, has about the same number of nerve endings as the head of the penis.

The vestibule is the area of the vulva inside the labia minora. It is rich in blood vessels and nerve endings. Its tissues are also sensitive to touch. Both the urinary and the vaginal openings are located within the vestibule.

The urinary opening is also called the urethral opening. Urine passes from the bladder through the body via this opening. The **urethra** is the short tube connecting the bladder to the urinary opening, located between the clitoris and the vaginal opening.

The vaginal opening is located between the urinary opening and the anus. The **hymen**, a thin piece of tissue, partially covers the opening. It is typically present at birth and usually remains intact until first penetration, although the vaginal opening is partially open and flexible enough to insert tampons before the hymen has been broken. Although the hymen may protect the vaginal tissues early in life, it has no other known function. Nevertheless, many cultures have traditionally placed great significance on its presence or absence. A common misconception is that a woman's virginity can be proved or disproved by the pain or bleeding that may occur with initial coitus. Although

Figure 4.3

External female sexual anatomy.

Clitoral hood
Clitoris
Labium minora
Hymen
Vaginal orifice (introitus)

Mons veneris
Urethral orifice
Vestibular bulb
Labium majora
Perineum
Anus

discomfort and spotting sometimes occur with first coitus, the hymen can be partial, flexible, or thin enough that there is neither discomfort nor bleeding. This very sensitive tissue also may stretch or break while performing activities such as bike riding, horseback riding, and gymnastics.

The **perineum** refers to the area of smooth skin between the vaginal opening and the anus. This tissue is rich with nerve endings and is sensitive to touch.

Internal Structures

Several structures lie along the vaginal opening. The vestibule refers to the area of the vulva inside the labia minora. The vaginal walls are lined with a vast network of bulbs and vessels that engorge with blood during sexual arousal, causing the vagina to increase in length and the vulvar area

to become swollen. These bulbs are similar in structure and function to the tissue in the penis that engorges with blood during male sexual arousal and causes penile erection.

The **Bartholin's glands** are located on each side of the vaginal opening. They secrete a liquid that lubricates the tissues at the vaginal opening. The glands are usually not noticeable. Occasionally, the duct from the gland becomes blocked and enlargement results. Medical intervention may be indicated if the condition does not subside within a few days.

In addition to the glands, a complex musculature underlies the genital area. The pelvic floor muscles have a multidirectional design (**Figure 4.4**) that permits the vaginal opening to expand during childbirth and contract after delivery. These muscles can lose muscle tone during

Figure 4.4

Pelvic floor muscles.

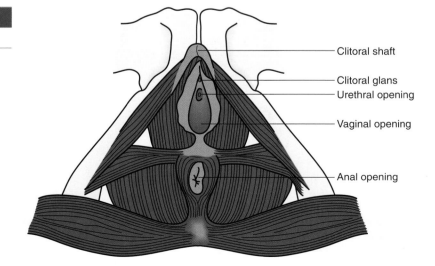

Clitoral shaft

Clitoral glans
Urethral opening

Vaginal opening

Anal opening

childbirth or over time. A series of exercises known as **Kegel exercises** can help restore the muscular tone, reduce involuntary urinary incontinence, and enhance sexual sensations (see **It's Your Health**).

Internal female sexual anatomy consists of the vagina, cervix, uterus, fallopian tubes, and ovaries (**Figure 4.5**). The **vagina** opens between the labia minora and extends upward into the body, angling toward the lower back. The vagina is approximately 3 to 5 inches in length when not aroused. The folded walls of the vagina, known as rugae, form a flat tube. These walls are warm, soft, and moist, and they produce secretions that help maintain the chemical balance of the vagina.

The vagina consists of three layers of tissue—mucous, muscle, and fibrous tissue—all of which are richly endowed with blood vessels. The mucosa is a layer of moist membrane inside the vagina. During sexual arousal, lubricating fluid exudes through the mucosa. The muscular tissue is concentrated around the vaginal opening. Fibrous tissue surrounds the muscular layer. This layer aids in vaginal contraction and expansion, and also serves as connective tissue to other structures in the pelvic cavity.

The **cervix**, located at the back of the vagina, is the mouth of the uterus and looks like a small, pink, glazed doughnut. Glands line the cervical canal and produce a constant downward flow of mucus to protect the uterine cavity from bacterial invasion. The cervix is composed of fibrous tissue that is capable of dramatic stretching. During childbirth, the cervical canal is 50 or more times its normal width.

The **uterus**, also known as the womb, is a thick, pear-shaped organ. It is approximately 3 inches long and 2 inches wide in a woman who has never had a child; after a pregnancy, it is somewhat larger. The uterus is suspended within the pelvic cavity by a series of six ligaments. The alignment of these ligaments permits some movement of the uterus within the cavity.

The uterine wall consists of three layers: the endometrium, the myometrium, and the perimetrium. The endometrium is the lining of the uterus. In preparation for fertilization, the endometrium thickens in response to hormone changes during the monthly menstrual cycle. The endometrium is also a source of hormone production. The myometrium, the middle layer, consists of the longitudinal and circular muscle fibers of the uterus. These muscle fibers are interwoven and enable the uterus to expand during pregnancy and contract during labor and childbirth. A thin membrane known as the perimetrium covers the

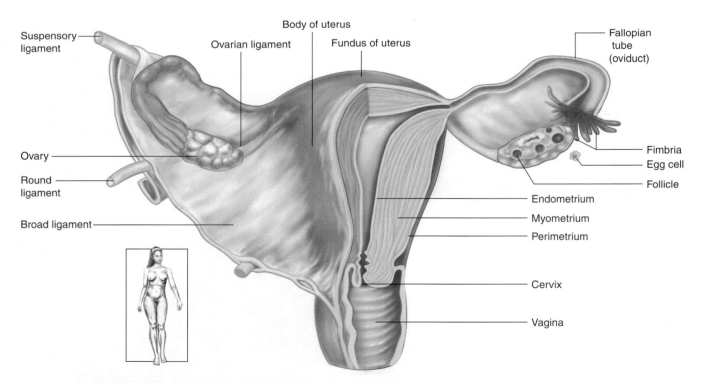

Figure 4.5

Internal female sexual anatomy.

myometrium. The perimetrium functions as the external surface of the uterus.

The **fallopian tubes**, which are thin, pale, pink filaments, connect the uterus with the ovaries. The outside end of each tube is like a funnel, with fingerlike projections called fimbriae that draw the egg from the ovary into the tube. The **ovaries** are located at the end of the fallopian tubes and are about the size of a small walnut in premenopausal women. The ovaries are endocrine glands that produce two classes of sex hormones: estrogens and progesterones. The estrogens influence the development of female physical sex characteristics and help regulate the menstrual cycle, while the progesterones help regulate the menstrual cycle and stimulate development of the uterine lining in preparation for pregnancy. During puberty, these hormones play a critical role in the maturation of the reproductive organs and the development of secondary sex characteristics, such as pubic hair and breasts.

The Menstrual Cycle

Women usually begin to menstruate in their early teens. During the **menstrual cycle**, the body prepares the uterine lining for implantation of a fertilized egg. If **conception** does not occur, the lining sloughs off and is discharged as menstrual flow. This menstrual discharge consists of blood, mucus, and endometrial membranes that sometimes present as small clots. The amount of menstrual flow varies, but is usually 6 to 8 ounces in volume per cycle (about half a can of soda). The cycle is often 28 days in length but can vary from 21 to 40 days.

A complex series of interactions between the hypothalamus and the pituitary gland in the brain, the adrenal glands on top of the kidneys, the ovaries, and the uterus regulates the menstrual cycle. The hypothalamus produces and secretes hormones and releasing factors that act directly on the pituitary gland. One such releasing factor, gonadotropin-releasing hormone (GnRH), is responsible for reproductive hormone control. GnRH varies in amount and frequency during each menstrual cycle. In addition, this hormone plays a role in the timing of puberty. Alterations in the GnRH pulse release may be the mechanism by which stressors such as athletic training or dieting influence menstrual cycles.

The menstrual cycle is a self-regulating and dynamic process in which the level of a particular hormone impedes or increases the production of the same and other hormones.

Problems with Menstruation

For most women, menstruation creates no medical problems, but some women experience certain physical and emotional difficulties. **Dysmenorrhea**, meaning "painful menstrual flow," is a term for what most women call "cramps." Dysmenorrhea may be caused by the normal production of prostaglandins that produce strong contractions of the uterus (primary dysmenorrhea) or by problems in

■ A wide variety of products are available for use during menstruation, including many different styles, sizes, and absorbencies of sanitary napkins or pads, tampons, and menstrual cups.

It's Your Health

Kegel Exercises

To identify the pelvic floor muscles:

1. Try stopping a flow of urine in midstream while urinating. The muscles that are tightened in this effort are the muscles of the pelvic floor.

2. Tighten the ring of muscles around the rectum, as if trying to stop a bowel movement. The muscles that are tightened in this effort are also muscles of the pelvic floor.

3. While lying down, place a hand over the abdomen. Tighten all of the muscles of the abdomen and pelvis. Notice that the hand will move. These are not muscles of the pelvic floor, and they should be relaxed during Kegel exercises. During the first few practice sessions, it is helpful to check with a hand to make sure that the abdominal muscles are relaxed.

To practice Kegel exercises:

1. Take deep breaths—do not forget to breathe.
2. Tighten the anal muscle, pulling inward and outward.
3. Tighten the vaginal muscle, pulling inward and outward.
4. Hold these muscles tight, counting slowly to 10, and then relax.

Do Kegel exercises in sets of 5 to 10 at a time, several times a day. Build up to being able to hold the contraction for 20 seconds at a time.

the uterus, fallopian tubes, or ovaries (secondary dysmenorrhea). Women with primary dysmenorrhea experience pain in the lower abdomen and back, while those with secondary dysmenorrhea often feel pain during urination and bowel movements. Relief from primary dysmenorrhea may be found through regular aerobic exercise; stress reduction techniques; adequate sleep; and decreased fat, caffeine, and sodium in the diet. Some women with primary or secondary dysmenorrhea may need anti-inflammatory medications or oral contraceptives to relieve the pain. Secondary dysmenorrhea is treated based on the underlying condition.

Premenstrual syndrome (PMS) is a group of symptoms linked to the menstrual cycle. PMS symptoms occur in the week or two weeks before the menstrual period, and they usually dissipate after menstruation starts. PMS can affect menstruating women of any age. It is also different for each woman. Most women of reproductive age have some physical discomfort, but about 5–8% of women suffer from severe premenstrual syndrome, where symptoms interfere with daily activities.[27] Although the root causes of PMS are not known, PMS is clearly linked to changing hormones during the menstrual cycle. Stress and emotional problems do not seem to cause PMS, but they may make it worse.

Diagnosis of PMS is usually based on a woman's specific symptoms, when they occur, and how much they affect her life. Symptoms include acne, breast swelling and tenderness, feeling tired, having trouble sleeping, upset stomach, bloating, constipation or diarrhea, headache or backache, appetite changes or food cravings, joint or muscle pain, trouble concentrating or remembering, tension, irritability, mood swings, crying spells, anxiety, and depression. Tracking the severity of these premenstrual problems daily on a calendar can assist clinicians with diagnosing PMS.[28]

PMS is more likely to present in women who are between their late 20s and early 40s, have at least one child, and have a family history of depression or a personal history of either postpartum depression or a mood disorder. Research also suggests that cigarette smoking, especially in adolescence and young adulthood, may increase the risk of moderate to severe PMS.[29]

A single universal treatment is not yet available for PMS. Experts recommend basic health measures such as a nutritious diet, adequate sleep, daily exercise, a daily multivitamin that includes 400 micrograms of folic acid, a calcium supplement with vitamin D, and cessation of cigarette smoking to reduce PMS symptoms. (All of these measures are also excellent steps for improving general health.) Over-the-counter pain relievers such as ibuprofen, aspirin, or naproxen may ease cramps, headaches, backaches, and breast tenderness. In more severe cases of PMS, prescription medicines can ease symptoms. One approach has been to use drugs such as birth control pills to stop ovulation from occurring. Women on the pill report fewer PMS symptoms, such as cramps and headaches, as well as lighter periods. Further research is needed to ascertain the efficacy of this approach.[30]

Premenstrual dysphoric disorder (PMDD) is a severe form of PMS. The condition can be disabling with emotional symptoms, such as intense sadness, despair, tension, anxiety, mood swings, irritability, anger, and physical symptoms consistent with PMS. There is evidence that a brain chemical called serotonin plays a role in PMDD. Studies have found continuous dosing regimens of selective serotonin reuptake inhibitors (SSRIs) to be effective in treating these symptoms.[31] Studies also suggest that cognitive behavioral therapy in the forms of individual counseling, group counseling, and stress management may also help relieve symptoms.[32]

Amenorrhea is the lack of menstrual flow. Primary amenorrhea occurs in women who have not yet begun menstruation and may result from hormone-related problems or extremely low body fat. Secondary amenorrhea is the lack of blood flow for 3 or more consecutive months, outside of pregnancy, breastfeeding, and perimenopause; it may result from conditions such as anorexia nervosa, ovarian cysts or tumors, substance abuse, stress, or use of oral contraceptives. Healthcare providers will want to work with a woman to first establish the cause of her amenorrhea and then consider options for treatment.

Physical Health and the Gynecological Examination

A gynecological examination usually begins with a medical history and a general physical examination, including a breast examination, and is followed by a pelvic examination. The pelvic exam provides the woman and her clinician with essential information about her gynecological health. It should be timed to avoid the menstrual period. It is also advisable to avoid douching at least 24 hours before an examination; some clinicians recommend avoiding vaginal intercourse for at least 48 hours before the examination as well. These precautions ensure a more accurate visualization of the cervix and greater likelihood of diagnosing an infection if it is present.

For the pelvic exam, the woman lies on her back with her bottom at the very end of the examining table and her

■ The speculum permits visual examination of the vagina and cervix during a gynecological visit.

© Elizabeth Dover/ShutterStock, Inc.

legs supported in foot stirrups. The pelvic examination consists of three phases:

- The external examination, in which the clinician inspects the vulva and perineum visually for any evidence of infection or injury.

- The use of a speculum, a device that holds the vaginal walls apart to permit visual inspection of the cervix, is the second phase. The provider inserts the speculum with the blade closed. Once inside the vagina, the provider opens the blades and locks them into place at the correct width. With the speculum open, the clinician inspects the vaginal walls and cervix for redness, irritation, unusual discharge, or lesions. The provider collects specimens for laboratory tests while the speculum is in place and then removes the speculum.

- The third phase of the examination is the bimanual examination, which involves the insertion of two gloved fingers of one hand into the vagina while the other hand presses downward on the abdomen. The purpose of this activity is to locate and feel the size, consistency, and shape of the uterus and ovaries and to check for any abdominal masses or tender areas.

A healthcare provider may also perform a rectal examination to evaluate the muscular wall separating the rectum

© Photodisc

■ The pelvic examination is an important part of a woman's health visit.

and vagina, the position of the uterus, and any possible masses or tenderness in the area.

Although they can be inconvenient and uncomfortable, pelvic examinations take only a few minutes and they provides a starting point to ascertain any gynecological or sexual health concerns. Pelvic examinations should be arranged at regular intervals throughout a woman's adult life (see **It's Your Health**).

Sexual Arousal and Sexual Response

Sexual arousal and response are physical, emotional, and mental processes that individuals experience very differently. The female sexual response is not a geographically isolated phenomenon of the vaginal area. Instead, the brain, senses, and hormones all play an integrated role in the response cycle.

The brain mediates thoughts, emotions, and fantasies that provide the psychological "stage" for the sexual experience. Hearing, touch, smell, sight, and taste influence the level of sexual arousal. In addition to performing their primary role of regulating the menstrual cycle, hormones also affect sexual arousal. The function of certain hormones in the sexual response cycle—specifically, estrogens and androgens—has been studied extensively for many years.

Estrogens promote cell growth and replication in the vaginal cells, increase blood flow in the vagina and urethra, and maintain vaginal lubrication in postmenopausal women. Androgens affect the brain by influencing sexual behavior and libido. Data are conflicting, however, regarding the role of androgens for improving libido and well-being in postmenopausal women.[33] Additional studies are needed to determine the specific roles of estrogen and androgen and the effects of estrogen–androgen therapy on a woman's health.

The sexual response cycle has been described in several ways, most notably by Masters and Johnson in the 1960s.[12] Masters and Johnson were primarily interested in studying the biology of sexuality. They focused their sexual response cycle on the physiological reactions occurring during sexual activity. They developed a linear four-phase model of sexual response: excitement, plateau, orgasm and resolution. Masters and Johnson reported three variations among women in the sexual response cycle (**Figure 4.6**): Pattern #1 demonstrates that some women are able to have one or more orgasms without dropping below the plateau level of sexual arousal; pattern #2, a variation of this response, includes an extended plateau with no orgasm; and pattern #3, which most closely resembles the typical male cycle, describes a rapid rise to orgasm with no definitive plateau and a quick resolution.

In the excitement phase of the female sexual response cycle, the clitoris swells with blood engorgement. This change ranges from slight to very distinct. The clitoral glans is highly sensitive. Some women find that the entire sexual response cycle can be set into motion and maintained to orgasm by light stimulation of the glans alone. In addition to clitoral swelling, the labia majora flatten and separate during the excitement phase. The labia minora increase in size, and lubrication begins.

Lubrication is a unique feature of the vagina and an important aspect of sexual arousal. It is often the first physiological sign of sexual arousal in women. Vaginal lubrication serves two primary functions. First, it enhances the possibility of conception by helping to alkalinize the normally acidic vaginal chemical balance; sperm are able to move faster and survive longer in an alkaline environment. Second, vaginal lubrication helps to increase sexual pleasure.

Many women cannot reach orgasm by penis insertion alone, and therefore prefer other forms of stimulation in addition to coital stimulation. The "G" spot, or Grafenberg spot, is a sensitive area that can lead to orgasm when stimulated. Orgasm is the shortest phase of the sexual response cycle, though female orgasms often last slightly longer than male orgasms. Orgasmic experiences vary widely in intensity, frequency, and duration among both men and women. The female physiological responses in the orgasmic phase include an elevated blood pressure, heart rate, and breathing pattern. These physiological responses are consistent whether they originate from direct clitoral stimulation or from coital stimulation, although women report wide differences in subjective feelings and preferences.[14,15]

Resolution is the final phase of the sexual response cycle. During this phase, the sexual systems return to the nonexcited state. A significant male–female response difference occurs in the resolution period. After orgasm, the male typically enters a refractory period—a time when no amount of additional stimulation will result in orgasm. This time

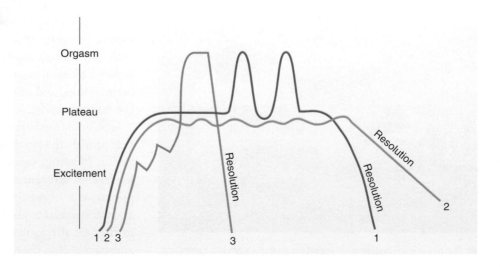

Figure 4.6

Masters and Johnson's model lists three variations among women in the sexual response cycle.

period has considerable variability among men and depends on physiological and psychological factors. In contrast to men, women generally experience no comparable refractory period, so they are physiologically capable of returning to another orgasmic peak during the resolution phase.

In the late 1970s, Helen Singer Kaplan introduced the concept of desire into her response cycle, which she condensed into three stages: sexual desire, followed by sexual arousal, and then orgasm. Both Master and Johnson's model and Kaplan's model have been criticized for the fact that the many women do not experience all of these stages or move through the phases sequentially.[34] Later models looked to encompass not only the biological processes, but the psychosocial and emotional elements as well. In the 1990s, Whipple and Brash-McGreer proposed a circular model, overlaying the phases of desire, excitement, plateau, orgasm, and resolution with the stages of seduction (creating the desire), sensations (which include excitement and plateau), surrender (orgasm), and time for reflection (during resolution).[35] The circular aspect of the model demonstrates the reinforcing effect that satisfaction and pleasure has on leading to another sexual experience. Upon reflection, a woman may or may not circle back to the seduction stage based on whether or not she has the desire to repeat the experience.

Another framework, proposed by Basson, is an intimacy-based cyclical model and incorporates the interaction between the mind and the body.[36] A woman may enter the sexual response cycle at various points; for example, she may not feel desire, but after being aroused through sexual stimulation, she may become desirous. The model acknowledges the importance of psychosocial issues, such as relationship satisfaction, need for emotional intimacy, and previous sexual experiences. Basson's model recognizes that intimacy needs may drive a woman's sexual response more than the need for physical sexual arousal. It also acknowledges that the goal of sexual activity may be physical satisfaction (orgasm) or a combination of physical and emotional satisfaction (connectivity with a partner).

The female sexual response cycles described here are simply frameworks for understanding the physiological events of sexual response. Sexual response cycles of individual women can vary considerably from these models. Also, as women age, physiological changes in the female sexual response cycle occur, such as diminished lubrication and decreased blood flow and thus decreased swelling of the clitoris and labia. In addition to a reduction in estrogen that may the cause of these changes, increased use of medications as well as incidence of medical conditions

may interfere with a woman's overall libido. Despite these issues, however, many women report being satisfied with their overall sexual relationship well into old age.

Forms of Sexual Expression

Society has traditionally restricted the "appropriate" forms of sexual expression. Missionary (vaginal intercourse with the male on top of the female) heterosexual sex is only one of many sexual expression options. Women may elect many different forms of sexual expression depending on their experience, life situation, and personal preferences.

Masturbation refers to erotic self-stimulation, usually to the point of orgasm. Historical records indicate that both genders have engaged in masturbation since ancient times. Masturbation practices begin early in life with infants exploring their genitals and receiving pleasure from touching them. Often self-stimulation continues throughout life, whether or not the individual is in an intimate relationship. Studies vary greatly regarding masturbation statistics, although all studies show that this practice is more common in males than females.

Even though masturbation is widespread, many women feel ashamed or embarrassed about the practice. Folklore has often labeled masturbation as sinful, evil, and even physically or mentally harmful. Such ideas are entirely false. Many therapists and sex experts believe that masturbation can be helpful as a sexual outlet and a means to become comfortable with one's own body.

Petting is the erotic stimulation of a person by a sexual partner, without actual sexual intercourse. Petting can include kisses, genital caresses, and oral–genital contact. Petting may culminate in orgasm. During adolescence, petting is often a way to experience intense sexual excitement without actually engaging in intercourse. Petting is carried over into adult sexual experiences as foreplay or for sexual variety.

Oral–genital stimulation, also known as oral sex, takes two basic forms. **Cunnilingus** is the act of sucking or licking the vulva, particularly the clitoris. **Fellatio** is the act of sucking or licking the penis and scrotum. A common sexual practice among both heterosexual and homosexual couples, oral sex is often believed to be a "safe" sexual activity. However, sexually transmitted infections such as genital herpes, human papillomavirus, and gonorrhea all can be transmitted through oral–genital sex.[37]

Anal intercourse is another form of sexual expression. Because the anal opening is richly endowed with nerves, this area can be very sensitive and sexually arousing. A

■ During adolescence, petting is a way to experience intense sexual excitement.

couple needs to be careful, however, in performing anal intercourse for many reasons. The anal sphincter tends to be tight and when stimulated can tighten even more, resulting in pain upon penetration. In addition, the anal region has no natural lubrication of its own, which increases the possibility of pain and injury. Usually anal intercourse can be accomplished without discomfort if precautions are taken. A water-based lubricant (not petroleum-based products, which weaken condoms) should be used. Care should be taken to avoid contamination of the vaginal area once anal penetration has occurred. However, unprotected anal intercourse has a high risk of transmitting many STIs, including HIV. Anyone engaging in anal intercourse should use a latex condom and never use a petroleum-based lubricant. In addition, after anal penetration, the genitals should be washed thoroughly before resuming vaginal or oral sex.

Sexual Dysfunction

Sexual dysfunction is the inability of an individual to function adequately in terms of sexual arousal, orgasm, or in coital situations. A recent national survey found about 40% of U.S. women report sexual problems, but only about 12% are distressed about it.[38] Older women experienced both the highest prevalence of sexual dysfunction and a reduced level of associated distress. The most distress occurred at midlife; younger women had the lowest prevalence of problems and associated distress.[38]

The medical and scientific community once classified women's sexual problems under the general label of "frigidity." These problems were severely misunderstood and thought to be symptomatic of a neurosis or some other psychological disorder that required long-term psychiatric

therapy. This traditional approach persisted despite the absence of a demonstrated relationship between the treatment and the alleviation of the sexual problem. More recently, however, the pharmaceutical industry has gained interest in understanding and treating female sexual problems with the hopes of uncovering a new market as lucrative as that for male-targeted medications such as Viagra.

Today, four major areas of sexual dysfunction are recognized among women: sexual desire disorders, sexual arousal disorders, orgasmic disorders, and sexual pain disorders. Treatments for each of these conditions require understanding the complex relationships between physiological and psychological considerations. Any form of sexual dysfunction or discomfort with intercourse or sexual stimulation should be evaluated to rule out underlying pathology (see **Self-Assessment 4.1**). In addition, the evaluation should include efforts such as counseling or therapy, if needed, to seek resolution of the condition.

Sex Therapy

Professional help may be indicated in cases where individual efforts, couple efforts, or both do not produce the desired effects. Sex therapy has evolved as a legitimate method for understanding sexual problems and increasing sexual satisfaction. Communication about sexual issues and finding ways to solve problems are critical but often difficult steps toward achieving a satisfying sex life; sex therapy can make such communication easier. Strategies with a therapist may range from expanding self-knowledge to sharing more effectively with a partner.

Therapy can also benefit individuals or couples by providing them with information. By providing specific, accurate, and reassuring information, a therapist is often able to address thoughts and feelings interfering with the person's ability to enjoy or respond to sexual activity. A therapist is also able to provide specific activities or homework "assignments" that enable the client to reduce anxiety, enhance communication, and learn new sexually enhancing behavioral techniques. Intensive therapy may be indicated in some situations in which personal emotional difficulties

I used to fake orgasms. I am not sure why, but somehow I felt it was necessary. My current partner figured it out, and we have spent a lot of time talking about this. I am seeing a therapist. With a few sessions, I was able to climax with masturbation, and I know that I am much more comfortable with my sexuality. I know that "faking it" was not fair to my partner or me.

35-year-old woman

■ A trained counselor or clinician can often provide valuable assistance for a woman who is experiencing sexual dysfunction.

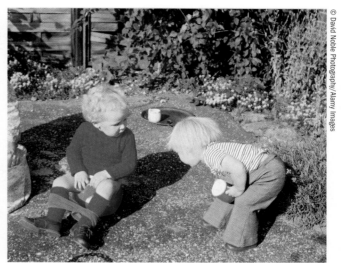

■ Children are innately interested in their bodies.

or significant relationship problems interfere with sexual expression.

Sexuality Through the Life Span

In many Western societies, childhood has traditionally been considered as a time of unexpressed sexuality and behavior, and adolescence has been viewed as a time to restrain immature sexual drives. However, current evidence suggests that sexuality and sexual capacity are not "awakenings" that suddenly appear at a definitive time in development, but rather that both male and female infants are born with the capacity for sexual pleasure and response.

Childhood

Individuals experience considerable variation in sexual development during childhood and adolescence. The

pleasures of genital stimulation are generally discovered in the first few years of life. Besides self-stimulation, prepubescent children may engage in play that has sexual elements. The activities range from exhibition and inspection to simulating intercourse by rubbing genital regions together. Both natural childhood curiosity and curiosity about what is forbidden probably play a role in these behaviors. As children get older, they become more keenly aware of and interested in body changes, particularly those involving the genitals and secondary sex characteristics.

Adolescence

Adolescence, the period from about 12 to 19 years of age, is the most dramatic stage for physiological changes and social-role development. The first few years of adolescence are known as puberty, and this is a time of dramatic physiological change. Over the past 20 years, the average age of puberty has decreased, with some girls seeing physical changes as young as the age of seven.[39] One study determined that the number of girls entering puberty at these early ages has increased markedly between 1997 and 2010. The onset of puberty generally occurs two years earlier in girls than in boys. Secondary sex characteristics appear at this time in response to higher levels of hormones. In females, estrogen levels result in pubic hair growth and breast budding. One study found that 10% of White girls, 23% of Black girls, 15% of Hispanic girls, and 2% of Asian girls had started breast development by age seven.[40] Early breast development, however, has not been accompanied by earlier ages of first menarche, which has remained nearly constant since the 1970s. A number of environmental

Self-Assessment 4.1

Self-Evaluation for Sexual Dysfunction

1. Do you experience pain or discomfort during intercourse?
2. Do you lack interest in or desire for sex?
3. Do you feel anxious when you begin to engage in sexual activity?
4. Do you lack pleasure when sexually stimulated?
5. Do you have difficulty achieving orgasm?

Answering yes to one or more of these questions may signify a sexual problem. Communication with one's partner may help resolve some of the issues. If not, women should seek medical attention to rule out any underlying causes and consider therapy to address ways to enhance sexual satisfaction.

factors may contribute to the earlier age of puberty, including higher rates of childhood obesity; increased intake of animal protein and meat; high dairy and soft drink consumption; and exposure to endocrine-disrupting chemicals found in plastics, pesticides, and other chemicals.

Hormone stimulation during adolescence causes additional internal changes. Vaginal walls gradually become thicker, and the uterus becomes larger and more muscular. The vaginal pH changes from alkaline to acidic as vaginal and cervical secretions increase in response to the changing hormone status. Eventually, menstruation begins. The first menstrual period is known as menarche. Initial menstrual cycles may be irregular and occur without ovulation. Most girls menstruate at about the age of 12 or 13, but considerable variation exists in this timing.[39,41]

The difficulties of adjusting to new physical characteristics pale in comparison to the psychological adjustments of adolescence. This period is characterized by evolving responsibilities and assimilation of societal expectations. In Western cultures, these expectations include inherent double standards for women. Sexual overtones are impossible to escape in society, appearing on everything from ads for jeans to magazine photos to television shows. However, society also communicates the message that young women should maintain their virginity and not be sexually adventurous. In contrast, society tends to be more tolerant of experimentation and overt sexual behavior in young men.

Young to Middle Adulthood

Both personal and cultural factors influence sexual behavior in adults. Several factors have contributed to a dramatic increase in single, sexually active adults over the past 50 years:

■ Many women are placing career goals before marriage.

■ Communication contributes greatly to the satisfaction of an intimate relationship.

- The trend toward marriage at a later age
- An increase in the number of women who never marry
- More women placing career goals before marriage
- An increase in the number of cohabitating couples
- A rise in divorce rates
- A greater emphasis on advanced education
- A greater number of women who no longer must depend on marriage to ensure their economic stability

Sexual relationships in adulthood can occur among single adults, within a marriage, or married people having interactions with people other than their own spouses. However, in the absence of definitive data, it is difficult to draw conclusions about how these arrangements affect and are affected by satisfaction, sexual behaviors, and other factors.

Older Adulthood

The term **climacteric** refers to the physiological changes that occur during the transition period from female fertility to infertility. At about age 40, the ovaries begin to slow the production of estrogen and androgens. **Menopause**, one of the climacteric events, refers to the cessation of menstruation and generally occurs at about 45 to 55 years of age (see Chapter 8). The hormonal changes of menopause affect the sexual response of most women. In general, all phases of the response cycle continue at a decreased intensity. The depletion of hormones associated with menopause can result in several vaginal changes, including dryness, thinning of the walls, and delayed or absent lubrication during sexual excitement. Hormone therapy may help some women cope with symptoms; however, hormone therapy may have side effects or health risks for some women (see Chapter 8). In some cases, prescription estrogen creams applied directly to the vagina may help prevent dryness and thinning. Water-soluble lubricants and vaginal moisturizers can help solve problems related to dryness, and Kegel exercises can help make sex more pleasurable by toning the pelvic floor muscles that support the bladder and uterus, which tend to relax as estrogen declines.

Although the general focus on sexual response in later years tends to highlight a decline in frequency and intensity of sexual activity, in fact the opportunities for sexual expression in a relationship often increase in later years, as pressures from work, children, and fulfilling life's goals may be reduced and more time becomes available for sharing with a partner. Couples may increasingly emphasize quality rather than quantity of sexual expression, and intimacy may find new and deeper dimensions in later years.

The perception that old age and sex are incompatible is erroneous. All too often, women dismiss sexual problems as a consequence of aging. In truth, most people can enjoy an active sex life no matter their age. Misconceptions about aging may have evolved for a number of reasons. Culturally, the United States still often equates sexuality with procreation. For older people who are neither capable of nor interested in the reproductive facets of life, this viewpoint offers little sensitivity or insight into their personal needs. Society also sends the message via the media that love, sex, and romance are only for the young and "sexy." The implicit message is that this scenario excludes older individuals.

Studies have found that sexual expression in older adults can provide relaxation, reassurance, and companionship, and can reduce depression and social isolation.[42] A comprehensive national survey of seniors found that most people

from the ages of 57 to 85 think of sexuality as an important part of their lives. The study also found that many older adults are sexually active, with sexual activity closely related to overall health.[43] Societal expectations can complicate sexual communication with older adults. Elders who are single may meet with disapproval from their family and friends when dating or engaging in sexual relations, and people in long-term care facilities may feel deprived of their right to privately engage in sexual behavior.

Sexual Violence as a Public Health Problem

Sexual violence violates a person's fundamental human rights and freedoms. Sexual violence can occur against men or women of any age. The perpetrator is often someone the person knows and can be a family member or friend, a respected member of the community, a colleague at work, or someone in a health facility or educational institution. Sexual violence can also occur in the highly organized and lucrative form of forced prostitution or trafficking.

Sexual Assault and Rape

Sexual assault and rape are crimes of aggression. **Sexual assault** often refers to forced sexual contact, while **rape** is usually defined as an event occurring without consent, involving the use of force or the threat of force to sexually penetrate the victim's vagina, mouth, or rectum. Rape may occur among strangers or intimates; it can also happen in a marriage, during a legal separation, or after a divorce. In addition, rape can occur between people of the same sex. Women are disproportionately affected by such sexual violence. One out of every six U.S. women and 1 in 33 men will be sexually assaulted in their lifetimes. College-age women are four times more likely to be sexually assaulted than the general population of women. These numbers translate into someone in the United States being sexually assaulted every 2 minutes.[44]

Rape and sexual assault crimes occur throughout the world. Many women who are raped or assaulted blame themselves for the attacks. In some cultures, especially in countries where women have a low place in society, families blame the girl or woman who is raped. Every year, as many as 5,000 women and girls around the world are murdered by members of their own families in honor killings, for the "dishonor" that the rape has brought to the family.[45] Chapter 14 provides more information on sexual violence, abuse, and harassment.

■ Sexuality is an important dimension of aging.

© Photodisc

Female Genital Mutilation

Female genital mutilation (FGM) is also known as female circumcision or female genital cutting. These procedures involve partial or total removal of the external female genitalia or other injury to the female genital organs for nonmedical reasons. The practice is usually performed on women by traditional circumcisers, who often play other central roles in communities, such as attending childbirths. Increasingly, however, medically trained personnel perform FGM. FGM is nearly always carried out on minors without their consent or under coercion.[46]

These practices, which destroy or cripple a woman's ability to feel sexual pleasure, are usually performed for cultural or religious reasons. Girls or infants suffer short-term and long-term consequences, including infections and other conditions ranging from lasting psychological harm to death. Globally, between 100 million and 130 million women have suffered FGM as young girls, and every year, an estimated 2 million girls are at risk, most often in Africa and South and East Asia, but also in parts of Europe, North America, and Australia. FGM is now illegal in the United States, but more than 100,000 women have undergone FGM or are currently at risk.[47]

Forced Sterilization

Forced sterilization, performed throughout the world for population control and eugenics (the Darwinian notion of producing a "perfect" race of humans), is a violent crime against the reproductive rights of women and men. People have been targeted for surgeries for being poor and/or illiterate; or for suffering from alcoholism, chronic disease, or mental and physical challenges. In countries with high rates of poverty, forced sterilization has been used to control population growth. Women have been bribed with payments of food, clothing, or money. Women also have also been unknowingly sterilized during childbirth or other medical procedures. Over the past 100 years, forced sterilizations have occurred all over the world, including Germany, Sweden, Japan, Peru, China, and the United States.

■ ■ ■ ■

Informed Decision Making

Sexual well-being encompasses more than sexual arousal and response. It includes effective decision making across the spectrum of issues affecting sexual health. A gynecological checkup is a good place to start for guidance in reproductive and sexual health matters, as well as preventive health screening. A woman can maximize the benefits of a gynecological examination by selecting a clinician who is sensitive to her needs. Often that means changing clinicians until the "right" one is found. Even so, it is better to "shop" while feeling well than to wait until a pressing medical problem requires immediate attention.

Understanding personal feelings, thoughts, and symptoms and articulating concerns and questions are essential for effective personal communication and preventive health. Communication is critical for promoting sexual health and responsible sexual behavior. Being able to talk about needs, feelings, concerns, and fears is an essential component of a healthy relationship. Sexual communication can contribute greatly to the satisfaction of an intimate relationship. Unfortunately, American language lacks a comfortable sexual vocabulary. Available language seems to be either "clinical" or "medical" in nature, which may be perceived as too cold and unfeeling, or "street language," which may be perceived as too crass or juvenile. Beyond the handicaps imposed by socialization and language limitations, difficulties in sexual communication may be rooted in fears of too much self-exposure. Any sexual communication involves a degree of risk and vulnerability to judgment, criticism, or rejection. The willingness to take risks may be related to the amount of trust that exists within a relationship.

Responsible sexual behavior is also essential for promoting positive sexual health. Children look to their parents as a first resource; a healthy, loving, committed relationship can serve as a blueprint for children. Although communication between parents and children can be helpful, many parents find it difficult to discuss sexual health issues. Some parents are unsure of their own knowledge about sexual health and therefore they fear that they may not benefit the child by sharing their own experiences and information.

As girls grow up, they begin picking up information from television, movies, books, magazines, and friends. Although this is a natural behavior, parents should maintain an open dialogue with their children to ensure that they continue to learn accurate information and are have the maturity and emotional control to make good decisions. Although television and radio often suggest sexual behavior, the media typically depict sexual behavior in short-lived romances without the use of contraception. According to the Institute of Medicine, "The Code of Silence has resulted in missed opportunities to use the mass media to encourage healthy sexual behavior."[48] It is important to realize that sexual relationships should include negotiation and communication skills, safe sex practices, and healthy and positive relationships.

Healthcare providers also can be a good source of information for adolescent girls and women. Women should articulate the reason for their doctors' visits (such as fears about STIs) and address their specific questions or concerns. Clinicians will not necessarily ask a standard set of questions or ascertain by examination the nature of a sexual concern or automatically detect an underlying fear or anxiety. Insisting that all questions be answered and persisting when answers are not clear are equally important avenues for a satisfactory visit. Women are often eager to please their healthcare providers and will nod as if understanding when they actually do not. This behavior results in more confusion and an increased likelihood of problems. Many women find it helpful to write down their questions and concerns and deal with them one by one with the clinician in the office before clothes are removed and the examination begins. Unfortunately, many healthcare providers do not address important topics regarding sexual health and appear uncomfortable when questions are asked of them.

Healthcare providers need to find ways to broach the subject in a respectful, culturally sensitive manner.

■■■■
Summary

Sexuality pervades every aspect of a person's life. It evolves throughout the life span, from the beginnings of sexual urges in girlhood to maintaining a fulfilling sexual life into old age. Understanding the biological, psychological, power, and sociological dimensions of sexual health enhances total wellness. Women must understand the unique facets of their own sexuality, from their physiology to their desires. Both positive and negative sexual experiences can affect a woman's overall well-being. Communication and awareness of sexuality are key factors to resolving these experiences in a healthful way. Incorporating open communication and awareness of sexuality into personal relationships, informed decision making, and preventive health care can enhance a woman's sexual health throughout her life span.

Profiles of Remarkable Women

Eve Ensler (1953–)

© Featureflash/ShutterStock, Inc

Eve Ensler is a playwright, performer, and activist whose work grows out of her own personal experiences with violence. Ensler's Obie-Award-winning play, *The Vagina Monologues*, is based on her interviews with more than 200 women about their intimate anatomy. The piece celebrates women's sexuality and strength and exposes the violations that women endure throughout the world. The play has been translated into more than 48 languages and has been performed in more than 140 countries. Ensler's performance in *The Vagina Monologues* can be seen in the 2002 HBO original documentary.

Ensler is also the founder of V-Day, which grew from her conversations with women who approached her after performances of *The Vagina Monologues* to tell her of their own experiences of violence. Today, V-Day is a global movement that helps antiviolence organizations continue and expand their core work on the ground, while drawing public attention to the larger fight to stop worldwide violence (including rape, battery, incest, female genital mutilation, and sexual slavery) against women and girls. V-Day has raised more than $80 million over 12 years and funded more than 10,000 community-based antiviolence programs and safe houses in the United States, Democratic Republic of Congo, Haiti, Kenya, Egypt, and Iraq.

In 2010, V-Day and UNICEF opened the City Of Joy, a facility for the survivors of sexual violence in Democratic Republic of Congo (DRC). Conceived, created and developed by the women on the ground, the City of Joy supports women survivors of sexual violence to heal and provide them with opportunities to develop their leadership through innovative programming of educational training and political activism. The women experienced extensive literacy and communications courses as well as civics and politics training that teach them about human rights, women's rights, and psychotherapy to help them recover from their trauma.

In November 2009, Eve was named one of *US News & World Report*'s "Best Leaders" in association with the Center for Public Leadership (CPL) at Harvard Kennedy School, and in 2010 she was named one of "125 Women Who Changed Our World" by *Good Housekeeping Magazine*.

Topics for Discussion

1. How have sexual norms affected you as an individual? Have there been positive as well as negative influences?

2. Should sex education be taught in the nation's public schools, and, if so, what kind of education should be provided? Which topics do you think are appropriate for school-based sex education courses?

3. Explain the terms gender and sex in your own words. Can a person be of female sex but have a male gender identity?

4. Gender-neutral parenting is a form of raising a child without letting others around the child to know his or her sex. Proponents of gender-neutral parenting point out that a child can choose clothes, toys, and behaviors freely, without the constraints imposed by society. Opponents of this type of rearing are concerned with isolation, bullying, or other social concerns among peers, as well as confusion for the child in other organized settings. Is gender-neutral parenting beneficial or detrimental to a child and why?

5. A paradox is that women appear to have a greater capacity for orgasm and can experience orgasm from a wider range of stimulation, yet seem to have more difficulty experiencing orgasm than men. Is this true? If so, which factors may contribute to this paradox?

6. How is homophobia displayed in modern society?

7. Many researchers have proposed nonlinear models of sexual response patterns. Identify two of these models.

8. What are ways to maintain healthy relationships while being aware of risks of sexually transmitted disease, pregnancy, and rape?

Key Terms

Amenorrhea: Absence of the menstrual period in a woman by age 16 (primary amenorrhea) or absence of the menstrual period for 3 to 6 consecutive months in a woman who has had regular periods since the onset of menstruation (secondary amenorrhea). It often is caused by stress, acute weight loss, or excessive strenuous exercise

Androgyny: A blending of typical male and female qualities in an individual.

Bartholin's glands: Two small glands located just inside the vaginal opening that help lubricate the vagina.

Bisexual: A person having a sexual orientation to persons of both sexes.

Cervix: The small end of the uterus extending into the vagina.

Climacteric: Physiological changes that occur during the transition period from fertility to infertility in both sexes.

Clitoris: A highly sensitive structure of the female external genitalia, the only purpose of which is sexual pleasure.

Conception: Formation of a viable zygote by the union of the male sperm and the female ovum; fertilization.

Cunnilingus: Oral stimulation of the clitoris or vulva.

Dysmenorrhea: Pain or discomfort just prior to or during menstruation.

Fallopian tubes: Tubes or ducts that allow for the passage of ova from the ovary to the uterus.

Fellatio: Oral stimulation of the penis or scrotum.

Gender dysphoria: The overall psychological term used to describe the negative or conflicting feelings about one's sex or gender roles.

Gender identity: How one psychologically perceives oneself as either male or female.

Gender role: The public expression of one's gender identity as well as the cultural expectations of male and female behaviors.

Heterosexual: A person with sexual orientation to persons of the opposite sex and/or sexual activity with another of the opposite sex.

Homophobia: Irrational fears of homosexuality, the fear of the possibility of homosexuality in oneself, or self-loathing toward one's own homosexuality.

Homosexual: A person whose primary social, emotional, and sexual orientation is toward members of the same sex.

Hymen: Tissue that partially covers the vaginal opening.

Intersexuality: The sexual physiology of an individual in which the person is born with sex chromosomes, external genitalia, or internal reproductive organs that are not considered "standard" as male or female.

Kegel exercises: Exercises that help strengthen the vaginal and pelvic floor muscles to help prepare the muscles for delivery, aid in a speedy recovery from delivery, help prevent or treat urinary incontinence, and help prevent or treat the loss of pelvic support.

Labia majora: The outer lips of the vagina.

Labia minora: The inner lips of the vulva, one on each side of the vaginal opening.

Masturbation: Excitation of one's own or another's genital organs, usually to orgasm, by manual contact or means other than sexual intercourse.

Menopause: The cessation of regular menstrual periods by surgical or natural means. Also known as the climacterium, the "change of life."

Menstrual cycle: A recurring cycle (beginning at menarche and ending at menopause) in which the endometrial lining of the uterus prepares for pregnancy. If pregnancy does not occur, the lining is shed at menstruation. The average menstrual cycle is 28 days.

Mons veneris: A triangular mound over the pubic bone above the vulva.

Ovaries: Reproductive organs that produce ova, estrogen, and progesterone.

Perineum: The area of smooth skin between the vaginal opening and the anus.

Premenstrual dysphoric disorder (PMDD): A condition associated with severe emotional and physical problems that are linked closely to the menstrual cycle; a more severe form of premenstrual syndrome (PMS).

Premenstrual syndrome (PMS): A group of cyclic symptoms that occur in some women about a week before menstruation, including breast tenderness, abdominal bloating, fatigue, fluctuating emotions, and depression.

Rape: Any unwanted sexual act, including forced vaginal or anal intercourse, oral sex, or penetration with an object.

Sexual assault: Conduct of a sexual or indecent nature toward another person that is accompanied by actual or threatened physical force or that induces fear, shame, or mental suffering. The term is frequently used as an all-encompassing term for any type of unwanted sexual advance.

Sexual dysfunction: The inability of an individual to function adequately in terms of sexual arousal, orgasm, or in coital situations.

Sexual health: A state of physical, emotional, and social well-being in relation to an individual's sexuality.

Sexual orientation: One's erotic, romantic, and affectional attraction to people of the same sex, to the opposite sex, or to both sexes.

Transitioning: The process in which transsexuals work to change their appearance and societal identity so as to match their gender identity.

Urethra: The tube through which urine passes from the bladder to outside the body. In men, semen also passes through the urethra.

Uterus: A hollow, muscular organ located in the pelvic cavity of females in which the fertilized egg becomes implanted and develops; also called the womb

Vagina: A moist canal in females extending from the labia minora to the uterus.

Vulva: The external genital organs of the female, including the labia majora, labia minora, clitoris, and vestibule of the vagina.

Websites

Advocates for Youth: http://www.advocatesforyouth.org

American Civil Liberties Union (ACLU): http://www.aclu.org

American College of Obstetricians and Gynecologists (ACOG): http://www.acog.org

American Social Health Association: http://www.ashastd.org

American Society for Reproductive Medicine: http://www.asrm.org

Association of Reproductive Health Professionals (ARHP): http://www.arhp.org

Gay and Lesbian Alliance Against Defamation (GLAAD): http://www.glaad.org

Go Ask Alice: http://www.goaskalice.columbia.edu

Guttmacher Institute: http://www.guttmacher.org

Human Rights Campaign (HRC): http://www.hrc.org

Intersex Society of North America (ISNA): http://www.isna.org

Kinsey Institute: http://www.kinseyinstitute.org

National Gay and Lesbian Task Force: http://www.thetaskforce.org

Parents, Families and Friends of Lesbians and Gays (PFLAG): http://community.pflag.org

Planned Parenthood: http://www.plannedparenthood
.org

Sexuality Information and Education Council of the
United States (SIECUS): http://www.siecus.org

World Health Organization (WHO): http://www.who
.int/reproductive-health/

■■■■
References

1. World Health Organization [WHO]. (2006). *Defining Sexual Health. Report of a technical consultation on sexual health 28–31 January 2002*, Geneva, Switzerland: WHO. Available at: http://www.who.int/reproductivehealth/publications/en/

2. Centers for Disease Control and Prevention [CDC]. (2010). Youth risk behavior surveillance—United States 2009. Surveillance Summaries. *Morbidity and Morality Weekly Report* 2010;59 (No. SS-5).

3. Centers for Disease Control and Prevention [CDC]. (2002). *Cohabitation, marriage, divorce, and remarriage in the United States.* Series Report 23, Number 22. Available at: http://www.cdc.gov/nchs/pressroom/02news/div_mar_cohab.htm

4. Eisenberg, M. E., Bernat, D. H., Bearinger, L. H., et al. (2008). Support for comprehensive sexuality education: perspectives from parents of school-age youth. *Journal of Adolescent Health* 42(4): 352–359.

5. Duffy, K., Lynch, D., & Santinelli, J. (2008). Government support for abstinence-only-until-marriage education. *Clinical Pharmacology and Therapeutics* 10(15). Available at: http://www.nature.com/clpt/journal/vaop/ncurrent/full/clpt2008188a.html.

6. Ott, M. A., & Santelli, J. S. (2007). Abstinence and abstinence-only education. *Current Opinions in Obstetrics and Gynecology* 19(5): 446–452.

7. Kohler, P. K., Manhart, L. E., & Lafferty, W. E. (2008). Abstinence-only and comprehensive sex education and the initiation of sexual activity and teen pregnancy. *Journal of Adolescent Health* 42(4): 344–351.

8. Boonstra, H. (2010). Sex education: another big step forward—and a step back, *The Guttmacher Policy Review* 13(2): 27–28.

9. Guttmacher Institute. (2011). State Policies in Brief: Sex and STD/HIV education. <http://www.guttmacher.org/statecenter/spibs/spib_SE.pdf>, accessed March 2, 2012.

10. Kinsey, A., Pomeroy, W., & Martin, C. (1948). *Sexual behavior in the human male.* Philadelphia, PA: W. B. Saunders.

11. Kinsey, A., Pomeroy, W., Martin, C., et al. (1953). *Sexual behavior in the human female.* Philadelphia, PA: W. B. Saunders.

12. Masters, W., & Johnson, V. (1966). *Human sexual response.* Boston, MA: Little, Brown.

13. Hite, S. (1976). *The Hite Report: A nationwide study of female sexuality.* New York, NY: Dell Books.

14. Tavris, C., & Sadd, S. (1977). *The Redbook report on female sexuality.* New York, NY: Delacorte Press.

15. Blumstein, P., & Schwartz, P. (1983). *American couples: Money, work and sex.* New York, NY: William Morrow.

16. Laumann, E. O., Gagnon, J. H., Michael, R. T., et al. (1992). *National Health and Social Life Survey, 1992: [United States].* Ann Arbor, MI: Inter-university Consortium for Political and Social Research.

17. U.S. Department of Health and Human Services. (2001). *The Surgeon General's Call to Action to promote sexual health and responsible sexual behavior.* Hyattsville, MD: Department of Health and Human Services.

18. Bancroft, J., Loftus, J., & Long, J.S. (2003). Distress about sex: a national survey of women in heterosexual relationships. *Archives of Sexual Behavior* 32(3): 193–208.

19. ABC News. (2004). *Primetime Live Poll: The American Sex Survey.* Available at: http://abcnews.go.com/images/Politics/959a1AmericanSexSurvey.pdf.

20. Herbenick, D., Reece, M., Schick, V., et al. (2010), Sexual behavior in the United States: Results from a national probability sample of men and women ages 14–94. *Journal of Sexual Medicine* 7: 255–265.

21. Wizemann, T. M., & Pardue, M. L. (Eds.). (2001). *Exploring the biological contributions to human health: Does sex matter?* Washington, DC: National Academies Press.

22. Johnson, C. V., Mimiaga, M. J., & Bradford, J. (2008). Health care issues among lesbian, gay, bisexual, transgender and intersex (LGBTI) populations in the United States: introduction. *Journal of Homosexuality* 54(3): 213–224.

23. Kruijver, F. P., Zhou, J. N., Pool, C. W., et al. (2000). Male-to-female transsexuals have female neuron numbers in a limbic nucleus. *Journal of Clinical Endocrinology and Metabolism* 85(5): 2034–2041.

24. Gooren, L. (2001). Gender identity and sexual behavior. In: DeGroot, L. J., and J. Jameson, (Eds.). *Endocrinology* (p. 2039), Philadelphia, PA: W. B. Saunders.

25. Jackson, N. C., Johnson, M. J., & Roberts, R. (2008). The potential impact of discrimination fears of older gays, lesbians, bisexuals, and transgender individuals living in small- to moderate-sized cities on long-term health care. *Journal of Homosexuality* 54(3): 325–339.

26. Marrazzo, J. M. (2004). Barriers to infectious disease care among lesbians. International Conference on Women and Infectious Diseases. *Emerging Infectious Diseases* 10(11): 1974–1978.

27. Yonkers, K. A., O'Brien, P. M., & Eriksson, E. (2008). Premenstrual syndrome. *Lancet* 371(9619): 1200–1210.

28. Borenstein, J. E., Dean, B. B., Yonkers, K. A., et al. (2007). Using the daily record of severity of symptoms as a screening instrument for premenstrual syndrome. *Obstetrics and Gynecology* 109: 1068–1075.

29. Bertone-Johnson, E. R., Hankinson, S. E., Johnson, S. R., et al. (2008). Cigarette smoking and the development of premenstrual syndrome. *American Journal of Epidemiology* 168(8): 938–945.

30. Lopez, L. M., Kaptein, A. & Helmerhorst, F. M. (2008). Oral contraceptives containing drospirenone for premenstrual syndrome. *Cochrane Database System Review* Jan 23(1): CD006586.

31. Shah, N. R., Jones, J. B., Aperi, J., et al. (2008). Selective serotonin reuptake inhibitors for premenstrual and premenstrual dysphoric disorder. *Obstetrics and Gynecology* 111:1175–1182.

32. Busse, J. W., Montori, V. M., Krasnik, C., et al. (2008). Psychological intervention for premenstrual syndrome: a meta-analysis of randomized controlled trials. *Psychotherapy and Psychosomatics* 78(1): 6–15.

33. Garefalakis, M., & Hickey, M. (2008). Role of androgens, progestins and tibolone in the treatment of menopausal symptoms: a review of the clinical evidence. *Clinical Interventions of Aging* 3(1): 1–8.

34. Kaplan, H.S. (1979). *Disorders of sexual desire and other new concepts and techniques in sex therapy.* New York, NY: Brunner/Hazel Publications.

35. Whipple, B., & Brash-McGreer K. (1997). Management of female sexual dysfunction. In M.L. Sipski & C. Alexander (Eds.) *Maintaining sexuality with disability and chronic illness: A practitioners guide* (pp. 509–534). Frederick, MD: Aspen Publishers.

36. Basson, R. (2001). The new model of female sexual response. *Sex Dysfunction in Medicine* 2: 72–77.

37. American College of Obstetricians and Gynecologists. (2008). Addressing health risks of noncoital sexual activity. *Obstetrics and Gynecology* 112: 735–737.

38. Shifren, J. L., Monz, B. U., Russo, P. A., et al. (2008). Sexual problems and distress in United States women. *Obstetrics and Gynecology* 112: 970–978.

39. Hillard, P. J. (2002). Menstruation in young girls: a clinical perspective. *Obstetrics and Gynecology* 99: 655–662.

40. Biro, F.M. (2010). Pubertal assessment method and baseline characteristics in a mixed longitudinal study of girls. *Pediatrics* 126(3): e583–e590.

41. Kaplowitz, P. B., Slora, E. J., Wasserman, R. C., et al. (2001). Earlier onset of puberty in girls: relation to increased body mass index and race. *Pediatrics* 108(2): 347–353.

42. Laumann, E. O., Anirudda, D., & Waite, L. J. (2008). Sexual dysfunction among older adults: prevalence and risk factors from a nationally representative U.S. probability sample of men and women 57–85 years of age. *Journal of Sexual Medicine* 5(10): 2300–2311.

43. Lindau, S. T., Schumm, L. P., Laumann, E. O., et al. (2007). A study of sexuality and health among older adults in the United States. *New England Journal of Medicine* 357(8): 762–874.

44. Rape, Abuse, and Incest National Network [RAINN]. (2008). *Statistics.* Available at: http://www.rainn.org/statistics.

45. United Nations Population Fund. (2000). *The state of world population 2000 report. Lives together, worlds apart: Men and women in a time of change.* Available at: http://www.unfpa.org/swp/2000/english/index.html

46. World Health Organization [WHO]. (2008). *Female genital mutilation.* Factsheet #241. Available at: http://

www.who.int/mediacentre/factsheets/fs241/en/print.html.

47. United States Congress. Report on Female Genital Mutilation as required by Conference Report (H. Rept. 106-997) to Public Law 106-429 (Foreign Operations, Export Financing, and Related Programs Appropriations Act, 2001). *Prevalence of the practice of Female Genital Mutilation (FGM); laws prohibiting FGM and their enforcement; recommendations on how to best eliminate FGM*. Available at: http://www.state.gov/documents/organization/9424.pdf

48. Institute of Medicine [IOM]. (2001). *No time to lose: Getting more from HIV prevention*. Washington, DC: National Academies of Science.

Chapter Five

Reproductive Health

Chapter Objectives

On completion of this chapter, the student should be able to discuss:

1. The four primary mechanisms for achieving birth control.

2. Contraceptive efforts from a historical perspective.

3. How sociocultural and religious considerations influence contraceptive use.

4. The prevalence of contraceptive use among American women today and sociodemographic differences among women.

5. Economic perspectives associated with contraception.

6. The importance of family planning services to demographic segments of American women, including adolescents.

7. The concept of contraceptive efficacy.

8. The concept of fertility awareness for contraception.

9. The mechanisms, risks, benefits, side effects, and contraindications of hormonal, barrier, permanent, and other methods of contraception.

10. Emergency contraception options.

11. The options available for an unplanned pregnancy.

12. The difference between induced and spontaneous abortion.

13. Abortion from a historical perspective.

14. Abortion from legal and political perspectives.

15. The pro-life, pro-choice, and middle ground positions on abortion.

16. Abortion from an epidemiological perspective.

17. The major types of abortion procedures.

18. Reasons why the assessment of risks, benefits, and contraindications is an integral component of contraceptive decision making.

19. The strategies in effective contraceptive decision making.

20. The importance of careful decision making regarding abortion.

womenshealth.jbpub.com

Women's Health Online is a great source for supplementary women's health information for both students and instructors. Visit

http://womenshealth.jbpub.com

to find a variety of useful tools for learning, thinking, and teaching.

Introduction

From a personal perspective, the ability to control the body's reproductive function is a necessary part of a woman's health, career, and family management. National survey data reveal that virtually all (99%) sexually experienced women have used some method of contraception and approximately 62% of reproductive-age women in the United States are currently using some form of birth control.[1] The two most popular forms of birth control are female sterilization and the birth control pill (**Figures 5.1** and **5.2**). Many methods of contraception are available today, and no one method is perfect. Ultimately, contraception is a shared responsibility, so the best method is one that a woman and her partner feel comfortable using and one that they will use correctly and consistently. The risk of STIs, should also influence a couple's decision about what type(s) of contraception to use.

Contraception is also important from a public health perspective. The Centers for Disease Control and Prevention (CDC) recognize contraception as one of the 10 great public health achievements in the 20th century.[2] Family planning allows today's women to have fewer children than in centuries past and to space births more widely, resulting in healthier infants, women, and children. Family planning has also helped women advance in society by enabling them to more easily integrate their educational, career and maternal roles.

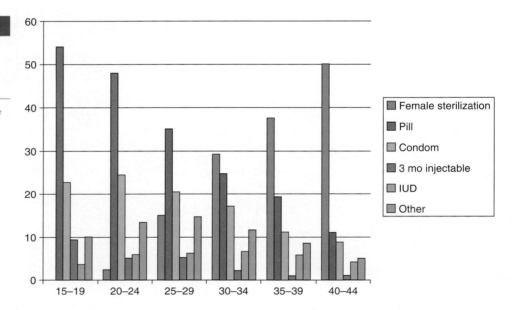

Figure 5.1

Percentage of U.S. women aged 15–44 who are currently using certain contraceptive methods by age group: 2006–2008.

Source: Data from U.S. Department of Health and Human Services. Centers for Disease Control and Prevention. (2010). *Vital and Health Statistics* 23(29): 27. Available from: http://www.cdc.gov/nchs/data/series/sr_23/sr23_029.pdf

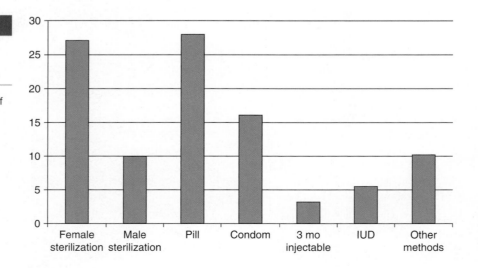

Figure 5.2

Contraceptive method choice among U.S. women 15–44 years, using contraception, 2006–2008.

Source: Data from U.S. Department of Health and Human Services. Centers for Disease Control and Prevention. (2010). *Vital and Health Statistics* 23(29): 27. Available from: http://www.cdc.gov/nchs/data/series/sr_23/sr23_029.pdf

■ Choosing the right contraception is a decision that couples should make together.

Perspectives on Contraception

Although the terms "birth control," "family planning," and "contraception" are often used interchangeably, each term has a distinct meaning. **Contraception** is a specific term for any procedure used to prevent fertilization of an ovum. **Family planning** is a term generally used to include the timing and spacing of children. **Birth control** is a broad term that refers to procedures that prevent the birth of a baby, so it would include all available contraceptive measures as well as sterilization, the **intrauterine device (IUD)**, and abortion procedures. With the exception of condoms, none of these methods provide protection against sexually transmitted infections (STIs).

There are four primary mechanisms by which birth control can be accomplished:

1. Preventing sperm from entering the female reproductive tract. Strategies that use this mechanism include abstinence, withdrawal, the condom, and male sterilization.

2. Preventing sperm from fertilizing an ovum once it has entered the female reproductive tract. Strategies that use this mechanism include the diaphragm, cervical cap, contraceptive sponge, and spermicides.

3. Preventing ovulation and/or preventing the ovum from reaching the sperm. Strategies that use this mechanism include oral contraceptives, hormone implants, hormone injectables, hormone patch, vaginal ring, and female sterilization.

4. Preventing progression or implantation of a fertilized ovum. Strategies that use this mechanism include the IUD, some forms of oral contraceptives, and

abortion. The Food and Drug Administration (FDA) labeling currently cites this mechanism for emergency contraception. However, scientific evidence suggests that emergency contraception actually works by preventing or delaying ovulation and does not inhibit implantation of a fertilized egg.[3]

Choosing when, if, and how to have sex or intercourse is a major decision for every person. The risks of unprotected sex include pregnancy and infections. Some couples may elect to practice **oral sex**, outercourse, or other forms of sexual intimacy before engaging in vaginal sex. Oral sex, or oral–genital contact, cannot result in pregnancy but can result in the transmission of sexually transmitted infections (see Chapter 7 for more information). **Outercourse** is the sharing of sexual intimacy through behaviors such as kissing, petting, and mutual masturbation without penile–vaginal penetration. These behaviors allow a couple to share pleasure and physical closeness without the risk of pregnancy; however, these activities can result in STI transmission if fluids are exchanged or if genital skin comes in contact with another person's genitals, mouth, or anus. Couples who practice outercourse require strong and motivated discipline to stay within limits: Ejaculation on, next to, or inside the vaginal opening has real risk for pregnancy and requires contraception if pregnancy is not desired. Contraceptive costs are another important consideration and can complicate decision making. Couples often face a choice between highly effective contraceptive methods that have side effects and other methods that have few side effects but may detract from sexual enjoyment and may have a higher failure rate.

Historical Overview

Throughout history and across global cultures, women have attempted to control their **fertility** by using many different methods. The biblical book of Genesis contains a reference to *coitus interruptus* (withdrawal), while records indicate that ancient Egyptian and Greek women made primitive diaphragms by inserting pastelike mixtures into their vaginas. Early attempts at spermicidal agents included mixtures of acid, juice, honey, alcohol, opium, and vinegar. Women from many ages and cultures have also consumed teas and sometimes septic solutions with the hopes that they would prevent unwanted pregnancy.

I am dependent on our local family planning clinic for birth control and my personal health care. We can't afford a private doctor.
—26-year-old mother of three

Until the introduction of the birth control pill in 1960, diaphragms and condoms were the primary forms of contraception. The earliest condoms were probably made from linen sheaths; later condoms were made from animal intestines. The cervical cap and diaphragm were introduced in the 1800s. In the mid-19th century, feminists in the United States began a birth control campaign with the slogan "Voluntary Motherhood." This campaign advocated birth control by abstinence. Margaret Sanger (1879–1966) and Mary Coffin Dennett (1872–1947) were early promoters of contraceptive birth control (sexual intercourse without pregnancy) in the United States, although the two advocated different means to achieve their goals. Birth control remained within the scope of national attention for many years. In the early 1900s, lower birthrates and changes in family structure among upper-class White Americans caused some to feel anxiety about "race suicide," in which the race's death rate would exceed its birth rate, leading to replacement in the nation's population by more fertile immigrants and poor people. Proponents of this elitist theory encouraged Anglo-Saxon women especially to have large families as a duty to their race and nation.

Today, many women take information on birth control and the availability of contraceptive devices for granted. However, for most of American history, contraceptives, as well as information about contraceptives, were illegal in parts or all of the country. Just 50 years ago, birth control pills were illegal in some states. In 1965 the Supreme Court's landmark decision, *Griswold v. Connecticut*, struck down a statute that banned the use of birth control and criminalized spreading information about its use. Justice William Orville Douglas based the decision on the fact that the case involved "the intimate relationship of husband and wife" and contraceptives were a logical extension of the marital relationship. In 1972, with *Eisenstadt v. Baird*, the Supreme Court established the right of unmarried people to possess contraception and invalidated a Massachusetts law that had made it a felony to give contraceptives to anyone other than a married person. Recent legal victories in the contraceptive movement have mandated increased women's access to more contraceptive options through their health insurers. The debate about insurance coverage, and particularly contraceptive options, continues to be a major political issue with the Patient Protection and Affordable Care Act of 2010.

Federal restrictions on contraceptive development have resulted in the United States having fewer contraceptive options than other developed nations. Since 2000, however, several new methods of birth control have become available in the United States, including the levonorgestrel-releasing intrauterine system (IUD), the hormonal contraceptive patch, the hormonal contraceptive ring, the hormonal implant, a 91-day regimen of oral contraceptives, two new barrier methods, and a new form of female sterilization.[4] U.S. women have a responsibility to stay informed as contraceptive technology evolves and to stay aware of the political and economic forces that might affect the availability of various devices or drugs.

Sociocultural Considerations

Birth control attitudes and practices and contraceptive availability vary widely among social classes and racial and ethnic groups. In some cultures, motherhood is the ultimate status a woman can reach and is considered a personal achievement. In male-dominated relationships and marriages, a woman may have considerable difficulty in expressing and asserting her concerns and need for contraception.

Religious beliefs often influence a woman's attitudes and practices about contraception. Many Protestant denominations endorse birth control as a marital option, although a growing number of ultraconservative Protestant denominations espouse limiting its use. Conservative and Reform Judaism teachings emphasize the individual choice of the married couple, with couples able to limit their family size for either health or social reasons. Orthodox Jews may practice contraception under special health circumstances by consulting with medical and rabbinical authorities. The Roman Catholic Church traditionally and still officially accepts only rhythm methods, involving periodic abstinence, for contraception. According to its teachings, the primary purpose of sexual intercourse is procreation, and any interference with procreation is considered to be a violation of natural law. However, a national study shows that 98% of Catholic women who have had sex have used a contraceptive method other than natural family planning.[5] This practice in violation of church teachings creates emotional difficulties for some Catholic women. The Muslim faith generally also forbids contraception, teaching that reproduction is both a sacred duty and a gift. However, although Muslims, on average, have the highest birth rates in the world, many Muslim couples use contraception, and some Islamic scholars approve of its use.[6]

In the United States, use of publicly funded family planning services has increased in recent years.[7] For many women, a family planning clinic is the entry point into the healthcare system and the one that they consider for their usual source of care. Studies have found use of family planning services varies with demographic factors. Women with lower levels of education and income, uninsured women, Latino women, and non-Hispanic Black women are less likely to have access to family planning services.[8] Inequalities in reproductive health service use are especially pronounced among young and socially disadvantaged women.[9] The underlying reasons for these differences are complex and the geographical distribution of clinics and private practitioners' offices may also help explain disparities in contraceptive use.

Birth control is a high priority for me. My family expects me to be a virgin when I marry. But we aren't ready to get married yet and I am not a virgin. I am afraid that my family will not understand this problem.

—20-year-old Hispanic American woman

As shown in **Figure 5.3**, specific contraceptive behaviors vary among racial and ethnic groups. Hispanic, White, and Black women differ in their use of the pill and male and female sterilization. There are significant differences

in the sterilization rates of the male partners, with male sterilization rates of 8% in the partners of White women, but only 3% of the partners of Hispanic women and 1% of the partners of Black women. The total sum proportion of each ethnic group's population using male sterilization or female sterilization was 23%, but the groups differed in whether they were more likely to use male or female sterilization. In addition, White women are more likely to use the pill compared to Hispanic and Black women.

Specific contraceptive behaviors also vary among age groups of women as **Figure 5.4** shows. In the 15–19 year range, 28% of women are currently using contraception, with the proportion of users rising in each successive age group through 44 years. A higher proportion of women under 30 use the pill as compared to other methods. Female sterilization is the leading contraceptive method among women from 30–44. Sexually experienced teens are currently more likely to use highly effective contraceptive methods compared to sexually experienced teens in the past; the increased use of these contraceptives may be a contributing factor to the national decline in teen birth rates.[10]

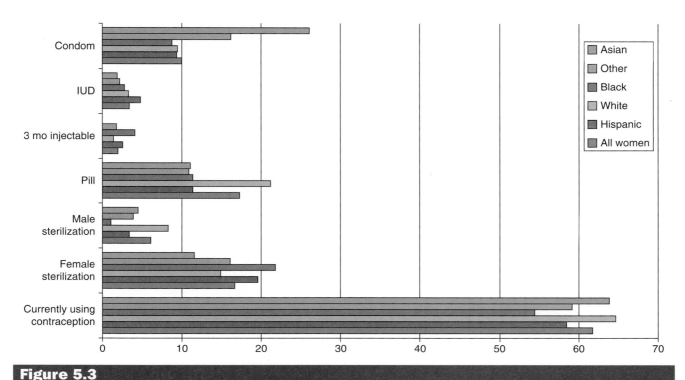

Figure 5.3

Current contraceptive status and specific method of women, 15–44 years, according to race and Hispanic origin: U.S., 2006–2008.

Source: Data from U.S. Department of Health and Human Services. Centers for Disease Control and Prevention. (2010). *Vital and Health Statistics,* 23(29): 27. Available from: http://www.cdc.gov/nchs/data/series/sr_23/sr23_029.pdf

Figure 5.4

Percentage of U.S. women who used any method of contraception at first intercourse, by mother's education, 2006–2008.

Source: Data from U.S. Department of Health and Human Services. Centers for Disease Control and Prevention. (2010). *Vital and Health Statistics* 23(29): 27. Available from: http://www.cdc.gov/nchs/data/series/sr_23/sr23_029.pdf

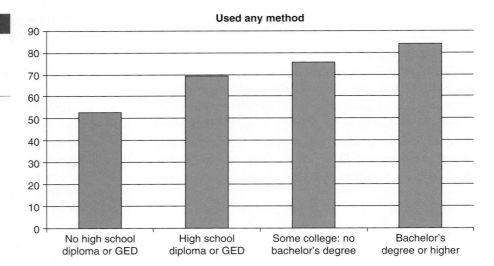

Economic Perspectives

Contraception and contraceptive use have three important economic conseqeuences: (1) contraceptive costs for the couple, (2) contraceptive issues with healthcare plans, and (3) the costs and benefits that contraception provides society compared to unintended outcomes, including pregnancies and STIs.

Contraceptive costs vary significantly, depending both on the method's initial expense and how often (if at all) the method needs to be repurchased. Birth control pills and diaphragms, for example, both have required office visit costs; however, pills may cost about $15–50 per month, while a diaphragm, which should last for about 2 years, has a one-time cost of about $100. Additional costs are associated with some methods. For example, contraceptive jelly or cream should be used each time with a diaphragm for greatest effectiveness, and insertion and removal fees should be considered with an IUD. Couples may be able to save on contraceptive costs by using a publicly funded facility. Publicly funded family planning clinics currently provide care for more than one-quarter of the more than 20 million women who obtain contraceptive services from a medical provider.[11] **Table 5.1** provides a comparative summary of contraceptive costs. The diaphragm is currently the most cost-effective method of preventing pregnancy; however, the diaphragm is not the most effective method, with a typical pregnancy prevention rate of 85%.[12] The associated pregnancy prevention rate as well as all the cost considerations should be part of any personal decision about contraceptive use.

While most contraceptives are prescriptive, not all insurance plans that provide coverage for prescription drugs include prescription contraceptive drugs and devices.

Legal victories in the contraceptive movement have mandated increased women's access to contraception through their health insurers. Twenty-six states require insurance policies that cover other prescription drugs to cover all FDA-approved contraceptive drugs and devices, as well as related medical services.[13] Federal employees achieved mandated coverage for contraception via an act of Congress in 1998. A 2010 national survey found coverage of contraceptives to be widespread but not universal, with 85% of large firms covering prescription contraceptives in their largest health plans.[14] In 2011, the U.S. Department of Health and Human Services (U.S. DHHS) adopted recommendations for women's preventive health care issued from the National Academies of Science and the Institute of Medicine. The Patient Protection and Affordable Care Act of 2010, based on these recommendations, requires new private health plans to cover contraceptive counseling and services and all FDA-approved methods of contraception without out-of-pocket costs to patients.

We are happily married, and someday we wish to have children, but right now our goal is to establish our careers. It would be really difficult for me to establish myself professionally if I become pregnant during the next 3 years.

—26-year-old attorney

The overall cost analysis of contraception should also include the societal costs of unintended pregnancies. Nearly one-half of the pregnancies in United States are unintended.[15] Unintended pregnancies, which present an increased risk of health problems for mother and baby, are more likely to occur in younger (18–24 years of age), economically disadvantaged, and cohabiting women with less than a high school diploma.[16] Two national studies have concluded that unintended pregnancies cost U.S. taxpayers about $11 billion per year.[17] Because these estimates are limited to public insurance costs for pregnancy, they are likely to be conservative and underestimate the true cost of unintended pregnancies. Subsidized family planning programs, such as those funded by Title X, could provide additional savings, but estimates of these savings vary widely. Existing family planning services clearly save money by preventing costs associated with unplanned pregnancies. The Guttmacher Institute estimates that without publicly funded family planning services, the number of unintended pregnancies and abortions occurring in the United States would be nearly two-thirds higher among women overall and among teens and poor women, the number of unintended pregnancies would nearly double.[18] In terms of public expenditures, for every $1 spent on family planning clinic services, an estimated $4.02 is saved.[19]

Additional cost considerations of unintended pregnancy include possible emergency contraception that may have associated prescription and office costs. The risks and costs of screening and treatment for STIs also contribute to the costs of some types of contraceptive failure. For individual women and men, contraceptive failure also has personal and emotional costs. If a woman knows she is not prepared to handle an unwanted pregnancy or STI, her behavioral and contraceptive choices should reflect these personal priorities.

Epidemiology Perspectives

Contraceptive Use

Contraception is an integral dimension of a woman's life. The "typical" American woman wants two children; she will spend about 5 years of her adult life being pregnant, postpartum, or trying to become pregnant; and she will spend three decades of her reproductive life trying to avoid being pregnant.[20] Virtually all (99%) of women who have had sexual contact with men have used some method of contraception at some time.[21] Among women currently using contraception, the oral contraceptive pill and sterilization are the most popular methods. The National Survey of Family Growth (NSFG) is conducted regularly and includes data on trends and sociodemographic group differences in births, pregnancy, and contraceptive patterns. As Figures 5.1, 5.2, 5.3, and 5.4 show, contraceptive use among women varies by age, race, and ethnicity. Use of contraception at first premarital intercourse is an important historical indicator of future contraceptive use. Compared to earlier generations of women, young women today are more likely to use contraceptives when they begin intercourse; this probability increases with greater maternal education and higher socioeconomic status.[22] Data from the NSFG survey indicate that 56% of women whose first intercourse occurred before 1985 used a method of contraception. That proportion increased to 76% in 2000–2004 and reached 84% in 2005–2008. As Figure 5.4 shows, about 84% of women whose mother had a college education used a contraceptive method at first intercourse, while only 53% of women whose mothers did not finish high school, used contraception at their first intercourse.

The 38% of women of reproductive age who are not currently using contraception includes women who are currently pregnant or postpartum, trying to become pregnant; have never had intercourse or no intercourse in the last 3 months, and are sterile for reasons other than contraceptive choice.

Contraceptive decision making is a complex task for a woman and her partner. Men and women may have somewhat different priorities when choosing a contraceptive method. Women consider the following characteristics to be "very important" when choosing a contraceptive method:[23]

Table 5.1 Contraceptive Costs*	
Low Reliability Options	
Abstinence	free
Fertility awareness	free
Better Reliability Options	
Cervical cap	$35–60/year
Condoms	$150/year
Diaphragm	$60/year plus doctor visit
IUD	$500–1,000 initial cost, but can last up to 12 years
Vaginal sponge	$500/year
Best Reliability Options	
Birth control pills or patch	$160–600/year
Injectables	$220–460/year
Sterilization	$1500–6,000 cost but effective for many years
Vaginal Ring	$160–600/year plus doctor visit

*These are approximate costs for public-sector settings. Private settings have significantly higher costs.

Source: Data from The Real Cost of Birth Control. Available at: http://money.usnews.com/money/blogs/alpha-consumer/2010/08/27/the-real-cost-of-birth-control-

- Effectively prevents pregnancy (90%)
- Effectively protects against sexually transmitted infections (77%)
- Provides no health risk (77%)
- Is easy to use (51%)
- Requires no advance planning (45%)

Together, these factors influence which contraceptive method women choose, how regularly they use it, and ultimately how effective contraceptive strategies are.

Contraceptive Services

Contraceptive services remain an unmet need for many women. More than one-half of the reproductive-aged women in the United States are in need of contraceptive services and supplies. These women are sexually active and able to become pregnant, but do not wish to become pregnant. Publicly funded services provide free or reduced-cost services, including the provision of contraceptives to the general public. Such sites include public health departments, Planned Parenthood facilities, hospitals, and community health centers. About 75% of poor, uninsured, African American, Latina, or immigrant women obtain their care from a family planning center and consider the center to be their usual source of medical care.[24]

Contraceptive Efficacy

Consistency and correct use are the two most important factors that determine contraceptive efficacy—how well a particular method is likely to work. However, even if used consistently and correctly, some methods are more likely to work than others, and contraceptive failure rates should have an important role in the selection of a birth control method. Failure rates are determined by following large groups of couples who use specific methods of birth control for a specified time and then counting the number of pregnancies that occur with couples using a given method. The larger the number of study participants, the more reliable the study results. A failure rate of 2% means there were 2 pregnancies per 100 women per year studied.

Two types of failure rates exist:

- The lowest observed failure rate represents a method's absolute top performance, the highest efficacy ever achieved in a reputable clinical trial. This rate is often referred to as the failure rate with perfect use.

- The failure rate for typical users is an average rate based on an analysis of a range of reputable studies. The failure

Table 5.2   Contraceptive Failure Rates

Method	Number of pregnancies expected per 100 women
Sterilization—female	<1
Sterilization—male	<1
Implant	<1
IUD	<1
Injection	<1
Oral contraceptives	5
Skin patch	5
Vaginal ring	5
Male condom	11–16
Diaphragm with spermicide	15
Sponge with spermicide	16–32
Cervical cap with spermicide	17–23
Female condom	20
Natural family planning	25
Spermicide alone	30
Emergency Contraception	1

Source: Adapted from U.S. Department of Health and Human Services, Office on Women's Health. (2011). *Frequently asked questions: Birth control methods*. Accessed at: http://www.womenshealth.gov/publications/our-publications/fact-sheet/birth-control-methods.cfm

rate for typical users is usually higher than the best-observed failure rates (**Table 5.2**).

Avoiding contraceptive failure is a goal of Healthy People 2020's national Health Objectives. Data from 2002 show that 12.4% of females experience a pregnancy despite using a reversible contraceptive method; the 2020 goal is to reduce this rate to 9.9%.[25]

While, in theory, abstinence is a very effective method of contraception, it is not a reasonable option for most women and has a high "typical use" failure rate. Several other methods have demonstrated high levels of "typical user" effectiveness, such as intrauterine contraception (IUDs), female and male sterilization, and hormonal implants. Very effective levels of contraception can be achieved with combined hormonal contraceptives such as the patch, pill, or ring; progestin-only pills or injections; and LAM (lactational amenorrhea method.) Other effective contraceptive methods include the diaphragm and the female and male condom. Moderately effective methods include the cervical cap, fertility awareness methods, spermicides, vaginal sponges, and withdrawal. The effectiveness of a birth control method depends in large part on how carefully and consistently it is used. A diaphragm does not work when it is left in a drawer, pills do not work if a woman forgets to take them, and condoms may break or leak, especially if improperly stored or worn.

Special Population: Adolescents

A sexually active female teen who does not use a contraceptive has a 90% chance of becoming pregnant within a year.[26] Teens and young adults often harbor many myths and misconceptions about contraception (see **Table 5.3**). Teenage girls tend to rely on their male partners for contraceptive implementation (withdrawal and use of condoms) during early sexual intercourse experiences and only later adopt prescription methods. The average delay between first intercourse and the first visit for medical consultation is about one year, and this visit is often motivated by a pregnancy scare. Condoms are the most common contraceptive method among sexually experienced teen females, with 95% having used the condom at least once; the second most common method was withdrawal, followed by the pill.[27] In recent years, states have expanded minors' authority to consent for health care, including care related to sexual activity. Teens are able to access contraceptive health services in all states without parental involvement. However two states, Texas and Utah, require parental consent for contraceptive services paid for with state funds.

Contraceptive Methods

Fertility Awareness Methods

Methods of fertility awareness include the calendar method, basal body temperature, "natural family planning," and the cervical mucus or ovulation method. These methods are based on avoiding sexual intercourse during a woman's most fertile time of the month, which includes the days previous to, during, and immediately following ovulation. Understanding the female menstrual cycle is an essential foundation for using fertility awareness methods. Couples using fertility awareness tend to have more accidental pregnancies than couples using most other contraceptive methods (Table 5.2).

All fertility awareness methods require identifying the fertile days in a woman's menstrual cycle. On fertile days, the couple abstains from intercourse or uses a barrier method of contraception. The calendar method requires determining when ovulation occurs by calculating the average length of consecutive menstrual cycles and then predicting when ovulation is most likely to occur. This is a difficult method to use effectively, especially for women with irregular menstrual cycles. One of the most

Table 5.3	Myths and Misconceptions About Contraceptives

There are perhaps as many myths and misconceptions about contraceptives as there are facts. A few of the more common ones are summarized below:

Myth: Birth control pills make a woman fat.

Some women may gain a few pounds while taking the pill; some women may lose weight.

Myth: A woman cannot get pregnant the first time.

A woman can become pregnant as soon as she begins to ovulate.

Myth: A woman needs to take a break from the pill every year.

There is no medical reason to have a break from the pill; it can be taken for many years without a break.

Myth: IUDs make sex uncomfortable for men.

IUDs are rarely felt by the male partner.

Myth: Wearing two condoms will provide twice as much protection.

Using more than one condom actually increases the risk of tearing due to friction.

Myth: Condoms detract from sexual pleasure.

Some condoms are designed to increase sensitivity. Not using a condom increases the risk of sexually transmitted infections.

Myth: Male withdrawal before ejaculation prevents pregnancy.

Pre-ejaculate fluid can contain sperm and timing of withdrawal is very difficult.

Myth: Plastic wrap can be a substitute for a condom.

Plastic wrap, balloons, and plastic bags do not work as protection during sexual intercourse. They do not fit and can be easily torn or displaced during sex.

Myth: A woman can't get pregnant while she is breastfeeding.

Breastfeeding will delay ovulation and will reduce the chance of getting pregnant, but it is not a guarantee. Nursing mothers who are sure they do not want to become pregnant should use an additional form of birth control.

Myth: Douching, showering, or urinating after sex will prevent pregnancy.

Douching is not effective, and there is some evidence that it may increase the risk for pregnancy by propelling the semen toward the cervix. Showering or urinating will not stop the sperm that have already entered the uterus through the cervix.

Myth: A woman can't get pregnant during her period.

A woman is usually not ovulating during her period, but sperm can live a long time inside a woman's body and women with irregular cycles often do not know when they are ovulating.

important changes during the menstrual cycle is the variation of hormones from the anterior pituitary and the ovaries. These hormonal variations cause biological alterations throughout the cycle, which lead to fluctuations in basal temperature patterns and variations in the type of cervical mucus produced. Many women are able to observe these changes during their fertility cycles and use methods of fertility awareness as birth control or a signal to use barrier methods of contraception.

Measuring the body's daily temperature (basal body temperature) can help to determine that ovulation has occurred. When progesterone is released immediately after ovulation, the body's temperature increases a small amount; however, women need to be certain that other factors, such as sexual activity, illness, or infection, are not causing these temperature fluctuations. Also, women can conceive a few days before or after ovulation, as sperm can be viable for up to 5 days and eggs are viable for 24 hours. Women also can sometimes determine the most fertile phase of the menstrual cycle by monitoring the change in the quality of the cervical mucus. During the most fertile phase around the time of ovulation, women experience an increase in discharge, with the mucus becoming more clear in color and slippery in consistency (often compared to egg whites).

Well, I am proof that you need to follow directions. I thought that using a diaphragm was enough. I don't like that spermicidal stuff, and I thought a diaphragm alone was good protection. So I am pregnant. I can't believe that this is because I didn't follow directions.
—21-year-old pregnant woman

Fertility awareness methods have the advantage of causing no side effects, no inherent risks, no contraindications or precautions, and anyone can use them. This method may be used with other barrier forms of contraception. Couples using fertility awareness with another contraception method have a lower risk of unintended pregnancy than couples using either method alone. These methods

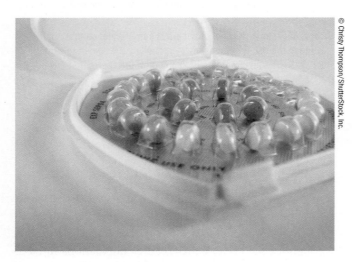

■ One type of birth control pills.

also help a woman understand her body and her cycles and empower her with practical knowledge.

Fertility awareness methods have many drawbacks, however, including limited effectiveness, challenges determining fertile days, the need to abstain from sexual intercourse during many days of the month, and the lack of protection against sexually transmitted infections. For a woman who absolutely does not wish to become pregnant, fertility awareness methods for contraception have inherent liabilities: Fertility awareness methods depend on partner compliance, careful observations and calculations, personal discipline, and good luck. Couples who rely solely on fertility awareness methods should plan on eventual failure of these methods.

Hormonal Methods

Hormonal Contraception

Combined hormonal contraception refers to contraceptive methods that include both an estrogen and progestin component. These methods include pills, patches, and vaginal rings. Single hormone contraception includes progestin pills, implants, and injectables.

Combined Oral Contraception Pills

The oral contraceptive pill has changed considerably since its initial launch into the marketplace in 1962. Today, more than 30 formulations are available to American women. Although the specific hormones are the same or similar, the dosages and formulations have undergone tremendous change. Oral contraceptives are now available in packets of 21, 28, or 91 pills to be taken once a day, preferably at the same time each day—it is important to take the pills as prescribed. There are many brands, which can have different hormone levels. Different women find that they prefer different formulations of pills. Talking with a healthcare provider about symptoms and concerns may help a woman find the pill that best suits her individual needs. Pills are usually started on the first or fifth day of a menstrual cycle. Sometimes women need to use a backup contraceptive for the first few days after starting the pill. Backup contraception should also be used when a pill user has extended vomiting or diarrhea or is taking certain medications, including some types of antibiotics.

Birth control pills suppress a woman's natural reproductive hormone cycle, and the synthetic estrogen and progestin of the pill produce an artificial cycle to replace it. Without the natural signals, the egg follicle in the ovary cannot mature, and ovulation cannot occur. Another way

© Christy Thompson/ShutterStock, Inc.

the pill prevents pregnancy is by inducing development of thick cervical mucus, in contrast to the profuse, slippery mucus associated with ovulation. The thick cervical mucus impedes sperm movement through the cervical canal and inhibits chemical changes in sperm cells that would permit them to penetrate the outer layer of the egg. The pill also acts as a contraceptive by preventing the uterine lining from thickening as it normally does in the menstrual cycle. Thus, even if ovulation and conception did manage to occur, successful implantation would be quite unlikely.

Overall, birth control pills are highly effective in preventing pregnancy: Effectiveness rates of 99% can be expected when they are taken properly.

Side Effects

Several side effects, both positive and negative have been associated with birth control pills, including:

1. Shorter, lighter, and more regular menstrual periods. The reduced amount of uterine lining results in reduced blood loss.

2. Reduction or elimination of menstrual cramps. Cramping is often associated with ovulation; because ovulation does not occur with use of birth control pills, cramping is reduced or eliminated. Steady progestin exposure with birth control pills tends to reduce or eliminate cramps and menstrual discomfort.

3. Mood changes. Some women may experience diverse reactions to birth control pills, such as irritability, depression, or mood swings. Some women, particularly those with a history of depression or premenstrual syndrome (PMS), may find these mood-related changes intolerable and choose to discontinue the pill.

4. Reduction or elimination of premenstrual symptoms. In many women, PMS tends to be significantly less severe or disappear with birth control pills.

5. Decreased libido. For some women, birth control pills may increase sex drive by reducing anxiety about pregnancy and alleviating discomfort or distaste at having to "get ready" for sex. From a biochemical perspective, however, some women may experience adverse reactions to birth control pills and experience a decrease in sex drive.

6. Spotting or bleeding between periods. The estrogen level maintained in the body by the pill is often lower than the natural level produced by the ovaries. This lower level may trigger slight uterine bleeding, which is generally referred to as "breakthrough bleeding." Such bleeding is more likely to occur when a pill is taken late or forgotten.

7. Weight changes. Some birth control pill users gain weight with the pill; others lose weight with its use.

8. Acne improvement. Most women who have acne notice significant improvement when they take birth control pills. In fact, some brands of pills are used to treat acne in some patients. However, birth control pills may cause chloasma, the darkening of skin pigment on the upper lip, under the eyes, and on the forehead. These pigmentation effects are not common and disappear when use of the birth control pills is discontinued.

Other effects associated with birth control pills include nausea, tender or larger breasts, headaches, and fluid retention.

Risks and Complications

Risks and complications are a major concern for oral contraceptive users, although many of these fears are unfounded. Safety issues concerning oral contraceptives are mainly based on the use of the original pills that contained high levels of hormones (although the original formulation of Enovid contained 150 mcg, current brands contain less than 50 mcg of estrogen) and the risks associated with smoking combined with use of oral contraceptives.

One concern about oral contraceptives has been that they may increase the risk of venous thromboembolism, the formation of abnormal blood clots within veins; these clots can sometimes break apart and cause blockages in a blood vessel. Venous thromboembolism, although rare, remains one of the serious possible adverse consequences of hormonal contraception. It has been estimated that venous thromboembolism rates in nonusers of reproductive age approximate 4–5/10,000 women per year, while rates in oral contraceptive users are in the range of 9–10/10,000 women per year. For comparative purposes, venous thromboembolism rates in pregnancy approach 29/10,000 overall and may reach 300–400/10,000 in the immediate postpartum period.[28] Thus, the absolute risk of this side effect is very small, and there is less danger of it occurring while on the pill than if a woman were to become pregnant and deliver.

An increased risk of high blood pressure, especially for older women and obese women, also has been associated with use of birth control pills. Other concerns identified by earlier studies of high-dose oral contraceptives include an increased risk of stroke and heart attack, though more recent studies show that there is no increased risk for either condition in women without preexisting risk factors, regardless of age. There is, however, an increased risk if the woman smokes or has hypertension. For women with cardiovascular risk factors or for women who smoke, nonhormonal methods of birth control may be the best option.[29]

Concerns have been raised about a possible connection between the pill and cancer in women. Since the pills were introduced five decades ago, sufficient time has elapsed to permit long-term studies on the possible association between the pill and cancer. Because some cancers depend on naturally occurring sex hormones, researchers have asked if the hormones in oral contraceptives affect cancer risk. To date, hundreds of studies have been conducted; the results have not always been consistent. Studies have revealed that taking oral contraceptives *reduces* a woman's chances of getting endometrial and ovarian cancers but slightly *increases* her chances of getting breast cancer, cervical cancer, and benign liver tumors. Because all cervical cancers are caused by high-risk HPV, a sexually transmitted virus, the association between oral contraceptive use and cervical cancer is likely to be indirect.[30]

Some evidence has shown that long-term use of birth control pills is associated with changes in the surface of the cervix. These changes may make pill users more vulnerable to cervical cancer and sexually transmitted infections of the cervix, particularly chlamydia. Confounding factors, however, make it very difficult to draw conclusions based on this evidence. Contradictory studies have shown no significant alterations of the cervix that would lead to associated risks. Women who have more than one sexual partner or who are at risk of transmission of sexually transmitted infections should consider using condoms in combination with birth control pills.

Several drugs can reduce the contraceptive effectiveness of the pill and increase the risk of bleeding between periods. These drugs include barbiturates, some anticonvulsants, antifungal medications, phenytoin (Dilantin), and certain antibiotics such as isoniazid, rifampin, and possibly tetracycline. It is probably wise for any woman using birth control pills to employ a backup form of contraception while taking any of these medications. Oral contraceptives also may prolong the effects of caffeine, theophylline, and benzodiazepines (e.g., Librium, Valium, and Xanax).

Advantages

In addition to offering the maximum protection possible against unwanted pregnancy with a temporary contraceptive method, oral contraceptives provide additional advantages over other methods. They are woman-controlled and discreet. They do not require any additional supplies or equipment, and they do not interfere with the spontaneity of lovemaking. Also, they provide regular menstrual cycle certainty, freedom from heavy cramps and excessive menstrual bleeding, and often relief of premenstrual symptoms. Menstrual periods become regular and predictable. The hormones in birth control pills provide some long-term health benefits as well as pregnancy prevention. For example, women who take birth control pills have a lower prevalence of ovarian and endometrial cancers[31] and benign breast disease.[32] Ovarian cysts are less common in women who have taken birth control pills and the pills may be prescribed to reduce the chance of developing new cysts.[33] Women who take the pill also are at lower risk for developing PID.[34] Oral contraceptives may also be prescribed to help treat iron-deficiency anemia because they lighten heavy menstrual flow.[35] For many years, scientists believed that oral contraceptives provided protection against osteoporosis because population data showed that long-term premenopausal use allowed women to enter menopause with higher bone densities than non-pill users.[36] Now, some evidence suggests that oral contraceptive use in young women may have an adverse effect on peak bone mineral density and osteoporosis.[37] More research on the relationship between pill use and osteoporosis is needed.

Contraindications

A contraindication is a medical condition that renders a treatment or procedure inadvisable or unsafe. Women who are contemplating use of birth control pills should carefully review and evaluate the contraindications before deciding to proceed. Absolute contraindications—meaning that the pills absolutely should not be taken—include:[38]

- A known cardiovascular disorder, now or in the past, such as thrombophlebitis, stroke, heart attack, coronary artery disease, or angina pectoris
- Impaired liver function
- Known or suspected cancer of the breast, uterus, cervix, or vagina
- Known or suspected estrogen-dependent neoplasia (abnormal tissue growth)
- Current or suspected pregnancy
- Abnormal vaginal bleeding
- Jaundice during previous pill use or pregnancy
- Malignant melanoma, now or in the past

■ Smoking in women older than 35 years of age

Oral contraceptive use when breastfeeding has generated concern for infant safety. Although there is no current evidence of harm, the question cannot yet be definitively answered. Experts believe that the risks of combined hormone contraceptive products usually outweigh the benefits before 4 weeks postpartum. Between 4 weeks and 6 months postpartum, the advantages of using the combined contraceptive method appear to outweigh the risks, although data are lacking for definitive conclusions.[39] The National Institutes of Health (NIH) advises that progestin-only oral contraceptives are safe for use by breastfeeding mothers. A mother who is fully breastfeeding (not giving her baby any supplemental food or formula) may begin taking this medication 6 weeks after delivery; if the mother is partially breastfeeding (giving the baby some food or formula), she should begin taking this medication by 3 weeks after delivery to prevent another pregnancy.[40]

Types of Birth Control Pills

Pill packaging options are available in monophasic (each cycle provides 21 identical hormone-containing pills), biphasic (each cycle contains two levels of hormones), and triphasic (each cycle contains three levels of hormones) formulations. Triphasic pills, the most recently introduced combination pills, contain three different progestin doses

■ The mini-pill can be an effective form of birth control, but it must be taken every day, preferably at a consistent time.

for different parts of each pill cycle. The primary advantage of triphasic pills is that the overall amount of progestin in a cycle is lower than it is with regular, identical-dose pills.

Traditionally, oral contraceptives have been prescribed in 21-day cycles of active hormone pills followed by a 7-day placebo or pill-free interval that produces predictable withdrawal bleeding in most users. Some women who follow this regimen, however, experience nuisance breakthrough bleeding, spotting, or amenorrhea. New formulations of continuous oral contraceptive therapy provide continuous hormonal dosing without monthly periods of menstrual flow. Clinicians agree there is no biological basis for the original pill cycle regime, as monthly bleeding is not necessary either for contraceptive efficacy or patient safety reasons.[41] The most commonly prescribed regimen for extended therapy is 84 days of active pill use followed by a 7-day hormone-free interval. Patient satisfaction studies indicate that many women prefer continuous therapy, as it provides fewer and lighter bleeding days and less bloating and menstrual pain.[42]

Estrogen dose is generally considered to be the most important factor in selecting a pill. Side effects and complications are reduced with lower estrogen doses. Minipills are estrogen-free (also called progestin-only) birth control pills that provide a continuous, low dose of progestin. These pills may be a better option for women who have certain health problems, such as blood clots, and cannot take pills with estrogen. They are slightly less effective than the phasic pills and have a higher likelihood of breakthrough bleeding in the early months of use. Minipills do not totally suppress hormone production, so the natural estrogen and progesterone production usually remains sufficient to trigger menstrual periods. There is less margin of error with these oral contraceptives, however—the likelihood of pregnancy increases substantially with just one or two missed tablets. Although menstrual periods tend to be less predictable with the minipills, women who use them generally experience fewer premenstrual symptoms, lighter or absent menstrual periods, decreased menstrual cramps, and less pain during ovulation. The minipill may also be prescribed to help treat sickle cell disease or dermatitis that seems to be related to menstrual cycles or to reduce iron-deficiency anemia.[43]

The minipill must be taken at the same time every day, and it may be less effective when taken with some drugs.

Hormonal Implants

A hormonal implant is a matchstick-like, small, flexible rod that releases a low, steady dose of hormones under the skin. Implants work like oral contraceptives, providing progestin that prevents ovulation. **Progestin** also thickens cervical mucus, preventing sperm from traveling through the cervix to the uterus. The implant is usually inserted under the skin of the upper arm, and it provides contraceptive protection for up to 3 years or until it is removed. The insertion procedure usually lasts about 5 minutes. A local anesthetic is used, and the procedure is normally painless. Hormonal implants are more than 99% effective in preventing pregnancy, but like other hormonal birth control products, they do not provide any protection against STIs. Hormonal implants are not as widely available as other forms of hormonal contraception because of the training that is needed for insertion and removal.

Irregular menstrual bleeding is the most common side effect reported with the implant. This usually occurs in the first few months of use. After 1 year on the implant, most

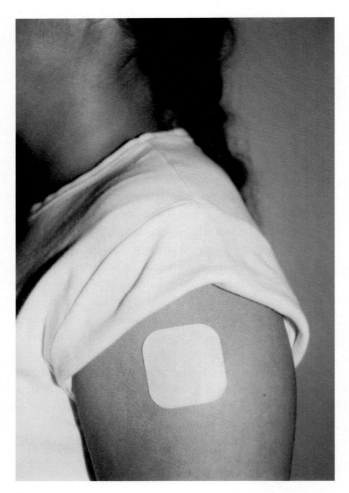

■ The contraceptive patch is worn on the skin for one week and replaced on the same day of the week for three consecutive weeks.

women report that they have fewer and lighter menstrual periods, and some women stop having periods entirely, though some women will report longer and heavier periods. Another possible side effect is difficulty in removing the implants, but this is minimized with an experienced practitioner. Fertility is not affected after the implant is removed. Benefits, cautions, and contraindications for implants are similar to those for the minipill. Studies have shown that the implant is safely tolerated and does not increase the risk for cardiovascular disease.[44]

The hormonal implant is highly convenient. Candidates for a hormonal implant include those women who do not desire children for at least 3 to 5 years and who are seeking a highly effective and convenient form of birth control. Women for whom other methods may be contraindicated or for whom daily, regular pill-taking or monthly refills would be an issue may find the implant appealing. Women who are pregnant, or who have unexplained vaginal bleeding, serious liver disease, or a history of breast cancer should not use a hormonal implant. Although the initial cost of the implant can be several hundred dollars, this cost provides pregnancy protection for 3 years, making it a cost-effective solution in the long run. Many insurers will cover the cost of the hormonal implant.

Hormonal Delivery Methods: Injectables, Patches, and Vaginal Rings

Other hormonal forms of contraception besides the pill and the implant include injectables, patches, and vaginal rings. They all provide steady and predictable doses of contraceptive hormones that prevent ovulation and thicken the cervical mucus.

The most common hormonal injectable, or "shot," is Depo-Provera. This injection of progestin is given intramuscularly, and it lasts 3 to 4 months. It has both a theoretical and actual-use effectiveness of almost 100%. It works best with a regular schedule of getting the injection every 12 weeks. In a study comparing the injectable and the pill, the injectable protected against bloating and mood swings but had an increased association with weight gain, bleeding episodes of more than 20 days, and missed periods.[45] Some women experience a delayed return to fertility after discontinuing the injections. Women who cannot take estrogen or who are breastfeeding are not good candidates for the injectable. As with other hormonal methods of contraception, the injection does not protect against sexually transmitted infections, and women with multiple risk factors for cardiovascular disease should consider other contraceptive options. Many women and teenagers have shown a decrease in bone density while using hormonal injections, but bone density appears to return to levels that are normal for the woman's age when the injections are stopped.[46]

The contraceptive patch is an adhesive patch that delivers hormones to the body. An advantage to the patch is that it does not require daily application: It is worn on the skin for 1 week and then is replaced on the same day of the week for 3 consecutive weeks. The fourth week is patch-free, and then the patch-use cycle resumes. The patch is durable and does not break away from the skin during warm weather, bathing, or vigorous exercise. Contraceptive patch users are exposed to higher doses of estrogen than pill users. Side effects to the patch are similar to oral contraceptives, although patch users report increased transient breast tenderness. Studies show an increased risk of venous thromboembolism (VTE) among patch user compared to oral contraceptive users.[47] A few years ago, the patch was shown to be less effective in women weighing 198 pounds (90 kilograms) or more.[48] A more recent analysis, however, concluded that there was no decrease in the effectiveness of the implant in overweight or obese women and that it should be offered as a first-line contraceptive method to any woman seeking a reversible and reliable birth control method.[49]

A vaginal ring, brand name NuvaRing®, is a relatively new hormonal contraceptive. It is a flexible, plastic ring that a woman inserts into the upper vagina. A provider is not needed for insertion or removal of the ring but a clinician must prescribe it. The ring is inserted in the vagina for 3 weeks and then removed for a week of menstruation, with a new ring inserted after the menstrual week. If a woman wishes to have continual protection without a menstrual week, she can insert a new ring every 3 weeks as a continuous form of birth control. The ring releases a

gradual and steady dose of hormones. Women must learn to correctly insert the ring and most women do not feel the ring when it is properly inserted. It can occasionally dislodge when a tampon is removed, but the ring can be rinsed and reinserted if this happens. Side effects to the ring are similar to those of the combination pill with additional possible effects of vaginal irritation or swelling and vaginal discharge.

Barrier Methods

Barrier methods of contraception were the primary forms of contraception before the pill and IUD. After the introduction of more recent, "high-tech" birth control measures, barrier methods were seen as messy, unromantic, and less sophisticated. Barrier methods, however, do offer several advantages over other contraceptives. The condom has reemerged, particularly as a result of the AIDS epidemic, as a major form of protection against HIV infection as well as other sexually transmitted infections, such as herpes and gonorrhea. In addition, the diligent, consistent, and proper use of condoms with a spermicide has demonstrated pregnancy protection rates fairly comparable to those seen with the pill and IUD.[50] Another major compelling reason for the return to barrier methods is that they have virtually no associated health risks, with the exception of rare allergic responses or localized irritation.

Barrier methods, as the name implies, provide a physical or chemical barrier that prevents sperm from fertilizing eggs. All barrier methods (except the female condom) are ideally used with **spermicide**, a chemical that breaks down the cell membranes of sperm for pregnancy prevention. Most barrier methods are used inside the vagina to cover the cervix and prevent sperm from entering the uterus. Male condoms are protective sheaths that enclose the penis during intercourse and ejaculation, while female condoms line the inside of the vagina and prevent semen from coming in contact with the vagina.

Barrier methods are very safe for the user, and problems and risks tend to be rare. One rare but important risk from barrier methods is toxic shock syndrome (TSS), which may be associated with the diaphragm, cap, and sponge. Although the TSS risk is small, the diaphragm, sponge, or cervical cap should not be used during a menstrual period or when any type of vaginal bleeding occurs. Further recommendations include delaying using these devices for 4 to 6 weeks after having a baby or until all postpartum bleeding completely stops. Toxic shock syndrome risk also can be

© michellegibson/iStockphoto.com

■ Barrier methods of birth control have virtually no associated health risks, but must be used every time a couple has sex.

minimized by not leaving the devices in place in the vagina for longer than the recommended time period.

Vaginal birth control devices are also associated with some other complications. A diaphragm, sponge, or cervical cap may cause a vaginal bacterial infection if it is left in place for more than 24 hours. A foul-smelling discharge indicates such an infection and should be evaluated by a clinician. The diaphragm and cervical cap also may increase the risk of urinary tract infections, indicated by painful and frequent urination.

Although the diaphragm and cervical cap require fitting by a clinician, women (and men) may purchase other barrier methods in pharmacies. With the exception of abstinence, condoms are the only contraceptive method that can reliably reduce the risk of transmission of STIs. Barrier methods are seen as noninvasive contraceptive measures by those women who do not want to have an IUD and who do not want to manipulate their hormonal system. They may also be used as backup contraceptive measures for a woman who has forgotten a pill or who questions an IUD's effectiveness. Some couples have intercourse sporadically or infrequently and find barrier methods appealing because they are effective and can be used only when necessary. Barrier methods are typically more effective among older women and careful users, compared to younger women, women who have frequent intercourse, and those who are not careful users.

Spermicides

Spermicidal agents are available as creams, foams, films, suppositories, or gels that are inserted into the vagina. Foams, creams, and jellies are thick liquids inserted via an applicator (**Figure 5.5**), while suppositories are soft capsules that melt into a thick spermicidal liquid after being inserted by hand. Contraceptive film contains spermicide in a small, thin sheet of glycerine that is placed over the cervix, which melts in response to body temperature, and the spermicide in the film is released into the vagina. Spermicides are available without a prescription in drugstores or from online retailers. Spermicides provide some protection as mechanical barriers, by spreading over the surface of the cervix and blocking access to the cervical opening. More importantly, though, the active ingredient in most spermicides, nonoxynol-9 (N-9) inactivates sperm by breaking down the surface of the sperm cells on contact. To be effective, spermicides must be inserted deep into the vagina.

Spermicidial agents have the advantage of being effective immediately upon use, and they may provide some protection against STIs. They do have time limits, however, and their effectiveness varies. For spermicidal agents to be effective, a woman must carefully read and and comply with the specific instructions for the agent she is using. An additional application of spermicide is needed for each round of lovemaking, and women should leave the product in place with no douching for at least 6 hours after each round. Women may use spermicidal agents alone or with diaphragms, cervical caps, or condoms. The agents are more effective when used with a barrier method. Spermicides are safe to use for extended periods of time. However, there are possible side effects with nonoxynol-9. These include irritation, itching, or the sensation of burning of the sex organs (either partner); in women, urinary tract infections, yeast infections, and bacterial vaginosis are possible.[51] These side effects are quite uncommon; one study found that only

Figure 5.5

Spermicidal agents.
Tips: (1) Woman should lie down after insertion; spermicide will leak out and have reduced effectiveness if she is in a vertical position. (2) No douching for 6 hours. (3) Keep extra supplies available—it is not possible to measure residual amounts of foam in containers. (4) Repeat intercourse requires repeat application of spermicide. (5) Wash reusable applicators with soap and water after use. Follow directions carefully for amounts and frequency of use.

(a)   (b)

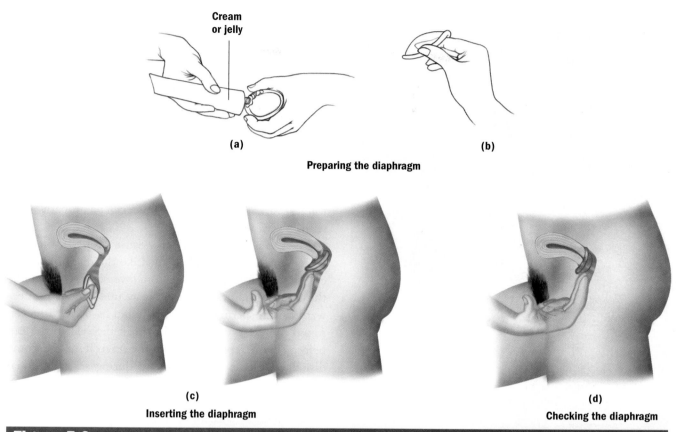

Cream or jelly

(a)

(b)

Preparing the diaphragm

(c)

Inserting the diaphragm

(d)

Checking the diaphragm

Figure 5.6

Diaphragm.

Tips: (1) Apply 1 to 2 tsp of spermicide to diaphragm rim and inside dome. (2) Insert the diaphragm by holding it in one hand, squeezing rim together in center. With other hand, spread labia and insert diaphragm. (3) Diaphragm is inserted deep into vagina with the anterior rim tucked into place last. (4) Check for proper placement of the diaphragm. Cervix is felt through dome—feels like tip of the nose. (5) To remove the diaphragm, assume the squatting position and break the suction by placing index finger between diaphragm and pubic bone. Hook finger behind anterior rim, bear down, and remove.

3–5 % of women who try spermicides discontinue use due to side effects.[52]

Diaphragm

A **diaphragm** is a dome-shaped latex cup rimmed with a firm, flexible band or spring (**Figure 5.6**). It should be filled with a spermicidal agent before being inserted into the vagina prior to intercourse. The spermicidal agent creates a tighter seal around the cervix and inactivates sperm on contact. The pubic bone anchors the diaphragm in place. Because the diaphragm must fit the cervix it is to cover, this contraceptive method requires clinician examination, fitting, and prescription. During the fitting, women should evaluate the comfort of the diaphragm as well as to practice its insertion and removal. Refitting of the diaphragm is necessary after a pregnancy, abortion, or significant weight change. A diaphragm should be replaced every 2 years.

Diaphragm effectiveness depends on proper fit and diligent use. A diaphragm that is too small may not stay in place and slip off the cervix; one that is too large may press on the urethra and cause a urinary tract infection. Application of the spermicidal cream or gel and insertion of the diaphragm can occur up to 6 hours before intercourse. If intercourse occurs more than once, women should use an additional application of spermicide for each event, regardless of how short a time the diaphragm has been in place. The diaphragm should not be removed or dislodged to add the cream or gel for a follow-up round of lovemaking; spermicide can be inserted directly into the vagina.

A woman may insert a diaphragm up to 6 hours before intercourse; the diaphragm need not interrupt or interfere with lovemaking. It should be left in place for a minimum of 6 hours after intercourse to allow the spermicide to inactivate all of the sperm. Douching should not occur

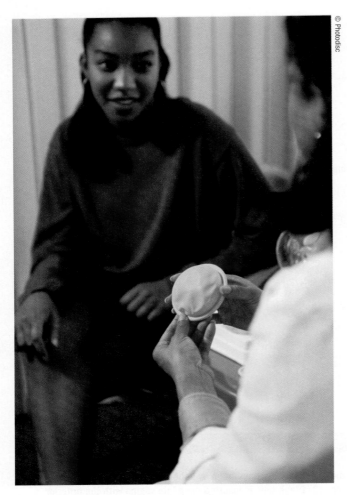
© Photodisc

■ A diaphragm is a dome-shaped latex cup rimmed with a firm but flexible band or spring.

during that time. A diaphragm is not recommended during menstruation.

The diaphragm should not remain in place longer than 24 hours. After removing the diaphragm, a woman should wash it with warm water and soap, rinse it, and dry it with a towel. Women should not use petroleum jelly or oil-based lubricants with a diaphragm for lubrication because these products will weaken the latex of the diaphragm. Women who desire additional lubrication may use a water-soluble lubricant, such as K-Y Jelly or Astroglide.

Side effects with the diaphragm are infrequent. Urinary tract infections, or an allergic response to the latex of the diaphragm or to the spermicide are possible, but rare. Some diaphragm users feel bladder pressure, rectal pressure, or cramps when the diaphragm is left in place 6 hours after intercourse. A smaller diaphragm or a different rim type may relieve this side effect. Women with poor muscle tone

of the vagina, a vaginal or cervical infection, vaginal bleeding, allergies to latex or spermicides, or a history of toxic shock syndrome should not use a diaphragm.

Cervical Cap

The **cervical cap**, shown in **Figure 5.7**, looks and works like a small, deep diaphragm. It is made of latex and is used with a spermicidal agent. The cap fits snugly over the cervix and suction holds it in place. Caps require a clinician's examination, fitting, and prescription, and they should be replaced each year for best protection. Due to normal anatomical variances, not every woman can be properly fitted with a cervical cap.

The cap's effectiveness depends on proper fitting and placement each time it is used. Like the diaphragm, the cap may be inserted hours before lovemaking, but unlike the diaphragm, it can be left in place up to 48 hours afterward. Fresh spermicidal agent should be used with each round of sex. Women should check the seal of the cap before sex and reposition it over the cervix if it has become dislodged. If the cap has moved during sex, additional spermicide should be used. A woman should not douche while the cap is in place, and a cervical cap should not be used during menstruation.

Side effects of the cervical cap are rare, but some women or their partners are allergic to latex. After childbirth, weight loss or gain of 10 pounds or more, pelvic surgery, a miscarriage, or an abortion, women should have their cervical caps refitted to ensure proper sizing. The cap is not recommended for women who have a history of toxic shock syndrome or a history of reproductive tract infections. Unlike the diaphragm, women with poor vaginal

■ The cervical cap looks and works much like a small, deep diaphragm.

Figure 5.7

Cervical cap.

Tips: (1) Fill cap approximately two-thirds full of spermicide. (2) Insert the cap by holding it in one hand, squeezing rim together in center. With other hand, spread labia and insert cap. (3) Cap is inserted deep into vagina. Use the index finger to press cap around the cervix until dome covers the cervix. (4) To avoid odor and reduce the risk of complications, remove within recommended time. (5) To remove the cap, break the suction by placing index finger between cap and pubic bone. Grasp dome and pull down and out.

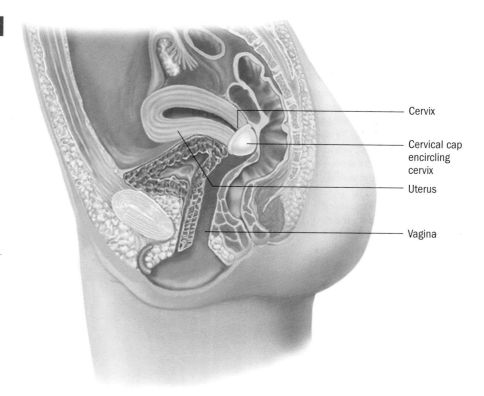

Cervix

Cervical cap encircling cervix

Uterus

Vagina

muscle tone or a history of urinary tract infections can use a cervical cap.

Condom

Condoms (**Figure 5.8**) are a popular barrier contraceptive. The male condom is a thin sheath, usually made of latex, but sometimes made of a natural animal membrane, or a synthetic material, that fits over an erect penis. Condoms are available with lubricants and spermicides and come in a variety of colors and textures. Condoms are portable, disposable, and easy to purchase. They may be discreetly carried and are, therefore, easily available when necessary. Women do not experience any post-intercourse vaginal leaking when condoms are used, and condoms permit the male partner to take an active role in birth control. Condoms made from latex or polyurethane are also the only methods that effectively prevent STIs. For couples wishing to be especially diligent in their birth control efforts, condom use can supplement other forms of contraception.

Condoms should be stored in a cool, dry place. Condoms stored in a heated area (such as a glove compartment) can deteriorate and be less effective. Because oil-based lubricants (such as Vaseline), weaken latex, water-soluble lubricants (such as K-Y Jelly or Astroglide) should be used

with latex condoms, if extra lubrication is desired. Prelubricated condoms may also help to reduce friction during intercourse and reduce the risk of vaginal or penile irritation.

Couples using condoms for birth control should use them for every act of sexual intercourse. Effective use of this contraceptive method requires commitment and discipline. A spermicide-coated condom affords the most effective birth control protection and may offer additional protection from STIs. The clear fluid that collects on the

■ Condoms can be latex, polyurethane, or lambskin.

Figure 5.8

Condom use.

Tips: (1) Avoid prolonged heat or pressure—condoms should not be stored in glove compartments or wallets. (2) Use only once and throw away. (3) If condom should break, use an extra dose of spermicide. (4) Put condom on an erect penis before it comes into contact with the vagina, pinching the tip of the condom to prevent air from becoming trapped. (5) Hold onto the rim of the condom as the penis is withdrawn from the vagina. (6) Do not use petroleum-based lubricants with condoms. (7) Latex condoms are better protection against the AIDS virus, though some individuals are sensitive or allergic to latex.

(a)   (b)

(c)   (d)

end of an erect penis may contain live sperm, so the condom should be placed on the penis before the penis comes near the vagina. When placing a condom on the penis, room should be left at the end of the condom to collect the semen. A person should pinch the tip of the condom before putting it on; this will ensure that there is room for the semen and will prevent air bubbles, which increase the risk for breakage, from forming. A condom that is stretched very tightly over the head of the penis is more likely to break or to force the seminal fluid along the shaft of the penis and out the end of the condom. The penis should be withdrawn from the vagina before the erection subsides, and the condom should be held during this withdrawal of the penis. As the penis begins to lose its erection, the condom will collapse and the contents of the condom may spill within the vagina. A quick visual inspection to ensure that the contents are inside and that no spill or leakage has occurred is a good idea.

Couples should use condoms both during and after treatment for any reproductive tract infection as a precaution against reinfection. Use of a latex or polyurethane condom is encouraged for women who are at risk for sexually transmitted infections—even for those who are using an effective form of birth control, such as the pill. Lambskin and novelty condoms do not protect against diseases. Condoms also should be used on any items that are used during sexual activity that penetrate both partners—examples would include shared sex toys, such as vibrators and dildos. In such cases, condoms should be changed between insertions if penetrating both vaginal and anal regions. Couples should not use more than one condom at a time, and never reuse a condom.

Female Condom

The **female condom** is another form of barrier contraception. It is the only female-initiated contraceptive method

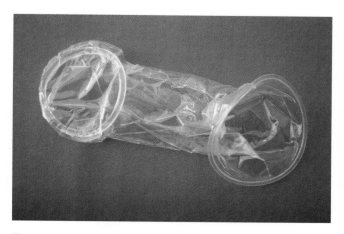

■ The female condom works by lining the entire vagina.

that can prevent both pregnancy and sexually transmitted infections. The female condom, approved by the FDA in 1993, is now available in many countries and is often promoted as a woman-controlled device for HIV protection. In spite of the educational details necessary for individual use, the female condom has enormous potential for improving women's choices for contraception and STI prevention, both in the United States and around the world. The female condom was originally made of polyurethane, but a newer version made of nitrile became available in 2007; an even newer version is being made of natural latex and is pending FDA approval for use in the United States.[53] The newer versions reduce some of the crinkling sounds associated with the original polyurethane version. The condom lines the entire vagina, preventing the penis and semen from coming in direct physical contact with the vagina. It consists of a sheath with a closed ring at one end and an open ring at the other. The female condom covers part of the external genitals, providing extra protection from semen leakage. Although lubricant is contained inside the female condom, additional lubricant is provided, and it should be used.

The female condom gives the woman more control and a sense of freedom with her personal protection. A woman does not need to see a clinician because the female condom is available in some drugstores and through online retailers; however, it is not as widely available as the male condom and costs more. The female condom is fairly effective in preventing both pregnancy and sexually transmitted infections. The female condom can make rustling noises during sex, but additional lubricant will help diminish this effect. The size and shape of the condom are unappealing to some women. Proper insertion of the penis into the condom is essential for the condom's effectiveness. Because the female condom is made of polyurethane, not latex, it may appeal more to individuals who have latex allergies, and because polyurethane transmits heat well, some couples find increased pleasure with the female condom. The female condom can be inserted up to 8 hours before sex. A study comparing the efficacy of the male and female condoms found that although mechanical problems are more common with the female condom, both devices involve a similar risk of semen exposure.[54]

Use of the female condom requires paying attention to details, as well as patience and practice (see **Figure 5.9**). Before insertion, rub the sides of the female condom together to evenly distribute the lubrication inside the pouch. The female condom should be stored in a cool, dry place and it should be used only once. It should not be used with a male condom, diaphragm, cervical cap, or sponge. The only side effect to the female condom is possible allergy to the lubricant.

Contraceptive Sponge

The **contraceptive sponge** is a one-time-use barrier method that acts as both a cervical barrier and a source

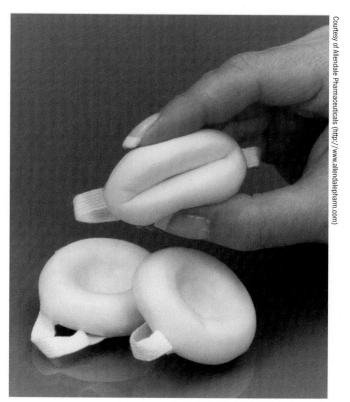

■ The contraceptive sponge acts as both a cervical barrier and a source of spermicide. It absorbs ejaculated semen.

■ Inner ring is
squeezed for
insertion

Inner ring

Open end

(a)

■ Sheath is inserted,
similarly to a
tampon

Uterus
Cervix
Vaginal canal
Inner ring
Open end

(b)

■ Inner ring is pushed
up as far as it can
go with index finger

Inner ring

Open end

(c)

■ Female condom
in place

Inner ring

Open end

(d)

Figure 5.9
The Female condom.

of spermicide; it also absorbs semen. The sponge is a soft, disk-shaped device made from polyurethane foam. One side of the sponge has a dimple that fits up against the cervix, and the other side has a nylon loop that facilitates removal. The sponge is relatively inexpensive, does not require a fitting or a prescription, and is available in drugstores and online retailers. The sponge is portable, disposable, and can be inserted a few hours before having sex. It does not interrupt lovemaking. The sponge is designed for 24 hours of use, and it should remain in place for 6 hours after the last round of sex. It does not require repeat applications of spermicide for additional sex. The effectiveness of sponge birth control, like all methods, varies depending on how it is used. The sponge is more effective in women who have never given birth than in women who have. Individual sponges cannot be reused.

Intrauterine Devices

An intrauterine device (IUD) is a small object that a clinician inserts into a woman's uterus. Today, the IUD is the most widely used contraceptive in the world. Even though the effectiveness of the IUD is superior to that of contraceptive pills, patch, or ring,[55] the device is not as popular in the United States as it is in the rest of the world. For example, a study in California found that although the IUD is available at no cost from the state family planning program for low-income women, only 1.3% of female patients obtain IUDs annually.[56] Modern forms of the IUD provide very effective and reversible long-term protection from unwanted pregnancy without increasing the risk of reproductive tract infections. Although initial costs for an IUD may be higher than other forms of contraception, their long-term effectiveness is an important consideration, and IUDs yield a very low cost over time.

Because it is extremely challenging to study the exact mechanism of contraceptive action with the IUD in humans, there is not yet scientific consensus about how IUDs prevent pregnancy. Their different designs present different theories for their effectiveness. The horizontal arms of some designs gradually release small amounts

An intrauterine device (IUD) is a small object placed in the uterus through the cervix by a clinician.

of copper into the uterine cavity, preventing sperm from successfully reaching eggs from a woman's ovaries. Other types slowly release a progestin hormone, causing a thickening of the cervical mucus, preventing sperm migration to the egg. All IUDs establish a chronic sterile inflammatory reaction in the uterus that interferes with sperm function so that fertilization is less likely to occur; they may also interfere with implantation.

Two highly effective forms of IUDs are available in the United States. One form is the Copper T-IUD, which is effective for at least 10 years and may be effective for up to 20 years.[57] This long-term effectiveness presents a good alternative to a younger woman who might be contemplating sterilization. The other available IUD is a hormonal device, LNG IUS (brand name Mirena®), which may be left in the uterus for up to 7 years. More effective than the copper IUD, it is sometimes used to treat endometriosis or as an alternative to hysterectomy for menorrhagia, a condition characterized by abnormally heavy and prolonged menstrual periods at regular intervals. Both IUD forms rival surgical sterilization in their effectiveness in preventing pregnancy. Less than 1% of users will experience an accidental pregnancy in the first year.[58] Menstrual bleeding is typically longer and heavier in the first 3–6 months for the Copper T device, while bleeding decreases, with

lighter and fewer days of bleeding with the LNG-IUD.[59] Provider education and training issues may prevent some healthcare providers from offering young women IUDs as often as hormonal contraceptives.

Permanent Methods

Healthy men and women usually have many years of fertility left after they have completed their childbearing. Surgical **sterilization** offers permanent birth control for individuals who are certain that they do not wish to have any more children. Female sterilization is second only to oral contraceptives in overall popularity as a method of birth control (see Figures 5.1 and 5.2). Advantages of sterilization for men and women include a very high rate of effectiveness and relatively quick, simple procedures that have minimal complications and side effects. Sterilization procedures do not disrupt either partner's hormones. An important disadvantage of sterilization as a form of birth control is that although it can sometimes be surgically reversed (a much more complicated procedure than sterilization), it should be considered a lifetime permanent choice to end childbearing. Also, sterilization, for men and women, provides no protection against STIs.

Perhaps the most important decisions for a couple is which partner will undergo permanent sterilization. Women have the option of having a tubal ligation (tubes "tied"), and men have the option of vasectomy. The most common choice is for a tubal ligation. This may be due to several factors. Many couples don't realize that a vasectomy poses far less risk to men than the risks associated with tubal ligation for women. Men may also be reluctant to have the procedure that surgically disrupts the passageway of sperm into the semen; as a result, semen no longer contains sperm, so conception cannot take place. A vasectomy is usually performed in a physician's office and a ligation requires a hospital setting.

Female Sterilization (Tubal Ligation)

Trends among older, reproductive-age U.S. women using contraception show a dramatic increase in sterilization rates. Sterilization of women has been made much easier in recent years by the development of new instruments and new techniques that have replaced laparotomy, which involves surgically opening the abdomen and tying off the fallopian tubes. Because unwanted pregnancies occasionally occurred after this procedure, newer techniques now often destroy or remove part of the fallopian tube.

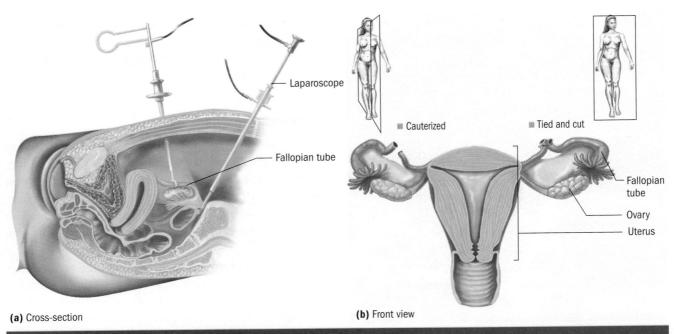

(a) Cross-section   **(b)** Front view

Figure 5.10

Female sterilization.
Tips: (1) Resume normal daily activities slowly after procedure. (2) Most sutures are dissolvable. (3) Take mild analgesic for discomfort.
(4) Resume sexual activity when comfortable. (5) Seek medical attention if temperature rises above 100°F, or if acute pain, discharge from incision, or bleeding is experienced.

We have three children and that is our family. The decision for sterilization was not difficult once we realized that we did not wish to become pregnant again. Our sex lives have improved—there is no need to worry about birth control anymore.

—35-year-old woman

Laparoscopic sterilization, also known as "band-aid" surgery, is one of these techniques. A laparoscope, a tube equipped with light and magnification lenses (see **Figure 5.10**), is inserted into the abdomen to provide a view of the uterus and tubes. The doctor uses a cauterizing instrument, rings, or clips to seal the fallopian tubes.

Minilaparotomy is the latest technique for tubal ligation. It requires a small abdominal incision and is performed under local or general anesthesia. A doctor lifts the fallopian tubes out of the incision, and then cuts, seals, and replaces them. The entire procedure takes a few minutes; the woman is able to go home after a few hours of recovery and observation.

A newer, less invasive procedure for female sterilization, called Essure, has been available for a decade. It is performed in an ambulatory clinic setting. The procedure requires the insertion of a small plug through a hysteroscope into each of the fallopian tubes. The plugs cause a local inflammatory process that results in tubal occlusion within 3 months of insertion. A backup form of birth control is needed for this period; a radiologic confirmation test can then confirm if the tubes are completely blocked. The method offers high sterilization efficacy without incisions, general anesthesia, or a prolonged recovery period for the woman.[60] The procedure is also more cost-effective than laparoscopic tubal ligation.[61]

Male Sterilization (Vasectomy)

A **vasectomy**, a 30-minute surgical procedure usually performed under local anesthesia in a physician's office, can permanently sterilize a man. In most cases, one or two small incisions are made just through the skin of the scrotum. The vas deferens is lifted through the incision and the two ends are tied or cauterized to seal them so that new sperm cannot enter the semen. Most men are able to return to work and normal activities the day after surgery but are advised to avoid strenuous activities, such as straining and lifting, for the first week after surgery. Vasectomy does not provide immediate contraceptive protection. Live sperm may remain in semen temporarily because mature sperm are stored in the vas deferens above the surgical site. As a consequence, men often are advised to use backup contraception for approximately 15 to 20 ejaculations.

Vasectomy offers several advantages. It is extremely effective as a permanent form of birth control and has a very low risk of complications compared to temporary forms of birth control or tubal ligation for women. Vasectomy does not cause any change in hormone levels or in the appearance or volume of semen. It also permits the male partner to take an active role in contraceptive responsibility.

Other Forms of Contraception

Not all contraceptive methods are appropriate for general use. Some methods are valid approaches to birth control, yet are associated with fairly high failure rates. **Abstinence** refers to no penis-in-vagina intercourse and depends on a couple's sustained willpower. In theory, abstinence is 100% effective for both preventing pregnancy and protecting against STIs; unfortunately, this method requires considerable personal sacrifice and has a high rate of failure in real life. Some couples consider oral sex or mutual masturbation, which do not result in pregnancy, a form of abstinence. However, oral sex can still transmit many sexually transmitted infections.

He told me that he knew what he was doing. It was the first time that I had sex. He pulled out but I still got pregnant. I was so foolish to think that I would not or could not get pregnant.

—16-year-old student

Withdrawal, also known as *coitus interruptus*, refers to interrupting lovemaking before ejaculation of semen. Although it may seem logical that conception requires semen and therefore requires ejaculation, withdrawal often fails as a form of birth control when the man is unable to remove his penis in time or because the penis releases some sperm before ejaculation. The failure rate for withdrawal as a form of birth control is fairly high because it is difficult for a man to know exactly when ejaculation will occur. The pregnancy failure rate in withdrawal has historically been attributed to the belief that preejaculatory fluid contained sperm. While some studies have shown no sperm in pre-ejaculatory fluid,[62] other studies contradict this finding,[63] so a couple should assume that there is some potential for preejaculate sperm to be present. It also is mentally and physically difficult to suddenly stop in the midst of lovemaking. Withdrawal does not protect either partner from sexually transmitted infections.

Lactational Amenorrhea Method (LAM)

Lactational (means breastfeeding) amenorrhea (means no monthly period) is a temporary family planning option for nursing women. Breastfeeding women may use this method, alone or with other forms of contraception, for the first 6 months postpartum. For LAM to be effective, the woman must be breastfeeding exclusively (no infant supplementation) on demand, be amenorrheic (no vaginal bleeding after 8 weeks postpartum), and have an infant younger than 6 months. This method works by preventing the release of eggs from the ovary. The failure rate of this contraceptive method is reported to be less than 2% if these criteria are met.[64] If pregnancy is not desired, another method of contraception must be used as soon as menstruation resumes, breastfeeding is decreased, or the baby reaches 6 months of age.

Emergency Birth Control

Emergency contraception (EC) is known by several other names, including emergency birth control (EBC), the morning-after pill, and postcoital contraception. These terms all relate to a therapy or procedure used to prevent pregnancy after an unprotected or inadequately protected act of sexual intercourse. Emergency contraception is a critical clinical resource for sexual assault survivors. In addition, contraceptive accidents can occur with any method or any couple. As seen in **Table 5.4**, a number of conditions warrant the consideration of EC. Women, their partners, and clinicians have often had a need for measures that can provide immediate additional backup pregnancy prevention. In the United States, the availability of emergency contraception has been a political story as much as a medical one. Conservative groups have organized heavy resistance to the availability and use of the product. Plan B was the first product approved for use in the United States as emergency contraception by the FDA. While the FDA approved Plan B in 1999, it was not available for over-the-counter (OTC) sales until 2006. In 2010, the FDA approved a newer form of EC, known as Ella, that is more effective and gives women more time to prevent an unintended pregnancy than the Plan B option. While these two hormonal options are available in the United States, other options are available for women in other regions of the world. A Cochrane Group review found several interventions are available and effective globally for emergency contraception. Of the hormonal methods, the group concluded that 25–50 mg of mifepristone was superior to other hormonal regimens. Their review also concluded that the copper IUD inserted after unprotected intercourse was effective in providing emergency contraception.[165] The copper IUD option is also currently available for women in the United States for EC use.

> I did not know that my regular birth control pills could be used for emergency contraception. I had missed a couple of them because I forgot to take them with me on a weekend trip. My pharmacist was very helpful in explaining my EC options.
> **—20-year-old college student**

It is important to understand how EC drugs work. Emergency contraception is not intended for routine use, but as a backup in the event of unprotected sex or a contraceptive failure. It provides no protection against STIs or HIV. Emergency contraception should not be confused with medical abortion. A medical abortion is used to terminate an existing pregnancy; EC is effective only *before* a pregnancy is established. While EC is *not a medical abortion drug*, the topic has been a source of debate over abortion and contraception. Some have argued that EC is equivalent to abortion because it works by preventing implantation of a fertilized egg into the lining of the uterus. Recent analysis of scientific data shows that EC works by stalling an egg's release from the ovary until sperm can no longer fertilize it or by thickening cervical mucus, hampering the upward motility of the sperm.[66] Emergency contraception is ineffective after implantation occurs.

Plan B, also known as Next Choice® in its generic form, is the most widely used form of EC in the United States. It was originally a two-pill process, but now Plan B One-Step® is available as a single pill EC. Plan B reduces the likelihood of pregnancy by 81 to 90% when taken within 72 hours of intercourse. It continues to reduce the risk of pregnancy up to 120 hours after intercourse, but effectiveness rates are reduced after 72 hours.[67] Ella is also a single-dose pill that is effective in preventing pregnancy up to 5 days after intercourse. A copper IUD can be used as EC up to 5 days after intercourse. If a woman can estimate her time of ovulation, she can place it up to 5 days after ovulation, even if that time is more than 5 days after intercourse. In addition to these two hormonal options and the IUD, sometimes regular birth control pills can also be used for EC. A woman can take birth control pills in two doses in a 12-hour interval. The same brand must be used for both doses and the active pills, not the placebo pills, should be used from the packets. However, the number of birth control pills required to effectively work

as emergency contraception varies from brand to brand, and not all brands can be used for EC. Additional information on birth control pills that can be used for EC is available on the Emergency Contraception website (http://www.not-2-late.com).

In 2010, the federal Emergency Contraception Education Act was introduced by Congresswoman Louise Slaughter (D-NY) (see Profiles of Remarkable Women in this chapter) to fund national campaigns to educate women and healthcare providers about EC, but the bill was not passed. The bill would have addressed the reality that many women and their healthcare providers do not understand available options for EC. Today, many women are unaware of EC, misunderstand its use and safety, do not have convenient and prompt access to it, or do not use it when a need arises. Some groups believe that EC availability would lead to increased sexual behavior risk taking; others have argued that EC would lead to fewer unintended pregnancies. While long-term studies cannot yet fully answer these important concerns, existing evidence indicates that most women who use EC use it responsibly. One study compared women seeking EC and women seeking family planning to be quite different. The EC group

Table 5.4   Emergency Contraception

Emergency contraception is indicated when a woman does not wish to become pregnant after she has had sex without using birth control or if the birth control method failed. The following examples warrant consideration of emergency contraception:

- Birth control was not used during intercourse
- Sex was forced
- Condom broke or came off
- Diaphragm or cervical cap tore or slipped out of place
- Two or three consecutive active birth control pills were missed
- Two week or longer delay in getting hormonal injection
- Contraceptive patch or vaginal ring is placed too late or removed too soon
- Spermicide tablet did not have time to melt before sex
- IUD comes out
- Failure to abstain from sex during fertile days when using natural family planning
- Any reason to believe that regular birth control may have failed

Source: U.S. Department of Health and Human Services, Office on Women's Health. (2011). *Frequently asked questions: Emergency contraception (Emergency birth control).* Accessed at: http://womenshealth.gov/publications/our-publications/fact-sheet/emergency-contraception.cfm had higher levels of education; they were more likely to have been protected at their last intercourse; and were less likely to have a previous STI.[68] A study of college students found their knowledge levels about EC to be poor. Less than one-third knew the prescription status of EC, common side effects, or mechanisms of EC. Only 16% knew that EC was available at their college health center.[69]

According to Planned Parenthood, costs vary from $10 to $70 for the hormonal pills; insertion of an IUD can cost up to $500. A woman who is not yet 17 will need a prescription, which requires an office visit that may cost up to $250. Twenty-eight states mandate health insurers to cover all FDA-approved prescription contraceptive drugs and devices, including EC. Two states, North Carolina and Arkansas, specifically exclude EC from the mandated contraceptive coverage.[70] Emergency contraception hormonal options are available in pharmacies but are kept behind the counter, requiring consumers to request them from a pharmacist.

Time is critically important for EC to be effective. Given the potential of any contraceptive method to fail due to unexpected circumstances, many women prefer to have a standby supply of EC "just in case."[71] Providing EC in advance of need gives women rapid access to it in case of unprotected intercourse or contraceptive failure. Studies have examined the availability of an advance supply of EC to see how it would affect contraceptive use and pregnancy rates. A meta-analysis found that advance provision of emergency contraception did not reduce pregnancy rates and did not negatively affect sexual and reproductive health behaviors. The authors acknowledge that many variables need further study to better understand the behavioral and social issues surrounding the failure to use emergency contraception even when it is readily available.[72] Additional information about emergency contraception is available online from the Office of Population Research at Princeton University and from the Association of Reproductive Health Professionals at http://ec.princeton.edu The site has no connection with any pharmaceutical company or for-profit organization, and the information is peer-reviewed by a panel of independent experts.

Handling an Unplanned Pregnancy

Women who experience an unplanned pregnancy must face a difficult decision. They may decide to terminate the pregnancy, to carry the baby to term and keep the child, or to carry the baby to term and have the child adopted. A woman must consider the implications of each decision to feel comfortable with her choice. Having a baby brings major changes to a woman's life, and it may cause many difficulties for women who are young and single. Plans for future education, careers, or relationships may have to be sacrificed to raise a child. All of these issues must be considered so that a woman does not resent her child based

---

Gender Dimensions: Health Differences Between Men and Women

Contraception

Historically, contraceptive options have been largely for women. This may be due in part to the reality that women, not men, get pregnant, or the fact that family planning research and contraceptive services have focused disproportionately on women. The female reproductive system has been extensively studied for centuries. Studies on male contraceptives have been seriously limited. Today, options for the male range from mildly effective (withdrawal) to highly effective (vasectomy). It could be argued that the remarkable effectiveness of modern hormonal contraceptives for women has given women high levels of protection, but that it has absolved men from participating in contraceptive protection and decision making. Men are often silent partners in preventing unwanted pregnancies.

Several factors contribute to the dominant role women play in contraceptive decision making and the availability of services for them. Modern medical care services provide ready access to contraceptive information and options for women. Women are taught and encouraged to see a gynecologist regularly in their teens; there is not a parallel system of routine health care for men. Society educates girls and young women early that the penalty of unprotected sex will be an unwanted pregnancy, personal and family shame, and economic hardships. The educational message to boys and young men is not the same, although legal issues surrounding paternity and child support in recent years have introduced the penalty concept to an unwanted pregnancy.

Multicultural surveys demonstrate that men are willing to participate in contraception, and their female partners trust them to do so.[88] Male contraceptive research includes hormonal and nonhormonal methods. Today the most significant barriers for expanded use include limited delivery methods and perceived regulatory obstacles. Novel combinations of reversible hormonal contraceptives in oral, implant, and injectable androgen methods are promising options for men.[89] International clinical studies have shown greater than 90% efficacy rates without serious adverse events for male hormonal methods.[90] Nonhormonal male contraceptives include products that target sperm motility. Although considerable progress has been made in clinical research on male contraception, no new product is currently available.

on a decision she has made. A woman may be concerned about financial and emotional support during the pregnancy, especially if she does not have support from the baby's father or from family and friends. Many family planning clinics, crisis pregnancy centers, and health departments have programs to meet the needs of these women.

Unplanned pregnancies are not always unwanted pregnancies. Often, a couple is not planning to have a child at the time that they become pregnant, but they want a child and happily decide to proceed with the pregnancy.

If a woman decides that she would like to carry the baby to term but not raise the child, she should look into adoption. Adoption can be "open," where the birth mother has some role in the child's future, or "closed," where the whole process remains confidential. Both public and private adoption services are available. Public adoption services are usually less costly but may be very competitive and require long waits for the adoptive parents. Parents often have to be more flexible about the age, gender, or race of child they are willing to adopt. Private adoptions usually involve a financial arrangement negotiated by an agency or lawyer between the adoptive parents and the birth mother. Private adoptions can be faster and allow adoptive parents and birth mothers to have more options in selecting each other. Adoptions also can be domestic or international, though adoption laws vary from country to country. In all adoptions, the parties involved must consider a host of legal and ethical factors. Many adoption agencies can help match the child with an adoptive family and may be able to arrange for the adoptive parents to pay for the mother's healthcare costs during the pregnancy.

Other women choose to terminate their pregnancies. In these cases, a decision should be made as early as possible to ensure a safe abortion.

Perspectives on Abortion

Abortion may be defined as the spontaneous or induced expulsion of an embryo or fetus before it is viable or can survive on its own. This can occur without human interference. Natural complications of fetal development, perhaps due to genetic, medical, or hormonal problems, can result in the spontaneous termination of the pregnancy. This termination of pregnancy is called a miscarriage or a spontaneous abortion (see Chapter 6). In contrast to a spontaneous abortion, an induced abortion involves a decision to terminate a pregnancy by medical procedures.

Abortions are one of the most common medical procedures undergone by women of reproductive age. In 2008, about 1.2 million women in the United States ended their pregnancies through abortion. Nearly one-half of American pregnancies are unintended, and about 22% of all pregnancies (excluding miscarriages) end in abortion.[73] As **Figure 5.11** shows, the number of annual abortions has decreased since peaking in the 1980s.

I am an organized and responsible person, but apparently contraceptive failure really can happen to anyone. It was impossible for me to raise a child at that time in my life. It would have destroyed everything that I had worked years for and my family could not help me. So I gave the baby up for adoption. I am not proud of it, but I am grateful that the child will have an opportunity for a decent life.
—32-year-old woman

Figure 5.11

Legal abortions, United States, selected years 1973–2007, per 100 live births.

Source: Data from Centers for Disease Control and Prevention (2010). Legal abortions and legal abortion ratios. *Health, United States, 2010.* Accessed June 26, 2012 at: www.cdc.gov/nchs/data/hus/hus10.pdf

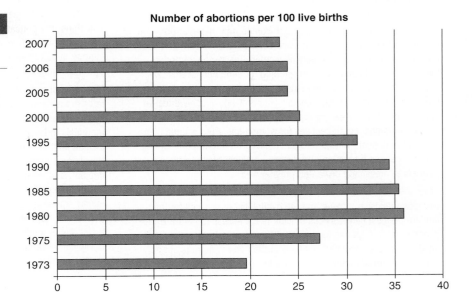

Number of abortions per 100 live births

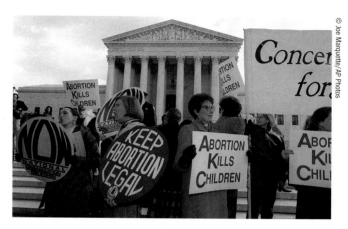

© Joe Marquette/AP Photos

■ Abortion continues to be one of the greatest debates in American society.

Historical Overview and Legal Perspectives

Women have ended unwanted pregnancies for thousands of years. The earliest methods used to induce an abortion were often either dangerous or used in ways to control women: Chinese legends attribute the prescription of mercury to induce abortion to emperor Shennong (c. 2737 B.C.E.), and in the Western world, ancient Greeks and Romans generally considered abortion acceptable during the early stages of pregnancy—so long as the prospective father did not object. St. Augustine (354–386 A.D.) agreed with Aristotle that abortion could be considered lawful before the fetus takes on a human-like shape and shows signs of movement, or during about the first 40 days of pregnancy. Through the 1800s, midwives and community healers in Western Europe and the United States used a variety of techniques to end pregnancies, making use of herbal abortifacients, mechanical methods (such as constriction of a girdle or introduction of foreign objects into the uterus), heat applied externally, strenuous physical activity, and starvation.[74]

Toward the end of the nineteenth century, physicians began leading movements to ban abortions, and by 1910, many states had passed legislation that prohibited abortion during all stages of pregnancy, with the exception of pregnancies that endangered the mother's health. Legal prohibition did not have its intended effect of reducing the incidence of abortions, however. Estimates of the number of illegal abortions performed annually in the 1950s and 1960s range from 200,000 to 1.2 million.[75] Without a legal method of obtaining abortions, many women sought out unlicensed and unskilled abortionists or to attempted to perform the procedure on themselves. Approximately 50%

of all maternal deaths resulted from illegal abortion during the first half of the 20th century.[76] During this time, the issue of equity mortality emerged as an abortion public policy consideration. Women with greater personal financial resources were able to arrange for safer, more "legal" abortions by traveling to less rigid jurisdictions or by persuading physicians to make exceptions for "therapeutic reasons," while women with fewer financial resources were more likely to suffer from unsafe abortions and incompetent abortionists.

The landmark Supreme Court decision *Roe v. Wade* legalized abortion in the United States on January 22, 1973. This decision declared unconstitutional all state laws that prohibited or restricted abortion during the first trimester of pregnancy. The decision stated that the "right of privacy . . . founded on the Fourteenth Amendment's concept of personal liberty . . . is broad enough to encompass a woman's decision whether or not to terminate her pregnancy." That right to privacy, however, had to be balanced against a state's interest in protecting prenatal life and women's health. Arguing that the state interests become stronger over the course of a pregnancy, the court sought balance by tying state regulation of abortion to pregnancy trimester. The ruling limited state interventions in second-trimester abortions and left the issue of third-trimester abortions up to each individual state. By dividing the ruling between a woman's interest and the state interest, the Court created a heated national debate that continues today. The debate has shaped national political agendas and polarized interests into opposing camps with intense grassroots support for each perspective.

In 1976, Congress introduced and passed the Hyde Amendment. This legislation banned Medicaid funding for abortion unless a woman's life was in danger. This amendment disproportionately affected low-income women, who were (and remain) less likely than other women to be able to pay for abortion services or to receive contraception. A compromise version of the Hyde Amendment eventually added exceptions for promptly reported rape and incest cases in which two physicians would testify that the woman's health would be seriously impaired by maintaining the pregnancy.

The 1991 case of *Rust v. Sullivan* upheld the constitutionality of the "gag rule," which prohibited federally funded clinics from providing information about and referrals for abortion. In 1992, the Court's ruling in the case of *Planned Parenthood of Southeastern Pennsylvania v. Casey* reaffirmed the central holdings of *Roe v. Wade*, but allowed states to restrict abortion access. This decision prompted many states to require parental consent, mandatory waiting periods, and counseling.

Some state laws have also limited antiabortion demonstrators' proximity to abortion clinics. These laws attempt to ensure the safety and privacy of women seeking abortions after many attacks on abortion clinics, women seeking abortions, and abortion providers took place.

Over the past decade, the Supreme Court has held more conservative views regarding the legal rights to abortion. In the 2007 case of *Gonzales v. Carhart*, the Court upheld a federal ban on a rare abortion procedure known as dilatation and extraction, despite the fact that the law did not allow an exception to the ban when the procedure was necessary to protect a woman's health. Along with the shifting balance of the Supreme Court, socially conservative state governments have enacted stronger limitations on abortion. In South Dakota, for example, a law implemented in 2008 requires doctors to tell women that abortion "terminates the life of a whole, separate, unique human being" and to cite medically inaccurate information linking abortion to suicide and other risks.[77] Since then, other states have further restricted abortion access. Just over two-thirds (68%) of the state reproductive health provisions are abortion restrictions.[78] **Table 5.5** provides a summary of the categories of state abortion restrictions.

The ramifications of abortion being a political issue are complex and widespread. Trained and available abortion care providers are limited, and these provider shortages may delay abortion services that are safest when provided early. A study found that 87% of U.S. counties had no abortion provider.[79] Another ramification of the intensity of the polarized views has resulted in provider murders, clinic bombings, death threats, acts of vandalism, harassment of clinic personnel, and postings of clinic patients online.

I am haunted by a story my mother told me of her friend who died years ago from a botched abortion. Her friend was desperate. It makes me realize that women will seek abortions whether they are legal or not. They should have access to safe facilities.
—27-year-old woman

Current Perspectives

Today legal abortions are very safe—markedly safer than childbirth.[80] Legal abortions are credited with decreasing both maternal and infant mortality. Abortion is both one of the most common gynecological procedures women experience and ranks among the most controversial and

Reasons women have an abortion

Conflict with education, work, or care for other dependents

Cannot afford to have a child

Desire not to be a single mother or relationship problems

Not ready to have a child

Source: Data from Finer, L. B., Frohwirth, L. F., Dauphinee, L. A., et al. (2005). Reasons U.S. women have abortions: quantitative and qualitative perspectives. *Perspectives on Sexual and Reproductive Health* 37(3): 110–118.

passionately debated topics in the United States. Traditionally, people who believe that abortion should be illegal have described themselves as "pro-life," whereas people who believe that women should be able to choose abortion to end their pregnancies have described themselves as "pro-choice." Journalists, who wish to appear neutral and not imply that either group is against life or choice, use the terms "antiabortion" and "abortion rights" to describe

Table 5.5 Categories of State Laws Restricting Access to Abortions

Parental approval or involvement required before a minor's abortion

Extended waiting period before abortions can be performed. Patients must make two visits to the facility—one for pre-abortion counseling, and another 18–72 hours later to receive the procedure

- Medicaid cannot be used to pay for abortion except in cases of life endangerment, rape, or incest

- Patients required to receive "preabortion counseling," often with medically inaccurate or misleading information, before receiving procedure

- Abortion facilities may have additional building requirements unrelated to patient safety (a small clinic may legally be classified as a hospital, with requirements to keep a large number of parking spaces or build wide hallways)

- Patients must receive ultrasounds before receiving abortions, regardless of medical need

- Private health insurance plans may not cover, or place large restrictions on covering, abortion procedures

- Legal restrictions on how medication abortion may be given that have no medical basis

Source: Adapted from Guttmacher Institute (2012). Troubling trend: More states hostile to abortion rights as middle ground shrinks. *Guttmacher Policy Review* 15(1). Accessed at: http://www.guttmacher.org/pubs/gpr/15/1/gpr150114.html

activists on either side. Legal issues continue to evolve at the personal, state, and national level about abortion and the challenges are likely to remain for some time.

Women choose to end their pregnancies for a variety of reasons. Women are most likely to choose abortion when facing an unwanted pregnancy, but may also choose abortion when they learn that they have a potentially deadly ectopic pregnancy, or that the fetus has a genetic disorder, neural tube defects, or some type of malformation. In a survey of more than 1,000 abortion patients, 74% of women said that having a child would reduce their ability to work, finish their education, or care for existing dependents; 73% said they could not afford to have a baby at the time; and 48% said they were either having relationship problems or did not want to be a single mother. Other commonly cited reasons were that the woman had completed her childbearing (38% of women), was not ready for another child (32%), or did not want people to know she was pregnant or that she had had sex (25%).[81]

The Antiabortion Perspective

The antiabortion (or "pro-life") position is typically based on the belief that a fertilized ovum is a human being from the moment of conception onward. From this perspective, a fetus has a right to live, and a woman does not have the ability to override that right by choosing an abortion. Antiabortion efforts to overturn abortion public policy have taken three major approaches: amendments to the U.S. and state constitutions that define human life beginning at conception; legislation and government action that defines human life beginning at conception; and efforts to slow or restrict access to abortion services. By defining a fetus as "human," antiabortion groups hope to afford fetuses the same legal rights and protection as adults and children and ultimately outlaw (or put severe legal restrictions on) all abortions.

The Abortion-Rights Perspective

Abortion-rights (or "pro-choice") advocates favor full legalization and ready availability of abortions. Abortion-rights advocates believe that women facing unwanted pregnancies will usually try to find a way to end them, and that legalizing abortion at least provides these women with safe services rather than putting their lives at risk. Additionally, abortion-rights activists typically do not believe that a fertilized ovum qualifies as "human life." Instead, they see abortion as part of a spectrum of a woman's reproductive health care.

Abortion-rights advocates believe that a woman should be able to choose whether or not to end a pregnancy because the fetus is ultimately still within and sustained by the woman's body.

Middle Ground

Most Americans' opinions about abortion have elements of both the antiabortion and the abortion-rights perspectives. Poll trends in recent years show a gradual decline in the percentage of Americans who now identify themselves as "pro-choice." The most recent poll shows 41% self-identify as "pro-choice" and 50% call themselves "pro-life."[82] Finding a suitable compromise on such a divisive issue remains a political and personal challenge.

However, research has found ways to safely prevent many abortions without increasing or decreasing women's access to safe services. The easiest of these methods may be to increase access to contraception and prevent the need for abortions of unwanted pregnancies. Allowing women and their partners to control when and if they want to have children will prevent enormous psychological and financial burdens for families as well. Increasing public assistance and access to family planning may also reduce abortion levels, because funds and aid will allow women living in poverty to better care for unintended pregnancies that do occur. In addition, allowing women access to abortion services does not necessarily increase the abortion rate; women who are determined to end their pregnancies may instead seek underground, possibly unsafe, services.

Epidemiology

Abortions have been legal throughout the United States since 1973. State laws, however, make abortion services more difficult to obtain in some states than in others. **Figure 5.12** depicts the rate of abortions in the United States over the past four decades. After an initial rise in the 1970s following legislation (**Figure 5.13**), the number of induced abortions stabilized in the 1980s and then declined and leveled off.

Several factors also appear to have affected this decline of abortion rates. Changes in U.S. demographics meant that a lower proportion of the female population was of childbearing age and at risk for having to consider abortion. The drive to educate girls about teen pregnancy and contraceptive options has also helped to reduce teen pregnancy. Other factors affecting the decline in abortions over time may include reduced access to abortion services, changing

Figure 5.12

Rate of abortions by race: 1990–2007

Source: Data from U.S. Department of Commerce, United States Census Bureau (2012). *The 2012 Statistical Abstract: The National Data Book.* Accessed June 27, 2012 at: http://www.census.gov/compendia/statab/2012edition.html

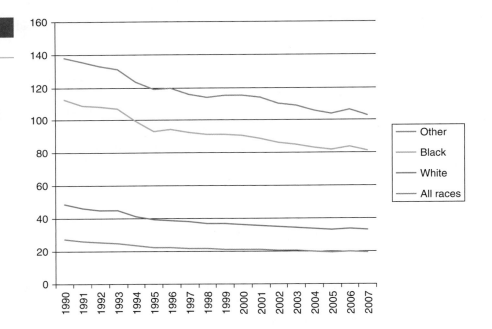

Figure 5.13

The number of legal abortions in the United States per 1,000 women ages 15–44, by year.

Source: Data from Centers for Disease Control and Prevention (2011). *Health United States, 2010, Health Trends.* Accessed June 25, 2012 at: http://www.cdc.gov/nchs/hus/contents2010.htm

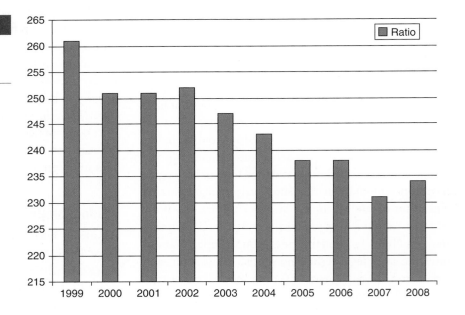

attitudes toward abortion, or more frequent decisions to continue unplanned pregnancies.

The profile of the typical abortion seeker has also changed in the last 20 years (**Figure 5.14**). In addition to young women who experience an unintended pregnancy, the growing number of women who get pregnant over the age of 35 has led to an increase in women who find out that their developing babies are at very high risk of birth defects or have a chromosomal abnormality like trisomy 18. Women living in poverty continue to be much more

likely than wealthy women to have abortions, in large part because poor women are more likely to experience unwanted pregnancies. The average cost of an abortion between 6 and 10 weeks' gestation is about $350 at an abortion clinic and $500 at a physician's office.[83] Additional characteristics of U.S. abortion patients include:[84]

- Majority are in their 20s
- Black and Hispanic women are overrepresented
- Most women having abortions have at least one child

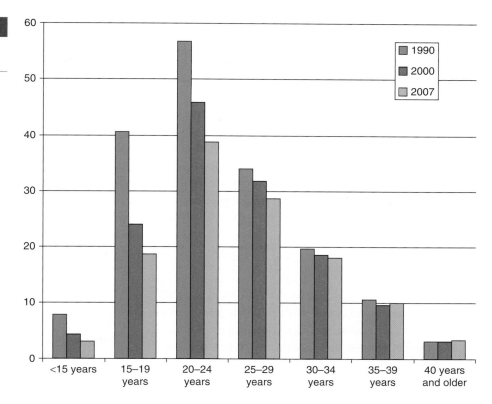

Figure 5.14

Abortion rate per 1,000 women by age group, 1990–2007

Source: Data from U.S. Department of Commerce, United States Census Bureau (2012). *The 2012 Statistical Abstract: The National Data Book.* Accessed June 27, 2012 at: http://www.census.gov/compendia/statab/2012edition.html

- Most women pay for abortions out of pocket even when they have health insurance

Abortion Procedures

Elective abortions in the United States can be either in-clinic surgical procedures or a medical prescription that causes abortion. The type of procedure used primarily depends on how far a woman is into her pregnancy.

In-Clinic Surgical Abortions

There are two primary procedures for in-clinic abortions: vacuum curettage and dilation and evacuation (D&E). **Vacuum curettage**, sometimes called Manual Vacuum Aspiration (MVA), is the most widely used abortion technique; about 75% of all legal abortions done in the United States use vacuum curettage.[85] This procedure is performed while the woman is under local anesthesia. It involves dilating the cervix and then inserting a vacuum curette, an instrument consisting of a tube with a scoop attached for scraping away tissue, through the cervix into the uterus. The other end of the tube is attached to a suction-producing apparatus, and the contents of the uterus are aspirated into a collection vessel. This procedure is

usually performed during the first trimester of pregnancy, or until 13 weeks, but can be done up to 20 weeks following conception. The length of pregnancy is determined from the onset of the last menstrual flow or the last missed period. Through 13 weeks of pregnancy, this procedure can be performed in a clinical office setting with appropriate backup facilities for unexpected medical problems. The actual procedure takes about 10 to 15 minutes after the cervix is dilated.

Dilation and curettage (D&C) is a technique used for many gynecological procedures but rarely in abortions. It can be used up to 16 weeks from the last period. A sharp curette is used to scrape out the contents of the uterus. The procedure requires that the woman be under general anesthesia. Dilation and curettage is rarely used in abortions in the United States because it is more painful than the vacuum curettage method, causes more blood loss, and requires larger cervical dilation.

Dilation and evacuation is a procedure that combines the D&C and vacuum curettage approaches. It is usually done between 13 and 15 weeks' gestation, but may be done through week 22. At this time, the cervix needs to be dilated to a greater extent because the products of conception are larger. This procedure is performed in the operating room of a clinic or hospital.

Oxytocin, a product produced in the posterior pituitary and also commercially manufactured, is often used to facilitate uterine contractions. It is commonly used with the D&C method and with hypertonic saline during second-trimester abortions.

As with all medical procedures, abortions carry some health risks. Abortion-related health risks are greatly reduced if the pregnancy is terminated as early as possible, the woman is healthy, and if the woman receives care in a competent facility. The most common postabortion problems include infection, retained products of conception in the uterus, continuing pregnancy, cervical or uterine trauma, and bleeding.

Medical Abortion

A medical abortion (sometimes referred to as a medication abortion or "abortion with pills") is an abortion performed with medication instead of surgery. Medical abortion offers women the opportunity to end pregnancies safely and in a way that is less invasive than surgical

Image provided by Olympus ACMI. Used with permission.

■ Most abortions in the U.S. are performed using vacuum curettage.

abortion procedures. Two drugs called mifepristone and misoprostol, used in succession, can end an early pregnancy. The drug combo is also known as RU-486 or Mifeprex. Since FDA approval of mifepristone, the proportion of medical abortions has grown and the proportion of surgical procedures has declined. About 14.6% of abortions performed in the United States in 2008 were with medical abortion.[84]

Mifepristone is a hormone pill that blocks the action of progesterone, which is necessary for ending a pregnancy. The FDA approved mifepristone in 2000 as a safe and effective alternative to surgical abortion in the United States. A woman first takes mifepristone at a provider's office; this causes the uterine lining to break down. Days later, a woman takes misoprostol to induce contractions and expel the fetal tissue. In some cases, a provider may use a medication called methotrexate instead of mifepristone.

A physician must perform medical abortions. Heavy bleeding and cramping ensue as a result of the misoprostol. These symptoms may last from a few hours to 2 weeks. The entire abortion is therefore considered to take anywhere from a few days to a few weeks and requires several visits to the healthcare provider's office. Possible side effects may include nausea, vomiting, diarrhea, headaches, hot flushes, and mouth sores.

Medical abortions may be performed as soon as a pregnancy is confirmed, and they must be performed within 7 weeks after a woman's last menstrual period. Women who are older than 35 years of age or who smoke should not use methotrexate or mifepristone. Other conditions that may preclude a woman from having a medical abortion include history of asthma, cardiovascular disease, uncontrolled hypertension, diabetes, ovarian cysts or tumors, and severe anemia.

Currently, lawmakers in many states are moving to restrict medical abortion. At both the federal and state levels, some have proposed legislation designed to curtail the availability of mifepristone and limit the number of doctors who can prescribe it.

Global Perspectives

Every year problems caused by pregnancy or childbirth kill more than 500,000 women. Ninety-nine out of 100 of these deaths occur in the developing world.[87] The World Health Organization (WHO) reports that in 2008, an estimated 21.6 million unsafe abortions took place, mostly in the developing world. Deaths due to unsafe abortion account for about one in eight (13%) of all maternal deaths.[88] It has been estimated that one in three deaths related to pregnancy and childbirth could be avoided if women who wanted effective contraception had access to it.

Despite the magnitude of this problem, the solutions to ending it are simple: Provide women with skilled attendants (such as doctors or midwives) when they give birth, provide family planning so that women and their partners can choose when and if they want to have children, and allow women access to safe abortion services. However, poor health systems, a lack of organized political willpower, and, in the case of abortion, legal restrictions and religious opposition have limited progress in this arena. Reductions in maternal mortality have been extremely slow over the past 20 years. Lessons can be learned from the international landscape. Countries with highly restrictive abortion laws are not associated with lower abortion rates. Abortions are generally safe in countries where abortion is permitted on broad legal grounds; in countries where abortion is prohibited or difficult to access, it is typically unsafe.[89]

Informed Decision Making

Contraception

Many effective, yet imperfect, birth control methods are available to women today. The decision-making challenge is to determine which method or combination of methods best meets each woman's unique needs. Safety and reliability are always the first concern. Other factors, such as health status, lifestyle, financial considerations, and patterns in sexual activity, also determine which method is preferred. Many women will decide to change to a different birth control method as their preferences and situations change. Communication is an essential component

■ Several contraceptive choices are available today.

of contraceptive decision making—couples should talk about their feelings, needs, and fears.

Determining Personal Needs

Sexual urges and sexual activity are normal, and pregnancy is a very real possible consequence of heterosexual intercourse. Both homosexual and heterosexual relationships also carry the risk of sexually transmitted infections, including HIV. For both technological and sociological reasons, women have traditionally shouldered the major responsibility for contraception. This has been unfair for women. Although most of the current contraceptives require primary use by women, couples can share the responsibility for contraception in many ways. Open and honest communication, sensitivity to each other's needs and feelings, and awareness of each method's strengths and weaknesses are essential components for effective decision making.

Specific strategies for informed contraceptive decision-making include the following (also see **Self-Assessment 5.1**):

1. Review needs.
   - Consider when or if you may desire a pregnancy. If you are sure that you never want to become pregnant, perhaps sterilization is the most logical option. If you would like to become pregnant in a few years, the more effective hormonal methods may be preferable. If you desire pregnancy later within the year, one of the barrier methods may be a better choice. If you not want to become pregnant and an abortion is out of the question, you may wish to consider a combination of two good birth control methods, such as foam and condoms, or pills and condoms.
   - Frequency of intercourse is another major consideration to review. If intercourse occurs frequently, barrier methods may prove to be inconvenient.
   - Number of partners should be considered. If a woman has more than one partner, or if her partner has another partner, she is at a greater risk for infection. In this case, a condom with spermicide in addition to birth control pills would provide the best protection against both sexually transmitted infections and pregnancy.
   - Emotional, behavioral, and psychological needs should be considered. A method may appear logical from a medical point of view, but if it is distasteful or undesirable, chances are that compliance with that method will be poor. The degree of partner

Strategies for Contraceptive Decision Making

Contraceptive decision making is a personal and private matter between a woman and her partner. The couple should consider several factors before deciding on what method to use. These factors include:

1. Evaluate needs:

   When/if a pregnancy will be desired

   How disruptive or difficult an unplanned pregnancy would be

   Frequency of intercourse

   Number of partners

   Risk of STIs

   Personal preferences for lovemaking

   Level of partner cooperation and interest

   Significance of spontaneity

   Comfort with touching one's own body or partner's comfort level of touching or being touched

   Manual dexterity for certain methods

   Financial considerations

2. Review medical history:

   Cardiovascular risk factors

   History of cancer

   Certain disabilities or chronic conditions

   Smoking status

   Allergies

   Circulatory disorders

3. Review reproductive health history:

   History of abortion or pregnancy scare

   Vaginal or cervical infections

   History of STIs

   Number of sexual partners or partner's number of partners

   Drug use (including alcohol)

   Past use of contraceptives

4. Put risks and benefits of methods in perspective:

   Weigh the advantages and disadvantages of each method in a personal perspective (see **Table 5.6**)

5. Reevaluate decision periodically:

   Each partner should assess level of compliance

   Each partner should assess level of satisfaction

---

cooperation is another important consideration, because barrier methods are more likely to succeed with partner cooperation and support.

- Couples should be honest and realistic when deciding which kinds of contraception they will use. Couples who are unable or unwilling to use condoms every time they have sexual intercourse may wish to consider another form of contraception to supplement or replace condoms. Birth control pills will not be effective unless a woman remembers to take them every day.

- Perhaps one of the most important considerations is an evaluation of partner feelings and support. Ideally, the contraceptive choice will be a joint decision made by a couple following open, honest discussion of all the considerations and issues. In a less than ideal situation, a woman would be unwise to depend on her partner for contraceptive decision making or use.

2. Consider medical factors. Carefully review risk factors for cardiovascular disease, smoking status, circulatory disorders, and other medical factors before deciding on birth control pills. A history of vaginal or cervical infections may rule out the use of diaphragms or cervical caps.

3. Review failure rates: the higher the failure rate, the greater the risk of an unwanted pregnancy. The difference in failure rates between "typical" and "perfect" use provides an estimate of the role human error plays for most couples. Some contraceptive methods, such as sterilization, are effective for virtually all couples; for other methods, failure rates for the average couple may be several times higher than for a consistent and diligent couple. Remember that typical failure rates are only an average, and that failure rates for couples who are less than diligent may be even higher.

4. Put the risks and benefits of the various methods in perspective. Weigh all dimensions and issues of the relationship carefully against the advantages and disadvantages of each birth control method. Carefully assess the risks and benefits of each method in terms of the individuals involved and their relationship. Some couples find rank different options based on convenience, failure rates, and other factors to determine the best contraceptive that meets their unique needs.

5. Periodically reevaluate the decision. Regular gynecological check-ups are opportunities to discuss contraceptive needs, options, and concerns with a clinician. At regular intervals, contracepting couples should reexamine the level of effectiveness and their individual levels of satisfaction with the selected method. A couple may want to reconsider both partners' needs, feelings, and family planning goals.

When to See a Healthcare Provider

It is necessary to see a clinician for prescription of the diaphragm, cervical cap, any hormonal methods, IUD, or sterilization. Other forms of birth control do not require a clinician's prescription, but conditions associated with these forms may warrant a clinic visit. In general, a woman should consult a clinician any time she experiences pain during intercourse or any unusual bleeding, spotting, discharge, or odor. Any burning or itching associated with spermicide use may be an indication of an allergy to the agent.

With a diaphragm, it is wise to check with a clinician any time the diaphragm does not seem to be fitting properly or there is discomfort, pain, or recurring bladder infections. After having a baby, it will be necessary to be refitted for a different-sized diaphragm because vaginal depth and muscle tone are usually altered by full-term pregnancy.

Abortion

Decisions regarding an unwanted pregnancy are private, personal, and difficult. They should not be rushed, and all options should be carefully weighed. Being able to talk through the process with a trusted person is essential. Options include terminating the pregnancy, continuing the pregnancy and raising the child, or continuing the pregnancy and relinquishing the child for adoption. Many supportive services are available for each of these options.

If a woman elects to have an abortion and is confident in her decision, she can reduce her risk of medical complications from the procedure by making arrangements in a timely fashion. In selecting an abortion facility, a primary concern should be the availability of around-the-clock emergency care services. Infection, bleeding, and other complications can almost always be treated successfully if treatment begins promptly. Other ways to minimize risks from an abortion include making sure the surgeon who performs the procedure is well trained and experienced and verifying the facility provides comprehensive care including postoperative instructions, education, and supportive services. Abortion counseling services are perhaps one of the most important features of a comprehensive facility.

■■■■
Summary

Being able to control reproductive functioning is a necessary component of women's health, career preparation, and family growth management. Many methods of contraception are available today, but no method is perfect. **Table 5.6** compares the methods discussed in this

---

Table 5.6	Comparisons: Contraceptive Options

Fertility Awareness Methods	
"Perfect use" effectiveness	96%
Typical effectiveness	75%
How it works	Prevents sperm from reaching egg
Advantages	No costs; causes no health problems; no side effects or contraindications; no supplies or advance preparation; partner shares responsibility; no delay immediately before sex or extra steps during lovemaking
Disadvantages	Requires considerable discipline and partner cooperation and regular menstrual periods: does not reduce STI risk
Availability	No purchase required
Comments	Unreliable form of contraception
Withdrawal	
"Perfect use" effectiveness	96%
Typical effectiveness	73%
How it works	Prevents sperm from reaching egg
Advantages	No costs; causes no health problems; no side effects or contraindications; no supplies or advance preparation; partner shares responsibility; can be used as a backup method of contraception

(continues)

Table 5.6   Comparisons: Contraceptive Options *(continued)*

Disadvantages	Requires consistent discipline and partner cooperation; compromises spontaneity; may decrease pleasure; does not reduce STI risk
Availability	No purchase required
Comments	Unreliable form of contraception

Birth Control Pills

"Perfect use" effectiveness	99%
Typical effectiveness	92%
How it works	Prevents release of eggs from the ovaries; thickens cervical mucus; causes uterine lining changes
Advantages	Fairly inexpensive; lighter and less painful periods; decreased PMS symptoms; improved skin conditions; protective for some chronic diseases; does not interfere with sexual activity; no delay or interference with spontaneity; protection against ovarian and endometrial cancer; some forms may be used for emergency contraception
Disadvantages	No protection against STIs; may be contraindicated for women with cardiovascular risk problems or women who smoke; must be taken daily; inconsistent studies for breast cancer risk
Availability	Requires clinical examination and prescription
Comments	Most effective form of temporary contraception; combination pills contain both synthetic estrogen and progesterone; minipill contains only progesterone and may cause some irregular bleeding

Hormonal Implants

"Perfect use" effectiveness	99%
Typical effectiveness	99%
How it works	Prevents release of eggs from the ovaries; thickens cervical mucus; causes uterine lining changes
Advantages	Fairly inexpensive; provides protection up to 3 years or until it is removed; highly convenient—nothing to remember; protective for some chronic diseases; no delay or interference with spontaneity
Disadvantages	Must be removed by clinician; irregular menstrual bleeding may occur; no protection against STIs; may be contraindicated for women with cardiovascular risk problems or women who smoke
Availability	Must be inserted by clinician; not all clinicians are trained for insertion and removal
Comments	Highly effective contraceptive; reversible once implant is removed

Injectable Contraceptives

"Perfect use" effectiveness	99%
Typical effectiveness	97%
How it works	Prevents release of eggs from the ovaries; thickens cervical mucus; causes uterine lining changes
Advantages	Fairly inexpensive; lasts 3 to 4 months; less bloating and mood swings than with pill; convenient—nothing to remember; protective for some chronic diseases; no delay or interference with spontaneity
Disadvantages	Must be prescribed by clinician; more weight gain and bleeding issues than with pill; no protection against STIs; may be contraindicated for women with cardiovascular risk problems or women who smoke
Availability	Clinical exam required; must be injected by clinician; not as widely available as the pill
Comments	Highly effective contraceptive; reversible once injections wear off, although there may be a waiting period; contains only progesterone so it is an option for women who cannot take estrogen

Hormonal Patches

"Perfect use" effectiveness	99%
Typical effectiveness	92%
How it works	Prevents release of eggs from the ovaries; thickens cervical mucus; causes uterine lining changes
Advantages	Fairly inexpensive; convenient; weekly schedule is easier than daily pill; similar side effects and benefits as pill; no delay or interference with spontaneity
Disadvantages	Less effective in women weighing more than 198 lbs.; no protection against STIs; may be contraindicated for women with cardiovascular risk problems or women who smoke
Availability	Requires clinical examination and prescription
Comments	Highly effective and convenient contraceptive

Table 5.6	Comparisons: Contraceptive Options *(continued)*

Vaginal Ring	
"Perfect use" effectiveness	99%
Typical effectiveness	92%
How it works	Prevents release of eggs from the ovaries; thickens cervical mucus; causes uterine lining changes
Advantages	Inexpensive; convenient; requires removal every 3 weeks; weekly schedule is easier than daily pill; similar side effects and benefits as pill; no delay or interference with spontaneity
Disadvantages	Requires clinical visit; women must learn to correctly insert and remove the ring; no protection against STIs; may be contraindicated for women with cardiovascular risk problems or women who smoke
Availability	Relatively new form of contraception; not all clinicians may be prescribing it
Comments	Highly effective and convenient contraceptive
Spermicide	
"Perfect use" effectiveness	82%
Typical effectiveness	71%
How it works	Kills sperm; absorbs ejaculate; blocks sperm from entering vaginal tract
Advantages	Inexpensive; no clinical visit; able to use it only as needed; few side effects and contraindications; provides some protection against some STIs; provides additional lubrication; effective immediately
Disadvantages	Required for each sex act; messy; must be applied just before intercourse; effective for 30–60 minutes; may be awkward or disruptive to use
Availability	Easily available in drugstores and online pharmacies in creams, foams, gels, film, or suppositories
Comments	Best contraceptive results are achieved when spermicide is used with a barrier method such as a condom or diaphragm
Diaphragm	
"Perfect use" effectiveness	94%
Typical effectiveness	84%
How it works	Blocks sperms from reaching egg; spermicide inactivates sperm
Advantages	Used only when needed; no side effects or contraindications (latex allergies are rare); can be inserted up to 6 hours ahead of time; reusable
Disadvantages	Moderately expensive one-time cost; clinical visit, fitting, and prescription required; must be used with a spermicide; may be awkward or inconvenient; may increase risk of urinary tract infections; dependent upon proper fit and diligent use
Availability	Clinical visit and fitting required
Comments	Spermicide must be used with each act of intercourse; diaphragm should be refitted when weight changes +/– 10 lbs.
Contraceptive Sponge	
"Perfect use" effectiveness	
Parous women (women who have had children)	80%
Nulliparous women (women who have not had children)	91%
Typical effectiveness	
Parous women	68%
Nulliparous women	84%
How it works	Kills sperm; absorbs ejaculate; blocks sperm from entering cervix
Advantages	Easy to use; spermicide is contained in sponge; may be inserted up to 24 hours before sex; provides continuous protection for 24 hours; relatively inexpensive; available without a fitting or prescription; less messy than other forms of spermicides; may provide some protection against STIs; disposable
Disadvantages	Less effective in women who have had children; requires some practice to insert and remove
Availability	Available in drugstores and online pharmacies
Comments	Sponges should not be reused

(continues)

Table 5.6	**Comparisons: Contraceptive Options *(continued)***

Cervical Cap

"Perfect use" effectiveness	82%
Typical effectiveness	76%
How it works	Blocks sperms from reaching egg; spermicide inactivates sperm
Advantages	Easy to use once technique is mastered; may be inserted up to 48 hours before sex; some protection against STIs; few side effects (latex allergies are rare); reusable
Disadvantages	Fairly expensive one-time cost; clinical visit, filling, and prescription required; not all women can be fitted with a cap; due to smaller size it may be more difficult to insert and remove than a diaphragm; effectiveness is dependent upon proper fitting, proper placement, and spermicide use each time
Availability	Generally available, although not all clinicians are skilled in educating women about insertion and removal
Comments	Should be replaced each year; should be refitted when weight changes +/− 10 lbs.

Male Condom

"Perfect use" effectiveness	98%
Typical effectiveness	85%
How it works	Provides a physical barrier between the penis and vagina; prevents sperm and ejaculate from entering vagina
Advantages	Inexpensive; provides strong protection against most STIs; no clinical visit, fitting, or prescription required; can be used with other methods; can be used as a backup method for other contraception; no hormonal or systemic effects
Disadvantages	Can be used for only one act of intercourse; can tear or slip during use; may decrease sexual pleasure; may interrupt lovemaking; requires cooperation of male partner; latex allergies may require use of polyurethane condoms
Availability	Widely available over-the-counter and from online sources; available with lubricants and spermicides, in a variety of colors, textures, and flavors
Comments	More effective when used with a spermicide; can degrade with heat, light, and oxidation, so should be stored in a cool, dry place

Female Condom

"Perfect use" effectiveness	95%
Typical effectiveness	79%
How it works	Prevents sperm from entering vagina; provides best level of protection for women from STIs by covering vagina and perianal area
Advantages	Used only when needed; no hormonal or systemic effects; empowering to women; clinical visit, fitting, or prescription not needed
Disadvantages	More expensive than male condom; may feel awkward; tendency to be noisy; requires partner cooperation; can be used for only one act of intercourse; requires attention to details for woman and her partner
Availability	Widely available over-the-counter and from online sources
Comments	More effective when used with a spermicide

Female Sterilization

"Perfect use" effectiveness	99%
Typical effectiveness	99%
How it works	Prevents egg from traveling between ovaries and uterus
Advantages	Permanent—lifelong freedom from contraception after procedure for the woman; no interruption of lovemaking; highly effective; no need for partner compliance
Disadvantages	Expensive one-time fee; no protection from STIs; surgical risks; not reliably reversible
Availability	Widely available
Comments	Even though actual risks with female sterilization are low, vasectomies pose far less risk to men; ideal option for women who do not desire more children

Male Sterilization

"Perfect use" effectiveness	99%
Typical effectiveness	99%
How it works	Prevents sperm from being in the ejaculate

Table 5.6	**Comparisons: Contraceptive Options** *(continued)*
Advantages	Lifelong freedom from contraception worries for the male; no interruption of lovemaking; shared responsibility by the male
Disadvantages	Expensive—one-time fee; not always reversible; surgical experience; no protection from STIs
Availability	Outpatient procedure
Comments	Vasectomies pose far less risk to men than tubal ligation does for women

Lactation Amenorrhea Method (LAM)

"Perfect use" effectiveness	Uncertain
Typical effectiveness	80%
How it works	Lactation suppresses ovulation
Advantages	No clinical visit; no costs; easy for nursing mother
Disadvantages	Only effective with direct breastfeeding on demand, meeting all nutritional needs of baby; not effective when any menstrual bleeding returns or after 6 months postpartum
Availability	Only for nursing mothers
Comments	Can be used with other forms of contraception

Intrauterine Device (IUD)

"Perfect use" effectiveness	99%
Typical effectiveness	99%
How it works	Inhibits fertilization; thickens cervical mucus; inhibits sperm function; thins and suppresses the endometrium; copper ions may disrupt sperm motility
Advantages	Highly effective; does not interfere with sexual activity; no hormonal impact; long-acting; nothing to remember; decreased risk of endometrial cancer; reduced menstrual flow; reversible
Disadvantages	Clinical visit required; high insertion and removal costs; no STI protection; few days of mild cramping and light bleeding upon insertion
Availability	Dependent upon provider willingness and training for insertion; generally available
Comments	IUDs are the most widely used reversible form of contraception in the world—used by 12% of women; are much less common in the United States

No Method

"Perfect use" effectiveness	15%
Typical effectiveness	15%
How it works	Dependent upon good luck
Advantages	No clinical visit; no costs
Disadvantages	Risky for unwanted pregnancy; no protection against pregnancy or STIs
Availability	
Comments	Couples using no method of contraception should plan on a pregnancy

chapter. The best method is one that a woman and her partner feel comfortable using, and one that they will use correctly and consistently. Although ideally contraception is a shared responsibility between both partners, in today's world a woman is likely to bear the burden of an unexpected pregnancy. All women in relationships where there is the possibility of pregnancy should therefore make informed, well-thought-out decisions regarding contraception.

Abortion is something that no woman wants to face, but it a choice that many women facing unwanted pregnancies will consider. Whether her personal beliefs about abortion,

a woman should be sensitive to the difficulties unwanted pregnancies bring. Abortion is not just an issue for young, unmarried women; many women who have planned a pregnancy turn to abortion when they discover their developing fetus has a serious birth defect or chromosomal abnormality. Questions around abortion continue to be a focus for much of the women's health and women's rights movements, as well as for conservative and religious political movements.

Preventing unwanted pregnancy is a primary responsibility of all sexually active couples. In the event of an unwanted pregnancy, understanding all options and risks is a critical prerequisite for effective decision making.

Profiles of Remarkable Women

Louise Slaughter

Courtesy of Congresswoman Louise M. Slaughter

Congresswoman Louise Slaughter has been serving in the U.S. House of Representatives since 1986 and holds several leadership positions in the House. She is a former microbiologist and holds a master's degree in public health. She has been a long-time champion of science, health and, particularly, women's health issues.

Rep. Slaughter played a leadership role in crafting and passing the Patient Protection and Affordable Care Act, ensuring that the bill would not contribute to the national deficit. She has been a leader in addressing livestock antibiotic use and is a leading Congressional expert on genetics issues. She wrote cutting edge legislation to protect Americans from genetic discrimination, which has now become law. As one of the leading advocates in Congress for women's rights, Rep. Slaughter served as co-chair of the Congressional Caucus for Women's Issues in the 108th Congress and continues to serve as co-chair of the Bipartisan Congressional Pro-Choice Caucus. She was a co-author of the historic Violence Against Women Act in 1994 and wrote legislation to make permanent the Department of Justice's Violence Against Women Office. She is leading the fight against sexual assault in the military. Rep Slaughter has championed historic increases in funding for women's health in breast cancer research. She fought for legislation guaranteeing the inclusion of women and minorities in federal health research and for the establishment of the Office of Women's Health at the National Institutes of Health (NIH). She has introduced legislation to direct the NIH to fund up to six national centers to focus on women's health and the environment as well as a bill to increase research on the impact of hormone disruptors on women's health.

■■■■

Topics for Discussion

1. What are some of the trends in contraceptive use over the past decades since the introduction of the pill?

2. What are some explanations for the higher contraceptive failure rate among younger women compared with older women?

3. What are some of the common reasons for birth control failure?

4. What are some examples of the influence of sociocultural, sociodemographic, or socioeconomic factors on birth control choices?

5. How do politics play in the availability or options for birth control or emergency contraception?

6. What factors should be considered when calculating the cost of a contraceptive?

7. How have the trends with contraceptive use changed for first intercourse over the past decades?

8. Describe the differences between types of failure rates for contraceptives.

9. Describe some common myths and misconceptions about contraception.

10. Select one method of birth control and describe the advantages and disadvantages of it as a contraceptive method.

11. What health conditions are contraindicated for hormonal methods of contraception?

12. Describe the issues that surround a decision for sterilization.

13. What are the laws in your state about emergency contraception? Is EC available locally for all women?

14. Are abortion services available locally in your state? What obstacles are in place for a woman who is seeking an abortion locally?

■■■■

Key Terms

Abortion: The spontaneous or induced expulsion of an embryo or fetus before it is viable or can survive on its own.

Abstinence: In terms of sex, the practice of refraining from sexual activity.

Birth control: An umbrella term that refers to procedures that prevent the birth of a baby, including all contraceptive measures, sterilization, and abortion procedures.

Cervical cap: A contraceptive device made of latex and individually customized to fit snugly over the cervix.

Condom: A barrier contraception method consisting of a sheath, preferably latex, that covers the penis during intercourse. It prevents pregnancy by collecting the semen in the receptacle tip.

Contraception: Intentional prevention of conception or impregnation through the use of various devices, agents, drugs, sexual practices, or surgical procedures.

Contraceptive sponge: A contraceptive device that acts both as a cervical barrier by absorbing ejaculated sperm and as a source of spermicide. It is available without fitting or prescription.

Diaphragm: A latex, dome-shaped cap inserted over the cervix to prevent conception.

Dilation and curettage (D&C): A minor surgical procedure in which the cervix is expanded enough (dilated) to permit the cervical canal and uterine lining to be scraped with a spoon-shaped instrument called a curette.

Family planning: Planning of when and if to have children, including the use of birth control and other options.

Female condom: A form of barrier contraception that lines the entire vagina, preventing the penis and semen from coming in direct physical contact with the vagina.

Fertility: The state of being fertile; the capacity to produce offspring.

Intrauterine device (IUD): A small, flexible, plastic, T-shaped device that contains either copper or the hormone progesterone and is inserted into the uterus by a clinician to prevent pregnancy. The IUS can be left in place for 1 to 10 years, depending on the type of device.

Oral sex: Stimulation of the genital or anal areas with the mouth or tongue. Unprotected oral sex can transmit sexually transmitted infections.

Outercourse: The sharing of sexual intimacy through behaviors such as kissing, petting, and mutual masturbation without penile–vaginal penetration.

Progestin: A natural or synthetic progestational substance that mimics some or all of the actions of progesterone. It has can be used as a form of birth control or emergency contraception (EC).

Spermicide: A chemical that breaks down the cell walls of sperm. It often is used in conjunction with barrier contraception methods.

Sterilization: The permanent, often surgical, end to fertility by interrupting the mechanisms of normal reproductive action.

Vacuum curettage: The most widely used abortion technique in the United States. In this procedure, the cervix is first dilated. A vacuum curette—an instrument consisting of a tube with a scoop attached for scraping away tissue—is then inserted through the cervix into the uterus. The other end of the tube is attached to a suction-producing apparatus, which aspirates the contents of the uterus into a collection vessel.

Vasectomy: A male sterilization method whereby one or two small incisions are made just through the skin of the scrotum. The vas deferens is lifted through the incision, and the two ends are tied or cauterized to seal them.

■■■■
Websites

American Congress of Obstetricians and Gynecologists: http://www.acog.org/For_Patients

Association of Reproductive Health Professionals: http://www.arhp.org

Centers for Disease Control and Prevention (CDC): http://www.cdc.gov/reproductivehealth/unintendedpregnancy/contraception.htm

Center for Reproductive Rights: http://www.crlp.org

The Emergency Contraception Website: http://ec.princeton.edu

EngenderHealth: http://www.engenderhealth.org

Guttmacher Institute: http://www.guttmacher.org

International Planned Parenthood Federation: http://www.ippf.org

The Henry J. Kaiser Family Foundation: http://www.kff.org

NARAL Pro-Choice America: http://www.naral.org

National Abortion Federation: http://www.prochoice.org/

National Organization for Women: http://www.now.org/

National Right to Life: http://www.nrlc.org/

National Women's Law Center: http://www.nwlc.org/

Planned Parenthood Federation of America: http://www.plannedparenthood.org

Public Agenda Issues Guide on Abortion: http://www.publicagenda.org

WomensHealth.gov: http://www.womenshealth.gov/about-us/

■■■■

References

1. U.S. Department of Health and Human Services [U.S. DHHS], Centers for Disease Control and Prevention [CDC]. (2010). Use of contraception in the United States: 1982–2008. *Vital and Health Statistics* 23(29): 5. Accessed at: http://www.cdc.gov/nchs/data/series/sr_23/sr23_029.pdf

2. U.S. Department of Health and Human Services [U.S. DHHS], Centers for Disease Control and Prevention [CDC]. (1999). Achievements in public health, 1990–1999. Family Planning. *Morbidity and Mortality Weekly Report* 48(50): 241–243.

3. New York Times. (2012, June 6). *Abortion qualms on morning-after pill may be unfounded.* Accessed at: http://www.nytimes.com/2012/06/06/health/research/morning-after-pills-dont-block-implantation-science-suggests.html?nl=todaysheadlines

4. U.S. Department of Health and Human Services [U.S. DHHS], Centers for Disease Control and Prevention [CDC]. *Reproductive Health. Contraception.* Accessed at: http://www.cdc.gov/reproductivehealth/unintendedpregnancy/contraception.htm

5. Jones, R. K. & Draweke, J. (2011). *Countering conventional wisdom: New evidence on religion and contraceptive use. Guttmacher Institute.* Accessed at: http://www.guttmacher.org/pubs/Religion-and-Contraceptive-Use.pdf

6. Pew Research Center. (2011). *The future of the global Muslim population.* Accessed at: http://features.pewforum.org/FutureGlobalMuslimPopulation-WebPDF.pdf

7. Frost, J. J., Hemshaw, S. K., & Sonfield, A. (2010). *Guttmacher Institute. Contraceptive needs and services: National and state data, 2008 update.* Accessed at: www.guttmacher.org/pubs/win/contraceptive-needs-2008.pdf

8. U.S. Department of Health and Human Services [U.S. DHHS]. *Healthy People 2020. Family planning.* Accessed at: http://www.healthypeople.gov/2020/topicsobjectives2020/overview.aspx?topicid=13

9. Hall, K. S., Moreau, C, & Trussell, J. (2011). Determinants of and disparities in reproductive health service use among adolescent and young adult women in the United States, 2002–2008. *American Journal of Public Health* 102(2): 359–367. Accessed at: http://ajph.aphapublications.org/doi/abs/10.2105/AJPH.2011.300380

10. U.S. Department of Health and Human Services [U.S. DHHS], Centers for Disease Control and Prevention [CDC]. (2012). *Sexual experience and contraceptive use among female teens: United States, 1995, 2002, and 2006–2010.* Accessed at: http://www.cdc.gov/media/mmwrnews/2012/0503.html#A1

11. Guttmacher Institute (2010). *Facts on contraceptive use in the United States.* Available from: http://www.guttmacher.org/pubs/fb_contr_use.html#5

12. The Real Cost of Birth Control. (2010). Available at: http://money.usnews.com/money/blogs/alpha-consumer/2010/08/27/the-real-cost-of-birth-control-

13. National Conference of State Legislatures. (2012). *Insurance coverage for contraception laws.* Accessed at: http://www.ncsl.org/issues-research/health/insurance-coverage-for-contraception-state-laws.aspx

14. Henry J. Kaiser Family Foundation. (2012). *Insurance coverage of contraceptives.* Available at: http://healthreform.kff.org/notes-on-health-insurance-and-reform/2012/february/insurance-coverage-of-contraceptives.aspx

15. U.S. Department of Health and Human Services [U.S. DHHS], Centers for Disease Control and Prevention [CDC]. (2012). *Unintended pregnancy prevention.* Accessed at: http://www.cdc.gov/reproductivehealth/unintendedpregnancy/

16. Finer, L. B., & Henshaw, S. K. (2006). Disparities in rates of unintended pregnancies in the United States, 1994 and 2001. *Perspectives in Sexual and Reproductive Health* 38(2): 90–96.

17. Guttmacher Institute. (2012). *Nation pays steep price for high rates of unintended pregnancy.* Accessed at: http://www.guttmacher.org/media/nr/2011/05/19/index.html

18. Guttmacher Institute. (2012). *Facts on publicly funded contraceptive services in the United States.* Available at: http://www.guttmacher.org/pubs/psrh/full/4309411.pdf

19. Frost, J. J., Finer, L. B., & Tapales, A. (2008). The impact of publicly funded family planning clinic services on unintended pregnancies and government cost savings. *Journal of Health Care for the Poor and Underserved* 19: 778–796.

20. Gold, R. B., Sonfield, A., Richards, C. L., et al. (2009). *Next steps for America's Family Planning Program: Leveraging the potential of Medicaid and Title X in an evolving health care system.* Guttmacher Institute. Accessed at: http://www.guttmacher.org/pubs/NextSteps.pdf

21. Jones, R. K., & Dreweke, J. (2011). *Countering conventional wisdom: New evidence on religion and contraceptive use.* Guttmacher Institute. Accessed at: http://www.guttmacher.org/pubs/Religion-and-Contraceptive-Use.pdf

22. Centers for Disease Control and Prevention [CDC]. (2010). *Use of Contraception in the United States: 1982–2008.* Accessed at: http://www.cdc.gov/nchs/data/series/sr_23/sr23_029.pdf

23. Grady, W. K.-W. (1999). Contraceptive characteristics: the perceptions and priorities of women and men. *Family Planning Perspectives* 31(4): 168–175.

24. Guttmacher Institute. (2012). *Facts on publicly funded contraceptive services in the United States.* Accessed at: http://www.guttmacher.org/pubs/fb_contraceptive_serv.html

25. U.S. Department of Health and Human Services [U.S. DHHS], Office of Population Affairs. (2010). *Reproductive health and Healthy People 2020.* Accessed at: http://www.hhs.gov/opa/pdfs/reproductive-health-and-healthy-people-2020.pdf

26. Guttmacher Institute. (2011). *Facts on American teens sexual and reproductive health. In brief: Fact sheet.* Accessed at: http://www.guttmacher.org/pubs/FB-ATSRH.pdf

27. Abma, J. C., Martiniez, G. M., & Copen, C. E. (2010). Teenagers in the United States: Sexual activity, contraceptive use, and childbearing, National Survey of Family Growth. *Vital and Health Statistics* 23(30). Accessed June 5, 2012 at: www.cdc.gov/nchs/data/series/sr_23/sr23_030.pdf

28. Reid, R., Leyland, N., Wolfman, W., et al. (2010) Oral contraceptives and the risk of venous thromboembolism: an update. *SOGC Clinical Practice Guidelines* 252. Accessed at: www.sogc.org/guidelines/documents/gui252CPG1012E.pdf

29. Shufeit, C. L., & Merz,C. (2009). Contraceptive hormone use and cardiovascular disease. *Journal of the American College of Cardiology* 53: 221–231.

30. National Cancer institute. (2012). *Oral contraceptives and cancer risk.* Accessed at: http://www.cancer.gov/cancertopics/factsheet/Risk/oral-contraceptives

31. Hannaford, P. C., Selvaraj, S., Elliott, A. M., et al. (2007). Cancer risks among users of oral contraceptives: Cohort data from the Royal College of Practitioners oral contraception study. *British Medical Journal* 355(7621): 651.

32. Vessey, M, & Yeates, D. (2007). Oral contraceptives and benign breast disease: An update of findings in a large cohort study. *Contraception* 76(6): 418–424.

33. Mayo Clinic Patient Information. (2012). *Ovarian cysts: Treatments and drugs.* Accessed at: http://www.mayoclinic.com/health/ovarian-cysts/ds00129/dsection=treatments-and-drugs

34. Rubin, G. L., Ory, H. W., & Layde, P. M. (1982). Oral contraceptives and pelvic inflammatory disease. *American Journal of Obstetrics and Gynecology* 144(6), 630–635.

35. Mayo Clinic Patient Information. (2012). *Iron deficiency anemia: Treatment and drugs.* Accessed at: http://www.mayoclinic.com/health/iron-deficiency-anemia/ds00323/dsection=treatments-and-drugs

36. Corson, S. L. (1993). Oral contraceptives for the prevention of osteoporosis. *Journal of Reproductive Medicine* 38(12suppl): 1015–1020.

37. Ziglar, S., & Hunter, T. S. (2012). The effect of hormonal oral contraception on acquisition of peak bone mineral density of adolescents and young women. *Journal of Pharmacological Practice* 25(3): 331–340.

38. American College of Obstetricians and Gynecologists [ACOG]. (2006). Use of hormonal contraception in women with coexisting medical conditions. *ACOG Practice Bulletin* 73. Accessed at: http://guidelines.gov/content.aspx?id=10924

39. Farr, S., Folger, S. G., Paulen, M., et al. (2010). U S. medical eligibility criteria for contraceptive use, 2010: adapted from the World Health Organization medical

eligibility criteria for contraceptive use, 4th edition. *Morbidity and Mortality Weekly Report* 59(RR-4):1–86.

40. National Institutes of Health, National Library of Medicine. (2012). *Progestin-only contraceptives.* Accessed at: http://www.nlm.nih.gov/medlineplus/druginfo/meds/a602008.html

41. Wright, K. P., & Johnson, J. V. (2008). Evaluation of extended and continuous use oral contraceptives. *Therapeutic Clinical Risk Management* 4(5): 905–911. Accessed at: http://www.ncbi.nlm.nih.gov/pmc/articles/PMC2621397/

42. Krishnan, S., & Kiley, J. (2010). The lowest-dose, extended cycle combined oral contraceptive pill with continuous ethinyl estradiol in the United States: A review of the literature on ethinyl estradiol 20 ug/levonorgestret 100 ug + ethinyl estradiol 10 ug. *International Journal of Women's Health* 2: 235–239.

43. Mayo Clinic Patient Information. (2012). *Minipill (progestin-only birth control.* Accessed at: http://www.mayoclinic.com/health/minipill/MY00991/DSECTION=why-its-

44. Merki-Feld, G. S., Rosselli, M., Imthurn, B., et al. (2011). No effect of Implanon® on inflammatory cardiovascular parameters. *Gynecological Endocrinology* 11, 951–955.

45. Berenson, A. B., Odom, S. D., Breitkopf, C. R., et al. (2008). Physiologic and psychologic symptoms associated with use of injectable contraception and 20 mg oral contraceptive pills. *American Journal of Obstetrics and Gynecology* 10(1016), 351–362.

46. American College of Obstetricians and Gynecologists [ACOG]. (2012). *FAQ #159. Frequently asked questions: Implants, injections, rings, and patches: Hormonal birth control options.* Accessed at: www.acog.org/~/media/For%20Patients/faq159.ashx

47. Dore, D. D., Norman, H., Loughlin, L. J., et al. (2010). Extended case-control study results on thromboembolic outcomes among contraceptive users. *Contraception* 81(5): 408–413.

48. Xu, H., Wade, J. A., Peipert, J. F., et al. (2012). Contraceptive failure rates of etonogestrel subdermal implants in overweight and obese women. *Obstetrics and Gynecology* 120(1): 21–26.

49. U.S. Department of Health and Human Services [U.S. DHHS], Office on Women's Health. (2011) *Frequently asked questions: birth control methods.* Accessed at: http://www.womenshealth.gov/publications/our-publications/fact-sheet/birth-control-methods.cfm

50. Planned Parenthood. (2012). *Condom information.* Accessed at: http://www.plannedparenthood.org/health-topics/birth-control/condom-10187.htm

51. Mayo Clinic Patient Information. (2010). *Spermicide.* Accessed at: http://www.mayoclinic.com/health/drug-information/DR602375

52. Xu, J., Shi, L., Zhou, X., et al. (2003). Contraceptive efficacy of bioadhesive nonoxynol-9 Gel: Comparison with nonoxynol-9 suppository. *Zhonghua Fu Chan Ke Za Zhi* 38(10): 629–361.

53. AVERT. *What female condoms are available?* Accessed at: http://www.avert.org/female-condom.htm

54. Macaluso, M., Blackwell, R., Jamieson, D. J., et al. (2007). Efficacy of the male latex condom and of the female polyurethane condom as barriers to semen during intercourse: A randomized clinical trial. *American Journal of Epidemiology* 166(1): 88–96.

55. Winner, B., Peipert, J. F., Zhao, Q., et al. (2012). Effectiveness of long-acting reversible contraception. *New England Journal of Medicine* 366: 1998–2007.

56. Harper, C. C., Blum, M., de Bocanegra, H. T., et al. (2008). Challenges in translating evidence into practice: The provision of intrauterine contraception. *Obstetrics and Gynecology* 111(6): 1359–1369.

57. Sivin, I. (2007). Utility and drawbacks of continuous use of a copper T IUD for 20 years. *Contraception* 75(6Suppl): S70–S75.

58. Family Health International. (2012). *Mechanisms of the contraceptive action of hormonal methods and intrauterine devices (IUDs).* Accessed at: http://www.fhi360.org/en/RH/Pubs/booksReports/methodaction.htm

59. Harper, C. C., Blum, M., de Bocanegra, H. T., et al. (2008). Challenges in translating evidence into practice: The provision of intrauterine contraception. *Obstetrics and Gynecology* 111(6): 1359–1369.

60. Therous, R. (2008). The hysteroscopic approach to sterilization. *Journal of Obstetrical and Gynecological Nursing* 37(3): 356–360.

61. Thiel, J. A., & Carson, G. D. (2008). Cost-effectiveness analysis comparing the Essure tubal sterilization procedure and laparoscopic tubal sterilization. *Journal of Obstetrics and Gynecology Canada* 30(7): 581–585.

62. Researchers find no sperm in pre-ejaculate fluid. (1993). *Contraceptive Technology Update* 14(10): 154–156.

63. Killck, S. R., Leary, C., Trussell, J., et al. (2011). Sperm content of pre-ejaculatory fluid. *Human Fertility* (1): 48–52.

64. International Planned Parenthood Federation. (2012). *Contraceptive effects of breastfeeding.* Accessed at: http://www.ippf.org/our-work/what-we-do/contraception/breastfeeding

65. Cheng, L., Guimezoglu, A. M., Piaggio, G., et al. (2008). Interventions for emergency contraception. *Cochrane Database System Review* Apr. 16(2): CD001324.

66. Planned Parenthood. (2012). *Morning-after pill (emergency contraception).* Accessed at: http://www.plannedparenthood.org/health-topics/emergency-contraception-morning-after-pill-4363.asp

67. U.S. Department of Health and Human Services, [U.S. DHHS], Office on Women's Health. (2011). *Frequently asked questions: Emergency Contraception (Emergency birth control).* Accessed at: http://womenshealth.gov/publications/our-publications/fact-sheet/emergency-contraception.cfm

68. Phipps, M. G., Matteson, K. A., Fernandez, G. E., et al. (2008). Characteristics of women who seek emergency contraception and family planning services. *American Journal of Obstetrics and Gynecology* 199(2): 111e.1–5.

69. Miller, L. M. (2011). College student knowledge and attitudes toward emergency contraception. *Contraception* 83(1): 68–73.

70. Guttmacher Institute (2012). *State policies in brief: Insurance coverage of contraceptives.* Accessed at: www.guttmacher.org/pubs/spib_ICC.pdf

71. Langston, A. (2010). Emergency contraception: update and review. *Seminars in Reproductive Medicine* 28(2): 95–02.

72. Polis, C. B., Schaffer, K., Blanchard, K., et al. (2007). Advance provision of emergency contraception for pregnancy prevention: A meta-analysis. *Obstetrics and Gynecology* 110(6): 1379–1388.

73. Guttmacher Institute (2011). *Facts on induced abortion in the United States.* Accessed at: http://www.guttmacher.org/pubs/fb_induced_abortion.html

74. Shain, R. N. (1986). A cross-cultural history of abortion. *Clinics in Obstetrics and Gynaecology* 13(1): 1–17.

75. National Organization for Women. (2010). *History of abortion.* Accessed at http://www.prochoice.org/about_abortion/history_abortion.html

76. National Abortion Federation. (2010). History of abortion. Accessed June 25, 2012 at: http://www.prochoice.org/about_abortion/history_abortion.html

77. Bazelon, E. (August 19, 2008). Script doctors: The dilemma facing South Dakota's abortion providers: Mislead your patients or break the law. *Slate.* Available at: http://www.slate.com/id/2198114/

78. Guttmacher Institute. (2012). Troubling trend: More states hostile to abortion rights as middle ground shrinks. *Guttmacher Policy Review* 15(1). Accessed at: http://www.guttmacher.org/pubs/gpr/15/1/gpr15011

79. National Women's Law Center. (2011). Women in county without an abortion provider. *Health Care Report Card.* Accessed at: http://hrc.nwlc.org/status-indicators/women-county-without-abortion-provider

80. Raymond, E.G. & Grimes, D.A. (2012). The comparative safety of legal induced abortion and childbirth in the United States. *Obstetrics and Gynecology* 119(2): 215–219.

81. Finer, L. B., Frohwirth, L. F., Dauphinee, L. A., et al. (2005). Reasons U.S. women have abortions: Quantitative and qualitative perspectives. *Perspectives on Sexual and Reproductive Health* 37(3): 110–118.

82. Gallup. (2012). *"Pro-choice" Americans at record-low 41%.* Accessed at: http://www.gallup.com/poll/154838/Pro-Choice-Americans-Record-Low.aspx

83. National Abortion Federation. (2010). *Abortion facts. Economics of abortion.* Accessed at: http://www.prochoice.org/about_abortion/facts/economics.html

84. Jones, R. K., Finer, L. B., & Singh, S. (2010). *Characteristics of U.S. abortion patients, 2008. The Guttmacher Institute.* Accessed at: http://www.guttmacher.org

85. Centers for Disease Control and Prevention [CDC]. (2011). Abortion surveillance—United States, 2008. *Morbidity and Mortality Weekly Report* 60(15).

86. Centers for Disease Control and Prevention [CDC]. (2011). Abortion Surveillance—United States, 2008. MMWR 60(15). Accessed July 25, 2012 at http://

www.cdc.gov/reproductivehealth/data_stats/index
.htm#Abortion

87. United Nations Population Fund [UNFPA]. (2007).
No woman should die giving life. Fact Sheet. Accessed
at: web.unfpa.org/safemotherhood

88. World Health Organization [WH]. (2012). *Unsafe
abortion: Estimates and prevention*. Accessed at http://

www.who.int/reproductivehealth/topics/unsafe_
abortion/en/index.html

89. Guttmacher Institute. (2012). *Facts on induced abortion worldwide*. Accessed at: http://www.guttmacher
.org/pubs/fb_IAW.html

Chapter Six

Pregnancy and Childbirth

Chapter Objectives

On completion of this chapter, the student should be able to discuss:

1. Historical dimensions of pregnancy, childbirth, and breastfeeding.

2. Conception and the process of cell division after fertilization.

3. Hormonal changes and fetal changes during pregnancy.

4. Nutritional and weight gain recommendations for pregnancy and exercise concerns with pregnancy.

5. Detrimental effects of smoking, alcohol, drugs, and various environmental risks on pregnancy.

6. Techniques for prenatal testing and complications of pregnancy.

7. The significant issues surrounding childbirth preparation, labor and delivery, cesarean section, and vaginal birth after cesarean section.

8. Physiological changes of the breast for breastfeeding.

9. Benefits and complications associated with breastfeeding.

10. The concepts of fecundity and infertility.

11. Causes and diagnoses of infertility.

12. Treatment of infertility, including assisted reproductive technologies.

13. Emotional effects of infertility.

14. Trends in breastfeeding.

15. Prevalence of infertility, its major causes, and the types of treatments used.

womenshealth.jbpub.com

Women's Health Online is a great source for supplementary women's health information for both students and instructors. Visit

http://womenshealth.jbpub.com

to find a variety of useful tools for learning, thinking, and teaching.

Introduction

This chapter provides an overview of pregnancy, childbirth, breastfeeding, and infertility. In addition to the obvious biological aspects, social, cultural, historical, legal, and ethical dimensions influence pregnancy and childbirth.

Historical Dimensions

The academic examination of childbirth as a social phenomenon did not really begin until the 1960s. Before that time, academic knowledge about childbirth came principally from the writings of medical historians who stressed the progressive history of scientific advances in obstetrics. This medical and historical account provided little insight into how the management of pregnancy or birthing affected women's experiences of birth or about women's reactions to and participation in such changes. The accounts also failed to document how the birth experience felt to the woman.

Today there is considerably more focus on the social, racial, economic, and ethnic aspects of childbirth. Childbirth history is now studied in a variety of contexts—medical, demographic, cultural, social, economic, professional, and symbolic, among others. In the United States, however, the medical perspective continues to dominate. The term *childbirth* generally evokes an image of a medical environment, with physicians and nurses, surgical drapes,

intravenous poles, and fetal monitors. In contrast, in the early United States, childbirth did not have an association with medical personnel or equipment except when a woman's life was threatened. Both immigrant and native populations considered childbirth to be part of a woman's domestic responsibilities.[1] Although specific cultural and ethnic variations existed in the management of the birthing process, all shared the tradition that only women attended other women. Women were the experts on birthing.[1]

> There is a realization that women's attitudes toward and behavior during birth are shaped and conditioned by the demands and expectations of family, peers, community, and often religion. What a woman expects from her childbirth experience, what she will do, what she will fear and not fear, how she will interpret what is happening to her, and what in fact will happen when she gives birth, depend in large measure upon how her society defines what birth should be and where she fits in the various hierarchies of that society.
>
> —**Janet Carlisle Bogdan (1990). Childbirth in America, 1650 to 1990. In R. D. Apple (ed.),** *Women, health, and medicine in America.*

During the mid-18th century, the expertise of women in birthing began to be questioned. Women in France began to deliver babies in hospitals under the watchful eyes of not only traditional midwives, but also physicians. Although physicians had previously witnessed or participated in abnormal deliveries, the hospitalization practices

■ The twentieth century brought medicalization and hospitalization to the childbirth experience.

Courtesy of Library of Congress, Prints & Photographs Division, Gottscho-Schleisner Collection [reproduction number LC-G613-T-46669].

enabled them to study and understand the normal childbirth process. Through close observation, measurements, and recordings, French physicians attempted to explain what they saw as the mysterious process of childbirth.[2] During the same period, the English medical establishment became more oriented to surgical techniques—specifically, the development of instruments known as **forceps** to assist in the extraction of the fetus from the woman. The European obstetrical knowledge quickly crossed the Atlantic, and U.S. physicians began appearing at the births of middle- and upper-class urban women. At first, physicians attended along with traditional midwives, but soon physicians replaced midwives during birth. Medical schools began to certify men as birth attendants, leading to a decline in traditional midwifery. By the end of the 18th century, physicians had established roles in managing childbirth throughout urban areas, including those for poor women.

With the medical presence during childbirth came a widening array of interventions, including medications, anesthesia, and birthing instruments. Accompanying the newly introduced technologies were additional problems of birth accidents, including tears and infections. Physician attitudes had changed from observing and learning to affecting and controlling. Women continued to actively participate in determining the terms of their childbirths only as long as the home was the birthing environment. Once birthing moved to the hospital, however, women lost this power.[3] The U.S. medical management of childbirth originated in urban northeastern areas. In the South and in some religious communities, childbirth retained much of its traditional aspects during the 19th and early 20th centuries. Immigrant groups also were more likely to continue with traditional practices.

The 20th century brought additional medicalization and hospitalization to the childbirth experience, while midwives remained in the more inaccessible portions of the United States. Despite the increased technology and promises of greater safety, women were exposed to greater mystification of childbirth than they had ever known.[3] This trend was in some ways ironic because women were electing to control their fertility and have fewer children, thereby increasing the significance of the childbirth experience. At the same time, they understood less about the process and were less in control of birthing than their grandmothers had been. This trend continued until the late 1950s and 1960s, when women began to openly express dissatisfaction with medicalized births. Europe again was the leader in a new trend of childbirth experiences that suggested that childbirth should be anticipated with joy and knowledge, not fear and ignorance, and could be accomplished with less pain, less medication, and less of the medical and surgical control typical of U.S. births. These natural-birth relaxation techniques are the foundation of modern efforts toward "prepared childbirth."

Social scientists have studied many aspects of modern and traditional childbirth practices. Historically, the care pregnant women received focused on childbirth in the woman's home, and other women gave this support. But modern medical and hospital practices, while making childbirth safe in many regards, have also created situations where continuous support from physicians and nurses during labor has become routine rather than the exception. Some experts believe that childbirth has become an "overmedicalized" process as opposed to a natural process, leading to excessive health costs, extensive stays for mothers, and something to be feared and treated rather than experienced. A large meta-analysis of continuous support for women during childbirth found women who had medical support were likely to have a slightly shorter labor, more likely to have a spontaneous vaginal birth, and less likely to report dissatisfaction with their childbirth experiences. The authors concluded that all women should have medical support throughout labor and birth.[4]

Other social scientists have examined the popular lay term of *natural childbirth*. Traditionally referring to childbirth without use of medications for pain relief and with minimal mechanical monitoring, studies have found that the term natural birth also may refer to the social practices surrounding the birth. Three practices common to natural childbirth include: (1) activity during birth, (2) preparation before birth, and (3) social support.[5] A natural childbirth attempts to create a more active and supportive experience for the mother during the birth of her baby.

Breastfeeding also has seen many changes over the years. The first variation on the practice of breastfeeding was the substitution of the mother's breast with that of a wet nurse—another woman who was able and willing to breastfeed for the mother. In the 1700s, "dry nursing," the mixing of flour, bread, or cereal with broth or water, became popular, as this early form of infant formula was a cheaper option than "wet nursing." As women entered the workforce during the Industrial Revolution, substitutes for milk were produced, resulting in a decline in the practice of breastfeeding.[6] Formula substitutes remained popular for those women who could afford them, until reports surfaced on the benefits of breastfeeding in the 1970s. Since that time, breastfeeding rates have again fallen and risen as a result of various factors, ranging from a woman's place

Figure 6.1

Healthy People 2020 Breastfeeding Objectives

Source: Data from U.S. Department of Health and Human Services. Downloaded April 30, 2011, from http://healthypeople. gov/2020/topicsobjectives2020/objectiveslist.aspx?topicId=26

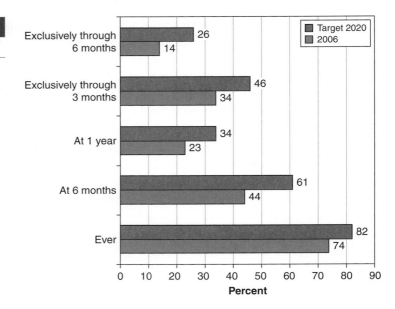

of employment to her personal finances, from her religious beliefs to her network of social support, and from her comfort with her own body to medical contraindications. Because breastfeeding has been shown to lower total healthcare costs by reducing sick care visits, prescriptions, and hospitalizations, the United States has identified breastfeeding as a major goal of the Healthy People 2020 National Health Objectives. As **Figure 6.1** shows, some progress has been made toward achieving these goals.

Pregnancy

Pregnancy lasts an average of 266 days from the time of fertilization or 280 days from the first day of the last menstrual period (often referred to as LMP). The gestational period is divided into three phases or trimesters of approximately 3 months each. Not all women have 28-day menstrual cycles, so due dates cannot be precisely determined (see **It's Your Health**).

Conception

Conception, also known as **fertilization**, is the union of the male sperm cell and the female egg cell. The sperm cell is one of the smallest cells in the body and is produced in enormous quantities: approximately 50 million each day by a healthy male. Sperm production is a continuous, lifelong process. Sperm are produced in the testicles; they are then moved through the epididymis to the seminal vesicles, where the sperm mature into motile sperm and are stored until they are needed in the semen. Mature sperm cells

It's Your Health

Calculating a "Due Date"

To calculate the expected due date of a pregnancy:

1. Determine the first day of the last menstrual period.
2. Add 1 week to the first day of the last menstrual period.
3. Subtract 3 months.
4. Add 1 year.

For example, if the first day of the last menstrual period was April 2, 2012, add 1 week (which is April 9, 2012), subtract 3 months (which makes it January 9, 2012) and then add 1 year, which is January 9, 2013.

It is important to remember that this is an estimate, although approximately 60% of births occur within 5 days of the dates predicted in this manner.

swim like miniature tadpoles with an undulating movement of a threadlike tail. During the process of ejaculation, these cells are combined with secretions from the male reproductive tract to form semen. If ejaculation occurs into or around the entrance of the vagina, fertilization is possible. It has been estimated that as many as 300 million sperm are deposited with ejaculation, but fewer than 20 actually arrive anywhere near the unfertilized egg.[7]

The human egg, or ovum, is far more rare than the sperm. Each woman is born with a supply of approximately 1 million egg cells, of which only about 300,000 eggs remain by the time a girl reaches puberty. One mature egg is released from a woman's ovaries each month during ovulation, usually resulting in 300 to 500 eggs being released during a woman's lifetime.

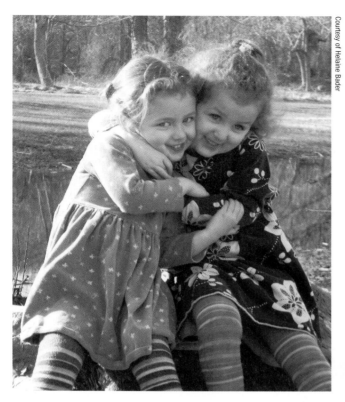

■ Dizygotic twins (fraternal twins) have different genetic traits and therefore different physical appearances.

After the sperm separates from the seminal fluid, it becomes more mobile as it travels toward the egg. If the woman is in the early or middle segment of her menstrual cycle, the cervical mucus is of a consistency to allow the sperm to pass into the uterus. If progesterone is the dominant hormone, as in the late segment of the menstrual cycle, the cervical mucus inhibits sperm penetration past the cervix. Conception usually takes place in the upper third of the fallopian tube. In a process called the acrosome reaction, the sperm releases an enzyme called hyaluronidase, which works to dissolve the outer layer of the egg cell and allows the sperm cell to advance toward the center of the egg to join with its nucleus. Only one sperm is able to penetrate the protective coating of the egg.

Two offspring born of the same pregnancy are called twins.

1. **Dizygotic twins** (also known as fraternal twins) result when two eggs are released from the ovary in one menstrual cycle and fertilized at the same time. Fraternal twins may be of the same or opposite sex and have different genetic traits and therefore different physical appearances. They are sustained through separate placentas and membranes.

- **Monozygotic twins**, also referred to as identical twins, result from a single fertilized egg splitting into equal halves. If both eggs become implanted within the uterus, two babies with identical genetic information will develop. Identical twins may share or have separate placentas and membranes.

At fertilization, the 23 **chromosomes** from the sperm combine with the 23 chromosomes of the egg to form the zygote. The **zygote**, or fertilized egg, contains the full complement of 46 chromosomes. This genetic information determines the unique characteristics of the individual, including eye and hair color, height, and all the other physical characteristics that are passed from one generation to the next. One pair of chromosomes determines the sex of the individual, with the usual arrangement of males having one X and one Y chromosome and females having two X chromosomes; however, chromosomal abnormalities

■ Monozygotic twins (identical twins) result from a single fertilized egg splitting into equal halves. As a result, these babies have identical genetic information.

can occur. Among the most common chromosomal abnormalities are those that involve missing or extra sex chromosomes. Abnormalities involving the X or Y chromosome can affect sexual development and may cause infertility, growth abnormalities, and other problems. (See **Table 6.1**.)

Cell division of the zygote usually occurs within 36 hours of fertilization and continues as the dividing cell mass moves through the fallopian tubes toward the uterus. It generally takes 3 to 5 days to reach the uterus; at this stage, the cell mass is known as a **blastocyst**. The blastocyst freely floats within the uterus for 1 to 2 days before implanting itself into the lining of the uterus. **Implantation** is often the marker for the beginning of a pregnancy, and the products of conception are generally referred to as the **conceptus**. For the first 8 weeks of gestation, the material is known as an **embryo**; from week 9 until birth, it is known as a **fetus**.

Table 6.1 Selected Sex Chromosome Abnormalities

Chromosomal Arrangement for Girls	Description
Turner syndrome (monosomy X; XO)	■ Short stature and possible certain physical features, such as a webbed neck ■ Lack ovarian development and infertile ■ Possible heart or kidney abnormalities ■ Impaired intelligence
Triple X (XXX)	■ Increased height ■ Normal fertility ■ At risk for language and motor delay

Chromosomal Arrangement for Boys	Description
Klinefelter syndrome (trisomy XXY)	■ Increased height ■ Effeminate ■ Decreased testicular size, normal sex function, but usually infertile ■ Possible slight breast development during adolescence ■ At risk for learning disabilities
XYY male	■ Increased height ■ Normal sexual function, genitalia, and fertility ■ Increased risk for motor delay, developmental delay, and learning disabilities

---

My niece was very short and she had some unique characteristics. It took a while for the doctors to diagnose her as having Turner syndrome. We have learned that this affects about one in every 2,500 females.

—27-year-old woman

Confirming Pregnancy

The benefits of early diagnosis of pregnancy are immeasurable. When pregnancy is desired, good prenatal care can begin immediately, and efforts can be made to protect the vulnerable embryo from chemical and physical agents. When pregnancy is not desired, early detection permits early decision making; if the woman elects to have an abortion, risks of complications are reduced at this stage.

It's Your Health

Early Signs of Pregnancy

Symptoms of pregnancy that often occur in the first 6 weeks:

    Missed period(s)

    Breast swelling and tenderness

    Fatigue

    Queasiness or nausea, vomiting

    Slightly elevated body temperature

    Mood swings

    Need to urinate frequently

Several symptoms often occur in the first 6 weeks of pregnancy (see **It's Your Health**). Most women begin to have symptoms 2 or 3 weeks after conception. An overdue period is usually the first definitive sign of pregnancy, although it is important to note that there are many reasons for missed periods other than pregnancy. Also, some women may bleed in early pregnancy and mistake the bleeding for a normal period.

Confirming a pregnancy involves a pregnancy test and a pelvic examination. **Human chorionic gonadotropin (hCG)**, a hormone specific to pregnancy, is easily detectable in blood and urine throughout the first 3 months of pregnancy. All pregnancy tests use chemical procedures to detect its presence.

Home pregnancy tests can be purchased without a prescription and are simple to use. Tests give the most reliable results when the urine is highly concentrated; hence, women are advised to use early morning urine as the testing sample. Some studies have also found that digital over-the-counter home pregnancy tests offer significant advantages over the more traditional nondigital methods.[8]

■ Home pregnancy tests are fairly expensive but quite simple to use.

Although home pregnancy tests are valuable sources of information, they are merely the beginning. If the findings are positive, it is important to set up an appointment for a pelvic examination. If the findings are negative, there is a need to determine why the menstrual period is late or missed. Urine or blood tests performed in a doctor's office are virtually 100% accurate and can be used to validate the pregnancy.

Hormonal Changes During Pregnancy

During pregnancy, a woman's hormone levels and physical characteristics change dramatically. The secretion of certain hormones, such as follicle-stimulating hormone (FSH) and luteinizing hormone (LH), produced by the anterior pituitary gland, is suppressed throughout pregnancy. Pregnancy-specific hormones, such as hCG and human placental lactogen (HPL), are responsible for influencing the course of the pregnancy. Likewise, the production of estrogen and progesterone is important for pregnancy.

Shortly after implantation, specific cells in the outer portion of the developing embryo secrete hCG. The presence of this hormone in the woman's system produces a positive pregnancy test result because, as noted earlier, hCG can be detected in the woman's blood and urine. The body produces large amounts of hCG during the first trimester to stimulate the **corpus luteum**, a structure formed on the wall of the ovary that secretes estrogen and progesterone to prepare the body for pregnancy. The corpus luteum is essential for the maintenance of early pregnancy. If it regresses, a spontaneous abortion, or miscarriage, results.

After the first 3 months of pregnancy, the corpus luteum is no longer essential to maintain the pregnancy and hCG

levels drop off. This change occurs because the placenta begins producing large amounts of estrogen and progesterone. The fetus also plays a role in maintaining the pregnancy. The fetal adrenal glands produce a precursor hormone during the first 3 months of pregnancy that is converted to estrogen in the placenta. The growing fetus and placenta contribute increasing quantities of estrogen and progesterone to the maternal blood system as the pregnancy progresses; the levels of both hormones rapidly decline at birth. Estrogen helps to regulate progesterone, thereby protecting the pregnancy, and initiates one of the major processes of fetal maturation; without estrogen, fetal lungs, liver, and other organs and tissues cannot mature. Estrogen also promotes the growth of ducts in the breast to prepare for lactation. Progesterone suppresses uterine contractions during pregnancy and stimulates the alveoli of the breasts.

Another hormone unique to pregnancy is human placental lactogen, also called human chorionic somatomammotropin. The structure and function of HPL are similar to that of human growth hormone. Human placental lactogen modifies the metabolic state of the mother during pregnancy to facilitate the energy supply of the fetus. It is also believed to stimulate breast growth during pregnancy and to prepare the breasts for lactation. Human placental lactogen levels rise throughout pregnancy. As birth approaches, the levels decline.

Physical and Emotional Symptoms

A woman's body experiences significant changes throughout pregnancy, with each trimester bringing new physical and emotional symptoms. **Figure 6.2** shows many of the

Photographed by Chris Bolduc

■ A woman's body experiences significant changes throughout pregnancy.

(a) First trimester   **(b)** Second trimester   **(c)** Third trimester

Figure 6.2

Changes in a woman's body during pregnancy. Through the three trimesters, the shape of the pregnant woman's body changes dramatically.

physical changes that occur during pregnancy. The first trimester is characterized by enlarged and tender breasts and, for many women, nausea and vomiting (commonly referred to as morning sickness). Women also may experience extreme fatigue, decreased interest in sex, moodiness and irritability, and skin changes such as darkening of the nipple and areola.

During the second trimester, morning sickness usually subsides, but is replaced for many women with other gastrointestinal problems such as heartburn, gas, and constipation. The second trimester is the period in which women gain most of their weight, usually between 12 and 14 pounds. The growing fetus can lead to breathing problems, due to pressure of the uterus and fetus on the bottom of the rib cage, and backache, caused by changes in posture to accommodate the growing fetus. Some women experience muscle and leg cramps, numbness and tingling of the hands, swollen or bleeding gums, and **Braxton–Hicks**

contractions (false labor). Swelling of the feet, ankles, and hands is common and is caused by the increased weight of the uterus slowing down blood and fluid circulation. Many women have significant changes in their skin's appearance during the second trimester. Striae gravidarum (known as stretch marks) begin to appear on the abdomen, breasts, and thighs; for some women, varicose veins appear in the legs. Other skin changes may include chloasma (brown patches on the face or neck) and linea nigra (a dark line from the belly to the pubic area) caused by increases in melanocyte-stimulating hormone. Changes in estrogen levels may cause redness of palms and red spots on the upper body. The second trimester also may be a time of renewed interest in sex.

In the third trimester, many of these symptoms—for example, heartburn and constipation, leg cramps, backache, breathlessness, and Braxton–Hicks contractions—continue. Women often experience an increase in leukorrhea (a whitish vaginal discharge) and colostrum (pre-milk) leaking from the breasts. Hemorrhoids, pelvic and buttock discomfort, and an itchy abdomen also are common complaints. A woman's interest in sex may decrease.

It's Your Health

Common complaints during pregnancy:
- Morning sickness
- Leg cramps
- Sleep issues
- Colds and flu
- Braxton-Hicks contractions
- Bladder infections
- Backaches
- Hemorrhoids
- Skin problems
- Mouth and gum discomfort
- Dizziness and faintness
- Indigestion
- Difficulty breathing
- Headaches
- Vaginal discharge and itching

I didn't need a pregnancy test to tell me I was pregnant. I just knew it. My breasts were tender and I had some vague queasiness. Sure enough—my home pregnancy test confirmed what I knew. I realize that some women aren't as sure, but I was totally positive that I was pregnant.

—25-year-old mother

Fetal Development

The process of development for the fertilized egg is both fascinating and complex. When the cluster of cells reaches the uterus, it is smaller than the head of a pin. Once the cells become embedded into the uterine lining, they are collectively known as an embryo. A sac known as the **amnion** or fetal sac envelops the embryo. As water and other small molecules cross the amniotic membrane, the embryo floats freely. The **amniotic fluid** protects the embryo from shocks and bumps and helps maintain a homeostatic, or constant, environment for the developing embryo. A primitive placenta soon forms. The **placenta** is the organ that supplies the growing fetus with oxygen and nutrients from the maternal bloodstream and serves as a conduit for the return of waste products back to the mother for disposal.

Major changes occur with the developing embryo as it evolves into a fetus (**Figure 6.3**).

First Month The embryo grows to about one-tenth to one-fourth of an inch in length and one-seventh of an

Figure 6.3A

Fetal development. Top left, human embryo between four and five weeks of development. Top right, human fetus about 11 to 12 weeks of development. Bottom left, human fetus about five months (20 weeks) of development. Bottom right, human fetus nearly full term—eight to nine months.

© Ngo Thye Aun/Dreamstime.com

Figure 6.3B

Fetal development. Top left, human embryo between four and five weeks of development. Top right, human fetus about 11 to 12 weeks of development. Bottom left, human fetus about five months (20 weeks) of development. Bottom right, human fetus nearly full term—eight to nine months.

© Miroslav Ferkuniak/Dreamstime.com

Figure 6.3C

Fetal development. Top left, human embryo between four and five weeks of development. Top right, human fetus about 11 to 12 weeks of development. Bottom left, human fetus about five months (20 weeks) of development. Bottom right, human fetus nearly full term—eight to nine months.

© Ngo Thye Aun/ShutterStock, Inc.

Figure 6.3D

Fetal development. Top left, human embryo between four and five weeks of development. Top right, human fetus about 11 to 12 weeks of development. Bottom left, human fetus about five months (20 weeks) of development. Bottom right, human fetus nearly full term—eight to nine months.

© Amitai/Dreamstime.com

ounce in weight. Foundations form for the nervous system, genitourinary system, circulatory system, digestive system, skin, bones, and lungs. The embryo has a two-lobed brain and a spinal cord. The arm and leg buds start to appear. The heartbeat appears on the 25th day.

Rudiments of the eyes, ears, and nose appear. The head is disproportionately large because of the early brain development.

Second Month The embryo's length is about 1 to 2 inches, and it weighs about one-sixth of an ounce. Ears, eyelids, fingers, and toes are distinct. At 8 weeks, all the major organs are formed. The circulatory system is closed, and the placenta starts working. The neural tube closes. After 8 weeks the embryo is called a fetus.

Third Month The length of the fetus is 2 to 3 inches and it weighs about an ounce. The sex of the fetus is defined, and it starts growing fuzzy hair, buds for future teeth, and soft fingernails and toenails. Kidneys begin to excrete urine. Other organs further develop. The nose and palate take shape, and the ears and earlobes are developed. At this time, the fetal heartbeat can be heard with a Doppler device.

Fourth Month The fetal length is 5 to 6 inches, and the weight is 2 to 5 ounces. The mother will start to discern fetal movements. The fetus can hear, move, kick, swim, sleep, and swallow. At this point, ultrasound can recognize external genitalia. The skin is pink and transparent, and eyebrows have formed.

Fifth Month Fetal length is 7 to 11 inches, and it may weigh up to 1.5 pounds. The skin is loose and wrinkled. Vernix, a white, greasy substance, and lanugo, a soft, fine hair, cover the skin for protection. Ultrasound can examine the baby's anatomy in detail.

Sixth Month The fetus weighs about 2 pounds. The skin is red and eyelids remain sealed. The fetus becomes active by kicking, punching, stretching, and turning over. It also coughs, hiccups, and responds to sudden noise. If born, the infant will cry and breathe, and it can survive with intensive neonatal care.

Seventh Month The fetal length is about 15 inches, and it weighs about 3 pounds. The eyes open and close, and the baby sucks its thumb. If born, the infant can usually survive. Eyelids are open, and fingerprints are set.

Eighth Month The fetus now gains about one-half pound per week and will most likely settle into position for birth. It is now about 17 inches long and weighs 4 to 5.5 pounds. The face and body have a loose and wrinkled appearance. Bones harden.

Ninth Month By the end of 37 weeks, the fetus is considered mature and ready to breathe. By 38 to 40 weeks, the baby weighs 6 to 9 pounds and is 19–21 inches in length. In the final month, the fetus gains about an ounce per day. The skin is filled out and smooth. The skull bones have hardened, and the baby is ready for survival outside the womb. The lanugo hair and most of the vernix have disappeared.

Preconception Care

Preconception care is the collective name for the steps a woman can take before she decides to become pregnant to ensure she is in good health when conception occurs. Many healthcare providers recommend that a woman see a clinician before getting pregnant and take a few basic steps to reduce the risk of certain problems during pregnancy. These steps include:

1. *Ensuring an adequate intake of folic acid.* The U.S. Public Health Service recommends that women of childbearing age get at least 400 mcg of folic acid daily, through food or dietary supplements. Many healthcare providers suggest supplementing the diet with folic acid for the 3 months before getting pregnant.

2. *Proper immunizations.* Women who are thinking of getting pregnant should be immunized against the communicable diseases that can harm a developing fetus, such as chicken pox and rubella, before conceiving.

3. *Healthy behaviors.* The preconception period is a good time for a woman to assess her health behaviors—smoking, alcohol use, caffeine intake, drug use, and medications. Items that should be avoided or limited during pregnancy should be minimized or eliminated in the preconception period.

4. *Nutrition.* Scientific research has shown that good nutrition is important for male and female fertility. A balanced diet including regular servings of fruits, vegetables, whole grains, lean meats, and dairy products will optimize the preconception period. Women should also get at least 1,000 mg of calcium daily (three 8-ounce glasses of milk) in the preconception period. (See Chapter 9 for more information.)

Prenatal Care

A pregnant woman should take good care of herself to ensure proper development of her unborn child. Good prenatal care encompasses a spectrum of topics from proper nutrition to regular prenatal health care.

Nutrition

Pregnancy increases a woman's need for nutrients and calories, making a balanced diet essential for women of childbearing age (**Table 6.2**). Sensible eating during pregnancy includes the basic concepts discussed in Chapter 9. It is important not to diet during pregnancy but rather to eat sensibly. Pregnant women do not need to eat twice as much food or calories, but rather consume the essential nutrients required for healthy development of the fetus.

Although it is recommended that a woman try to meet her vitamin and mineral requirements by eating a balanced diet, many healthcare providers recommend prenatal supplements to ensure adequate intake in addition to this diet. **Folate** is a B vitamin that is essential for the healthy development of the fetus; it is found naturally in green, leafy vegetables; nuts; beans; citrus fruits; and some fortified cereals. **Folic acid**, the synthetic form of the B vitamin folate, appears to help prevent **neural tube defects** such as spina bifida. As a result of folic acid's role in preventing neural tube defects, the Food and Drug Administration (FDA) has required enriched grain products, such as breads, pasta, and bagels, to be fortified with folic acid. This fortification has prevented many cases of neural tube defects, but the effects have not been equally seen across all racial and ethnic groups. Non-Hispanic White and Hispanic births have shown significant decreases in neural tube defects, but researchers emphasize that efforts to increase folic acid consumption should be continued for all racial and ethnic groups.[9]

Calcium and iron are important minerals for all women, including pregnant women. Calcium is essential to the formation of bone and teeth in the fetus, and it prevents the pregnant woman from losing her own bone density while providing for the growing fetus. Iron helps carry oxygen in the blood and reduces the risk of pregnancy-induced hypertension. Women often require iron supplements, because most female iron stores are not adequate to supply both mother and unborn child given the large demand for iron throughout the pregnancy. Iron supplements should be taken with vitamin C to facilitate their absorption.

Women should drink plenty of fluids throughout pregnancy. A woman's blood volume and blood fluids increase significantly during pregnancy, and drinking enough fluids will help to prevent dehydration and constipation. Pregnant women should also avoid certain foods during pregnancy, to help prevent infections that may harm the fetus (see **It's Your Health**).

Table 6.2   Healthy Food Choices for a Pregnant Woman

The foods below are the best sources of nutrients needed by pregnant and breastfeeding women. (For more information on nutrition, see Chapter 9.)

Vegetable Group (choose fresh, frozen, canned, or dried)

- Carrots
- Sweet potatoes
- Pumpkins
- Spinach
- Cooked greens (such as kale, collards, turnip greens, and beet greens)
- Winter squashes
- Tomatoes and tomato sauces
- Red sweet peppers

Dairy Group

- Fat-free or low-fat yogurt
- Fat-free milk (skim milk)
- Low-fat milk (1% milk)
- Calcium-fortified soymilk (soy beverage)

Fruit Group (choose fresh, frozen, canned, or dried)

- Cantaloupes
- Honeydew melons
- Mangoes
- Prunes or prune juice
- Bananas
- Apricots
- Oranges and orange juice
- Red or pink grapefruit

Grain Group

- Fortified ready-to-eat cereals
- Fortified cooked cereals

Protein Foods Group

- Beans and peas (such as pinto beans, soybeans, white beans, lentils, kidney beans, and chickpeas)
- Nuts and seeds (such as sunflower seeds, almonds, hazelnuts, pine nuts, peanuts, and peanut butter)
- Lean beef, lamb, poultry, and pork
- Oysters, mussels, crab
- Salmon, trout, herring, sardines and pollock

NOTE: Shark, swordfish, king mackerel, or tilefish contain high levels of mercury and should not be eaten when pregnant or breastfeeding. Limit white (albacore) tuna to no more than 6 ounces per week.

Source: Reproduced from U.S. Department of Agriculture. Health and nutrition information for pregnant and breastfeeding women. Available online: http://www.choosemyplate.gov/pregnancy-breastfeeding/making-healthy-food-choices.html

It's Your Health

Foods to Avoid During Pregnancy

Sushi and other raw fish, especially shellfish (oysters, clams).

Hot dogs or luncheon meats (such as ham, turkey, salami, and bologna) unless they are reheated until steaming hot.

Unpasteurized milk, unpasteurized fruit and vegetable juices, or foods made from unpasteurized milk, including soft cheese (feta, brie, Camembert, Roquefort, queso blanco, queso fresco). Soft cheeses may be eaten if they are made with pasteurized milk.

Refrigerated pates, meat spreads, or smoked seafood. Canned versions of these products are safe to eat.

Raw vegetable sprouts (alfalfa, clover, and radish), which can carry *Salmonella* or *E. coli.*

Raw or undercooked meat, poultry, and eggs, as well as products made with raw or partially cooked eggs (such as eggnog, hollandaise sauce, and some Caesar salad dressings).

Some herbal supplements and teas.

Swordfish, shark, king mackerel, and tilefish, which have high levels of mercury.

- According to the FDA/Environmental Protection Agency (EPA), women who are pregnant can eat up to 12 oz. (two average-sized fish meals) per week of fish or shellfish that are lower in mercury, such as shrimp, salmon, catfish, and canned light tuna. White (albacore) tuna contains more mercury than canned light tuna, so women should limit their consumption of canned white tuna and tuna steaks to no more than 6 oz. per week.

- Women should check for local advisories about any fish caught in waters by family and friends. If no advice is available, women should limit their consumption to less than 6 ounces per week of this type of fish and not eat any other fish during the week.

Table 6.3 — Pregnancy Weight Gain Distribution

	Pounds
Baby	8
Placenta	2–3
Breasts	2–3
Amniotic fluid	2–3
Blood supply	4
Fat stores	5–9
Uterus	2–5
Total	25–35 pounds

a woman's body. Failure to gain adequate weight is associated with higher infant morbidity, lower birth weight, and preterm deliveries.[10]

© Creatas

■ Folic acid appears to be a protective factor against neural tube defects, which develop in the first month of pregnancy. It is important for a woman to begin increasing her folic acid intake before she becomes pregnant.

Weight gain is another important prenatal nutritional issue. It is not necessary to "eat for two," but extra nutrients and calories are needed in the prenatal period. A woman should consult with her healthcare provider about how much weight to gain during her pregnancy. A woman of average weight is generally advised to gain 25 to 35 pounds during her pregnancy; an underweight woman should gain more, between 28 and 40 pounds; and overweight women may need to gain only 15–25 pounds. Obese women should have a total weight gain of 11–20 pounds. Women who are expecting multiple births will need to gain more weight than a single pregnancy. Women often average a weight gain of 4 to 6 pounds in the first trimester and 1 pound per week in the second and third trimesters. As shown in **Table 6.3**, pregnancy weight gain is distributed throughout

Exercise

Proper exercise during pregnancy can have many benefits. Studies show that women who exercised in the 3 months before pregnancy felt better during the first trimester than did those who did not exercise; similarly, women who exercised in the first and second trimesters felt better in the third trimester than those who did not exercise. Well-conditioned women often have shorter labor, less need for obstetric intervention during pregnancy and childbirth, and speedier recovery after childbirth. The American College of Obstetricians and Gynecologists (ACOG) recommends at least 30 minutes of daily active exercise during pregnancy to reduce backaches, constipation, bloating, and swelling. Exercise also helps prevent or treat gestational diabetes; improves energy and mood; improves posture; promotes muscle tone, strength, and endurance; and helps

© Photos.com

■ Proper exercise during pregnancy can have many benefits. Walking, swimming, and low-impact aerobics are particularly good choices for pregnant women.

the pregnant woman sleep better. The ACOG, however, does not recommend exercise for weight reduction while a woman is pregnant.[11]

The exercise program of a pregnant woman must be geared to her current level of fitness, medical history, past pregnancies, stage of fetal development, and maternal complicating factors. Walking, swimming, and low-impact aerobics are particularly good exercise choices for pregnant women. Classes or exercise videos made specifically for pregnant women are also good options.

Activities that involve bouncing, jarring, twisting, or any activity that places the abdomen in jeopardy should be avoided during pregnancy. Examples of activities that should be avoided include horseback riding, scuba diving, and downhill skiing. Contact sports are too risky, as is any activity that requires rapid stops and starts or an extreme range of motion. The center of gravity for the body changes during pregnancy, increasing the risk of loss of balance. Exercises that require lying on the back, particularly after the fourth month, can be dangerous because this position can block the blood supply to the uterus and depress fetal heart rate. A resting position on the side does not compromise fetal blood supply.

Many questions regarding the safety and benefits of exercise during pregnancy remain unanswered. Although women with medical or obstetric complications should avoid rigorous physical activity, healthy women should continue exercising under their healthcare provider's supervision.

Another form of exercise, known as pelvic muscle or Kegel exercises, is important during pregnancy. Increasing the strength of the pelvic muscles decreases urine loss during late pregnancy and may speed up the rehabilitation of the pelvic floor after vaginal delivery.

Avoiding Toxic Substances

Maternal exposure to many substances during pregnancy has been shown to have detrimental effects on the developing fetus. Many of these topics are discussed in detail elsewhere in this book. Note, however, that cigarettes, alcohol, and drugs have specific detrimental effects on the fetus.

Not smoking is essential to a healthy pregnancy and birth. The Centers for Disease Control and Prevention (CDC) reports that smoking before and during pregnancy is the single most preventable cause of illness and death among mothers and infants.[12] Women who smoke before pregnancy are twice as likely to experience a delay in conception and have a 30% increased risk of being infertile compared to nonsmoking women. Women who smoke during pregnancy are also twice as likely to experience complications including premature rupture of membranes, early separation of the placenta from the uterus, and blockage of the cervix by the placenta. The CDC also reports that babies born to women who smoke during pregnancy have a 30% increased risk of being born premature, of low birth weight, and of being more likely to die of sudden infant death syndrome (SIDS). Unfortunately, about 13% of women still smoke during pregnancy. As **Figure 6.4** shows, younger, less educated, non-Hispanic White, and American Indian women are more likely to smoke during pregnancy.

Alcohol also is detrimental for both the mother and her developing baby. Alcohol consumption during pregnancy is known to cause alcohol-related defects among infants and **fetal alcohol syndrome (FAS),** which is characterized by growth retardation, facial malformations, and central nervous system dysfunctions, including mental retardation. Alcohol appears to act in concert with several other factors to promote the development of FAS in infants:

- Differences in the degree of prenatal exposure to alcohol
- Maternal drinking patterns
- Possible genetic susceptibility to FAS
- Differences in maternal metabolism of alcohol
- Time of gestation during heavy alcohol consumption
- Interactions of alcohol use with other drugs and medications
- Maternal nutritional status

The fetus is especially vulnerable to the effects of alcohol during the first trimester of pregnancy, when the development of the central nervous system occurs. Research also links maternal drinking during pregnancy with an increased risk of early stillbirth.[13] In spite of campaigns to reduce alcohol consumption during pregnancy, usage levels still remain fairly high. About 1 in 8 pregnant women in the United States reports alcohol use, and about 1 in 50 pregnant women reports binge drinking (having five or more drinks at one time).[14]

Consumption of other drugs also can adversely affect a developing fetus. No medications or over-the-counter

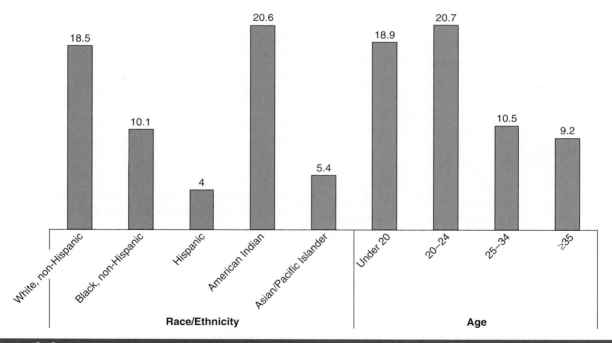

Figure 6.4

Prevalence of smoking during the last three months of pregnancy by race/ethnicity, education and age.

Source: Data from Tong, V., Jones, J., Dietz, P., D'Angelo, D., and Bombard, J. (2009). Trends in Smoking Before, During, and After Pregnancy—Pregnancy Risk Assessment Monitoring System (PRAMS), United States, 31 Sites, 2000-2005. *Morbidity and Mortality Weekly Report* 58(SS04);1-29

preparations should be taken during pregnancy without first consulting with a clinician. Illicit drug use—most notably the use of cocaine—is associated with fetal distress, low birth weight, and impaired fetal growth. The consequences of drug use during pregnancy include severe damage to the baby's brain and nervous system as well as other birth defects. Compared with mothers who did not smoke marijuana, smokers had smaller, sicker babies and a higher risk of stillbirths. Also, babies may be prone to excessive crying and trembling. Drug use may lead to neurochemical birth defects by disrupting normal development of the brain, and, in turn, cause long-term effects on intelligence, mental development, and learning.

Based on national survey data, substance use among pregnant women between 2002 and 2010 varied by race. Data indicate that 4.4% of pregnant White women used illicit drugs such as marijuana, cocaine, Ecstasy and other amphetamines, and heroin, while 7.7% of pregnant Black women did.[16] These and other illicit drugs may pose various risks for pregnant women and their babies. It is difficult for scientists to ascertain which birth defects are attributable to which illicit substance. Because many pregnant women who use illicit drugs also use alcohol and tobacco, which also pose risks to unborn babies, it often is difficult to determine which substance causes the adverse outcomes. Additionally, illicit drugs may be prepared with impurities that may be harmful to a pregnancy. What is known is that some of these drugs can cause a baby to be born too small or too soon, or to have withdrawal symptoms, birth defects, or learning and behavioral problems. Women who are pregnant and using heroin should work with a physician to quit using, as abruptly stopping use of the drug can cause miscarriage.[17]

Many over-the-counter prescription medications can prove dangerous during pregnancy as well. The antibiotic streptomycin can cause deafness, and the antibiotic tetracycline can lead to bone abnormalities and discolored teeth. Even aspirin and acetaminophen may affect a developing fetus. Clearly, it is important for pregnant women to consult their physicians before taking any type of medication.

Environmental Risks

Although not all environmental hazards can be avoided, a pregnant woman should take some precautions to protect herself and her baby. Although data are scarce, it is believed that the rapidly developing fetus is especially vulnerable to pollutants, toxic wastes, heavy metals, pesticides, gasses, and other hazardous compounds. For example, the element lead can cross the placenta and has been associated with intrauterine death, prematurity, and low birth weight.[18] Air pollution, such as secondhand smoke, can be detrimental to both a woman's health and the developing fetus. Scientists also have concluded that prenatal exposure to tobacco and environmental lead is a risk factor for attention deficit hyperactivity disorder (ADHD) in children.[19] Diagnostic X-rays should be avoided if possible throughout the pregnancy or if there is the possibility of pregnancy. X-ray exposure is associated with respiratory diseases and blood disorders in the fetus, as well as miscarriage.

Another environmental risk to consider during pregnancy is heat exposure. Women who use hot tubs and saunas or who have high fevers early in pregnancy have been found to be at greater risk of having children with neural tube defects such as spina bifida. Although more research is needed on this subject, it appears that the greatest risk arises early in the pregnancy when the fetal central nervous system is developing.[20]

Prenatal Testing

Prospective parents often worry whether their baby will be born normal and healthy. Most of the time, these worries are unfounded: Almost all children born in the United States are healthy. However, the CDC reports that 1 of every 33 babies is born with a birth defect.[21] A birth defect can affect almost any part of the body. The well-being of the child depends mostly on which organ or body part is involved and how much it is affected. Most birth defects occur during the first three months of pregnancy. Birth defects can be genetic in origin, or they can be caused by exposure to harmful agents.

Risk factors that increase the likelihood of birth defects include family or personal history of birth defects, a previous child with a birth defect, certain medications used around the time of conception, diabetes before pregnancy, and women being age 35 years or older when the baby is due.

Screening tests are performed during pregnancy to assess the risk of certain birth defects. If a screening test shows an increased risk for a certain defect, further diagnostic tests can confirm whether it actually exists. Screening tests include:

- *First-trimester screening tests* combine the result of special **ultrasound** tests and blood tests to detect **Down syndrome** and trisomy 18. Ultrasound is a noninvasive procedure that uses high-frequency sound waves to project an image or sonogram of the fetus. This type of ultrasound exam, called nuchal translucency screening, measures the thickness of the translucent space at the back of the fetus' neck. Babies with Down syndrome, trisomy 18, or other chromosomal problems tend to accumulate more fluid than babies without chromosomal abnormalities, causing a larger space. The exam must be performed between 11 and 14 weeks, when the base of the neck is still translucent. Increased levels of pregnancy-associated plasma protein A and human chorionic gonadotropin, found by testing the blood, also may indicate Down syndrome.

- *A second trimester screening test*, called "multiple marker screening," examines blood for abnormal levels of substances linked with certain birth defects such as Down syndrome and neural tube defects. This test, referred to as triple or quadruple screening, measures the level of three or four substances:

  - **Maternal serum alpha-fetoprotein (MSAFP)**, a substance produced by the fetal kidneys between the 13th and 20th weeks of pregnancy and found in the mother's blood.

  - Estriol, a hormone made by the liver of the fetus and the placenta.

  - Human chorionic gonadotropin, a hormone made by the placenta.

  - Inhibin-A, another hormone produced by the placenta.

- *Detailed ultrasound exams* are usually done after 18 weeks of pregnancy and allow for a more extensive view of the baby's organs and features.

Diagnostic tests try to detect a genetic disorder or birth defect. They are offered to women at risk of genetic disorder based on family history or the results of screening tests. Diagnostic tests include:

- **Amniocentesis** (**Figure 6.5A**) is usually performed at 15 to 20 weeks of pregnancy. The doctor guides a thin needle through the abdomen and uterus and withdraws a small amount of amniotic fluid. Cells from the fluid are analyzed for chromosomal defects. Complications from the procedure are rare. One large study found that the procedure-related fetal loss rate after mid-trimester amniocentesis performed on patients in a contemporary prospective clinical trial was 0.06%. There was

■ Performed at various times during pregnancy, ultrasound uses sound waves to show a picture of the baby. Ultrasound can check the age, growth, and size of a fetus; identify multiple pregnancies; and diagnose complications or birth defects.

Figure 6.5A

Amniocentesis is a test for fetal abnormalities that involves withdrawing amniotic fluid and inspecting the cells contained within it.

Prenatal Testing

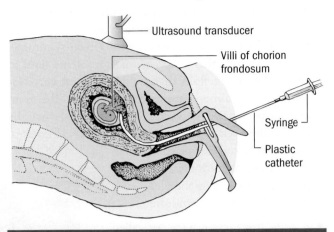

Figure 6.5B

In chorionic villus sampling, fetal cells from the chorionic villi (fingerlike projections on the developing placenta) are suctioned out through the cervix.

no significant difference in loss rates between those undergoing amniocentesis and those not undergoing amniocentesis.[22]

- **Chorionic villus sampling (CVS)** (**Figure 6.5B**) detects some of the same chromosomal abnormalities as amniocentesis; however, it can be performed earlier, at 10 to 12 weeks of pregnancy. The doctor guides either a small tube through the vagina and cervix or a thin needle through the abdomen and uterine wall to take a small sample of tissue from the placenta. The chorionic villa contain cells with the same genetic makeup as the fetus. The sample is studied for chromosomal or other defects. Complications from CVS are rare.

- *Fetal blood sampling*, also known as cordocentesis, tests fetal blood for chromosomal defects and other problems. This procedure involves the insertion of a needle through the abdomen and uterine wall to take blood from a vein in the umbilical cord. Cordocentesis is usually performed when amniocentesis or CVS is not possible because results are needed quickly. There is a small chance of fetal loss after fetal blood sampling.

If the results are abnormal, counseling and supportive services can help the parents make decisions that best meet their needs.

Women also should be tested for **Rh incompatibility** through a simple blood test. Most people produce Rh factor, a protein located on the surface of a red blood cell. A person who does not produce Rh factor has Rh-negative blood. Rh incompatibility occurs when an Rh-negative mother and an Rh-positive father conceive a baby who inherits the father's Rh-positive blood type. If the fetal Rh-positive blood cells enter the mother's bloodstream, the mother forms antibodies against the fetal blood cells in a process called maternal sensitization. This situation often occurs in a first pregnancy with an Rh-positive fetus, but because of the small amount of antibodies produced, it does not cause problems with the fetus. Future pregnancies, however, are at greater risk of antibodies crossing the placenta and causing Rh disease in the fetus. Rh-negative mothers should receive an injection of Rh immune globulin after delivery, during pregnancy, after a miscarriage, and after certain procedures such as amniocentesis. Without treatment, the most severely affected fetuses will be stillborn. In the newborn, Rh disease can result in jaundice, anemia, brain damage, heart failure, and death. Rh disease does not affect the mother's health.

Complications of Pregnancy

Five common complications of pregnancy—ectopic pregnancy, gestational diabetes, preterm delivery, stillbirth, and preeclampsia—are responsible for one-quarter of maternal and neonatal morbidity and mortality.[23]

I had some rather severe abdominal pain and some bleeding. I knew my period was late, but I was shocked to learn from my doctor that I had had a miscarriage. I didn't even know that I was pregnant.

—24-year-old woman

Ectopic Pregnancy

Ectopic pregnancy occurs when the fertilized egg implants outside the uterus, usually in the fallopian tube. The egg begins to grow outside the uterine cavity and presents a risk for rupture and hemorrhage. This problem occurs in about 1% to 2% of pregnancies.[24] Increased awareness and improved technologies that identify early ectopic pregnancies have greatly decreased maternal deaths; however, ectopic pregnancy-related deaths still account for 6% of all pregnancy-related deaths.[24]

Several factors increase the risk of an ectopic pregnancy by causing disruption of fallopian tube function (see **Table 6.4**). Pelvic inflammatory disease (PID), commonly caused by gonorrhea or chlamydia, is the most common risk factor. (See Chapter 7 for more information.) Symptoms of ectopic pregnancy usually begin in the seventh or eighth week of gestation. The most common symptoms are abdominal pain and tenderness and a missed menstrual period. The abdominal pain can be subtle at first, sometimes localized on one side, and increase in severity if tearing of the fallopian tube causes internal bleeding. Abnormal vaginal bleeding or spotting occurs in most ectopic pregnancies. Blood tests and vaginal or abdominal ultrasound tests can effectively diagnose an ectopic pregnancy. In some cases, an ectopic pregnancy may degenerate and require no intervention. In most cases, however, laparoscopic surgery may be performed to remove the fertilized egg that cannot survive outside the uterus.

Gestational Diabetes

Gestational diabetes usually occurs in the second half of pregnancy. Two to ten out of every 100 pregnant women in the United States will develop gestational diabetes.[25] Most women can control their blood sugar levels with diet and exercise, but some women with gestational diabetes or women who had diabetes before pregnancy need insulin injections to control their blood sugar levels. A woman is considered to be at high risk for gestational diabetes if she is very overweight, previously had gestational diabetes, has a strong family history of diabetes, or has glucose in her urine. The baby of a mother with gestational diabetes is at risk of being born very large and with extra fat, making delivery difficult and more dangerous, with an increased risk of cesarean section. The baby is also at greater risk of having breathing problems and low blood glucose after birth. For most women, glucose levels return to normal after pregnancy, but they have a 35% to 60% chance of developing type 2 diabetes in the next 10 to 20 years.[25]

Preterm Delivery

Pregnancy usually lasts from 38 to 42 weeks. Labor that begins before week 37 of pregnancy is considered **premature labor**. Babies born prematurely may have problems with breathing, eating, and temperature control, and they are more likely to die within the first month of life than a full-term baby. Approximately 12% of babies in the United States are born preterm, a decrease of 5% since 2006.[26] Women are at higher risk of preterm birth if they have had a previous preterm birth, are pregnant with twins or more, have certain uterine or cervical abnormalities, or have certain medical conditions. Women who seek late prenatal care or no care at all, as well as women who smoke, drink alcohol, use drugs, or experience stress, are also at greater risk. Women can decrease their risk of premature birth by recognizing the warning signs of preterm labor (see **It's Your Health**).

Table 6.4 Ectopic Pregnancy Risk Factors

- Pelvic inflammatory disease (PID)
- Previous ectopic pregnancy
- Previous tubal or pelvic surgery
- Endometriosis
- Infertility or infertility treatments
- Utero or tubal abnormalities
- DES (a drug once prescribed to prevent miscarriage) exposure
- Cigarette smoking

It's Your Health

Warning Signs of Preterm Labor

A healthcare provider should be contacted immediately if any of the following symptoms develop during pregnancy:

- Contractions every 10 minutes or more frequently
- Vaginal bleeding
- Vaginal fluid leakage
- Pelvic pressure
- Low, dull backache
- Cramps that feel like menstrual cramps
- Abdominal pain or vomiting

Stillbirth

Stillbirth is a common term for death of a fetus in the middle of the second trimester or later, while the fetus is still in the uterus. It is also called intrauterine fetal death or demise. There are multiple causes of stillbirth, including a mother with diabetes or high blood pressure, infection in the mother or in the fetal tissue, congenital abnormalities, and Rh disease. In addition, twin-to-twin transfusion (when twin circulations connect in a shared placenta); umbilical cord problems such as knots, tightened cord, cord wrapped around the fetal body or neck, cord prolapse (the cord falling down through the open cervix during labor); and placental problems, including poor circulation, can lead to a stillbirth.

Symptoms of a stillbirth vary but they may include the following common signs: stopping of fetal movement and kicks, spotting or bleeding, no fetal heartbeat heard with stethoscope or Doppler, and no fetal movement or heartbeat seen on ultrasound. Treatment of the woman following a stillbirth depends on many factors such as the number of weeks gestation, the size of the fetus, and how long since the fetal heartbeat stopped. Stillbirth is often very difficult for parents and other family members. Often, the fetus is fully formed and is delivered just as any baby. It may be very hard emotionally for a woman to go through labor, yet not have a baby to take home. Counseling is important for all parents with a stillbirth to help them understand their feelings and begin the work of grieving.

Miscarriage

A **miscarriage**, or spontaneous abortion, is defined as a pregnancy that ends before the twentieth week of gestation. An estimated 10–15% of clinically recognized pregnancies end in spontaneous abortion,[27] though experts acknowledge challenges in estimating rates. Miscarriages often occur early in the pregnancy, even before women are aware that they are pregnant. Factors associated with miscarriage include advanced maternal age, chromosomal abnormalities, single gene mutations, structural uterine abnormalities, endocrine abnormalities, immunologic factors, genital infections, cigarette smoking, alcohol use, and various environmental and occupational exposures. Some of these, such as chromosomal abnormalities, are clearly related to the embryo and others, such as uterine abnormalities, are clearly related to the mother. Karyotyping of the products of conception after miscarriage indicates that about two-thirds are chromosomally abnormal.[28]

A miscarriage is usually characterized by bleeding and cramping. Generally, when a woman experiences bleeding or cramping early in the pregnancy, bed rest is recommended. In some cases, the symptoms subside and the pregnancy proceeds normally. In other cases, the bleeding increases, the cervix dilates, and the embryo is released from the body. If the miscarriage is complete, the bleeding stops, and the uterus returns to its normal shape and size. If the miscarriage is incomplete, any remaining fragments must be removed in a procedure known as a dilatation and curettage (D&C). The risk for miscarriage decreases after the first trimester of pregnancy.

The causes of miscarriage vary and are not always clear. This uncertainty is a source of frustration for many couples who feel the need to understand why the miscarriage happened. Grief associated with miscarriage is often underestimated, leaving many affected women with inadequate support from their partners, friends, family, and healthcare providers.[29] The intensity of a woman's emotional distress may be related to the desirability of the pregnancy, late gestational age of the fetus, lack of social support, a lengthy period of trying to get pregnant, and use of infertility treatments. Women also may feel that they have disappointed their partners or families.

Preeclampsia

Preeclampsia is pregnancy-related high blood pressure. It can also be called **toxemia**. Preeclampsia usually occurs after about 30 weeks of pregnancy. In addition to having high blood pressure, mothers with preeclampsia often experience protein in their urine, swelling of the hands and face, sudden weight gain (a pound a day or more), blurred vision, severe headaches, dizziness, and intense stomach pain. The only real cure for preeclampsia is delivery, which may not be best for the baby. Labor is usually induced if the condition is mild and the woman is near-term (37 to 40 weeks gestation). If a woman is not ready for labor, she and the baby will be monitored, often in a hospital setting, until her blood pressure stabilizes or the baby is born.

Genetic Disorders and Congenital Abnormalities

Genetic disorders are diseases caused in whole or in part by a variation or mutation of a gene. Scientists are learning that thousands of diseases have genetic components. Genetic disorders are responsible for a significant number of miscarriages, often without being diagnosed, so calculating the total number of disorders is a complicated process.

Today more than 6,000 abnormalities have been identified, ranging from mild differences (as in certain hemoglobin abnormalities) to fatal or overwhelmingly disabling conditions, such as trisomy 18 (Edwards's) syndrome and trisomy 13 (Patau's) syndrome. The risk of a single gene disorder is estimated at 1 in 200 births.

Genetic diseases result from single-gene alterations, chromosomal abnormalities, or multifactorial errors. Single-gene disorders are caused by a mutation in a single gene. (Each chromosome contains thousands of individual genes.) The mutation may be present on one chromosome or two chromosomes where one is inherited from each parent. Sickle cell disease, cystic fibrosis, and Tay–Sachs disease are single-gene disorders. Chromosome disorders are caused by extra or missing chromosomes or chromosome parts. Down syndrome, for example, is caused by an extra copy of chromosome 21, but no individual gene on the chromosome is abnormal. Multifactorial inheritance disorders are caused by a combination of small variations in genes, often in concert with environmental factors. Heart disease and most cancers are examples of these disorders. Another multifactorial example is albinism, an inherited inability to generate the protective pigment melanin. Albinism greatly increases susceptibility to skin cancer after excessive exposure to sunlight. Behaviors are also considered to be multifactorial. Behaviors are complex traits involving multiple genes that are affected by many other factors. Researchers are learning more about the genetic contribution to behavioral disorders such as alcoholism, obesity, certain mental illnesses, and Alzheimer's disease.

Because early detection of these conditions is essential, states and territories mandate newborn screening of all infants born within their jurisdiction for certain disorders that may not otherwise be detected before developmental disability or death occurs. Newborns with these disorders typically appear normal at birth. A recent expert panel has identified 29 conditions for which screening should be mandated.[30]

Infections

Any infection in the mother can potentially cause harm to an unborn fetus. Sexually transmitted infections, including HIV, can be particularly dangerous during a pregnancy. (For more information, see Chapter 7.)

- Gonorrhea, chlamydia, and syphilis can cause preterm delivery and miscarriage.

- Bacterial vaginosis (BV), an infection of the vaginal area that is usually benign and asymptomatic, can lead to preterm delivery as well as low-birth-weight babies. The presence of BV also is associated with an increased risk of HIV infection.

- Perinatal transmission of HIV can occur during pregnancy, labor and delivery, or via breastfeeding. Since medications can reduce the risk of perinatal HIV transmission, testing of pregnant women and subsequent treatment of those who are infected have dramatically reduced transmission rates. Perinatal transmission is the most common route of HIV infection in children, and it is now the source of almost all AIDS cases in children in the United States.[31] The actual number of AIDS cases associated with perinatal transmission has decreased dramatically in recent years, though the disease burden remains disproportionately high for racial and ethnic minorities.

The CDC recommends that all pregnant women be tested for HIV as early in pregnancy as possible. Pregnant women should also be screened for chlamydia, gonorrhea, hepatitis B, and syphilis.[32]

The most common prenatal infection today is **cytomegalovirus (CMV)**, a viral infection. Cytomegalovirus causes mild flulike symptoms in adults, but in newborns, it can cause small birth size, brain damage, developmental problems, enlarged liver, hearing and vision impairment, and other malformations. Each year in the United States, about 1 in 150 children is born with CMV infection and 1 in 750 children has permanent disabilities as a result of CMV infection. About 80% of babies born with CMV never have symptoms or problems.[33]

A blood test can ascertain if a woman already had a CMV infection. More invasive tests, such as amniocentesis, can help determine if the fetus is infected. Because CMV is found in body fluids, including urine, saliva, breast milk, blood, tears, semen, and vaginal fluids, a woman can become infected with CMV when she comes in contact with them. Good hygiene by pregnant women is still the best way to protect unborn babies against CMV infection.

Rubella is also linked with birth defects. A rubella infection is usually mild and often asymptomatic. The biggest danger of rubella is if a woman gets it during the first 20 weeks of pregnancy: She may lose the pregnancy, or the virus could cause problems to her unborn baby such as cataracts, deafness, or damage to the heart or brain. There is no treatment for rubella, but the measles-mumps-rubella

(MMR) vaccine can prevent it. All women of reproductive age should be immunized against rubella if they have not had this formerly common childhood illness.

Group B streptococcus (GBS) is a bacterium that can cause illness in newborn babies and pregnant women. It is the most common cause of life-threatening infections in newborns, and it is a frequent cause of newborn pneumonia. On average, about 1,200 babies less than 1 week old get early-onset group B strep disease.[34] In most cases, this disease can be prevented in newborns by administering IV antibiotics to women in labor who had a baby with group B strep disease in the past, or who now have a urinary tract infection caused by group B strep. Pregnant women who carry the bacterium, as confirmed with a positive test during pregnancy, should also be given antibiotics during labor.

Other Considerations

Women should be aware of postpartum issues, such as depression. Many women will experience postpartum "blues," mood swings, and slight depression for several days after a baby's birth. These feelings are normal and will go away in the first few weeks. Some women experience more severe symptoms, however, which will warrant treatment. Women who are more susceptible to postpartum depression include those women who suffer from depression, have experienced postpartum depression in a previous pregnancy, have severe premenstrual syndrome (PMS) or premenstrual dysphoric disorder (PMDD), and/or are experiencing other stressors in their family, marriage, or life at the time of the birth. (See Chapter 12 on mental health.)

Women with disabilities and chronic conditions who want to become pregnant may have special considerations to discuss with their healthcare providers. Certain conditions that are common in pregnant women, such as vaginal and urinary tract infections, fluid retention, and decreased mobility, may create even more significant problems for women with preexisting conditions or disorders. Other difficulties may also impair the mobility of women with physical disabilities. As her body changes with pregnancy, a woman with impaired mobility may experience balance problems and new pressure points if she is in a wheelchair. Each disability or condition may present with different issues, just as each pregnant woman may present with different complications and issues. Throughout the pregnancy, from preconception to postpartum, women with disabilities or chronic conditions should work with a team of healthcare providers to ensure favorable pregnancy and postpregnancy outcomes.

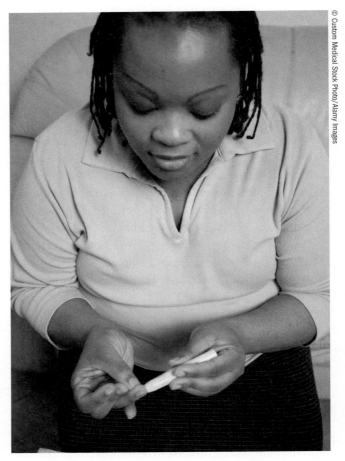

■ Women with diabetes are at an increased risk for complications with pregnancy.

I knew that having a baby would be difficult, but I was not prepared to feel so numb, miserable, hopeless, and worried. I learned that I was one of the 10–15% of mothers who experience postpartum depression. Fortunately my doctor was really helpful. I would encourage any new mom to talk to her doctor if she is feeling really sad or "down." Sometimes it is just normal "baby blues." But sometimes it can be serious. Getting help early can make a huge difference.
—30-year-old mother

Childbirth

Many women have special concerns about their childbirth experience. Experts agree that interfering with the normal physiological process of labor and birth in the absence of medical necessity increases the risk of complications for the mother and baby. Unfortunately, hospital routines and procedures have often taken priority over the needs of the laboring mother and her baby. Some experts argue that many modern medical interventions, including cesarean surgery, labor induction, electronic fetal monitoring, ultrasound examinations, episiotomies, unnatural birthing positions, pubic shaving, enemas, IV lines, drugs, and forced mother and baby separations, are too normative, and often do not improve birth outcome or the labor and delivery process.[35] Today, many birthing centers encourage the following practices to promote an optimal physiological birth experience for the mother and her baby:[36]

- Avoiding medically unnecessary induction of labor
- Allowing freedom of movement for the laboring woman
- Providing continuous labor support
- Avoiding routine interventions and restrictions

- Encouraging spontaneous pushing in nonsupine positions
- Keeping mothers and babies together after birth without restrictions on breastfeeding

In many areas, women can decide what type of healthcare provider they want for the birth of their baby. High-risk mothers or mothers with high-risk infants have fewer options because they may require specialists who are familiar with their particular conditions. The preferences of the mother and her partner are important considerations for making many childbirth decisions. **Self-Assessment 6.1** provides a checklist for childbirth considerations. The

Self-Assessment 6.1

Childbirth Considerations

Birthing issues	Very Important	Not Important	Don't Want	Birthing issues	Very Important	Not Important	Don't Want
Hospital delivery room	___	___	___	**Second-stage labor:**			
Hospital birthing room	___	___	___	Labor room	___	___	___
Birthing center	___	___	___	Delivery room	___	___	___
Home	___	___	___	Birthing room	___	___	___
Obstetrician	___	___	___	Family present	___	___	___
Family practitioner	___	___	___	Delivery position flexibility	___	___	___
Certified nurse-midwife	___	___	___	Episiotomy	___	___	___
Partner/coach:				**After delivery:**			
Present during labor	___	___	___	Prolonged holding of baby	___	___	___
Present during delivery	___	___	___	Warm-water bath for baby	___	___	___
Present for all procedures	___	___	___	Breastfeeding in birthing area	___	___	___
Present during cesarean	___	___	___	**Postpartum:**			
Present during recovery	___	___	___	Private room	___	___	___
Early labor:				Baby rooming in with mother	___	___	___
Stay home as long as possible	___	___	___	Breastfeeding	___	___	___
Arrive early and settle in	___	___	___	Bottle-feeding	___	___	___
Wear own clothes	___	___	___	Length of stay in facility	___	___	___
Perineal shave	___	___	___	Sibling/family visitation	___	___	___
Enema	___	___	___	Postpartum depression concerns	___	___	___
Intravenous tube	___	___	___				
First-stage labor:							
Labor room	___	___	___				
Birthing room	___	___	___				
External fetal monitor	___	___	___				
Internal fetal monitor	___	___	___				

Decisions on places of birth, birthing positions, pain relief, and breastfeeding can be made based on this checklist.

After completing the assessment, women should discuss their issues of concern with their partner and their healthcare provider.

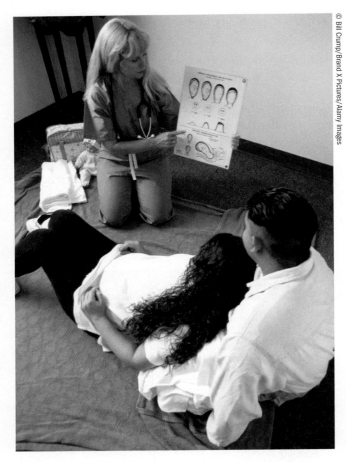

■ Childbirth education classes help a couple prepare for delivery by teaching relaxation and pain management techniques. The classes also provide the opportunity for the couples to discuss their concerns and excitement.

list can serve as a basis for further questions and decision making between a woman and her childbirth healthcare providers.

Labor and Delivery

Labor and delivery can be rewarding and satisfying when a woman anticipates the sequence of events and is prepared for the process. Long before actual labor begins, the uterus changes to prepare itself to function efficiently during labor and delivery. By the end of the pregnancy, the uterus measures about 10 to 14 inches. Its capacity has increased nearly 500 times during the pregnancy, and it increases in weight from 1.5 ounces to 30 ounces. The uterine muscle fibers grow to 10 times their original thickness. The uterus is one of the strongest muscles in a woman's body, and it contracts powerfully during labor. Throughout pregnancy, the uterus contracts at slightly irregular intervals. These irregular contractions, known as Braxton–Hicks contractions, differ

from "real" labor contractions in that they do not gradually increase in frequency, intensity, or duration. Instead, they serve to increase the blood circulation and help the uterus to accommodate the growing baby.

Three distinctive signs indicate that labor is beginning:

- Regular, progressive uterine contractions that occur every 5 minutes or so and last from 45 seconds to a minute. The contractions gradually become longer, stronger, and closer together.
- Rupture of the membranes, or "bag of waters." This rupture may be a slow leak or a gush. The fluid is usually clear.
- The "bloody show." It involves the passage of a small amount of bloodstained mucus, which serves as a plug in the cervix to protect the fetus from infection. As the cervix begins to dilate, this plug is released.

Other less distinctive signs of approaching labor include diarrhea, backache, and an increase in Braxton–Hicks contractions. The only confirmation that labor has begun is a pelvic examination that reveals a softening, thinned-out, and dilating cervix.

Many factors affect the progress of labor, including the position of the baby and the shape of the mother's pelvis. Although all experiences are different, each labor progresses through three distinct stages (**Figure 6.6**).

Stage I is from the onset of labor to full dilation of the cervix. The cervical canal shortens until the cervix is as thick as the uterine wall. This process, in which the cervix is "taken up" into the uterus, is known as **effacement**. Once the cervix is effaced, the force of the uterine contractions begins to dilate the cervix, although effacement and dilation may occur simultaneously. Dilation refers to the size of the round opening of the cervix. It is measured in centimeters or finger widths. Full dilation is 10 cm or 5 finger widths (**Figure 6.7**).

Stage II of labor begins when the cervix is completely dilated and ends with the birth of the baby. The presentation of the baby—the part of the body positioned to emerge first—is usually by the top of the head, known as a vertex presentation. When the feet or buttocks present first, it is known as a **breech** presentation. The breech position occurs in about 3% of deliveries and usually results in a longer labor. Because a breech delivery presents greater risks to the mother and baby, a cesarean delivery is often performed.

As the baby's head appears, or crowns, an episiotomy may be performed. An episiotomy is an incision in the

(a) Early first-stage labor

Placenta

Symphysis pubis

Urinary bladder

Vagina

Cervix

Rectum

(b) Later first-stage labor: the transition

Ruptured amniotic sac

(c) Early second-stage labor

Placenta

(d) Third-stage labor: delivery of afterbirth

Placenta

Uterus

Umbilical cord

Figure 6.6

Labor and delivery. Stage I: the cervix becomes fully dilated; stage II: the infant is born; stage III: the afterbirth is delivered.

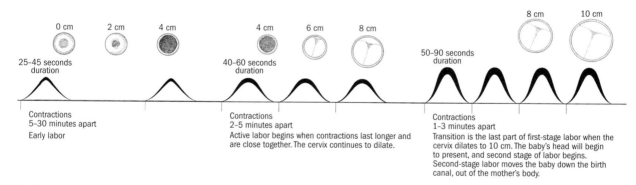

0 cm   2 cm   4 cm   4 cm   6 cm   8 cm   8 cm   10 cm

25–45 seconds
duration

40–60 seconds
duration

50–90 seconds
duration

Contractions
5–30 minutes apart

Early labor

Contractions
2–5 minutes apart

Active labor begins when contractions last longer and
are close together. The cervix continues to dilate.

Contractions
1–3 minutes apart

Transition is the last part of first-stage labor when the
cervix dilates to 10 cm. The baby's head will begin
to present, and second stage of labor begins.
Second-stage labor moves the baby down the birth
canal, out of the mother's body.

Figure 6.7

Dilation through stages of labor.

perineum that enlarges the vaginal opening for birth. The traditional argument for performing this procedure is that a surgical incision heals better and faster than a jagged tear. Once routine with vaginal deliveries, the practice of episiotomies has been seriously questioned as to its necessity and benefits for all pregnancies. Recent studies show that episiotomies were linked with more pain, more difficulty healing, and a longer wait for resuming sex after childbirth, with no obvious benefits for most women. Only women requiring a quick delivery for babies in distress should receive an episiotomy. Rate of episiotomies decreased from 29% of vaginal births in 1997 to 12% in 2008.[37]

Stage III lasts from the completion of delivery of the baby to completion of delivery of the **afterbirth**, or placenta. In this final stage of labor, the uterus contracts firmly after the delivery of the baby. The placenta separates from the uterine wall and is expelled. If an episiotomy has been performed, it is sutured at this time.

Pain Relief in Childbirth

Women experience different levels of pain during childbirth. The reality of childbirth is that it usually involves some physical hurt. The physical and psychological techniques promoted in childbirth preparation classes can dramatically influence the perception of pain and the confidence in dealing with labor difficulties. These pain relief measures have the inherent advantage of not producing any chemical disruption in the mother's body, which could then affect the baby or the birthing process.

Good labor support helps a woman throughout labor. Physical and emotional comfort, information, guidance, and communication with the healthcare staff are invaluable to the laboring woman and can greatly reduce her anxiety and need for pharmacological interventions. Nondrug options include:

- *Comfort measures:* These are things that a woman can do for herself, that her companion can do for her, or that can be done to the laboring environment to increase her personal comfort level.

- *Mental strategies:* Many women employ a variety of techniques including special breathing, meditation, prayer, music, focal points, and singing to reduce anxiety and create a sense of calm during labor.

- *Medications:* A variety of pain-relieving medications are available for childbirth. Most decisions about medications are actually personal choices, not medical decisions. For this reason, it is important for the pregnant woman to learn about possible medications before she goes into labor. Tranquilizers and analgesics are often used together for general relaxation and to take the edge off of contractions.

Anesthetics used during labor and delivery may be given in different forms. **Epidural anesthesia** is the most popular choice among pregnant women, and it allows the mother to be awake during the delivery. The anesthetic is injected through a catheter that is placed in a space adjacent to the spinal cord. Spinal anesthesia is injected directly into the spinal canal. Like the epidural, it prevents a woman from being able to move around in labor and often inhibits a woman from pushing. Pudendal anesthesia is injected into the area around the vagina and perineum. This method is least likely to affect the baby.

Cesarean Delivery

A **cesarean delivery** (also known as a cesarean section) is the birth of a baby through surgical incisions made in both the wall of the mother's abdomen and her uterus. Anesthesia is required for the procedure. Clearly, a cesarean birth is sometimes necessary for the safety of the mother or the baby—for example, when there are problems with the baby, problems with the woman's passage area, or problems with the delivery process. However, considerable controversy exists today over whether this type of delivery is being performed too often. The rate of cesarean sections had increased dramatically between 1970 and 1988, rising from 5.5% of all births in 1970 to a high of 24.7% in 1988. Between 1991 and 1996, however, the U.S. cesarean rate dropped by 8%, but then increased again by 50% between 1996 and 2009 to 32.9% of all births (**Figure 6.8**).[39]

One cause for cesarean section is **fetal distress**, a condition in which some aspect of labor or the baby's environment places the baby at risk. For example, the baby's oxygen supply might be cut off owing to **abruptio placentae**, in which the placenta separates prematurely from the wall of the uterus. This event threatens not only the baby, but also the mother with a risk of hemorrhage. A **prolapsed cord** is another risky situation in which the umbilical cord comes through the pelvis before the baby and can disrupt the flow of oxygen to the baby due to a compressed cord.

Problems with the birth passage also influence the decision for a cesarean delivery. **Cephalopelvic disproportion**, in which the baby is too large for the pelvis, is a common reason for choosing this type of delivery. A woman in labor whose baby is in a transverse lie, a crosswise position in the uterus, will need a cesarean delivery because neither the head nor the buttocks are in the pelvis. When a baby is in a breech position, the buttocks emerge before the head. The head has a larger diameter than the buttocks, and the risk is that it will not fit well through the passage because it has not had the opportunity to mold and nestle into the pelvis throughout the labor process. Multiple births are also more likely to require cesarean delivery. A relatively rare complication of the passageway is obstruction by a fibroid, a benign tumor, or even the placenta (**placenta previa**). Usually these obstructions or other problems with fetal passage can be diagnosed before labor and delivery, which permits time to discuss various options with the healthcare provider.

Other conditions may also indicate the need for cesarean delivery. For example, the term "failure to progress" describes cervical failure to dilate adequately despite regular uterine contractions. To avoid prolonged distress to mother and baby in this situation, a cesarean delivery may be performed. Herpes is another reason for a cesarean delivery: If a woman has active lesions in the birth canal, a cesarean delivery is indicated to avoid infecting the baby.

Vaginal Birth After Cesarean Delivery

For many years, a widely held philosophy about childbirth was "once a cesarean, always a cesarean." This philosophy may be partially responsible for the overall increase in cesarean birth rates in the United States during recent years. National data indicate a steady decline in cesarean sections through 1996, owing in part to the movement encouraging vaginal birth after cesarean delivery (VBAC). By the late 1990s, however, studies revealed that some women should not attempt VBAC for fear of uterine rupture or the need for an emergency cesarean section. Many smaller hospitals stopped offering VBAC out of medical liability concerns.[40]

The American College of Obstetricians and Gynecologists (ACOG), as well as many hospital boards, have taken a strong position on VBAC to help control the morbidity associated with major abdominal surgical procedures and to help reduce the spiraling costs of health care. A trial of labor

is recommended for most women who underwent a previous cesarean section and have no unusual circumstances or conditions. ACOG has found that the mother usually experiences fewer complications with VBAC than with cesarean birth in terms of infection, bleeding, and anesthesia. Other advantages of VBAC include a shorter hospital stay and recovery period as well as significant cost savings. Women giving birth in hospitals that are not equipped for emergency cesarean sections and women with certain medical contraindications should not undergo VBAC.[40]

Breastfeeding

Physiological Changes of the Breast

During pregnancy, hormones prepare the breasts for lactation (milk production). The breasts enlarge as the cells that produce milk increase in number and the ducts that carry milk develop (**Figure 6.9**). The nipple and areola become more elastic and are protected by a natural lubricant secreted from tiny glands under the skin. After delivery, levels of estrogen and progesterone in the body rapidly decrease, triggering the production of milk. Two hormones are released in response to a baby's suckling:

- *Prolactin*, which stimulates lactation.
- *Oxytocin*, which is responsible for the transportation of milk from the producing cells to the milk ducts to the nipple.

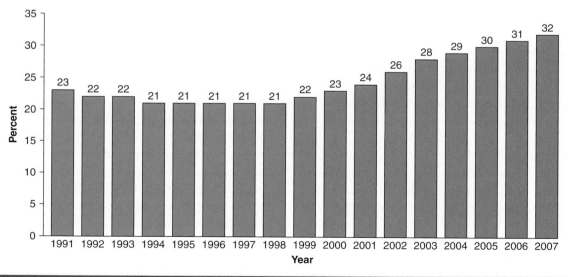

Figure 6.8

Total Cesarean rates for first births, United States, 1991–2007.

Source: Modified from Menacker, F., Hamilton, B.E. (2010). Recent trends in cesarean delivery in the United States. National Center for Health Statistics, no 35. Downloaded April 30, 2012 from http://www.cdc.gov/nchs/data/databriefs/db35.pdf.

Figure 6.9
The female breast.

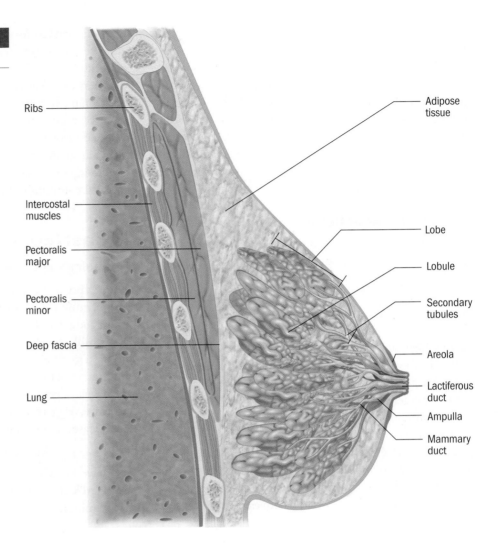

The composition of breast milk varies depending on the stage of lactation, the stage of feeding, and the mother's diet. Early milk, or milk produced during the pregnancy and for 3 to 5 days after birth, is called **colostrum**. Colostrum is yellowish in color, thicker than milk, and rich with protective antibodies and protein. Transitional milk leads to regular mature milk after about 10 days. During feedings, low-fat, thirst-quenching milk is released first, followed by higher-fat, more nourishing milk. The milk's vitamin content is representative of the mother's vitamin intake.

Benefits of Breastfeeding

Breastfeeding provides many benefits, including protection against many acute and chronic diseases as well as advantages for general health, growth, and development (see **It's Your Health**). Breast milk is highly nutritious,

providing all of the nutrients that a growing baby needs. It is ideal as a baby's sole source of nutrients for the first 6 months of life. In addition, breast milk contains enzymes to aid the infant's digestion as well as antibodies to protect against infection. Evidence has shown that breastfed infants have fewer and less severe episodes of diarrhea; fewer cases of upper respiratory, ear, and even urinary infections; and fewer hospitalizations and doctor's visits. Studies also show the possibilities of breast milk protecting against type 1 diabetes mellitus (childhood-onset diabetes), celiac disease, SIDS, obesity, and childhood cancers (such as lymphoma and leukemia). [41] Prolonged and exclusive breastfeeding is also believed to improve children's cognitive development.[42]

New mothers may also reap benefits from breastfeeding. Due to the increased levels of oxytocin from breastfeeding, the uterus returns to its normal size more quickly and

It's Your Health

Benefits of Breastfeeding

Infant's Benefits

- Fewer episodes and decreased severity of diarrhea and gastrointestinal difficulties
- Decreased incidence of ear infections, urinary tract infections, and upper respiratory infections
- Fewer hospitalizations and visits to the doctor's office
- Fewer food allergies
- Possible protection against diabetes, celiac disease, SIDS, chronic digestive disease, and childhood cancers
- Possible benefits of cognitive development

Mother's Benefits

- Less postpartum bleeding
- Faster return to pre-pregnancy weight
- Possible decreased incidence of ovarian and breast cancers

Benefits for Both

- Special bond between mother and infant

Table 6.5   Economic Benefits of Breastfeeding

- The U.S. Department of Agriculture's Economic Research Services estimates that at least $3.6 billion in medical expenses could be saved each year if the number of children breastfed for at least 6 months increased to 50%.
- Families spend $2.5 billion a year on breast milk substitutes such as infant formula.
- The U.S. Department of Agriculture's Special Supplemental Nutrition Program for Women, Infants and Children (WIC) spends $740 million per year to buy formula for babies who are not breastfeeding.
- Every 10% increase in the breastfeeding rate among WIC recipients would save WIC almost $1 million per year.
- For every 1,000 babies who are not breastfed, there are 2,033 more medical office visits, 212 extra days of hospitalization and 609 excess prescriptions.
- Given that Medicaid covers 41% of U.S. births, increasing rates of breastfeeding among infants covered by Medicaid may help state budgets.
- Insurers, including Medicaid, spend $1.6 billion a year to cover sick-child office visits and prescriptions to treat the three most common illnesses—respiratory infections, otitis media (ear infections), and diarrhea—in the first year of life for formula-fed infants versus breastfed infants.
- From $4.6 to 9 billion excess are spent every year on conditions and diseases that are preventable by breastfeeding.

Source: Health Resources and Services Administration (HRSA) Maternal and Child Health Bureau, and the Centers for Disease Control and Prevention (CDC). (2002). [Adjusted for inflation for 2009 dollars] and National Conference of State Legislatures. (2010). The economic benefits of breastfeeding. *Legisbrief* 18(1).

the woman experiences less postpartum bleeding. Breastfeeding also helps a woman to return to her pre-pregnancy weight more quickly, although she is less likely to lose her last 5 pounds of weight. Women who breastfeed may have a lower risk of rheumatoid arthritis, cardiovascular disease, and ovarian and premenopausal breast cancer.[41] Besides all of the physical health benefits, breastfeeding can create a special bond between mother and infant. Additionally, breastfeeding has the economic benefit of saving money that would otherwise be spent on formula and the medical conditions that breastfeeding can prevent (**Table 6.5**).

Although any length of breastfeeding is better than no breastfeeding, research indicates that exclusive and prolonged breastfeeding has a greater protective effect than short-term nursing or nursing along with supplemental formula feeding. Experts recommend that mothers breastfeed their babies exclusively for 6 months, and that they continue to breastfeed while supplementing with solid foods until the baby's first birthday.

Optimizing Breastfeeding

Even though breastfeeding offers many advantages for children and mothers, society, and the environment, nursing mothers still must face social and cultural barriers. Education is a primary challenge, especially for first-time mothers, who benefit from antenatal and postpartum breastfeeding instruction and support.[43] Breastfeeding is not always easy, especially for first-time mothers, but experienced guidance and care can solve problems in many cases. Worksite support also influences breastfeeding decisions and a woman's ability to continue breastfeeding upon returning to work.

Complications of Breastfeeding

Breastfeeding is not always the best option for some infants. Women who are infected with HIV; have untreated active tuberculosis; are users of alcohol, tobacco, or other recreational drugs; are undergoing cancer chemotherapy or radiation treatment; or are using certain necessary medications that may not be healthy for the developing infant should not breastfeed. Infants with **galactosemia** (an inherited disease caused by a lack of enzyme for processing galactose that can lead to organ enlargement, cataracts, and mental retardation) should not be breastfed.

■ Breast pumps are useful to mothers who work or who have difficulty breastfeeding.

Women may experience difficulties with feeding, including the following problems:

- Inverted or flat nipples
- Raw or cracked nipples
- Severely swollen breasts
- Problems with the infant latching on
- Pain during latch-on

These problems often can be resolved by changing positions, massaging the breasts, or using a nipple shield to protect the breast. Other complications may require medical attention, such as **mastitis** (bacterial infection of the breast) or **thrush** (yeast infection that affects the mouth of the baby). Women should talk to their healthcare provider or a nursing lactation specialist if they experience problems with breastfeeding.

Diet, Drugs, and Alcohol During Breastfeeding

Women who choose to breastfeed should consume a healthy diet to ensure adequate intake of the necessary vitamins and minerals. Caloric intake should be increased by 500 calories per day relative to a woman's pre-pregnancy diet. Women should maintain a sufficient calcium intake (1,000 mg per day) to rule out any possibility of long-term effects of breastfeeding on the mother's bone density. Note that any substance taken in by the mother can be passed to the infant through the breast milk, including harmful substances such as caffeine, alcohol, and certain drugs. For this reason, breastfeeding women should consult their healthcare providers before taking any medications.

Infertility

Fecundity refers to a woman's physical ability to have a child. Women with impaired fecundity include those who find it physically difficult or medically inadvisable to conceive or deliver a child. The term *impaired fecundity* is also used to describe women who, although having sexual intercourse on a regular basis without contraception for 36 months or more, fail to become pregnant. This definition of reduced ability to bear children differs from the medical definition of infertility, which is the inability of couples who are not surgically sterile to conceive after 12 months of regular intercourse without contraception.

Causes

Fertility-related difficulties can arise at many points, including the process of ovulation in women, sperm production in men, or the maintenance of the embryo after fertilization has taken place.

- In 25% to 35% of couples, the fertility problem is in the male.
- In 25% to 35% of couples, the fertility problem is in the female.

- For the remaining couples, infertility is a result of both a male and a female factor or unknown causes.

Many factors contribute to infertility. Problems with ovulation are responsible for most cases in women. Without ovulation, eggs are not present for fertilization. Symptoms that might indicate a woman is not ovulating include irregular or absent menstrual periods. Blocked or scarred fallopian tubes due to PID, endometriosis, or previous surgery for an ectopic pregnancy can all cause infertility in women. Physical or anatomical problems with a woman's uterus or uterine fibroids may also contribute to infertility.

Age and other factors can affect a woman's ability to conceive. Because more women are delaying childbirth until their 30s and 40s, age is becoming a more common infertility consideration. Poor diet, smoking, alcohol, sexually transmitted infections (STIs), and health problems that cause hormonal changes can also contribute to infertility.

Depression and stress may have a direct effect on hormonal regulation and ovulation. Weight is another important factor in infertility. Women who are overweight or obese often have irregular or infrequent menstrual cycles and are at increased risk of infertility. Underweight women also have infertility issues due to low body fat levels.

Diagnosis

Various tests can often determine the cause of infertility and thus the appropriate treatment method. Tests can be used to confirm if and when a woman ovulates, as well as evaluate ovarian function and uterine receptivity to implantation. A simple method of determining whether ovulation is occurring, for example, is to monitor a woman's basal body temperature to see whether a slight increase in her temperature occurs midway through her menstrual cycle.

Tests can also examine the quality of the mucus. The ferning test involves collecting mucus near the time of ovulation to see if, when smeared, it resembles the fronds of a fern. If so, the woman's estrogen levels are normal, and the mucus is creating a desirable environment for the sperm to travel.

A postcoital test may also be performed before ovulation. Mucus is collected within 6 hours after intercourse and is viewed under a microscope to see whether it contains multiple, active sperm.

Other tests used to diagnose infertility include the following:

- Blood tests for measuring hormone levels
- Radiograph studies such as a hysterosalpingogram, which outlines obstructions or abnormal growths in the uterus or fallopian tubes

Gender Dimensions: Health Differences Between Men and Women

Male Infertility

Problems with male fertility contribute to about one-third of cases of infertility. Many of the same factors that reduce fertility in women also affect male fertility. In most cases, producing too few sperm (oligospermia) or none at all (azoospermia) causes male infertility. Other sperm production problems include issues with sperm motility, such as abnormal structure that prevents sperm from moving correctly, or sperm ability to fertilize the egg, oftentimes caused by abnormal sperm shape. Other factors that can play a role in infertility include:

- Age
- Health problems, including sexually transmitted infections (STIs)

and various medical treatments, such as chemotherapy and radiation therapy.

- Emotional factors such as high levels of stress.
- Alcohol or drugs, smoking, and anabolic steroids. For example, studies have shown that smokers' sperm are less likely to bind tightly to an egg—a necessary step for fertilization.
- Environmental factors, such as prolonged exposure to high temperatures, radiation, or heavy electromagnetic or microwave emissions, which can decrease sperm count or affect the viability of the sperm.

- Laparoscopic surgery to view the uterus, fallopian tubes, and ovaries

A common test used to diagnose male infertility is semen analysis. Semen is evaluated for the number of sperm present, the volume of ejaculate, the motility of the sperm, and the size and shape of the sperm. If a man has a low sperm count, blood tests may be performed to measure various hormones and proteins. A physical examination and an ultrasound of the scrotum also may be performed to detect varicose veins that may need repair.

For a couple dealing with infertility, finding the cause can be a long, complicated, and trying process. It can take months, and for couples without health insurance that covers therapy, the process can be quite expensive.

Treatment

A variety of treatment approaches can be employed depending on the cause of the infertility. The most basic form of treatment relies on a change in sexual activity. By using a basal body temperature chart, for example, women can monitor their temperature changes and better determine their exact time of ovulation. About 85% to 90% of infertility cases are treated with drug therapy or surgical repair of reproductive organs. Medical approaches to infertility may involve hormones to treat cervical mucus problems or difficulties in ovulation, while ultrasound is used to monitor the response of the ovaries during treatment.

- To stimulate ovulation, a medication called clomiphene citrate (trade name Clomid) is often prescribed. It stimulates the release of luteinizing hormone and causes an increase in estradiol, thereby triggering ovulation.
- Gonadotropin-releasing hormone (GnRH) may be administered to improve a woman's response to ovulation stimulants.
- Follicle-stimulating hormone (FSH) stimulates egg follicles in the ovaries.
- Human chorionic gonadotropin (HCG) works with clomiphene citrate to help stimulate the follicle to release its egg.

Microsurgery is a useful technique for male and female problems that require surgical intervention. Using a laparoscope, doctors can open blockages in a woman's fallopian tubes or correct structural abnormalities of the uterus or ovary. Surgery may also be used in males to open blocked sperm ducts or to repair a **varicocele** (a mesh of varicose veins in and around the testicle), which is often associated with infertility.

■ Many couples who have had trouble conceiving use assisted reproductive technologies to assist them in getting pregnant.

Other techniques that have shown success to date include artificial insemination and **assisted reproductive technologies (ARTs)**. **Artificial insemination** is the process of implanting sperm from a donor into a woman near the time of her ovulation. Sperm donors are screened for HIV infection and various genetic disorders, as well as categorized by certain features to create as optimal a match as possible between the woman and the donor. Artificial insemination is often used when the infertility problem is based on a male factor.

Any treatment or procedure that involves the handling of human eggs and sperm for the purpose of helping a woman become pregnant qualifies as a type of ART. All ART procedures involve stimulating the ovary to produce eggs, harvesting the eggs with a microscopic needle, and then removing the eggs from the woman's body. The CDC estimates that ART accounts for slightly more than 1% of total U.S. births. More than 60,000 infants were born as a result of ART cycles performed in 2009.[44] ART methods are listed below.

- **In vitro fertilization (IVF)** involves removing the ova from a woman's ovary just before normal ovulation would occur. The woman's egg and her partner's sperm are placed in a special fertilization medium for a specific period of time and are then transferred to another medium for continued development. If the fertilized egg cell shows signs of development, it is returned to the woman's uterus within several days by means of a hollow tube placed through the vagina and cervix. The egg cell implants itself in the lining of the uterus, and the pregnancy continues as normal.

- **Gamete intrafallopian transfer (GIFT)** involves placing sperm and eggs into the fallopian tubes. This procedure is less time-consuming and less expensive than IVF. GIFT mimics nature by permitting fertilized eggs to divide in the fallopian tubes. It has a success rate similar to that seen with IVF, but is more invasive than IVF.

- **Zygote intrafallopian transfer (ZIFT)** is a similar process that involves adding the fertilized egg to the fallopian tube at an earlier point than GIFT.

- **Intracytoplasmic sperm injection (ICSI)** involves injecting sperm directly into the egg with a microscopic needle.

- **Egg donation** is used when a woman is unable to produce eggs or she has a genetic disorder that will be passed on to the child. Egg donors must be willing to dedicate an enormous amount of time to this process because of the amount of drug treatment and monitoring that they must undergo. It is not a simple procedure for either the donor or the recipient of the egg.

- **Embryo transfer** is a procedure in which the sperm of the infertile woman's partner is placed in another woman's uterus during ovulation. Approximately 5 days later, the fertilized egg is transferred to the uterus of the infertile woman, who then carries the developing embryo.

- **Host uterus** is a procedure in which the sperm from a man and the egg from a woman are combined in a laboratory. The fertilized egg is then implanted into the uterus of a second woman who agrees to bear the child, which is not genetically related to her.

- **Surrogacy** occurs when a woman is artificially inseminated with the sperm of an infertile woman's partner. She carries the baby to term, usually for an established fee and the provision of her health care. After delivery, the baby is turned over to the couple.

Each of these procedures, while offering hope to infertile couples, can raise ethical and legal questions.

Emotional Effects of Infertility

Infertility and the procedures used to treat it are extremely stressful for most couples. In some cases, women who undergo the often arduous tests experience anger and resentment toward their partners, especially if their partners do not provide adequate support and share in their experiences. If the cause of infertility is determined, the man or woman who is experiencing the medical problem may feel guilty and blame himself or herself for failing to become pregnant. The experience of becoming pregnant and miscarrying can also lead to excitement and anticipation followed by depression and frustration. Once involved in testing, couples may become hopeful again but hesitant. The mix of emotions often leads to confusion and miscommunication between the couple.

As a couple prepares to undergo an ART procedure such as IVF, more grief may be experienced. In addition to fearing that it is the last option available, couples must shoulder the exorbitant costs of infertility treatment and face the possibility that it may be unsuccessful. Women who fail to become pregnant following any type of fertility therapy experience grief and depression before, during, and after treatment. Women may feel despair, anger, and a loss of control as their hopes of becoming pregnant fade. Effective coping behaviors and a strong network of family and friends appear to reduce a couple's emotional stress. If treatment fails, some couples accept happiness without their own biological children in their lives, whereas other couples may opt for adoption.

We had been trying to have a baby for several years. It was so frustrating because all of our friends were having babies. We felt so many things—guilt, embarrassment, fear, and anger. Finally, after a lot of testing, we tried IVF and it worked! We have a little girl. It was a long and difficult journey to have her, but we are so pleased.
—35-year-old woman

Epidemiology

Traditional epidemiological data on pregnancy and childbirth have focused on issues of maternal and child morbidity and mortality. In recent years, an expanded focus has provided insight into other important considerations of pregnancy, childbirth, breastfeeding, and infertility.

Pregnancy

In 2009, a total of 4,130,663 births were recorded in the United States. Teenage birth rates fell to a new record low, continuing a decline that began in 1991. The birth rate fell to 39.1 births per 1,000 females 15–19 years of age in 2004, though significant variations exist in the birth rates for teenagers among racial groups; **Figure 6.10** compares 1991 and 2009 birth rates for White, Black, Hispanic, American Indian, and Asian/Pacific Islander teenagers. Birth rates for women in all age groups from 15 to 39 declined, while rates continued to rise for women 40 to 44 and were unchanged for 45 years and older mothers.[45]

Figure 6.10

Birth rates for teenagers 15–19 years of age by race and Hispanic origin.

Source: Reproduced from Martin, J. A., Hamilton, B. E., Ventura S. J., et al. (2011). Births: Final data for 2009. *National Vital Statistics Reports* 60(1). Hyattsville, MD: National Center for Health Statistics.

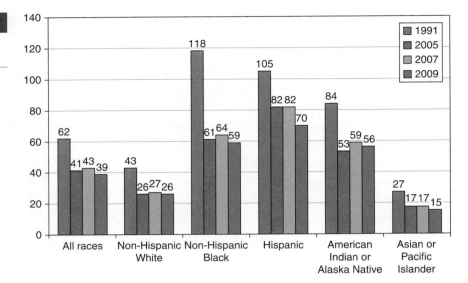

Pregnancy and childbirth are safe experiences for many women; however, any medical or obstetric complication is one too many. In the early 1900s, 1 in 150 women died from causes related to pregnancy, with the death rate among women of color being nearly double that of White women.[46] These deaths were typically caused by infection, toxemia, abortion, and hemorrhage. Today, leading causes of pregnancy-related deaths include cardiovascular disease, hemorrhage, and pregnancy-related hypertension. In 1900, there were approximately 850 maternal deaths per 100,000 live births in the United States. Today, U.S. maternal deaths are about 1% of that number. Although this reduction in maternal mortality is impressive, women of color are still three to four times more likely than White women to die of pregnancy-related causes, and the risk for Black women is the highest among all racial groups (**Figure 6.11**). The pregnancy-related mortality ratio for 2006 to 2007 was 15.1 deaths per 100,000 live births.[47]

The **infant mortality rate** (also called the infant death rate) is the number of children dying under a year of age divided by the number of live births that year. This rate is an important measure of the well-being of infants, children, and pregnant women because it is associated with factors such as maternal health, quality of and access to medical care, socioeconomic conditions, and public health practices. In 2008, the U.S. infant mortality rate was 6.61 infant deaths per 1,000 live births.[48] As **Figure 6.12** shows, the rates range from 4.51 deaths per 1,000 live births for Asian or Pacific Islander mothers to 12.67 for non-Hispanic Black mothers. Infant mortality rates were higher for infants who were born in multiple deliveries or whose

mothers were teenagers or aged 40 and older. Infant mortality was also higher for male infants and infants born preterm or at low birth weight. Congenital malformations, low birth weight, and sudden infant death syndrome (SIDS) accounted for 45% of the infant deaths.

Low birth weight is defined as a birth weight of less than 2,500 grams (5.5 pounds); this and the period of gestation are the most important predictors of an infant's subsequent health and survival. Because of their much greater risk of death, infants born at the lowest birth weights and

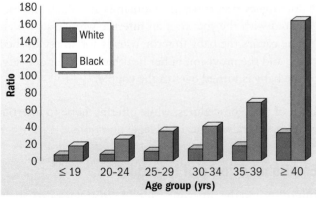

Deaths per 100,000 live births.

Figure 6.11

Pregnancy-mortality ratios, by age and race, United States, 1991–1999.

Source: Chang, J., et al. (2003). Pregnancy-related mortality surveillance—United States, 1991–1999. *Morbidity and Mortality Weekly Report* 52 (SS02): 1–8.

Figure 6.12

Infant mortality rates by race and ethnicity of mother: United States, 2008.

Source: Data from Mathews, T. J., and MacDorman, M. F. (2012). Centers for Disease Control and Prevention. Infant mortality statistics from the 2008 period linked birth/infant death data set. *National Vital Statistics Reports* 60(5).

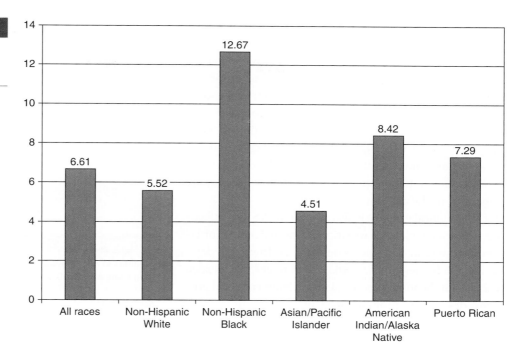

gestational ages have a large impact on overall U.S. infant mortality. In 2008, infants weighing less than 1,000 grams accounted for only 0.8% of births but nearly one-half of all infant deaths in the United States. A similar pattern is seen with infant gestation data. Only 0.8% of births occurred at less than 28 weeks of gestation, but they too account for nearly one-half of all infant deaths in the United States.[48]

I cannot remember much about the birth of my first baby. I was young and scared, and I only wanted to be "knocked out." Afterwards, I realized that I had missed one of the most important events of my life. With my second baby, we went to classes and I read everything I could. I really was prepared. I felt so much more in control of what was happening to me. Birth is something too wonderful to miss.

—30-year-old woman

Breastfeeding

Breastfeeding rates in the United States have increased since 1999, with the United States as a whole and 25 states achieving the Healthy People 2010 goal of 3 out of every 4 new mothers initiating breastfeeding in 2010. Rates of exclusive breastfeeding at 3 and 6 months and breastfeeding at 6 and 12 months, however, remain low. Among children born in 2008, 75% initiated breastfeeding, 44% were breastfeeding at 6 months, and 24% were breastfeeding at 12 months of age (**Figure 6.13**).[49] Only 35% were exclusively breastfeeding at 3 months and 15% were exclusively breastfeeding at 6 months.

Worksite support for working nursing mothers is an important challenge for many women. In one national study, the availability of employer-sponsored childcare was found to increase the likelihood of breastfeeding 6 months after birth by 47%. In addition, on average, working an additional 8 hours at home per week increased the probability of breastfeeding initiation by 8% and breastfeeding 6 months after birth by 16.8%.[50]

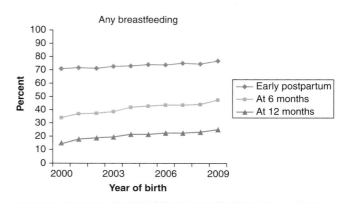

Figure 6.13

Percent of U.S. children who were breastfed by birth year, United States.

Source: Reproduced from Centers for Disease Control and Prevention. (2009). Breastfeeding among U.S. children born 2000–2009. CDC National Immunization Survey. Downloaded September 13, 2012 from: http://www.cdc.gov/breastfeeding/data/NIS_data/index.htm.

Studies on breastfeeding in the United States have historically shown substantial racial/ethnic and socioeconomic disparities. In a national study, immigrant women in each racial/ethnic group had higher breastfeeding initiation and longer duration rates than native women of the same racial/ethnic group. Acculturation was associated with lower breastfeeding rates among both Hispanic and non-Hispanic women.[51] In another study, researchers found that immigration status was strongly associated with increased breastfeeding initiation, suggesting that cultural factors are important in the decision to breastfeed.[52]

Geographical variance is also a factor in U.S. breastfeeding. There are wide state variations in breastfeeding initiation and duration, with the western and northwestern states having the highest rates.[53] Additional research is needed to ascertain the influence of state legislation and local programs designed to promote breastfeeding practices.

Fertility

Technically, fertility simply denotes successful production of offspring. The U.S. Census Bureau collects fertility data and provides reports showing historical trends with childbearing and associated sociodemographic data. Recent fertility data indicate the following trends:[54]

- More women in their early 40s are childless, and those who are having children are having fewer than ever before. In the last 30 years, the number of women ages 40 to 44 with no children has doubled.

- Women 40 to 44 years old will end their childbearing years with an average of 1.9 children each. Hispanic women will have an average of 2.3 children each, higher than that of White non-Hispanic, Black, or Asian women.

- About 36% of women who gave birth in the previous 12 months were separated, divorced, widowed, or unmarried.

- Unemployed women had about twice as many babies as working women, although women in the labor force accounted for the majority (57%) of recent births.

- One-quarter of all women who had a child in the past year were living below the poverty level.

Infertility

Infertility is usually defined as not being able to get pregnant after trying for 1 year. Of the 62 million women of reproductive age in 2002, about 1.2 million, or 2%, had an infertility-related medical appointment within the previous

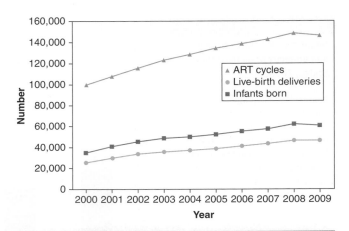

Figure 6.14

Numbers of ART cycles performed, live-birth deliveries, and infants born using ART, 2000–2009.

Source: Reproduced from Centers for Disease Control and Prevention. (2011). Assisted reproductive technology (ART) report: section 5—ART Trends, 2000-2009. Downloaded May 20, 2012 from http://www.cdc.gov/art/ART2009/sect5_fig51-63.htm#f51.

year, and 8% had an infertility-related medical visit at some point in the past. Infertility services include medical tests to diagnose infertility, medical advice and treatments to help a woman become pregnant, and services other than routine prenatal care to prevent miscarriage. Additionally, 7% of married couples in which the woman was of reproductive age (2.1 million couples) reported that they had not used contraception for 12 months and the woman had not become pregnant.[55] Assisted reproductive technology is associated with a substantial risk for multiple births. **Figure 6.14** shows the number of ART cycles performed, live-birth delivery, and infants born using ART from 1996 to 2005.

Informed Decision Making

Informed decision making about pregnancy should begin before conception. The newly conceived offspring depends on its mother for nutrition and well-being weeks before the mother may know that she is pregnant. If the mother is a smoker or is abusing alcohol or drugs during this critical early period of development, her child is at a decided disadvantage.

Pregnancy

A pregnant woman has to take good care of herself to provide the best care for her unborn child. Regular prenatal care that begins early in the pregnancy is essential and is associated with reduced infant morbidity and mortality.

Most women see their clinician once a month during the pregnancy until week 28. In the last trimester, this frequency increases to every other week until week 36, when weekly visits until delivery are indicated. Proper nutrition; adequate and appropriate exercise; and avoidance of alcohol, tobacco, caffeine, and illegal drugs are all essential components of good prenatal care.

Childbirth

Childbirth is a personal, special, and an irreplaceable event. Preparation for birthing helps to ensure the best possible experience. Childbirth education classes provide many valuable opportunities for learning, practical preparation, and building skills for a rewarding and facilitated childbirth experience. They also provide an opportunity to share concerns and discuss plans. Local resources for childbirth options, such as birthing centers or home deliveries, can be evaluated. Classes provide motivation to learn relaxation and pain management techniques. Strategies that are taught may include breathing techniques, such as **Lamaze**; relaxation techniques; muscle-strengthening exercises; and different positions that facilitate labor, thereby promoting an uncomplicated birth. Resources in childbirth preparation vary. Some communities offer many resources; in other communities, resources are rather few and far between. To maximize the benefits from a childbirth education class, the qualifications of the instructor, class size, and class focus should be carefully evaluated.

Breastfeeding

Breastfeeding can be a very rewarding experience. Women who have difficulty beginning the process are encouraged to "stick with it" as both the mother and the infant learn how to work with each other. Although suckling is instinctual for the infant, feeding from the breast is a learned behavior for the mother. Adjusting positions, anticipating the infant's hunger, and relaxing during the feeding are ways to make breastfeeding more pleasurable for both mother and infant. Breastfeeding assistance is usually offered postpartum at the hospital, and lactation specialists also are available for women when they return home with the baby. Aside from the bond created between mother and

© Michael Newman/PhotoEdit, Inc.

■ Hospitals and birthing centers often have lactation specialists on staff to help new mothers learn the ropes of breastfeeding.

Profiles of Remarkable Women

Martha May Eliot, M.D. (1891–1978)

Martha May Eliot, a pioneer in maternal and child health, graduated from Radcliffe College and the medical school at Johns Hopkins University. She taught at Yale University's Department of Pediatrics until 1935, while also directing the National Children's Bureau Division of Child and Maternal Health. As Bureau Chief, Eliot conducted community studies, exploring issues of social medicine and ways that public health measures could prevent disease. She also drafted most of the Social Security Act's language dealing with maternal and child health in 1934. During World War II, Eliot provided care for more than 1 million servicemen's wives through the Emergency Maternity and Infant Care program. She continued her involvement with women's and children's health after the war by working with the World Health Organization (WHO) and the United Nations Children's Fund (UNICEF) in significant capacities.

After leaving her position at the National Children's Bureau Division of Maternal and Child Health, Eliot became Department Chair of Child and Maternal Health at Harvard University's School of Public Health. She received many honors throughout her lifetime that recognized her work as a leading pediatrician and the force behind many maternal and child health programs. She was one of the first women admitted into the American Pediatric Society, the first woman elected president of the American Public Health Association (APHA), and the first woman to receive APHA's Sedgwick Memorial Medal. APHA now awards the Martha May Eliot Award to recognize others' achievements in maternal and child health.

child, breastfeeding offers significant health benefits to both parties.

Infertility

Infertility should be recognized as a problem of a couple, not the woman or her partner. Because the factors that reduce fertility are shared, both partners must be evaluated when initiating an infertility workup. Infertility services are widely available today, and evolving technologies have enabled many couples to have a child. Infertility clinics can offer couples information, support, and procedures to address their specific needs. Identification of infertility services is often facilitated through referral from a gynecologist.

■■■■
Summary

Pregnancy, childbirth, and breastfeeding are exciting, yet complex, dimensions of women's health. Cultural, historical, legal, and ethical factors influence how women deal with pregnancy, give birth, and care for their infants. Understanding the physiological causes for the physical and emotional changes that occur in a pregnant woman can often help make the pregnancy process more manageable. Prenatal care is a vital component of a healthy pregnancy, and usually includes nutritional counseling, genetic testing, ultrasounds, and ongoing monitoring of the mother and baby. Many women experience the changes of pregnancy and the birth of their child without complications. Others learn firsthand the emotional hardships of infertility, miscarriage, diagnosis of abnormalities in the fetus, premature delivery, or complications during the delivery. For couples who have difficulty conceiving, a host of medical and surgical options exist to achieve a pregnancy; however, these methods are imperfect and often carry a high financial (as well as emotional) cost. As with other areas of women's health, informed decision making is critical throughout the prenatal to postnatal periods.

■■■■
Topics for Discussion

1. What are the possible advantages and disadvantages of treating childbirth as a "medical" condition (i.e., constant medical care led by doctors and healthcare providers, hospitalization, etc.)?

2. Should pregnant women be restricted in their access to tobacco, alcohol, or drugs?

3. What should you do, if anything, if you see a young mother smoking? What if she is drinking or not wearing a seatbelt?

4. Should preparation for childbirth be required for all women?

5. Discuss the rights of pregnant teenagers as parents. What rights do a teen's parents have in regard to her pregnancy?

6. Does the father of the child have any say in pregnancy decisions if the mother and father are not married?

7. What are possible ethical and legal dilemmas associated with infertility techniques and treatments?

■■■■
Key Terms

Abruptio placentae: A complication of pregnancy in which the placenta separates prematurely from the wall of the uterus.

Afterbirth: The placenta and amniotic sac that are expelled from the womb after the baby is delivered.

Amniocentesis: Procedure between the 16th and 20th weeks of pregnancy intended to detect fetal defects. The amniotic sac is punctured with a needle and syringe, and amniotic fluid is obtained for analysis.

Amnion: The innermost membrane of the amniotic sac, which contains the amniotic fluid.

Amniotic fluid: Watery fluid that surrounds a developing embryo and fetus in the uterus.

Artificial insemination: Introduction of semen into the uterus or oviduct by unnatural means close to the time of ovulation. It is most often used when the infertility problem is male related.

Assisted reproductive technologies (ART): Any treatment or procedure that involves the handling of human eggs and sperm with the purpose of helping a woman become pregnant.

Blastocyst: A mass of embryonic cells that results from repeated divisions of the zygote.

Braxton–Hicks contractions: The contraction of the uterus at irregular intervals throughout pregnancy. These contractions are not like "real" labor contractions in that they do not gradually increase in frequency, intensity, or duration.

Breech: Birth presentation in which the feet, knees, or buttocks of the fetus present before the head.

Cephalopelvic disproportion: A complication of pregnancy in which the size of the baby's head is deemed too large or the mother's birth canal is too small to accommodate vaginal delivery. This condition is an indication for cesarean delivery.

Cesarean delivery: The surgical procedure in which an infant is delivered through an incision made in the abdominal wall and uterus.

Chorionic villus sampling (CVS): A procedure performed to detect fetal abnormalities in which samples of chorionic villi are removed and examined.

Chromosomes: The structures in the nucleus of each cell composed of DNA and protein that contain the genes that provide information for the transmission of inherited characteristics.

Colostrum: Early milk, or milk produced during the pregnancy and for 3 to 5 days after birth. Colostrum is yellowish in color, thicker than milk, and rich with protective antibodies and protein.

Conceptus: The products of conception or fertilization, including the fertilized egg and its enclosing membranes.

Corpus luteum: A yellowish body that forms on the ovary at the site of the ruptured follicle where the egg has been released. It secretes progesterone to help prepare the body for pregnancy.

Cytomegalovirus (CMV): A viral infection that causes mild flu-like symptoms in adults but that can cause small birth size, brain damage, developmental problems, enlarged liver, hearing and vision impairment, and other malformations in newborns. Babies with CMV are infected in utero, although only 10% of those so infected have symptoms. Pregnant women often acquire CMV from infected children with few or no symptoms. Cytomegalovirus is the most common prenatal infection today, and it is an opportunistic infection of HIV/AIDS.

Diagnostic tests: Medical tests used to detect a disease or condition.

Dizygotic twins: Two offspring developed from two eggs released from the ovary and fertilized at the same time. They may be the same or opposite sex and may differ physically and in genetic traits. Also called fraternal twins.

Down syndrome: A congenital condition characterized by various degrees of mental retardation and abnormal development. It is caused by the presence of an extra chromosome, usually number 21 or 22.

Ectopic pregnancy: The implantation of a fertilized egg outside the uterus.

Effacement: The thinning of the cervix before delivery.

Egg donation: A type of assisted reproductive technology used when a woman is unable to produce eggs or has a genetic disorder that will be passed on to her child. Egg donors must be willing to dedicate an enormous amount of time to this effort because of the drug treatment and monitoring that they must undergo.

Embryo: An organism in its early stage of development in humans. The embryonic period lasts from the second to the eighth week of pregnancy.

Embryo transfer: A fertility procedure in which the sperm of the infertile woman's partner are placed in another woman's uterus during ovulation. The fertilized egg is removed a few days later and transferred to the uterus of the infertile woman.

Epidural anesthesia: A type of anesthetic used during delivery that is injected through a catheter placed in a space beside the spinal cord. Epidurals are the most common choice of anesthesia made by pregnant women and allow the mother to be awake for the birth.

Fecundity: The physical ability of a woman to have a child. Women with impaired fecundity include those who find it physically difficult or medically inadvisable to conceive or deliver a child.

Fertilization: The union of an ovum and a sperm.

Fetal alcohol syndrome (FAS): Alcohol-related defects among infants caused by prenatal maternal alcohol consumption. They are usually characterized by growth retardation, facial malformations, and central nervous system dysfunctions including mental retardation.

Fetal distress: Signs of distress in the fetus, such as slowing of heart rate or acid in the blood.

Fetus: The unborn baby in the uterus from the eighth week of gestation until birth.

Folate: A B vitamin found in foods such as chickpeas, spinach, strawberries, kidney beans, and citrus fruits and juices.

Folic acid: A form of folate used to fortify grain-based foods, such as bread, flour, rice, pasta, and cereal.

It is vital for cell growth and function and for the development of a healthy neural tube in fetuses.

Forceps: Surgical instruments used for grasping. Obstetric forceps may be used to extract a baby from the birth canal during delivery.

Galactosemia: An inherited disease characterized by the lack of the enzyme needed for processing galactose (sugars in milk products); can cause mental retardation if not treated properly.

Gamete intrafallopian transfer (GIFT): A procedure for treating infertility that involves placing sperm and egg cells into the fallopian tubes.

Gestational diabetes: A form of diabetes that develops in 2% to 5% of all pregnancies, but usually disappears when the pregnancy is over.

Group B streptococcus (GBS): A type of bacterium that can cause illness in newborn babies and pregnant women. Pregnant women with GBS do not necessarily infect their babies; however, babies who develop signs and symptoms are at risk of sepsis, pneumonia, meningitis, long-term disabilities such as hearing or vision loss, and death. Obstetricians can test women for GBS and prevent disease by administering antibiotics intravenously during labor.

Host uterus: A procedure in which the sperm from a man and the egg from a woman are combined in a laboratory. The fertilized egg then is implanted into the uterus of a second woman, who agrees to bear the child who is not genetically related to her.

Human chorionic gonadatropin (hCG): A hormone produced by the chorionic villi in a pregnant woman.

Implantation: The embedding of the fertilized ovum in the uterine lining 6 to 7 days after fertilization.

In vitro fertilization (IVF): A procedure for treating infertility that involves removing the ova from a woman ovary. The ova and the sperm (from the woman's partner) are placed in a medium; if fertilization occurs, the conceptus is injected into the woman's uterus.

Infant mortality rate: The number of deaths of children less than 1 year old divided by the number of live births that year. The infant mortality rate is an important epidemiological indicator of the well-being of pregnant women, infants, and children.

Infertility: The inability to conceive a child.

Intracytoplasmic sperm injection (ICSI): A procedure for treating infertility that involves the injection of a single sperm directly into a mature egg.

Lamaze: A method of childbirth preparation in which the expectant mother is prepared psychologically and physically through breathing exercises and concentration to control pain during childbirth while maintaining consciousness.

Mastitis: An infection in the breast, usually caused by bacterial infection. It results in localized pain, redness, and heat with symptoms of fever, nausea, and vomiting.

Maternal serum alpha feto-protein (MSAFP): A prenatal screening test that measures a substance produced by the baby's kidneys found in the mother's blood between the 13th and 20th weeks of pregnancy.

Miscarriage: A pregnancy that terminates before the 20th week of gestation because of fetal defects or pregnancy problems.

Monozygotic twins: Two offspring developed from one fertilized egg that splits into equal halves. Monozygotic twins are of the same sex, share the same genes, and look nearly identical. Also called identical twins.

Neural tube defects: Defects of the spine and brain caused by failure of the neural tube to close during pregnancy.

Placenta: An organ that develops after implantation where the embryo attaches via the umbilical cord for nourishment and waste removal.

Placenta previa: A complication of pregnancy in which the birth canal becomes obstructed by the placenta.

Preeclampsia: A complication of pregnancy characterized by high blood pressure, swelling caused by fluid retention, and high levels of protein in the urine. Also called toxemia.

Premature labor: Labor that begins before the completed ninth month of fetal gestation.

Prolapsed cord: A complication of pregnancy in which the umbilical cord comes through the pelvis before the baby. It can result in a disrupted flow of oxygen to the baby due to a compressed cord.

Rh incompatability: A condition that occurs when an Rh-negative mother and an Rh-positive father conceive a baby who inherits the father's Rh-positive blood type. This situation may present problems during pregnancy, labor, and delivery if the fetus's Rh-positive blood cells enter the mother's bloodstream.

Rubella: An infectious disease often causing birth defects in pregnant women. Also called German measles.

Stillbirth: Death occurring before or during birth of a fetus of sufficient size and age to be otherwise expected to survive.

Surrogacy: A procedure for treating infertility in which a woman is artificially inseminated with the sperm of an infertile woman's partner. She then carries the pregnancy to term for the infertile couple.

Thrush: A yeast infection that infects the mouth.

Toxemia: A complication of pregnancy characterized by high blood pressure, swelling caused by fluid retention, and high levels of protein in the urine. Also called preeclampsia.

Ultrasound: A procedure that uses high-frequency sound waves to project an image of structures inside the body, such as an organ or a fetus during pregnancy.

Varicocele: A mesh of varicose veins in and around the testicle, which is associated with infertility and may have to be treated with surgery.

Zygote: A fertilized egg.

Zygote intrafallopian transfer (ZIFT): A method of assisted reproductive technology in which a fertilized egg is placed in the fallopian tube, allowing the zygote to continue its cell division and become implanted in the uterus naturally.

■■■■
Websites

American Academy of Pediatrics: http://www.aap.org

Centers for Disease Control and Prevention: Breastfeeding: http://www.cdc.gov/breastfeeding

Centers for Disease Control and Prevention: Reproductive Health Information Source: http://www.cdc.gov/reproductivehealth

La Leche League International: http://www.lalecheleague.org

March of Dimes: http://www.marchofdimes.com

National Campaign to Prevent Teen Pregnancy: http://www.teenpregnancy.org

Resolve: The National Infertility Association: http://www.resolve.org

■■■■
References

1. Bogda, J. C. (1990). Childbirth in America, 1650 to 1990. In R. D. Apple (ed.). *Women, health, and medicine in America.* New York, NY: Garland Publishers.

2. Wertz, R. W., & Wertz, D. C. (1977). *Lying-in: A history of childbirth in America.* New York, NY: Free Press.

3. Leavitt, J. W. (1986). *Brought to bed: Childbirthing in America, 1750–1950.* New York, NY: Oxford University Press.

4. Hodnett, E. D., Gates, S., Hofmeyr, G. J., et al. (2007). Continuous support for women during childbirth. *Cochrane Database of Systematic Reviews.* Jul 18;(3):CD003766.

5. Mansfield, B. (2008). The social nature of natural childbirth. *Social Science Medicine* 66(5): 1084–1094.

6. Barness, L. A. (1991). Brief history of infant nutrition and view to the future. *Pediatrics* 88: 1054–1056.

7. Ansley, D. (1992). Spermtales. *Discover* 13(6): 66–69.

8. Tomlinson, C., Marshall, J., & Ellis, J. E. (2008). Comparison of accuracy and certainty of results of six home pregnancy tests available over-the-counter. *Current Medical Research Opinion* 24(6): 1645–1649.

9. Williams, L. J., Rasmussen, S. A., Flores, A., et al. D. (2005). Decline in the prevalence of spina bifida and anencephaly by race/ethnicity: 1995–2002. *Pediatrics* 116(3): 580–586.

10. IOM [Institute of Medicine] and NRC [National Research Council]. (2009). *Weight gain during pregnancy: Reexamining the guidelines.* Washington, DC: The National Academies Press.

11. American College of Obstetricians and Gynecologists [ACOG]. (2011). *Exercise during pregnancy.* Available at: http://www.acog.org/~/media/For%20Patients/faq119.pdf

12. Centers for Disease Control and Prevention [CDC]. (2007). *Preventing smoking and exposure to secondhand smoke before, during, and after pregnancy fact sheet.* Available at: http://www.cdc.gov/nccdphp/publications/factsheets/Prevention/pdf/smoking.pdf

13. Aliyu, M. H., Wilson, R. E., Zoorob, R., et al. (2008). Alcohol consumption during pregnancy and the risk of early stillbirth among singletons. *Alcohol* 42(5): 369–374.

14. Centers for Disease Control and Prevention [CDC]. (2009). Alcohol use among pregnant and nonpregnant women of childbearing age—United States, 1991–2005. *Morbidity and Mortality Weekly Report* 58(19): 529–532.

15. Substance Abuse and Mental Health Services Administration. (2011). *Results from the 2010 National Survey on Drug Use and Health: Summary of national findings*. Rockville, MD: Office of Applied Studies. NSDUH Series H-41, DHHS, Publication No. SMA 11-4658.

16. March of Dimes. (2008). *Illicit drug use during pregnancy*. Available at: http://www.marchofdimes.com/pregnancy/alcohol_illicitdrug.html

17. Papanikolaou, N. C., Hatzidaki, E. G., Belivanis, S., et al. (2005). Lead toxicity update. A brief review. *Medical Science Monitor* 11(10): RA329–RA336.

18. Froehlich, T.E., Lanphear, B. P., Auinger, P., et al. (2009). Association of tobacco and lead exposures with attention-deficit/hyperactivity disorder. *Pediatrics* 123(60): 1054–1063.

19. Chambers, C. D. (2006). Risks of hypothermia associated with hot tub or spa use by pregnant women. Birth Defects Research. Part A. *Clinical and Molecular Teratology* 76(8): 569–573.

20. Centers for Disease Control and Prevention [CDC]. (2008). Update on overall prevalence of major birth defects—Atlanta, Georgia, 1978–2005. *Morbidity and Mortality Weekly Report* 57:1–5.

21. Eddleman, K. A., First and Second Trimester Evaluation of Risk (FASTER) Trial Research Consortium. (2006). Pregnancy loss rates after midtrimester amniocentesis. *Obstetrics and Gynecology* 108(5): 1067–1072.

22. Moore, L. E. (2008). Recurrent risk of adverse pregnancy outcome. *Obstetrics and Gynecology Clinics of North America* 35(3): 459–471.

23. Centers for Disease Control and Prevention [CDC]. (2003). Pregnancy-related mortality surveillance—United States, 1991–1999. *Morbidity and Mortality Weekly Report Surveillance Summary* 52:1–8.

24. Centers for Disease Control and Prevention [CDC]. (2011). National diabetes fact sheet: National estimates and general information on diabetes and prediabetes in the United States, 2011. Accessed at: http://www.cdc.gov/diabetes/pubs/factsheet11.htm

25. Martin, J. A., Hamilton, B. E., Ventura, S. J., et al. (2011). Births: final data for 2009. *National Vital Statistics Reports* 60(1).

26. Schieve, L. A., Tatham, L., Peterson, H. B., et al. (2003). Spontaneous abortion among pregnancies conceived using assisted reproductive technology in the United States. *Obstetrics and Gynecology* 101(5): 959.

27. Heffner, L. J. (2004). Advanced maternal age—how old is too old? *New England Journal of Medicine* 351(19): 1927–1929.

28. Côté-Arsenault, D. (2007). Threat appraisal, coping, and emotions across pregnancy subsequent to perinatal loss. Nursing Research 56(2): 108–116.

29. Watson, M. S., Mann, M. Y., Lloyd-Puryear, M. A., et al. (2006). Newborn screening: toward a uniform screening panel and system. *Genetics in Medicine* 8(Suppl 5): 1S–11S.

30. Centers for Disease Control and Prevention [CDC]. (2007). Mother-to-child (perinatal) HIV transmission and prevention. Available at: http://www.cdc.gov/hiv/topics//perinatal/resources/factsheets/pdf/perinatal.pdf

31. Centers for Disease Control and Prevention [CDC]. (2006). Sexually transmitted diseases treatment guidelines 2006. Available at: http://www.cdc.gov/std/treatment/2006/specialpops.htm#specialpops1

32. Centers for Disease Control and Prevention [CDC]. (2010). Congenital CMV infection trends and statistics. Available at: http://www.cdc.gov/cmv/trends-stats.html

33. Centers for Disease Control and Prevention [CDC]. (2008). Group B strep infection in newborns. Available at: http://www.cdc.gov/groupbstrep/about/newborns-pregnant.html

34. Klein, M. C., Sakala, C., Simkim, P. et al. (2006). Why do women go along with this stuff? *Birth* 33(3): 245–250.

35. Romano, A. M., & Lothian, J. A. (2008). Promoting, protecting, and supporting normal birth: a look at the evidence. *Obstetric, Gynecologic, and Neonatal Nursing* 37(1): 94–105.

36. Podulka, J., Stranges, E., and Steiner, C. (2011). *Hospitalizations related to childbirth, 2008. HCUP Statistical Brief #110*. Available online: http://www.hcup-us.ahrq.gov/reports/statbriefs/sb110.pdf

37. National Center for Health Statistics. (2011). Births: Final data for 2009. *National Vital Statistics Reports* 60(1).

38. American College of Obstetricians and Gynecologists [ACOG]. (2010). Vaginal birth after previous cesarean section. *ACOG Practice Bulletin* 115.

39. American Academy of Pediatrics. (2012). Policy statement: Breastfeeding and the use of human milk. *Pediatrics* 129(3): e827–e841.

40. Kramer, M.S., Aboud, F., Mironova, E., et al. (2008). Breastfeeding and child cognitive development: New evidence from a large randomized clinical trial. *Archives of General Psychiatry* 65(5): 578–584.

41. Keister, D., Roberts, K. T., & Werner, S. L. (2008). Strategies for breastfeeding success. *American Family Physician* 78(2): 225–232.

42. Centers for Disease Control and Prevention [CDC], American Society for Reproductive Medicine, Society for Assisted Reproductive Technology. (2011). 2009 assisted reproductive technology success rates: National summary and fertility clinic reports. Available at: http://www.cdc.gov/art/ART2009/

43. Martin, J. A., Hamilton, B. E., Ventura, S. J., et al. (2011). Births: final data for 2009. *National Vital Statistics Reports* 60(1): 1–70.

44. Rochat, R. W., Koonin, L. M., Atrash, H. K., et al. (1988). Maternal mortality in the United States: report from the Maternal Mortality Collaborative. *Obstetrics and Gynecology* 72(1): 91–97.

45. Berg C. J., Callaghan W. M., Syverson C., et al. (2010). Pregnancy-related mortality in the United States, 1998–2005. *Obstetrics and Gynecology* 116:1302–1309.

46. Mathews, T. J., & MacDorman, M. F. (2012). Infant mortality statistics from the 2008 period linked birth/infant death data set. *National Vital Statistics Reports* 60(5): 1–49.

47. Centers for Disease Control and Prevention [CDC]. (2011). Breastfeeding report card—United States, 2011. Available online: http://www.cdc.gov/breastfeeding/pdf/2011BreastfeedingReportCard.pdf

48. Jacknowitz, A. (2008). The role of workplace characteristics in breastfeeding practices. *Women's Health* 47(2): 87–111.

49. Singh, G. K., Kogan, M. D., & Dee, D. L. (2007). Nativity/immigration status, race/ethnicity, and sociodemographic determinants of breastfeeding initiation and duration in the United States, 2003. *Pediatrics* 119(Suppl 1): S38–S46.

50. Celi, A. C., Rich-Edwards, J. W., Richardson, M. K., et al. (2005). Immigration, race/ethnicity, and social and economic factors as predictors of breastfeeding initiation. *Archives of Pediatrics and Adolescent Medicine* 159(3): 255–260.

51. Centers for Disease Control and Prevention [CDC]. (2010). Racial and ethnic differences in breastfeeding initiation and duration, by state—National Immunization Survey, United States, 2004–2008. *Morbidity and Mortality Weekly Report* 59(11):327–334.

52. Dye, J. L. (2008). *Fertility of American women*. Current Population Reports. U.S. Census Bureau. Washington, D.C. Available at: http://www.census.gov/prod/2008pubs/p20-558.pdf.

53. Centers for Disease Control and Prevention [CDC]. (2008). *Assisted reproductive technology*. Available at: http://www.cdc.gov/ART/

Chapter Seven

Sexually Transmitted Infections

Chapter Objectives

On completion of this chapter, the student should be able to discuss:

1. Basic information about bacterial, viral, and parasitic sexually transmitted infections (STIs), how they are transmitted, and how they affect the body.

2. Relative infection rates of STIs in women, the United States as a whole, and different ethnic groups.

3. Biological and cultural reasons why STIs disproportionately affect and infect women and people of color.

4. How stigma associated with STIs hurts people who are infected and slows prevention and treatment efforts.

5. Routes of transmission, symptoms, and course of infection for each of the major sexually transmitted infections in the United States.

6. The links between HPV, cervical cancer, and genital warts, and the importance of screening for HPV.

7. National and global trends related to the AIDS epidemic.

8. The course of HIV/AIDS infection and how treatment works.

9. The role of open communication, both with clinicians and with partners, in regard to STIs.

10. The importance of personal responsibility and risk reduction in making decisions about one's sexual life.

womenshealth.jbpub.com

Women's Health Online is a great source for supplementary women's health information for both students and instructors. Visit

http://womenshealth.jbpub.com

to find a variety of useful tools for learning, thinking, and teaching.

Introduction

Infections passed from one person to another through sexual intimacy are known as **sexually transmitted infections (STIs)**. At least 20 distinct infections are transmitted through sexual contact. Sexually transmitted infections pose significant health risks for women: Women are not only at higher risk for acquiring STIs than men, but they also suffer greater complications from these conditions. Sexually transmitted infections include chlamydia, gonorrhea, herpes, hepatitis, human papillomavirus (HPV), and human immunodeficiency virus (HIV). Sexually associated infections, which may be acquired sexually or nonsexually, include trichomoniasis, yeast infections, and bacterial vaginosis.

The consequences of STIs depend on the organism causing the infection. Gonorrhea and chlamydia can permanently damage the reproductive system, even in the absence of symptoms. Herpes is an incurable disease with painful and often emotionally devastating symptoms, but it usually does not pose a long-term health risk. Infections such as bacterial vaginosis or yeast infections may be major annoyances, but they do not have serious life-threatening sequelae. AIDS, and in some cases syphilis and hepatitis, can threaten life itself. Some infections attack a single structure, such as the labia or cervix, while others can spread throughout the reproductive tract. Some bacteria and viruses may enter the bloodstream and result in systemic effects.

■ Historically, society has looked on STIs as punishment for immoral activity. In addition, women, or women's behaviors, have been viewed as the source of the disease.

Having one STI increases a person's risk of acquiring another STI. For example, an individual with herpes or gonorrhea may be up to seven times more likely than an uninfected person to acquire HIV through sexual contact.[1] STIs also increase a person's infectiousness: An HIV-positive individual infected with another STI is more likely to transmit HIV through sexual contact and to acquire other STIs if exposed.[2]

Sexually transmitted organisms know no class, racial, ethnic, or social barriers. All individuals are vulnerable if exposed to the infectious organism. Society, however, has a tendency to look on STIs as punishment for immoral activity. In addition, women have been viewed as either the source of disease or deserving of infection. Common reactions to finding out about a STI include disbelief, hurt, guilt, embarrassment, anger, fear, shame, and a feeling of loss of control over one's sexuality and health. The emotional effects of some infections are often as serious or worse than the physical consequences.

Viral STIs, which are incurable, bring the added pressure of worry over how the lingering virus will affect present and future relationships. Knowledge and prevention are the best defenses against STIs, followed by early diagnosis and treatment to reduce or eliminate the consequences of infection.

Perspectives on Sexually Transmitted Infections

Historical Overview

Although STIs are a modern epidemic, they are not modern infections. Historical references to STIs reach back thousands of years. The oldest books in the Bible describe diseases that probably were gonorrhea and syphilis. Ancient Greek and Roman physicians identified genital warts and sexually transmitted chancres in their writings; Hippocrates described the mechanism for gonorrhea transmission as "excesses of the pleasures of the Venus." Susruta, an ancient Hindu, also described gonorrhea. In ancient Rome, Tiberius issued a decree outlawing public kissing to curb a herpes epidemic. Spanish explorers may have brought syphilis to Europe from the New World; between 1495 and 1500, syphilis ravaged Europe. Several characters in plays by William Shakespeare's plays appear to have the disease.

Epidemiological Data and Trends

Sexually transmitted infections are a major public health problem, especially among young men and women. The

United States has the highest rate of STI infection in the industrialized world: More than 65 million Americans are now living with an incurable STI. One of every four women in the United States between the ages of 14 and 19—3.2 million adolescents—has a common sexually transmitted infection.[3] Young people make up one-fourth of the sexually experienced population, but have nearly 50% of the country's STIs.[4] There are many reasons for this. Adolescents and young adults are more likely to be sexually active; adolescents also appear to have a greater biological risk of infection. Other factors, such as difficulties accessing appropriate health care, the increased risk of multiple short-term sexual relationships, and inconsistent use of barrier contraception, also increase their risk of exposure.[2]

Measuring the scope of the STI epidemic is a difficult task. Some STIs are reportable conditions (diseases required by federal law to be reported to prevent and control their spread), and national data on them are available. Other STIs are not reportable, and actual incidence rates can only be estimated (**Figure 7.1**). Healthcare providers are required to report cases of chlamydia, gonorrhea, and syphilis, but healthcare facilities vary widely in the manner that they report these diseases. Many STIs are asymptomatic, so many infected individuals are not diagnosed.

Sexually transmitted infection estimates that do exist provide a startling picture of the epidemic. For example, 18% of women between the ages of 15 and 19 have HPV,

and 4% have chlamydia.[3] About one in five Americans has genital herpes. The Centers for Disease Control and Prevention (CDC) estimate that there are almost three million new cases of chlamydia each year in the United States.[4]

There are significant racial disparities in rates of STI infection (**Figure 7.2**). Chlamydia is more than seven times more common among Black females than among White females, and 69% of the recorded cases of gonorrhea in the United States occur among Black Americans.[4] Sexually transmitted infections also affect Hispanic and Native American women at higher rates than non-Hispanic Whites.

These disparities exist for many reasons. In general, people of color have reduced access to testing and care, and are more likely to live in poverty, reducing the chance of effective treatment and increasing the likelihood of complications and disease progression. In general, Americans are also more likely to choose a partner of the same race—and for people of color, this means that a person's sexual partner is more likely to have an STI and to face similar obstacles to testing and treatment. Taken together, these factors have a considerable synergistic effect. In addition to these legitimate disparities, reporting bias may also affect the data collected. Minorities are more likely than Caucasians to visit public clinics, which are often the main source of STI estimates, accounting for some increased reporting of disease among these groups.

Figure 7.1

Estimated incidence (new cases) of major STIs in the United States among American youth (ages 15–24) in 2000.

Source: Weinstock, H., Berman, S., and Cates, W. Jr. (2004). Sexually transmitted diseases among American youth: incidence and prevalence estimates, 2004. *Perspectives on Sexual and Reproductive Health* 36(1). Reprinted with permission from the Guttmacher Institute.

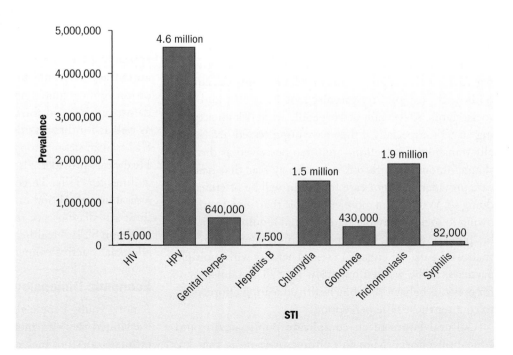

Figure 7.2

Race/ethnicity differences in rates of gonorrhea, chlamydia, and syphilis

Source: Data from Centers for Disease Control and Prevention. (2010). Sexually Transmitted Disease Surveillance.

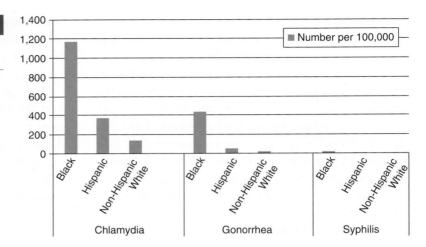

Social Issues and Dimensions

Sexually transmitted infections are biologically sexist, presenting greater risk and causing more complications for women than for men. Women experience most of the STI burden and complications, including infertility, perinatal infections, genital tract neoplasia, and death. In women, STIs are often silent, presenting as asymptomatic but remaining damaging and infectious. Sexually transmitted infections in pregnant women frequently place fetuses at risk of illness, congenital anomalies, developmental disabilities, and death. Because STIs are most prevalent among women aged 15 to 24, these women experience the greatest burden of chronic pelvic pain, pelvic inflammatory disease (PID), ectopic pregnancy, and infertility.[4] Women constitute the majority of individuals living at or below the poverty line in the United States, and people living in poverty are less likely to have access to comprehensive STI diagnostic, treatment, and follow-up services.

Considerable stigma accompanies an STI diagnosis, regardless of the culprit organism. Many people still equate STIs with immorality, promiscuous behavior, and low social status. All sexually active people are at risk for acquiring an STI, especially if they have unprotected sex. Sexually transmitted infections are often perceived as dirty or shameful, and an infected woman may fear that healthcare providers will not care for her or will be offended by doing so. Women are more vulnerable than men to stigma owing to society's double standard that requires women to be "pure" or virginal, while men are often expected to "sow their wild oats," or engage in sexual activity with multiple partners. Some women may view an STI as punishment for previous behavior. Public health education efforts need to counter these false perceptions.

Cultural issues often complicate public health and education efforts. Men in cultures or regions that are intolerant of homosexuality may identify themselves as "straight" while having secret, high-risk encounters with other men, ultimately infecting their girlfriends or wives. Many women are not in charge of contraceptive decision making and may unknowingly put themselves at risk by engaging in sexual activities with philandering or infected partners. Drug-related sexual behaviors (selling or trading sex for drugs), as well as risky sexual activity while under the influence of alcohol and other drugs, greatly increase the risk for STI transmission. Emotions often dominate logical behavior and rational thinking—for example, among sex workers who wear condoms with clients but not with boyfriends, and among teenage girls who believe that condoms are unnecessary when a boyfriend declares his love.

Healthcare providers may also neglect certain populations of women when it comes to screening for these diseases. Women whose sexual partners are exclusively women appear to have a lower prevalence of some STIs, but they are still at risk for infection and therefore should be advised on prevention guidelines. Latex barriers, such as dental dams, can be used for oral–genital or oral–anal contact, as well as for direct skin-to-skin contact, so as to prevent STI transmission among people of all sexual orientations. Healthcare providers also may not screen women with disabilities for STIs. To complicate matters, a woman with a disabling condition may have sensory impairments that limit self-diagnosis or may manifest altered symptoms of common STIs. Healthcare providers should be aware that all sexually active women are vulnerable to STIs.

Economic Dimensions

Among young people alone, the medical costs of STIs in the United States are more than $10 billion each year.[6] This estimate does not include lost wages, loss of productivity due to STI-related illness, out-of-pocket costs, or costs incurred by the transmission of STIs to infants, which can result in significant lifelong expenditures.

For bacterial STIs, complications of untreated chlamydia and gonorrhea present the greatest costs. Without medical attention, these STIs can lead to PID and future fertility problems, leading to even more costs and health concerns. Because viral STIs cannot be cured and may require treatment for years, they tend to cost more than bacterial STIs. The greatest expenses associated with viral STIs result from treatment of precancerous cervical lesions caused by HPV infection and treatment of sexually transmitted HIV infection. In addition to their economic dimensions, STIs carry a high human cost of pain, suffering, and grief. Chlamydia and gonorrhea complications can lead to chronic pain, infertility, and other complications, which can affect a woman's health and well-being throughout her lifetime.

HIV/AIDS creates enormous costs at both the societal and individual levels. The rapid spread of HIV in many parts of the world, especially sub-Saharan Africa, has brought catastrophic economic consequences as the primary wage earners have fallen ill or died. In the United States, the cost of the drugs required to keep HIV infection in check can approach $15,000 per year. People living with HIV/AIDS in the United States are thus a population with special needs for health insurance and prescription drug coverage, as the costs of the disease far exceed the ability of most individuals to pay for necessary services and treatments.

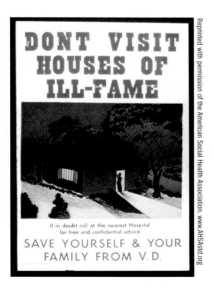

■ Although this public service announcement is more than 50 years old, people still equate STIs with immorality, promiscuous behavior, and low social status.

Over the past decade, global spending on HIV has grown dramatically, allowing more people to receive treatment, get tested, and reduce their chances of infection. From 2004 to 2010 the number of people receiving treatment for HIV in low- and middle-income countries grew by five million.[7] Increased access to treatment has helped to reduce AIDS-related deaths by 19% during the same time period. The mobilization of this money, as well as the logistical efforts to provide and distribute treatment, are a major global achievement. Yet this effort is only the beginning: an additional 10 million people living with HIV still need treatment, and the global recession of 2008–2009 has eliminated or threatened many sources of funding.[7] Continuing the fight against HIV will require a renewed commitment, as well as effective use of resources where they are most needed.

Clinical Dimensions and Treatment

Considerable variation exists in the course of infection, symptoms, and optimal treatment of STIs, depending on the responsible organism. This section reviews the clinical and treatment perspectives of each major STI.

Infection Process

Sexually transmitted infections can be caused by bacteria, viruses, or parasites. Each organism requires a unique diagnostic strategy and treatment.

Bacteria, which cause gonorrhea, chlamydia, syphilis, vaginitis, and many other infections, receive nourishment from the fluid or tissue in which they reside. Their waste products are released into these invaded tissues. The body's **immune system** senses the presence of the foreign bacteria and mobilizes white blood cells to attack them. The infected area becomes warm, red, and swollen owing to the increased circulation and the accumulation of **pus**. The local host cells may be destroyed directly from the bacteria, indirectly from the excessive swelling and waste products, or even by the body's own overzealous immune response. In many cases, bacterial waste products are toxic beyond the local area and may result in systemic conditions of aches, fever, chills, and malaise. An example of a systemic illness produced by bacterial waste products is **toxic shock syndrome**, which is caused by certain strains of *Staphylococcus aureus* bacteria.

Although the immune system routinely fights off invading organisms throughout the body, bacterial infections in the reproductive tract are particularly challenging. The pelvis contains ideal media for bacterial growth and proliferation, especially during menstruation and after a miscarriage or abortion. Bleeding seems to facilitate bacterial invasion, and blood enhances bacterial growth. In addition, many kinds of bacteria normally live in the intestine and vaginal area, so the normal ecosystem of these areas involves a delicate balance of organisms. Harmful bacteria that upset this balance can be killed by antibiotics, but taking such drugs to kill one organism often results in the death of the normal bacteria as well. When these bacteria levels are reduced, yeast colonies may proliferate, and additional treatment may be necessary.

Viruses, which cause herpes, HPV, hepatitis, and HIV, follow unique invasion patterns. These tiny organisms are made of DNA or RNA and are hundreds to thousands of times smaller than bacteria. Their attack mechanism also differs from that of bacteria. Viruses invade normal cells and take over the metabolic functions, replicating themselves thousands or millions of times in the process. As this replication occurs, viruses often destroy their host cells. The body's immune system eventually recognizes invading viruses and responds to them. The immune response is often effective at controlling a viral invasion, but in some cases viruses can stay dormant inside human cells, where the immune system cannot reach them. Viral STIs, especially HIV, present difficult challenges to medical researchers. HIV weakens and even subverts the host immune system, allowing **opportunistic infections** that the body normally fights off easily to invade and proliferate. Because antibiotics are ineffective against viral organisms, researchers are

constantly looking to develop effective antiviral drugs that do not cause harm to the human host.

Ectoparasitic infections are caused by tiny parasites that reside on the skin and survive on human blood and tissue. Although small or invisible to the naked eye, these parasites are many times larger than bacteria or viruses. Parasitic infections include scabies and pubic lice ("crabs"). Parasites cause itching and may cause bumps or a rash, but are easily treated with a topical cream. Parasitic infections are not considered major STIs; although they affect many people, they are more an annoyance than a serious health threat.

Bacterial STIs

Gonorrhea

Despite decades of knowledge about how **gonorrhea** is transmitted and an effective cure in the form of antibiotics, gonorrhea remains prevalent in the United States. In 2010, there were 309,341 reported cases of gonorrhea in the United States.[4] Women, adolescents, and young adults bear the highest burden of this disease. Many women with gonorrhea do not experience any symptoms; instead, gonorrhea is often detected at routine gynecological screenings or when a male partner develops symptoms that lead to clinical treatment. When symptoms do present in women, they may include unusual vaginal discharge or bleeding, painful urination, painful intercourse or bleeding after intercourse, pelvic pain or tenderness, or fever. The gonococcus bacterium thrives in moist, warm cavities. As a consequence, gonococcal infections may present in the reproductive tract, throat, eyes, and rectum. Accurate diagnosis of gonorrhea requires a culture taken from the cervix and urethra, and from the throat and anal area if those areas may have been exposed.

There are several treatment options for gonorrhea, but treatment is complicated by the frequent coexistence of unrecognized chlamydial infection and the increasing incidence of gonorrheal antibiotic-resistant strains. Because neither gonorrhea nor chlamydia may be apparent upon physical examination, gonorrhea treatment usually includes screening for antibiotic resistance and prescribing additional antibiotics to treat chlamydia effectively. The sequelae of gonorrhea are so severe and threatening to general health and reproductive capability that any woman exposed to a partner with gonorrhea, even in the absence of symptoms, should be treated. Symptoms may indicate gonorrhea has spread, so longer and more intensive

Courtesy of CDC

■ Magnified view of herpes simplex virus. About one in four young people in the United States will be affected by a viral STI.

antibiotic treatment is indicated. This often means hospital admission for intravenous antibiotic therapy. About a week after antibiotic treatment for gonorrhea, reculture is necessary for a woman and her partner(s). This follow-up is especially important because gonorrhea is now often resistant to certain antibiotics, and further treatment may be necessary to eliminate the disease.

Reinfection with gonorrhea is common, so sexual intercourse should be avoided until cultures on both partners confirm that treatment was successful. Untreated or unsuccessful treatment of gonorrhea may result in PID or a syndrome caused by disseminated gonococcal infection, which can include septicemia (blood poisoning), joint infection, skin problems, and heart and brain infections.

■ Magnified view of the bacteria that cause chlamydia. Bacterial sexually transmitted infections can be treated with antibiotics, but they often appear without symptoms.

Chlamydia

Chlamydia is the most commonly reported infectious disease in the United States. Young women are most likely to be infected (**Figure 7.3**). More than 1 in 35 women between 15 and 24 years of age in the United States has chlamydia.[5] Chlamydia infections, which are caused by sexually transmitted bacteria, are the leading cause of preventable infertility and ectopic pregnancy. Symptoms of chlamydia are often similar to symptoms of gonorrhea. Most women and about one-half of men with this STI do not have any symptoms. If symptoms are present, women usually experience a yellowish vaginal discharge, burning with urination, or general pain in the lower abdomen. Chlamydia can invade the uterus, fallopian tubes, cervix, urethra, and even liver without symptoms ever manifesting

themselves. When the chlamydia infection moves into the upper reproductive tract, the condition is known as pelvic inflammatory disease (PID).

Chlamydia screening remains one of the most important national efforts to maintain and improve fertility. Routine chlamydia screening could prevent up to 60% of the new cases of PID in the United States.[8] To screen for chlamydia, a healthcare provider may obtain a culture using a cotton swab in the genital area. Newer, more accurate urine-based tests that identify the genetic makeup of the chlamydia bacteria are becoming more common; these tests also make screening easier for men. Because gonorrhea and chlamydia often coexist, culture for gonorrhea is a standard procedure when chlamydia is suspected.

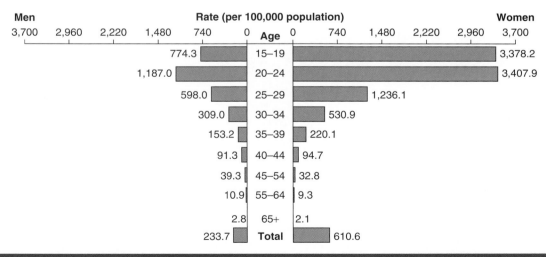

Men						Age	Women					

Rate (per 100,000 population)

Men	Age	Women
774.3	15–19	3,378.2
1,187.0	20–24	3,407.9
598.0	25–29	1,236.1
309.0	30–34	530.9
153.2	35–39	220.1
91.3	40–44	94.7
39.3	45–54	32.8
10.9	55–64	9.3
2.8	65+	2.1
233.7	Total	610.6

Figure 7.3

Chlamydia rates by age and sex, 2010

Source: Reproduced from Centers for Disease Control and Prevention. (2010). Sexually Transmitted Disease Surveillance.

A woman may be treated for chlamydia, even without a confirmed diagnosis, based on symptoms and physical examination. The affected woman's partner(s) should be treated at the same time, and a follow-up examination is usually performed about 4 weeks after treatment to ensure that the therapy was successful. Sexual intercourse should be avoided until after the chlamydia has been cured.

Aggressive treatment is necessary with chlamydia because uterine invasion occurs fairly rapidly, and the invasion process may be asymptomatic. Full PID treatment is undertaken if the organism has invaded the uterus. Treatment delay may result in the organism reaching the fallopian tubes with resultant scarring, tubal obstruction, infertility, and ectopic pregnancy. Pregnant women infected with chlamydia may be at increased risk for spontaneous abortions, stillbirth, preterm delivery, and delivery of low-birthweight infants. Transmission of the organism to the baby may result in eye infections and pneumonia in the infant.

Pelvic Inflammatory Disease

Pelvic inflammatory disease (PID) is a frequent, serious complication of the female reproductive tract (**Figure 7.4**). The infection process may be located in specific areas or spread throughout the pelvic cavity. About one million women in the United States experience PID every year.

Chlamydia and gonorrhea are responsible for most cases of PID, which is a major cause of infertility and hospitalization in young women; medical costs related to PID in the United States are more than $1.3 billion a year.[9] National efforts to screen women at risk seem to be helping to prevent PID, with documented decreases in hospitals, clinics, and doctor's offices over the past 15 years.[4]

Pelvic inflammatory disease symptoms vary considerably. Many women with PID have no symptoms at all, while some women have symptoms that can easily be overlooked or mistaken for something else, such as vaginal discharge, mild but persistent abdominal or back pain, or pain during intercourse. Other women experience sudden and severe pelvic pain, fever, shaking chills, or heavy vaginal discharge or bleeding. Chlamydial PID is more likely to present with the former, more subtle symptoms, and gonorrheal PID is more likely to present with the latter, more severe set of symptoms.

Clinical evaluation is necessary for PID diagnosis. The first step in confirming the presence of PID is eliminating

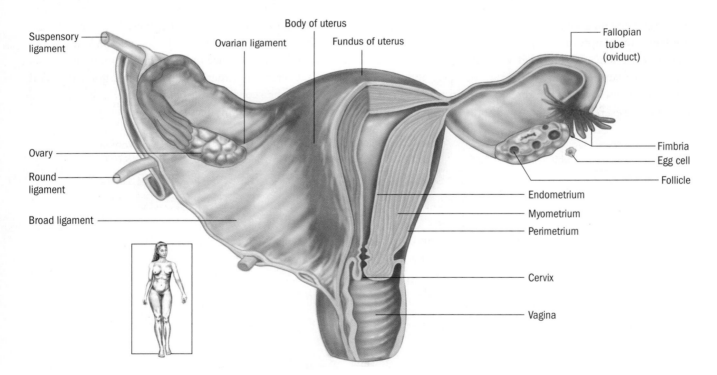

Figure 7.4

Pelvic inflammatory disease can affect any or all of a woman's reproductive organs.

the possibility of other serious conditions that may manifest themselves in a similar manner. Although uterine tenderness and discharge indicate possible infection, bacterial culture is necessary to identify the causative bacterium and determine the most appropriate treatment course.

The most serious complication of PID is infertility, which occurs in about 10–15% of cases.[4] Pelvic inflammatory disease from chlamydia is also a leading cause of ectopic pregnancies—pregnancies where the fetus develops outside of the womb and cannot survive.[9] If PID is limited to the uterus, antibiotic treatment can usually resolve the problem with little likelihood of permanent damage or future complications. In contrast, infection in the fallopian tubes, ovaries, or abdominal cavity is a cause for significant concern. Permanent damage from PID is especially likely if the infection has invaded the fallopian tubes, because the tubes are fragile and easily damaged by an infectious process. Infection causes swelling and scarring of the tubes, which can lead to blockage and distortion, impairing future fertility.

Women who have had PID should take extensive precautions to avoid reinfection. Present and previous sexual partners must be treated with the same antimicrobial regimen as the infected woman, whether or not the partners have symptoms.

Syphilis

After the introduction of antibiotics in the 1940s, **syphilis** rates fell for 60 years. Public health officials had hopes of completely eliminating syphilis in the United States, but in the year 2000, syphilis rates in the United States started to rise.[4] Since then, new syphilis cases have increased slowly but steadily, mostly among men, but also among women and infants. Although minorities are still more likely than their White counterparts to be infected with syphilis, these differences have shrunk over the past decade.[4]

Syphilis is caused by the bacterial organism *Treponema pallidum*. It is highly infectious and has a long, varied clinical course. If untreated, it may cause serious consequences, including cardiac and neurological damage and even death. Although the syphilis bacterium can be killed with antibiotics, the damage caused by long-term infection is permanent. There are three major stages of syphilis: primary, secondary, and tertiary.

Primary syphilis, the first disease stage, usually occurs 3 to 12 weeks after sexual contact with an infected individual. The first symptom is an open sore, called a chancre, at the site of sexual contact. The chancre is usually painless despite its appearance. The chancre heals and disappears without scarring within 2 to 6 weeks, whether or not the individual receives treatment.

The course of *secondary syphilis* is also variable and occurs from 1 week to 6 months after primary syphilis. There are a variety of secondary-stage symptoms, most notably a rash on the palms of the hands, the soles of the feet, and the external genitals; these rashes may develop into open sores. Individuals are highly infectious in this stage. Symptoms usually last 3 to 6 months but may reappear temporarily for several years. This latent phase of syphilis may be temporary or permanent.

A few people progress to the most dangerous phase, *tertiary syphilis*. Tertiary syphilis symptoms appear 10 to 20 years after initial exposure if the individual has not received treatment. These symptoms include heart disease, nerve and brain damage, spinal cord damage, blindness, and death.

Syphilis can pass from an infected woman to her developing fetus. Early screening and treatment of pregnant women are essential to prevent congenital syphilis. Untreated syphilis infection during pregnancy often results in miscarriage, stillbirth, or severe birth defects. Babies born with syphilis may suffer from skin sores, rashes, swollen liver and spleen, **jaundice**, and anemia, and if they are untreated after birth, damage to the heart, brain, and eyes may occur.

High doses of antibiotics are prescribed for early-stage syphilis; more prolonged, intensive treatment is indicated if the individual has been infected for a year or longer. Preventive measures for this STI are similar to those for other STIs (see "Informed Decision Making: Reproductive Tract Infections"). For all stages of syphilis, sexual partners must be concurrently treated. Effective treatment and follow-up in the primary and secondary stages of the disease can prevent further serious, permanent damage.

Vaginitis

Several kinds of vaginal infections can be transmitted through sexual interaction. Because they may also be transmitted through nonsexual means, however, they are not generally referred to as STIs. Trichomoniasis, yeast infections, and bacterial vaginosis are fairly common reproductive tract infections. Although they are responsible for physical and emotional discomfort, they do not typically pose long-term health problems.

Trichomoniasis

Trichomoniasis is caused by a one-celled protozoan and is usually transmitted via sexual contact, but the infectious organism is capable of surviving outside a human host in a wet environment, such as on a swimsuit or wet towel, and transmission between individuals can occur via these objects.

Some women do not experience any symptoms with trichomoniasis. When symptoms do occur, they typically include a frothy, thin, grayish, or greenish vaginal discharge; intense vaginal itching; an objectionable odor; pain during urination and intercourse; and urinary frequency. Diagnosis is confirmed with a wet smear of vaginal secretions.

Trichomoniasis can be effectively treated with antibiotics in either a single-dose or multiple-dose format. Because many women and most men infected with trichomoniasis do not experience symptoms, sexual partners should be treated at the same time, and condoms should be used until treatment is complete. Recurrent infections are common with trichomoniasis in pregnant women. This disease may result in premature rupture of membranes, preterm delivery, low birthweight, or a genital or lung infection in the newborn.

Yeast Infections

Yeast organisms (also known as *Candida albicans*, fungus infection, monilia, and candidiasis) normally exist in the microscopic ecosystem of a woman's body. A yeast infection occurs when the population of yeast organisms grows large enough to irritate the vagina and vulva. Yeast infections are very common—most women will have at least one during their lives. While yeast infections are usually only temporary, the symptoms can be painful and irritating, and include a thick, white, cottage cheese-type vaginal

discharge, redness, swelling, and itching. Diagnosis is generally made by microscopic examination of a sample of the vaginal discharge or a culture. Although yeast infections affect the female reproductive tract, yeast infections are usually not sexually transmitted.

Yeast infections are usually treated with antifungal vaginal cream (Monistat, Gyne-Lotrimin, Vagistat, Femstat) with dosage regimens of 1, 3, or 7 days, depending on the medication. Treatment of partners is usually unnecessary. Medications for yeast infections are available in over-the-counter forms; for women with chronic and recurrent infections, this has made treatment easier, cheaper, and faster by reducing the waiting time for a prescription and the expense of a clinical visit. For women who are not sure what type or kind of vaginal infection they may have, self-treatment is not a good idea, however.

Although yeast infections do not usually affect fertility, reinfection is common. Recurrent attacks may occur shortly after treatment or be delayed for a considerable period of time. What causes yeast to grow out of control is not always known. Women taking antibiotics may experience yeast infections when the antibiotics kill off the populations of "good" vaginal bacteria, allowing small populations of yeast to overgrow. Persistent yeast problems often present during pregnancy and in women who take oral contraceptives. Women with diabetes and women who are overweight also report higher frequencies of such infections. For women with recurrent infections, prolonged or intermittent treatment is often recommended to keep yeast growth under control. Concurrent treatment for yeast whenever antibiotics are prescribed may also help women with chronic yeast infections.

Bacterial Vaginosis

Bacterial vaginosis (BV) is known by many terms, including nonspecific vaginitis, *Gardnerella vaginalis*, bacterial vaginitis, *Haemophilus vaginalis*, *Corynebacterium vaginalis*, and anaerobic vaginosis. This condition is caused by an overgrowth of several species of vaginal organisms, which may be transmitted by sexual activity.[11] Bacterial vaginosis is considered a sexually associated condition but not necessarily a sexually transmitted infection. Although BV does not usually cause complications on its own, it is considered to be a cofactor in the acquisition of other sexually transmitted infections, including HIV.[12] Bacterial vaginosis is more prevalent among women with more than one sexual partner, intrauterine device (IUD) users, and women who have cervicitis.

The most common cause of abnormal vaginal discharge, BV is very common, usually detected in 10% to 40% of women worldwide.[12] Symptoms include a gray or white frothy discharge that may be thick or watery and that may have an objectionable odor. Painful urination, vaginal pain or burning during intercourse, redness, and itching may also be present.

While many women complain of vaginal odor, discharge, or irritation, as many as 50% of women with BV may be asymptomatic; thus, routine screening is recommended whenever STI testing is indicated.[2] Identifying bacterial vaginosis is relatively straightforward. Diagnosis may be made with microscopic examination of a discharge sample or a wet mount of vaginal cells. Pregnant women with bacterial vaginosis may have an increased risk of delivering preterm, low-birthweight infants. Bacterial vaginosis may coexist with other STIs and has been identified as a possible factor in HIV transmission. Because BV also may be associated with PID, definitive diagnosis is important to ensure adequate treatment.

Recommended treatment regimens consist of antibiotics. Treatment of sexual partners is not standard procedure, although it may be indicated if reinfection occurs after treatment or if sexual transmission is suspected.

Regular douching can increase a woman's risk of bacterial vaginosis. Douching may harm the vaginal flora and can increase the risk for bacterial vaginosis as well as other infections.[13]

Viral Sexually Transmitted Infections

Human Papillomavirus

Human papillomavirus (HPV) is an extremely common virus spread by skin-to-skin contact. There are more than 100 strains or types of HPV. Some strains of HPV are transmitted through nonsexual means and can cause warts on the hands, feet, and other parts of the body. About 40 strains of HPV, however, are transmitted sexually and affect the genital area. It is these sexually transmitted types of HPV that will be discussed in this chapter.

There are two broad types of sexually transmitted HPV. "High-risk" HPV can cause cervical dysplasia, a form of abnormal cell growth that can lead to cervical cancer. While most women who get HPV never develop cervical cancer, almost every single case of cervical cancer is linked to high-risk HPV. "Low-risk" HPV can cause warts on or around the genital area, but does not increase the risk for cervical cancer.

Each year, more than 6 million people in the United States, most of them in their teens or early 20s, are infected with HPV. Both high and low-risk HPV are present in 20% to 40% of women of almost all age groups (See **Figure 7.5**). Most people who are sexually active will acquire HPV at some point in their lives; most of these people will never know it.[3]

Cervical cancer is the second-most common cancer among women around the world. Fortunately, almost all cases of cervical cancer are preventable. Cervical cancer is typically preceded by abnormal cell growth called cervical dysplasia, which can be found during a routine Pap smear; in addition, a DNA test is available to detect whether a person has a high-risk strain of HPV. A screening program that includes Pap smears and HPV DNA testing (see **It's Your Health** on page XXX) can identify women at risk and almost always find cervical dysplasia before it becomes cancerous.

In addition, two vaccines, Gardasil and Cervarix, provide protection against the most common strains of HPV. The development of HPV vaccines represents a major, but incomplete step toward eliminating cervical cancer. Both vaccines prevent infection from HPV types 16 and 18, which are responsible for 70% of cases of cervical cancer. Additionally, Gardasil prevents infection from HPV types 6 and 11, which cause about 90% of cases of genital warts in men and women. The FDA has approved Gardasil and Cervarix, and both vaccines have been shown to be very safe and well tolerated. However, either vaccine requires a series of three injections to be effective and is most effective if given before a person becomes sexually active. In addition, neither vaccine prevents infection from the high-risk types of HPV responsible for the other 30% of cervical cancer cases. Gardasil and Ceravix are also both expensive compared to other vaccines, making widespread vaccination a relatively costly option.

Current medical knowledge has the potential to eliminate cervical cancer. Vaccination, if implemented widely, could prevent most cases of HPV infection, while widespread screening involving a combination of Pap tests and HPV testing could find the remaining cases of cervical dysplasia before they develop into cancer. However, while the potential to end this disease exists, a considerable challenge remains with educating the public about cervical cancer,

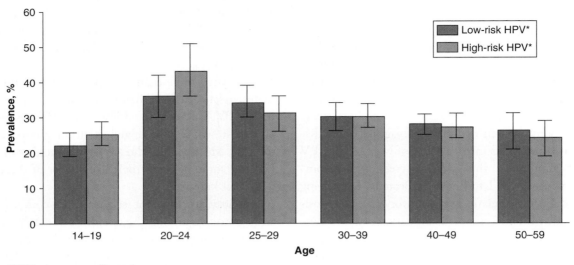

*HPV = human papillomavirus.

Note: Error bars indicate 95% confidence interval. Both high-risk and low-risk HPV types were detected in some females.

Figure 7.5

HPV—Prevalence of high-risk and low-risk types among women aged 14–59, 2003–2006.

Source: Adapted from Hariri, S., Unger, E., Sternberg, M., et al. Prevalence of genital HPV among females in the United States, the National Health and Nutrition Examination Survey, 2003–2006. *Journal of Infectious Diseases*, 2011.

overcoming misplaced fears about vaccination, and expanding women's access to screening and care.

There is no cure for HPV, but symptoms of both high-risk and low-risk HPV can be treated. Additionally, the body's immune system can often rid the body of the virus, effectively "curing" an individual. HPV infections are often asymptomatic, and a person can have HPV for years without the virus causing harm to the body. Left untreated, however, cervical dysplasia caused by high-risk HPV can cause serious harm or death, so prevention and screening efforts are extremely important for women's health.

For many women, the first indication of a high-risk HPV infection is a routine Pap smear. For a woman with an inconclusive Pap test, HPV DNA testing conducted on the residual material collected from a Pap can help identify the presence of HPV to determine if she is at risk for cervical dysplasia. Women who are 30 or older can get an HPV test along with their Pap tests. Women who are negative

Gender Dimensions: Health Differences Between Men and Women

HPV Vaccination: Who Should Get It?

HPV may be the most biologically sexist of all sexually transmitted infections. Low-risk HPV can cause genital warts in both men and women, but while both men and women can get or receive high-risk HPV, men are almost never affected by it. (Some strains of HPV have been linked to penile or anal cancer in men, but these cancers are extremely rare.) Gardasil, one of the vaccines available for HPV, appears to protect both men and women from most cases of genital warts in addition to preventing women from contracting most cases of high-risk HPV.

The CDC currently recommends that preteen girls and young women receive either vaccine, and that preteen boys and young men receive the Gardasil vaccine. Vaccination could prevent most cases of cervical cancer in women, and could dramatically reduce the number of cases of genital warts in both sexes. However, vaccinating both men and women for HPV would cost hundreds of millions of dollars. Leaving men (as well as women over 26, who are at substantially greater risk for acquiring HPV) unvaccinated and investing those funds in other forms of STI prevention could have a dramatically larger impact on the health of men and women. In addition, screening procedures would need to be continued to find cervical cancer caused by the high-risk strains of HPV unaffected by the vaccines. While the HPV vaccines are an important advance, they alone will not be the answer to eliminating cervical cancer.

on both tests can be reassured that they do not have HPV and they are not at risk for developing cervical cancer in the near future. If the HPV DNA test is positive, a gynecologist may look for evidence of warts or abnormal cell growth in the cervix or vagina. While Pap tests are routinely used in gynecological exams, it can also produce false positive results, indicating possible dysplasia while none is present, and it cannot identify the presence of high-risk HPV unless dysplasia is present. For this reason, a negative HPV test provides a degree and duration of reassurance not achievable by any other diagnostic method[14] (**Table 7.1**).

While many women with cervical dysplasia will never develop cervical cancer, some women may need aggressive treatment to prevent cancer development. Colposcopic examination and biopsy of suspicious areas are indicated. Women at risk for cervical cancer should be diligent about personal care, medical follow-up, and annual Pap smears and pelvic examinations.

HPV infection with low-risk HPV is usually characterized by single or multiple lesions or warts, which may first appear as small, round elevations in the skin but may grow in size and number and blend together in a cauliflower-like growth. Genital warts vary in size, may exist in single or multiple units, and may be raised or flat. In

| **Table 7.1** | Understanding Cervical Cancer Screening: Pap and HPV Test Results and What They Mean |

Normal and Abnormal Pap Test Result	What It Means
Normal Pap smear (Pap test)	Your cervical cells appear to be healthy.
Abnormal Pap smear (Pap test)	There appear to be changes in your cervical cells that need to be evaluated further.
Borderline or inconclusive Pap test result (officially called atypical squamous cells of undetermined significance, or "ASC-US")	Your cervical cells are not obviously normal, but they are not clearly abnormal either. Having an HPV test can help determine whether you need further evaluation.

women, these painless lesions may occur on the buttocks, anus, inner thighs, vulva, vagina, and cervix; depending on their location, symptoms can be present without a woman knowing about them.

When warts regress, HPV may still be present, just not readily apparent. Once contracted, the virus has a variable incubation period during which no symptoms are visible

---

It's Your Health

HPV Testing and Vaccination

Pap Tests (Pap Smears)

The Pap test is an examination that looks for signs of abnormal cell growth in the cervix. In the five decades they have been in use, Pap smears has prevented millions of women from dying of cervical cancer.

Strengths: A national screening program based on Pap tests is already in place. Pap tests find most cases of abnormal cell growth before they become cancerous.

Limitations: Pap tests sometimes produce positive results in the absence of dysplasia; because the tests look for abnormal cell growth, not the actual virus, frequent screenings are required. Because so many screenings are necessary, the Pap test is not an especially cost-effective solution. In addition, Pap tests can be painful and embarrassing for the women taking them.

HPV Testing

Instead of looking for cervical dysplasia, an early sign of disease, the HPV test looks for the DNA of the actual virus.

Strengths: Studies consistently show that HPV tests outperform Pap testing. A combined program of HPV testing and Pap tests is nearly 100% effective at identifying women at risk.

Limitations: The current screening infrastructure in the United States is based on Pap testing; implementing a new system will require political will and financial investment. The presence of high-risk HPV does not guarantee that cancer will develop.

HPV Vaccination

Two vaccines, Gardasil and Cervarix, each prevent infection from the two types of HPV that cause most cases of cervical cancer. Gardasil also prevents infection from the strains of HPV that cause most cases of genital warts. Both vaccines are given as a series of three injections over a six-month period. The CDC recommends vaccination with either vaccine for preteen girls and young women, and vaccination with Gardasil for preteen boys and young men.

Strengths: Gardasil and Cervarix both prevent infection from the high-risk strains 16 and 18, which are responsible for 70% of current cases of cervical cancer, and the low-risk HPV strains 6 and 11, which are responsible for 90% of current cases of genital warts. Studies have shown the vaccine to be safe and effective.

Limitations: Screening programs still need to be in place to find the other 30% of cervical cancers caused by high-risk strains of HPV not covered by the vaccine. The vaccine does not protect women who have already been infected, and it requires three doses to be effective. The vaccines are relatively expensive (about $400) to complete.

and the person is not yet infectious. Warts usually appear 1 to 8 months after exposure, but may not manifest themselves for years. Diagnosis of low-risk HPV is usually based on visual detection during clinical examination.

Although warts may regress spontaneously, they are frequently distressing. Treatment is often indicated to remove visible warts for psychological and aesthetic reasons, as well as to reduce the likelihood of transmission. HPV infections can be quite persistent and can recur regardless of which treatment method is selected. Treatment is easier and less painful in earlier stages. The particular treatment depends on the extent of HPV infection and its location. Options include topical agents applied by the patient or provider, cryotherapy (freezing of warts), laser surgery, electrosurgery, and surgical removal.

There is risk of recurrence after any therapy for external genital warts; however, recurrence rates may be the lowest with patient-applied topical therapies.

HPV can present problems in pregnancy, though this is relatively rare. A pregnant woman with low-risk HPV has a small chance of passing the virus to her child during vaginal delivery. In these cases, a doctor may treat warts before childbirth to reduce these risks.

Only a small percentage of the millions of women who contract high-risk HPV every year will ever develop cervical cancer. Although no treatment can "cure" HPV, most individuals' immune systems will eventually clear the virus even without treatment. At this point, a person would no longer have HPV, though he or she could be reinfected with an exposure to a new strain. The strength of the immune system appears to affect the course of infection: Conditions that alter or slow the immune response may encourage dysplasia. Men infected with high-risk strains of HPV may still transmit the virus, even if the virus never affects them or causes symptoms.

Special Precautions

Although latex condoms may reduce the likelihood of transmission, they probably do not provide reliable protection from HPV. HPV is spread by genital skin-to-skin contact, not bodily fluids—because a latex condom does not cover all of the genital skin, it cannot guarantee prevention of transmission, even if no visible symptoms are present. A female condom may provide more protection than a traditional condom that covers the penis, but there are no guarantees with either type of condom use.

Herpes Simplex Virus

Herpes simplex virus (HSV) is a very common sexually transmitted infection. Herpes can be caused by two distinct, closely related viruses: HSV-1 and HSV-2. HSV-1 is the main cause of recurring sores in the mouth known as cold sores or fever blisters, while HSV-2 typically causes similar symptoms that appear in the genital area and is responsible for most cases of "genital herpes." However, if HSV-1 is exposed to the genital area of an uninfected person (for example, through oral sex), HSV-1 can infect the genital area of that person; similarly, exposure to HSV-2 can infect the oral area of a person as well.

More than one-half of the U.S. population has an infection of HSV-1, and 16.2% has an infection of HSV-2.[15] Most people with herpes do not know they are infected. Herpes has become much more common over the past 50

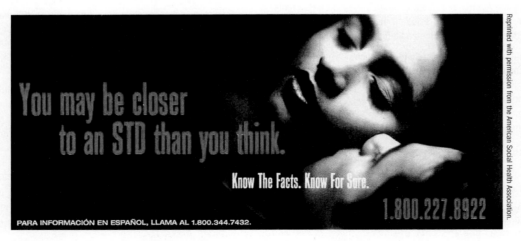

■ Honest communication before sexual intimacy is essential for assessing risk behaviors and avoiding transmission of disease.

years, as can be seen from the number of visits to physician's offices following an initial outbreak (**Figure 7.6**).

My husband of 22 years and I divorced recently, and so I'm new to the dating scene. I've started seeing a very sweet guy who later told me that he has herpes. I was very shocked at first, but now that I know about the disease, it's not nearly as bad as I first thought. My daughter, who's in college now, and I had a real heart-to-heart conversation about safer-sex practices afterward. She actually knew more than I did!

—50-year-old mother of two

Herpes is incurable, and it can be extremely painful and psychologically devastating. Yet for the vast majority of cases, herpes is not a serious medical condition. Symptoms of HSV are usually most severe just after acquiring the infection. Symptoms may appear anywhere from 1 day to 4 weeks after exposure. Lasting about 12 days, herpes generally presents as single or multiple small, painful blisters that appear in the vulva or buttocks of women. If sores are present on the cervix, they often go unnoticed. The blisters evolve into painful ulcers in a couple of days. These symptoms may be accompanied by vulvar swelling, fever, and enlarged and tender lymph nodes. Sores usually heal in 1 to 4 weeks with little or no scarring. The time between outbreaks is referred to as the latent or inactive phase. During this time, genital sores have healed but the infection remains.

A **prodrome** or warning phase often precedes a herpes outbreak. The warnings may consist of tingling or itching sensations in the area where sores later appear. It is not known what causes repeat outbreaks of herpes. Some people find that irritating stimuli to the infected area, such as tight clothing, menstrual changes, or exposure to sunlight or extreme heat or cold, can trigger an outbreak whereas others do not notice any such effects.

The human body can never rid itself of the herpes virus. Between outbreaks, the virus evades the immune system by lying dormant within host nerve cells, where the immune system cannot reach it; however, in most cases the immune system does get better at fighting the virus. Recurrent outbreaks are usually milder and shorter than the original outbreaks, and people with herpes generally have fewer outbreaks as time goes by. Although there is no surefire way to prevent all outbreaks, maintaining a healthy lifestyle helps the immune system keep the virus in check. Any stress on the body can also stress the immune system; indeed, many people report that outbreaks begin when they are already sick with a cold or flu, have gone a long time without getting enough sleep, or are experiencing stressful times in their lives—all things that can burden the immune system. Ironically, refraining from obsessing or worrying excessively about a herpes infection, while still remaining knowledgeable about the disease, may help prevent outbreaks.

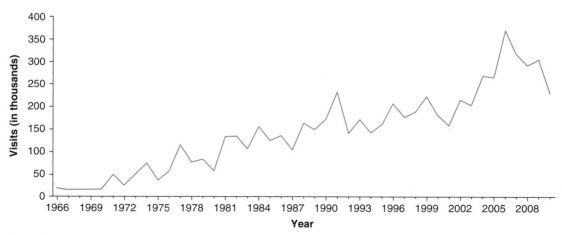

Note: The relative standard errors for genital herpes estiamtes of more than 100,000 range from 18% to 30%. See other surveillance data sources in the appendix and table 44.

Figure 7.6

Genital herpes—Initial visits to physicians' offices, United States, 1966–2010.

Source: Adapted from IMS Health, Integrated Promotional Services. IMS Health Report, 1966–2010.

Herpes outbreaks show considerable variability from person to person. Some outbreaks last as long as 3 weeks; others are as short as a few days. Outbreaks may involve many blisters, or just a few, or even a single blister. Some individuals experience outbreaks every few months; others have one or more each month. Some individuals never experience recurrent outbreak symptoms after the initial event, though this is an uncommon occurrence. Infectiousness remains an important concern, even for individuals who are unaware of their herpes symptoms.

Active herpes sores are very contagious during both the initial attack and the recurrences. Both HSV-1 and HSV-2 can be spread from sores to the eye, where serious infection is possible. An oral infection can be spread to infants and children via kissing or casual contact. People infected with herpes undergo periods of **asymptomatic viral shedding**. During these periods, active herpes virus is present on a person's infected area and may be infectious, whether or not symptoms are present. Viral shedding typically lasts for 2 to 20 days during an initial outbreak and for 2 to 5 days during recurrent outbreaks. Researchers have not been able to determine exactly how infectious an individual is when asymptomatic shedding occurs, but it is known that the risk of transmission is highest when active sores are present. Active sores contain hundreds of times more virus than viral sheddings from genital secretions. Diagnosing herpes is typically made based on the patient's history, or from a culture or examination of symptoms. Because clinical diagnosis is often inaccurate, viral culture and type-specific serology may be used as confirmation.

There is no cure for herpes. Prescribed antiviral medications may reduce or suppress symptoms, and antibiotic ointment may help prevent a secondary bacterial infection of the sores. Herpes medication may also reduce the chance of transmission between outbreaks.[16] Acyclovir, valacyclovir, and famciclovir are the current treatments of choice for herpes and can relieve symptoms and shorten healing time. All three medications inhibit the ability of the virus to use proteins, thereby interfering with its ability to replicate. Clinicians may prescribe acyclovir to women who acquire herpes during pregnancy or who have severe outbreaks around the time of delivery.[2] The FDA has approved three different treatment regimens for herpes: (1) therapy for an initial outbreak, (2) episodic therapy to speed healing and relieve discomfort during recurrences, and (3) suppressive therapy on a daily basis to attempt to prevent outbreaks. Because the effects of a herpes transmission are usually limited to symptoms and transmission, a woman with herpes should take an active role in deciding the treatment regimen, if any, that is right for her. Women with severe symptoms may wish to take suppressive therapy, whereas women who have outbreaks that are mild or not noticeable may opt for episodic therapy or seek to manage the virus without medication.

Special Precautions

Good personal hygiene is essential during a herpes outbreak. The infected individual should wash his or her hands thoroughly after touching a herpes sore to avoid possible transmission to another mucous membrane, such as the eyes or mouth. Care should be taken to avoid spreading the virus to others, including infants and children. If active herpes is present in or near the mouth, kissing should be avoided. As a precautionary measure, personal objects such as washcloths, toothbrushes, drinking cups, and towels should not be shared. Although clinical studies have not demonstrated effective indirect transmission, the virus can remain alive outside the body for several hours in a moist environment.

There are no guarantees of "safe sex" with herpes, but there are ways to reduce risk. At a minimum, sexual intercourse, including oral sex, should be avoided when active herpes sores are present. Because sores contain high populations of viruses, individuals should wait until the sores are completely healed before resuming sexual activity. Because it is difficult to tell when a herpes outbreak is beginning, open communication about risks and feelings are another key risk-reduction strategy. Condoms appear to provide some protection, with female condoms providing better coverage than male condoms.[17] Because herpes sores can be present in areas not covered by either condom, however, there are no guarantees against transmission. Condoms and other risk-reduction strategies are especially important in a situation in which the male partner has herpes and the female partner does not and is pregnant. An initial attack of herpes during pregnancy presents serious risks to the developing fetus, including possible pregnancy loss or preterm delivery.

Women with herpes should be diligent about protecting themselves from further infection by other STIs. Such women are at increased risk for acquiring HIV and other STIs because of the open sores associated with the herpes virus.

Pregnant women with herpes should begin prenatal care early. The risk is greatest for women who contract herpes during their pregnancy. If active lesions are present in the vaginal canal at the time of birth, a cesarean delivery may be undertaken to avoid exposing the infant to the virus. Infant exposure to the virus may cause infections of the eyes, skin, mucous membranes, and central nervous system, and even death. However, most pregnant women with herpes deliver vaginally and give birth to healthy babies.[2]

Although no one wants to get genital herpes, in most cases the stigma of the disease vastly outweighs its physiological effects. Herpes is closely related to the viruses that cause chickenpox and mononucleosis (mono), yet because herpes is sexually transmitted, people with herpes may describe themselves as "dirty" or "tainted" or feel that they will never be lovable or able to enter a sexual relationship again. The truth is that many people with herpes have strong relationships and healthy sex lives. Although there is no way to guarantee prevention of sexual transmission, there are many ways to reduce risk, from avoiding sex or wearing condoms between outbreaks, to taking suppressive therapy to reduce outbreaks and asymptomatic shedding. Some people decide to enter relationships with other people who have herpes to avoid infecting another person, although other STIs would still be a potential concern. Because the symptoms of herpes infections are transient and often ultimately quite mild, some couples with one infected partner decide that the benefits of a healthy, unique, loving relationship outweigh the drawbacks of possible herpes transmission.

Comfort Measures

Keeping the genital area clean and dry minimizes discomfort during a herpes flare-up. A hair dryer on a cool setting may be used to dry the area thoroughly without irritation or discomfort. Genital cleansing must be gentle because rubbing can cause lesions to break and bleed. Many women find **sitz baths** comforting during outbreaks of herpes. Domeboro solution or Epsom salts may be added to the sitz bath. Cold, wet compresses or cleansing pads containing glycerol and witch hazel applied to the sores may also provide temporary relief. In addition, some women find icepacks helpful during outbreaks.

Hepatitis

Hepatitis, an inflammation of the liver, is caused by infection with one of several viruses—type A, B, C, D, E, F, or G. Hepatitis B and C both may be spread through sexual intimacy or contact with infected blood (such as sharing needles to inject drugs).

Hepatitis B, the type of hepatitis most likely to be spread sexually, remains the one STI that can be entirely prevented

■ Both hepatitis A and B can be prevented with immunization.

via vaccination; a three-shot vaccine can provide lifetime immunity to both hepatitis A and hepatitis B. Since the early 1980s, infants have routinely been vaccinated for hepatitis A and B. Most individuals who have not been vaccinated as infants may safely receive the vaccines as adults.

Vaccination and other preventative efforts have dramatically reduced the number cases of hepatitis A and B. From 1989 to 2009, new cases of hepatitis A have fallen by 95%, and new cases of hepatitis B have fallen by 85%.[18]

Progression of hepatitis B varies from person to person. For some, hepatitis B is an acute infection, lasting for 6 months or less; for others, hepatitis B can be a chronic infection, lasting for years or decades. Chronic hepatitis B can lead to chronic liver disease, permanent liver scarring, and even death.

Hepatitis C is both the most common cause of chronic liver disease and the most common blood-borne disease in the United States. It is mostly transmitted through contact with infected blood, intravenous drug use, or contaminated blood transfusion, but may be spread sexually if exposure to blood occurs. Hepatitis C, like hepatitis B, can cause an acute or chronic infection, but hepatitis C is more likely to be persistent and cause complications.

HIV/AIDS

AIDS (acquired immune deficiency syndrome), a progressive disease caused by **HIV (human immunodeficiency virus)**, is characterized by the destruction of the immune system. There are no constant, specific symptoms associated with this condition, and no effective cure or vaccine is available. The best way to stop HIV is to prevent infection. Recent therapeutic advances have allowed people living with HIV to live long, full lives; however, HIV remains a serious, lifelong infection.

It's Your Health

AIDS Facts: Dispelling AIDS Myths

AIDS is not a disease of homosexual men.

Women are susceptible to AIDS.

AIDS may not be spread by casual contact.

AIDS cannot be transmitted to humans from insects.

There is no risk of acquiring AIDS by donating blood.

Information and education are the best weapons against AIDS.

Confidential, anonymous testing for AIDS is available.

HIV is a **retrovirus**, a virus that incorporates its genetic material into the genome of the cell it attacks. When HIV, also known as the AIDS virus, enters the bloodstream, it attacks specific white blood cells called CD4 or T lymphocytes. The virus also replicates. The CD4 cells are no longer able to stimulate a cellular defense response, and the body's systemic immune system is compromised. The number of CD4 cells in an infected person's body decreases as the number of HIV-infected cells increases. AIDS is the final stage of HIV; it is diagnosed when the person has a positive test for antibodies to HIV and a low T-lymphocyte count. An HIV-positive person also may be diagnosed with AIDS when one of 26 known infections, called opportunistic infections, is present. Opportunistic infections present a potentially fatal risk to individuals with AIDS.

HIV is transmitted from one person to another through sexual intercourse; shared intravenous needle use; contaminated blood or blood products; or from mother to child during pregnancy, birth, or breastfeeding. HIV is not spread by casual, social, or family contact. Although HIV is a sophisticated and elusive killer within the body, the virus quickly dies when exposed to the open air; unbroken human skin provides excellent protection from HIV.

An individual with HIV may have no physical symptoms, so it is impossible to tell whether a person is infected just by looking at him or her. In fact, one out of five people living with HIV do not know they are infected.[19] HIV-infected individuals can transmit the virus, however, even in the absence of symptoms. The HIV incubation period ranges from months to years. No individual or groups of individuals are immune to HIV/AIDS.

Perspectives on AIDS

Historical Overview

AIDS was first diagnosed in the United States in 1981. By the start of the 21st century AIDS had gone from being an unknown disease to a national and global epidemic. Over the past 15 years, scientists, health workers, doctors, and activists have united to fight this disease. These efforts have made an enormous difference: People are now living longer, healthier lives with HIV, and the rate of new infections in the United States and around the world has fallen. The challenge of the next generation will be to sustain these advances and make further progress.

For years, the origins of HIV were unknown. It is now believed that HIV is a mutated descendant of SIV, a virus in wild African chimpanzees. Genetic analyses of the oldest known specimens of HIV indicate that the virus probably first began spreading among humans between 1884 and 1924 in what is now the Democratic Republic of the Congo.[20] These cases went unnoticed because they spread at low levels among relatively unexamined populations, and because technology to identify the virus was nonexistent.

Men who have sex with men still constitute a disproportionate percentage of people infected with HIV. However, anyone who engages in risky sexual behavior or intravenous drug use is at risk. HIV epidemics in other countries have been spread primarily by intravenous drug users or heterosexual sex. A complicating factor is that, like many intravenous drug users, many men who have sex with men hide or deny their risky behaviors and pose as noninjecting, straight men.

Global Perspectives

In the 1980s and 1990s, HIV spread with alarming, destructive rapidity throughout the world. Developing countries—sub-Saharan Africa especially—were hit the hardest. In the year 2000 alone, three million people died from HIV/AIDS. Eighty percent of those deaths occurred in sub-Saharan Africa, home to just 10% of the world's population. Over the past 25 years, more than 12 million children in sub-Saharan Africa have lost their parents to AIDS, and sickness and deaths among the current generation of young adults will affect local economies for decades.[7]

The primary manner of transmission has varied from region to region. In the United States and much of Europe, AIDS was at first most common among gay and bisexual men. However, in Russia and parts of Asia, intravenous drug use has been a major mode of transmission, and heterosexual contact has been the primary mode of transmission in sub-Saharan Africa and many other regions.

As the epidemic has spread, governments, scientists, activists, health workers, humanitarian organizations, and others have worked to identify the areas in greatest need, improve access to treatment, provide better care, and encourage testing and prevention. This effort has curbed the growth rate of HIV. Since its peak in 1999, the number of global new cases has fallen by 19%; in many sub-Saharan African countries, new cases have fallen by more than 25%.[7] Over the past decade, millions of people have received access to life-saving treatment, and as a result, AIDS-related deaths have also fallen. However, these gains are fragile and incomplete. Close to 10 million people with HIV continue to lack access to treatment, and more than 2.5 million people are infected every year. The global fight to control this catastrophic disease is only getting started.

Today, more than 33 million people—95% of whom live in developing countries—are living with HIV (See **Figure 7.7**).[7] More than half of all people currently living with HIV are women and girls. In 2009, 2.7 million people were infected, and 1.8 million people died of HIV-related causes.[21]

Epidemiological Data and Trends

In the United States, about 48,000 people are infected with HIV each year, and about 1.1 million people are living with HIV.[22] About 85% of HIV-infected women acquire the virus through heterosexual contact; almost all of the rest acquire it through injection drug use.

AIDS and HIV infection rates present different epidemiological patterns by sex. Women did not constitute a sizable proportion of the total number of HIV cases in the United States until several years into the AIDS epidemic,

but this number has grown since then. In 1992, women accounted for 13.8% of people infected with HIV; by 1998, they represented 20% of this total. Over the past decade, this proportion appears to have stabilized at about 24%.[22] As **Figure 7.8** shows, Black and Hispanic women make up a disproportionately large percentage of people living with AIDS.

The number of people living with HIV and AIDS in the United States has steadily increased over the past 20 years, even as the number of infections has plateaued (see **Figure 7.9**). This is largely due to improved treatments and better access to treatment and care; with new infections continuing even as fewer people are dying of the disease, the total number of people with HIV/AIDS is growing.

> *I don't sleep around a lot. I have been with only three guys. But I have herpes. I can't tell where I got it ... I mean, it's like I have slept with not only those guys, but everyone else they have had sex with. How can a person really trust someone not to have an STI these days?*
>
> **—21-year-old woman**

Special Concerns for Women

Women are an at-risk, HIV-susceptible population. A focus on male homosexuality as a risk factor, along with a failure to focus on women as a unique high-risk group for HIV, have created significant obstacles in diagnosis,

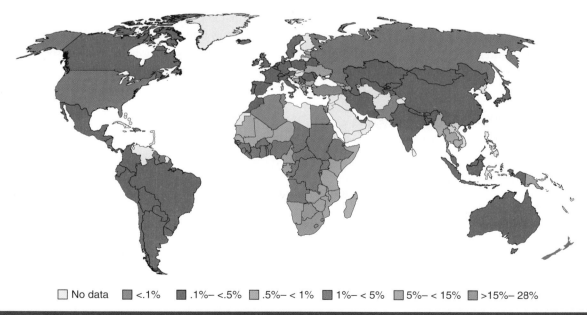

☐ No data   ■ <.1%   ■ .1%– <.5%   ■ .5%– < 1%   ■ 1%– < 5%   ■ 5%– < 15%   ■ >15%– 28%

Figure 7.7

Global Prevalence of HIV, 2009

Source: Reproduced from UNAIDS. (2010). UNAIDS Global Report.

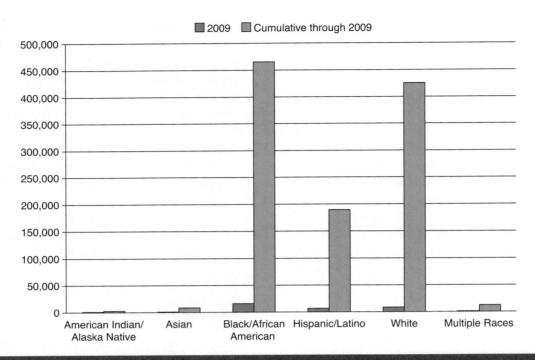

Figure 7.8

Estimated number of AIDS diagnoses in the United States

Source: Data from Centers for Disease Control and Prevention. (2011). HIV Surveillance—United States, 1981–2008.

prevention, and treatment, which leads to a delay in women receiving appropriate medical care. In the United States, women are more likely to die from AIDS than men; however, when both groups have equal access to health care, no differences in rates of survival are expected.

Women are far more likely to contract HIV from a man through heterosexual intercourse than a man is to contract the infection from a woman. This difference in part reflects

a woman's exposure to a greater quantity of secretions that carry the virus (i.e., semen) and the greater mucosal surface area of the vagina and cervix in which infection can occur. In addition, women are likely to experience small tears in the vaginal lining during intercourse, increasing their susceptibility to infection by HIV-positive semen.

Women who partner with women are not free from risk, however. Many women who consider themselves

Figure 7.9

Number of people living with HIV/AIDS and new infections of HIV, United States.

Source: Data from Hall HI, Song R, Rhodes P, et al. Estimation of HIV incidence in the United States. *JAMA* 2008;300: 520–529; CDC. HIV Prevalence Estimates—United States, 2006. *MMWR* 2008;57(39):1073-76.

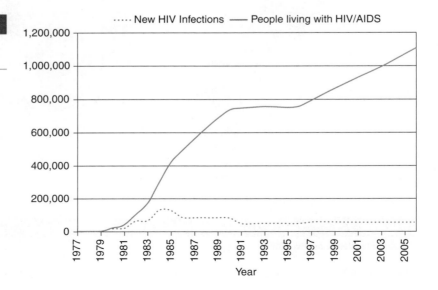

lesbians have had heterosexual intercourse and may have received HIV through that avenue without knowing it. Also, although woman-to-woman sexual contact does appear to be less risky for transmission of HIV, other STIs may be spread that way.

Social Issues

HIV and AIDS disproportionately affect men and women of color. Black women are more than 15 times more likely than White women to be infected with HIV, and Hispanic women are about five times more likely than White women to be infected.[21] As Figure 7.8 shows, the number of AIDS diagnoses also disproportionately affects Black and Hispanic women. More than 30 years after the disease was first diagnosed, AIDS continues to be a leading cause of death for black men and women aged 35–44.

There are many reasons for these disparities, many of them similar to the reasons for ethnic disparities for other STIs. As discussed earlier in the chapter, people of color are more likely to have reduced access to testing and treatment, and are more likely to choose a partner of the same race, increasing the chance of exposure. In addition, many of the first AIDS-related resources and treatment centers were geared toward a White, gay male audience. Reducing these continuing racial disparities will be an important public health challenge over the next decade.

Black women with HIV face the dual stigma of being neither White nor male. Black women who have HIV are less likely to receive treatment than other ethnic groups and are more likely to die early. About one-half the people in the United States who die from AIDS are Black.[22] Class undoubtedly plays a large role in this disparity. Women who are economically deprived often have inadequate access to healthcare facilities and are more likely to be unhealthy in general. Many do not have health insurance, are chronically underinsured, or lack information on how to access and use scarce public healthcare facilities.

It's Your Health

Anonymous Versus Confidential Testing*

Anonymous testing: The person receives an identification number, provides no name or personal information, and may provide information for demographic use only. An identification number is used to receive test results.

Confidential testing: Test results are kept in confidence (not disclosed to others); however, the patient is identified and results are part of the patient's medical records. These records may be made available to certain people under certain conditions.

*Some facilities may offer both confidential and anonymous testing.

Early limitations with the male-based CDC diagnostic criteria for AIDS prevented many women with AIDS from being correctly diagnosed. Even with the revised criteria, few studies have provided clear diagnostic criteria for women. As a consequence, women are sometimes ineligible for benefits and services available to others diagnosed early on with AIDS, and they may be excluded from clinical trials.

Epidemiological efforts at the beginning of the AIDS epidemic largely viewed women as vectors of AIDS transmission to their offspring and male sexual partners. Early studies were limited to perinatal assessment efforts and surveys of prostitutes. As a consequence, women were not considered as victims of transmission from their male partners. The identification of "high-risk groups" (homosexual and bisexual men, intravenous drug users, hemophiliacs, prostitutes, inmates, and people from specific geographical areas) both stigmatized the members of these groups and denied risk among nongroup members. Women are often unaware of the risks to themselves or others because they do not belong to these "high-risk" groups, even if they practice high-risk behaviors. Likewise, some women may not be aware of the high-risk behaviors or histories of their partners.

In 2010, the U.S. government launched a national strategy to reduce the rate of new infections, increase access to care, and reduce the continuing HIV-related health disparities in the United States. Accomplishing these goals will take a renewed, persistent effort on the part of federal, state, and local governments, as well as activists, medical organizations, and ordinary citizens.

Clinical Dimensions and Treatment Issues of AIDS

Diagnosis of HIV is extremely important both for early treatment and prevention of further transmission. Persons with HIV are contagious whether or not they have symptoms. In fact, the month just after infection is generally one of the most contagious periods in the course of infection. Many tests attempt to detect HIV antibodies, which are found in blood and other bodily fluids of an infected person. The **enzyme-linked immunosorbent assay (ELISA)** is an HIV screening test that determines whether a person's serum contains antibodies to one or more HIV antigens. It is used for screening large samples of blood and as a preliminary screening test for individuals because of its low cost and fast results. If an ELISA test gives positive results, a confirmatory **Western blot test** should be performed. When used together, the two tests are highly accurate. Other tests, such as fluorescent antibody tests, polymerase chain reaction (PCR), the

Single-Use Diagnostic System (rapid testing), and saliva and urine tests, may be used by some clinicians as well.

The ELISA test does not look for HIV itself, but rather for HIV antibodies—the body's unique immune response to HIV. The longer a woman waits after a risk to get tested, the more confidence she can place in a negative result. It takes about 25 days for the average person with HIV to develop detectable antibodies. An early negative HIV antibody test is not a guarantee against infection. Those at risk of HIV should have a repeat test at least 3 months after the initial test to confirm their results. HIV tests are available at local blood banks, AIDS research programs, physicians' offices, clinics, and health departments. The Food and Drug Administration (FDA) has approved four different rapid antibody tests for HIV. These tests have the advantages of offering testing at a lower cost and provide a patient with results on the same visit she got tested.

Home testing kits, which can be purchased at drugstores or ordered online, are available for people who are reluctant to visit a healthcare provider or have limited access to healthcare facilities. A woman can collect her own blood sample through a finger prick; the sample is then mailed to a laboratory. She can use an identification number to obtain anonymous results over the phone. After hearing her results, the caller can speak to a counselor to discuss the meaning of the test.

Once infected with HIV, symptoms vary. Some women experience a temporary flulike illness 1 to 2 months after exposure to the virus; these symptoms typically disappear on their own without treatment. Without treatment, a person will typically begin to experience symptoms of AIDS 5 to 10 years after infection. These symptoms may include swollen lymph nodes, fatigue, recurring yeast infections, weight loss, and chronic diarrhea. Although studies suggest that gynecological symptoms are often the first signs of HIV infection in women, symptoms in women have only recently been included in the CDC criteria for diagnosis. When women seek treatment for these gynecological conditions, HIV testing may be delayed or avoided because it is not suspected. Potential indicators of HIV infection in women include gynecological infections such as candidiasis (yeast infection), PID, HPV, genital ulcers, HSV, pneumonia, and sepsis. When AIDS develops, opportunistic infections often begin to further break down the immune system.

Early treatment of HIV delays or prevents the onset of AIDS and can reduce the virus to unmeasurable levels in the blood. AZT, also known as zidovudine, was the first anti-HIV drug approved in 1987. Since then, combination drug therapy—multiple medications that work together—has greatly improved the quality of life for many people. New types of drugs, including nucleoside analogs and protease inhibitors, are now used together as part of an "AIDS cocktail" or HAART (highly active antiretroviral therapy). HAART therapy usually consists of three medications that attack HIV in distinct ways; this "triple attack" helps prevent HIV, which mutates rapidly, from developing resistance to any one type of medication. These drugs still have significant limitations and side effects, however, and the search continues for more effective and more affordable treatment regimens.

Perinatal transmission of HIV is a special concern for women because the majority of HIV-infected women are of reproductive age. If an HIV-infected woman has a low T-cell count and becomes pregnant, she is more likely to develop HIV-associated illness during pregnancy. Without treatment, approximately one-fourth of all babies born to HIV-infected mothers will be infected with the virus.

Joe had a long-term relationship with this girl, and they broke up last year. I used to worry about that relationship, but now I am more worried about the insignificant encounters he had after they broke up. He doesn't know anything about them, and neither do I. How do I evaluate my risk?

—23-year-old woman

Prompt treatment can greatly reduce the chance of transmission; perinatal transmission of HIV has decreased over the past 20 years, but unfortunately it continues to exist. In one study of HIV-infected women, HAART therapy regimens prevented perinatal HIV transmission among all women who were compliant with their treatment regimens.[23]

Informed Decision Making

Making clear decisions about sexual intimacy can be very difficult. There are many reasons for this. Sexual arousal, the desire to be liked, societal expectations, drugs and alcohol, individual experiences, and other factors all affect how people think and make decisions. Even on a practical level, deciding what constitutes "sexual intimacy" and what form of intimacy would be comfortable and appropriate (kissing alone? Kissing and touching, with or without clothing? Oral sex? Vaginal intercourse? Something else?) depends on the preferences and morals of each partner and on the specific occasion (see Chapter 5 for a more in-depth discussion of sexual decision-making). Adding the possibility of receiving (or transmitting) a STI adds another layer of complexity to this process.

Women who choose to become sexually active are responsible for their decision. Every woman who engages in sexual activity should understand how to communicate what she wants (and what she does not want) and know about basic STI risks, symptoms to look out for, and prevention strategies. Prevention is especially important because many STIs are either incurable or can have permanent consequences.

Apart from abstinence, the most reliable prevention strategy for STIs is long-term mutual monogamy with a single partner. The most significant risk factor for any STI is the woman's partner(s). The risk of contracting an STI increases when a woman has more than one sex partner and when her partner(s) has more than one sex partner. Sexually transmitted infections should be considered a distinct possibility whenever a woman is not in a strictly exclusive, monogamous, long-term relationship.

Safer sex practices are important for any sexual relationship where there is any doubt about a partner's or one's own monogamy or status of HIV and other STIs. Safer sex entails any form of sex in which semen, blood, or vaginal secretions are prevented from passing from one person to another. Latex condoms (or a polyurethane female condom) with spermicide are the key ingredient of safer sex. Condoms must be used correctly each time a person has oral, anal, or vaginal intercourse. If a condom breaks or falls off, its protective effect is lost. Data show that latex condoms, when used consistently and correctly, greatly reduce the chances of transmission of HIV and many other STIs (female condoms also appear to be significant risk reducers, but the data on their effectiveness are comparatively new).[24] The risk of acquiring an STI increases with the number of partners a person has, but a person only needs to be exposed once to acquire an STI.

Sexually transmitted infections are transmitted by sexual intimacy. Intimacy includes "traditional" sex (vaginal intercourse), oral or anal sex, and other forms of intimate skin-to-skin and mucous membrane-to-mucous membrane contact. Sexually transmitted infections can be transmitted in both homosexual and heterosexual encounters. Although the notion of safe sex is misleading, safer sex practices can greatly reduce the overall risk of acquiring an STI. **Table 7.2** compares safer, risky, and dangerous sex practices.

Latex condoms prevent fluid exchange, and used properly, can greatly reduce the risk of transmission of HIV. However, latex condoms probably provide less protection for some STIs, such as herpes and HPV, which are spread by contact with symptoms or infected genital skin. Some practices are more risky for contracting some STIs than for others. A person is extremely unlikely to get HIV from receiving oral sex even without a condom, for example, but could easily get herpes or syphilis in this way.

Consistent condom use can greatly reduce risk, but there are no guarantees; viruses located at sites other than

Table 7.2 Some Sexual Activities and Their Relative Risk Levels

Activity	Level of Risk	Ways to Reduce Risk
Anal intercourse without a condom	High	Use a latex condom or female condom; only have sex with a mutually monogamous, tested partner
Vaginal intercourse without a condom	High	Use a latex or female condom; only have sex with a mutually monogamous, tested partner
Oral sex	High (however, risk for HIV is very low for receiving oral sex)	Use a latex condom for oral sex with a man or a dental dam or other moisture barrier for oral sex with a woman; only have sex with a mutually monogamous, tested partner
Mutual masturbation (hand-to-genital contact)	Very low, assuming no visible symptoms or cuts in the skin are present	Refrain from activity when there are symptoms or cuts in the skin
Kissing, no sores or broken skin	Very low; slight risk of oral herpes or syphilis infection	Refrain from activity when there are symptoms or cuts in the skin
All sexual activities with a mutually monogamous partner who is free from infection	None, assuming partner is truly negative	Refrain from kissing when possible symptoms are present
Abstaining from all sexual contact	None	Make sure partner has been tested for all STIs and is trustworthy

■ Home testing is an important option for those women who wish to be anonymous.

the penis, such as the scrotum, anal region, vulva, or inner thighs, are not covered by condoms, and transmission from these sites can still occur.

Frank, honest communication before sexual intimacy is essential. Although it may be difficult to have an honest discussion about infections and previous risk behaviors, the price of not communicating can be high. Honest communication is a mark of personal maturity. If a potential partner is unable or unwilling to discuss infections and intimacy concerns, it may indicate a lack of maturity that should be present in a trusted sex partner. Sexual closeness should be avoided if either partner has any symptoms of infection or if there are any suspicions of infection. Delaying activity for a few days and having symptoms evaluated may prevent lifelong consequences. Because many people with STIs honestly do not know they are infected, many couples now see a clinician together for examination and STI testing before initiating a sexual relationship.

Talking about incurable STIs such as herpes and HPV can be especially difficult. The timing of communication is important. Waiting until after sex to tell someone about a herpes infection may understandably upset a partner.

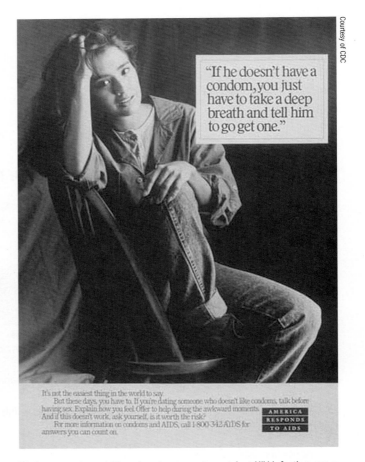

"If he doesn't have a condom, you just have to take a deep breath and tell him to go get one."

It's not the easiest thing in the world to say.
But these days, you have to. If you're dating someone who doesn't like condoms, talk before having sex. Explain how you feel. Offer to help during the awkward moments. And if this doesn't work, ask yourself, is it worth the risk?
For more information on condoms and AIDS, call 1-800-342-AIDS for answers you can count on.

AMERICA RESPONDS TO AIDS

■ Latex condoms, although not a guarantee against HIV infection, are a key consideration in prevention of HIV transmission.

Courtesy of CDC

However, because of the stigma of the disease, a person with herpes may want to wait until some level of trust has been established before informing a potential sex partner. Being calm and knowledgeable about an infection also aids in communication. Many people are ignorant about the course of infection of STIs or the means by which they are spread. Open and frank discussion benefits both partners; studies have found that sharing a herpes diagnosis with a supportive spouse or lover and avoiding denial as a coping mechanism helps people with herpes come to better and healthier terms with their infections.

I felt weird when Karen insisted that we go to the doctor together before we had sex. I guess I was afraid that one of us would have something. But we didn't and, you know, I think that our relationship is stronger because she insisted. I respect her for having the courage it took to do that. I wish that it had been my idea.

—22-year-old man

When to Get Tested or Treated

No one wants to have a sexually transmitted infection, but anyone who is sexually active has some risk of acquiring one. The decision to get tested can be a difficult one, but some form of treatment is available for all STIs. Many STIs can be cured easily with proper antibiotic regimens, and others can be treated to alleviate symptoms and reduce or prevent harm to the body. Women (and men) may visit a trusted clinician for testing, but health departments and Planned Parenthood facilities also offer confidential, low-cost testing and treatment for most STIs (see the "It's Your Health" box on this page).

Symptoms for STIs may be painful and obvious, entirely absent, or mistaken for other conditions. If a woman suspects that she *may* have an infection, she should be evaluated. Waiting for symptoms to go away is an exercise in futility, because although some symptoms may temporarily disappear, the disease may still be present, transmissible, and causing harm to the body.

If a partner has an infection or is suspicious of an infection, it is important to curtail sexual activity, and both individuals should seek clinical evaluation. Treating one partner and not the other often results in a "ping-pong" cycle of infection and re-infection. In addition, sharing one antibiotic prescription between two people usually means that neither partner receives adequate treatment and can contribute to antibiotic resistance.

Using leftover antibiotics from previous infections is equally foolhardy because supplies are usually inappropriate and inadequate, and may serve merely to mask the symptoms, complicating an accurate diagnosis later. Sexual

Self-Assessment 7.1

Assessing Sexual Practices—Safety First for Sexual Health

Answer each of the following questions:

1. I avoid having multiple sex partners. yes no
2. I avoid having anonymous sex partners. yes no
3. I avoid having sex with someone who has a high risk for having a STI. yes no
4. I avoid exchanging sex for money or drugs. yes no
5. I or my male partners use a latex condom with a spermicide. yes no
6. I avoid anal sex. yes no
7. I avoid sex with someone whom I don't know well. yes no
8. I avoid using intravenous drugs. yes no

9. I avoid sex with anyone who has genital sores or lesions. yes no
10. I take precautions to prevent unwanted pregnancy. yes no
11. I avoid sexual activity while under the influence of drugs or alcohol. yes no
12. If I am a woman, I get regular Pap tests or have been tested for HPV yes no

If you answered any of these questions with a "no," it is important to reconsider the risks involved with your personal sex behaviors. You should also be tested for STIs.

■ Latex condoms, although not a guarantee against infection, are a key component of risk reduction for STIs

Over spring break my boyfriend went skiing and he said he "slept around a little." So what should I do about protecting myself? I'm on the pill, but should we get tested or use a condom? I really am confused.

—**22-year-old woman**

If a woman has douched before the visit, the clinician may not be able to diagnose the condition accurately. A bimanual examination follows the internal examination. (See Chapter 4 for details of the gynecological examination.) Any suspicious lesion in the perineal area is cultured, and a rectal culture is obtained if the woman has had anal intercourse.

Treatment Concerns

Treatment regimens for STIs vary according to the specific pathogen involved, severity of infection, location of infection, previous infections, and personal medical history. A woman should inform her clinician if she is taking any prescriptions or over-the-counter medications. Previous drug reactions are also important, because previous reactions to one drug may contraindicate the use of other drugs. If a woman suspects that she may be pregnant, she should advise the clinician of that possibility as well. Pregnant women should avoid some antibiotics because they can stain the permanent teeth of the developing fetus or cause other side effects. It is of paramount importance that prescribed medications be taken as recommended. If antibiotics are prescribed for 10 days, then they need to be taken for 10 days, even if symptoms dissipate earlier.

Several STIs require follow-up examinations to ensure that the treatment regimen was successful. Failure to comply with follow-up guidelines may result in unsuccessful treatment and continued disease transmission and damage. Because reproductive tract infections may cause abnormal Pap test findings, after an infection has cleared up, may be a good idea to have a Pap test repeated in 6 to 12 weeks. A reading at that time will give a more accurate report of the cervical status than one conducted during a period of inflammation.

activity should be curtailed or condoms diligently used until both partners are certain of a cure.

Women are often embarrassed to mention their fears about STIs to a clinician. If there is a risk of infection, it is important to discuss this possibility. Although no woman wants to find out that she has an STI, it is always better to know than not to know: STIs can be spread and do serious biological damage even in the absence of symptoms, and all STIs are treatable, if not curable. Clinicians may not routinely test for STIs or look for them in a routine gynecological examination. If oral or anal sex has been part of a woman's sexual experience, the clinician should be advised so that a comprehensive examination may be conducted for an accurate diagnosis. Finally, it helps to be prepared. Writing down a list of questions to ask a clinician and practicing questions to ask with a friend beforehand are two strategies women can use to make sure they get all the information they need without making additional visits.

A physical examination for STIs is often like a routine gynecological examination, but it is not limited to the genital area. An examination of the mouth, throat, and lymph nodes usually precedes the genital examination. The genital examination is conducted in a lithotomy position, which requires that the woman lie on her back with her legs spread and positioned in stirrups. This position enables the healthcare provider to examine the perineal area. The examination begins with a careful visual inspection by the clinician. A speculum is inserted into the vagina for an internal examination. The clinician then examines the vagina for discharge, odor, ulcerations, or inflammation.

Summary

Sexually transmitted infections can pose serious health threats to women. By understanding these conditions (**Table 7.3**) and making informed decisions about personal behaviors and health-seeking behaviors, women can

Table 7.3	**Basic Information About the Major Sexually Transmitted Infections**
AIDS (Acquired Immune Deficiency Syndrome)	
Organism	Viral—HIV (human immunodeficiency virus)
Transmission	Blood or sexual fluids entering the body, usually through sexual intercourse, sharing needles, or from mother to child before or during birth
Symptoms	Flu-like symptoms such as fever, weight loss, fatigue, and enlarged lymph nodes may appear and disappear shortly after infection; identifiable opportunistic infections may take years to appear.
Diagnosis	AIDS diagnoses are made based on T-cell counts or the presence of opportunistic infections. HIV can be easily identified with antibody tests.
Treatment	No treatment will prevent HIV infection or rid the body of HIV; however, antiviral medications, when used properly, can delay the onset of AIDS and improve quality of life.
Special Concerns for Women	Increased reproductive health problems; possible perinatal (mother-to-child) transmission (can be dramatically reduced with treatment).
Potential Long-Term Consequences	If AIDS goes untreated, opportunistic infections can cause grave illness or death.
Chlamydia	
Organism	Bacteria—*Chlamydia trachomatis*
Transmission	Direct contact with infected mucosal membrane or sexual fluids
Symptoms	Most women are asymptomatic; symptoms may include vaginal discharge and excessive urination, pelvic pain, fever, and nausea.
Diagnosis	Urine tests or culture of symptoms or discharge; alternatively, a diagnosis may be made by examining symptoms and ruling out gonorrhea.
Treatment	Antibiotics will stop infection but may not be able to repair damage from long-term infection.
Special Concerns for Women	Pelvic inflammatory disease (see PID), possible co-infection with gonorrhea, reinfection with an untreated partner, perinatal (mother-to-child) transmission
Potential Long-Term Consequences	Infertility, ectopic pregnancy, chronic pelvic pain, possibility of systemic infection
Gonorrhea	
Organism	Bacteria—*Neisseria gonorrhoeae*
Transmission	Direct contact with infected mucosal membrane or sexual fluids
Symptoms	Most women are asymptomatic; symptoms may include vaginal discharge and excessive urination, pelvic pain, fever, and nausea.
Diagnosis	Urine tests or culture of discharge or the infected area
Treatment	Antibiotics will stop infection but may not be able to repair damage from long-term infection.
Special Concerns for Women	Pelvic inflammatory disease (PID), possible co-infection with chlamydia, reinfection with an untreated partner, perinatal transmission
Potential Long-Term Consequences	Infertility, ectopic pregnancy, chronic pelvic pain, possibility of systemic infection
Hepatitis B (HBV)	
Organism	Virus—hepatitis B virus
Transmission	Entrance of blood or sexual fluids into the body; most cases occur through unprotected sexual contact or shared needles.
Symptoms	Often asymptomatic; symptoms include nausea, fever, dark urine, jaundice (yellowing of the skin and eyes), and abdominal discomfort.
Diagnosis	Blood tests to identify virus or antibodies; liver tests and symptoms may also be used in diagnosis.
Treatment	No cure for hepatitis B exists, but antiviral medications may help in some chronic cases. A three-shot vaccine will prevent hepatitis B infection; most infants born in the United States after 1982 have received this vaccine.
Special Concerns for Women	Perinatal transmission
Possible Long-Term Consequences	Possible liver disease or liver cancer in chronic cases; most infections eventually resolve on their own.
Herpes Simplex Virus (HSV)	
Organism	Virus—herpes simplex (two types—1 and 2)
Transmission	Direct contact with symptoms; contact with the infected area carries a low but real risk even without symptoms.

(continues)

Table 7.3   Basic Information About the Major Sexually Transmitted Infections *(continued)*

Symptoms	Painful sores, blisters, or rashes on the genital area, rectum, or mouth that appear and disappear periodically; women may be asymptomatic or have symptoms in the cervical area that go unnoticed.
Diagnosis	Examination or culture of symptoms; blood tests can identify herpes antibodies.
Treatment	No cure or vaccine available; some antiviral medications can reduce duration or number of outbreaks.
Special Concerns for Women	Possible perinatal transmission, especially if herpes infection takes place during pregnancy; herpes sores may increase the likelihood of receiving HIV or other STIs if exposed.
Possible Long-Term Consequences	Rare in otherwise healthy adults; severity, duration, and frequency of symptoms usually diminish over time.

HPV (Human Papillomavirus)

Organism	Virus—human papillomavirus (almost 100 strains, about a dozen of which are sexually transmitted)
Transmission	Genital skin-to-genital skin contact
Symptoms	"High-risk" strains of HPV can cause abnormal cell growth on the cervix; if untreated this cell growth (dysplasia) can sometimes advance to cervical cancer. Other, "low-risk" strains can cause warts to appear on the external genital or anal areas in men or women.
Diagnosis	Warts may be diagnosed by physical examination; cervical dysplasia may be diagnosed with biopsy; DNA testing of the virus can identify the presence of HPV.
Treatment	Abnormal cell changes in the cervix may be treated by cryotherapy, loop electrosurgical excision (LEEP), cone biopsy, or laser surgery. Treatment for genital warts revolves around removing symptoms, not eliminating the virus, and consists of topical caustic agents, electrocautery, cryotherapy, and laser surgery.
Special Concerns for Women	Cervical changes, if untreated, may develop into cervical cancer; warts may interfere with pregnancy in rare cases.
Possible Long-Term Consequences	Cervical dysplasia can lead to cervical cancer if undiagnosed or untreated; most cases of HPV go away on their own eventually.

Pelvic Inflammatory Disease (PID)

Organism	Bacteria—usually *Chlamydia trachomatis* (chlamydia) or *Neisseria gonorrhoeae* (gonorrhea)
Transmission	PID itself is not transmitted but usually develops as a complication of gonorrhea or chlamydia.
Symptoms	Cases may be asymptomatic; abdominal pain or pain during intercourse, unusual vaginal discharge or bleeding, fever, and nausea.
Diagnosis	Clinical evaluation based on symptoms and possible presence of a causative bacterial agent
Treatment	Antibiotics; surgery may be necessary in advanced cases.
Special Concerns for Women	Reinfection of bacterial infection from untreated or undertreated partners; possible perinatal transmission of bacterial agent
Possible Long-Term Consequences	Infertility, ectopic pregnancy, recurrent infection, chronic pelvic pain

Syphilis

Organism	Bacteria—*Treponema pallidum*
Transmission	Skin-to-skin contact with infected area or symptoms; perinatal transmission
Symptoms	Primary stage: painless sore (chancre)
	Secondary stage: rash, hair loss, enlarged lymph nodes
	Tertiary stage: systemic damage
Diagnosis	Blood tests; microscopic verification of organism; examination of symptoms
Treatment	Antibiotics will stop infection but cannot undo systemic damage.
Special Concerns for Women	Perinatal transmission, possible reinfection from untreated or undertreated partners, sores may increase likelihood of receiving HIV or other STIs if exposed.
Potential Long-Term Consequences	Untreated infections can cause permanent damage to all major body systems or even death.

Trichomoniasis

Organism	Single-celled protozoan—*Trichomonas vaginalis*
Transmission	Direct sexual contact, less likely through contaminated wet objects (towels, swimming suits)
Symptoms	Many women and most men are asymptomatic; symptoms may include white or greenish yellow discharge, vaginal itching, or painful urination.
Diagnosis	Examination of symptoms or culture of infected area
Treatment	Oral antibiotics
Special Concerns for Women	Reinfection from untreated or undertreated partners
Possible Long-Term Consequences	Rare for otherwise healthy women

Profiles of Remarkable Women

Felicia Hance Stewart, M.D. (1943–2006)

Felicia Hance Stewart was an obstetrician/gynecologist who was also a distinguished clinician and researcher. Following her time as a practicing physician, Stewart served as Deputy Assistant Secretary for Population Affairs in the Department of Health and Human Services, making her the most senior official in the United States responsible for domestic and international policies on family planning and population issues. In this position, she had direct responsibility for management of the National Family Planning Program (Title X) and the Adolescent Family Life Program (Title XX).

In 1996, Stewart was appointed the Director of Reproductive Health Programs for the Henry J. Kaiser Family Foundation, where she focused on improving services for low-income women and preventing unintended pregnancy. In 1999, she joined the Center for Reproductive Health Research and Policy at the University of California, San Francisco. As a Co-Director of the Center, Stewart conducted U.S. and international projects that spanned the disciplines of contraception, abortion, and sexually transmitted infections.

Stewart served as the principal investigator on many research projects and published numerous articles and textbooks on contraception and family planning. She contributed greatly to issues concerning reproductive health and, consequently, served on many national scientific and professional advisory and review committees. Stewart authored *Understanding Your Body: The Concerned Woman's Guide to Gynecology and Health*, a nontechnical reference book, and co-authored *Contraceptive Technology*, a professional reference for family planning. Stewart may be most remembered for her leading role in the research establishing that the emergency contraceptive known as Plan B is both safe and effective when sold without a physician's prescription. Her published research led to the availability of over-the-counter Plan B in a number of states, including California.

reduce their risk of exposure and the effects of disease. Personal responsibility and informed decision making are essential to preventing and managing STIs.

■■■■

Topics for Discussion

1. Sexually transmitted infections are biologically "sexist." What does this mean?

2. How do cultural and emotional dimensions complicate STI public health and educational efforts?

3. Why is reinfection so common with some bacterial STIs?

4. Imagine that you are in a relationship and that you have an infection with HSV or HPV. How and when would you begin discussing your infection? How would you feel if the situation were reversed?

5. Describe three productive and three nonproductive ways to inquire about a person's past.

6. In spite of the knowledge base about AIDS, people still report a strong fear of AIDS. Why? What are some of the myths associated with AIDS?

7. What should a woman do upon learning of a positive HIV antibody test?

8. HIV is similar to HSV and HPV in that it is a sexually transmitted virus that has no cure. How is it different?

9. What would you tell a friend or loved one who suspected that she might have an STI but was afraid to get tested?

10. Balancing STI risk reduction with flexibility and intimacy in sexual relationships is a difficult task for many people. How do you balance these two needs? Are these two needs always in opposition to each other?

■■■■

Key Terms

AIDS (acquired immune deficiency syndrome): A progressive disease caused by HIV, which gradually destroys an infected person's immune system. AIDS is the final stage of HIV infection. Although there is no way for an infected person to get ride of HIV, modern medications can often slow the progress of the disease, or prevent AIDS from developing entirely.

Asymptomatic viral shedding: Most often associated with herpes simplex virus infections. Viral shedding occurs when active herpes virus, present in the nerve cells of an infected person, moves along the nerves to the surface of the skin. Shedding often occurs without any symptoms (asymptomatic), but the person may still be infectious, meaning that it can be passed on to others.

Bacteria: Single-celled organisms that multiply and cause disease by forcing the body to release poisons and germ-fighting antibodies. Unlike viral infections, bacterial infections usually can be treated by antibiotics.

Bacterial vaginosis (BV): Inflammation of the vagina, caused by an overgrowth of the normal bacteria found in the vagina and resulting in an imbalance. The most common cause of vaginitis, this infection is sometimes, but not always, sexually transmitted.

Chlamydia: A sexually transmitted infection that is caused by the bacterium *Chlamydia trachomatis*. Most people are asymptomatic and, therefore, are not aware of their infection. If left untreated, Chlamydia can cause serious damage to a woman's reproductive system. Chlamydia is the most frequently reported infectious disease in the United States.

Ectoparasitic infections: Infections caused by tiny parasites that reside on the skin and survive on human blood and tissue. Infections include scabies and public lice ("crabs"). Parasites cause itching and may cause bumps or a rash, but are easily treated with a topical cream.

Enzyme-linked immunosorbent assay (ELISA): Laboratory test used to detect antibodies produced in response to HIV infection. If HIV antibodies are found with this test, it is repeated. If antibodies are found on a second ELISA test, a Western blot test is performed.

Gonorrhea: A sexually transmitted bacterial infection that can cause dangerous complications leading to infertility, ectopic pregnancy, or persistent pain in the pelvic area. It can even spread to the bloodstream and cause arthritis or life-threatening heart or brain infections.

Hepatitis: Inflammation and destruction of liver cells.

Herpes simplex virus (HSV): A family of contagious viruses that infect humans. Viruses in the herpes family include HSV-1 and HSV-2, which can cause sores in the mouth or genital area (the latter infection is often referred to as "genital herpes") as well as the virus that causes chicken pox.

HIV (Human Immunodeficiency Virus): A virus that attacks and damages the white blood cells in the body's immune system that are needed to fight off infection. HIV eventually causes AIDS when so many white blood cells have been destroyed that the immune system can no longer fight off illness.

Human papillomavirus (HPV): An extremely common sexually transmitted virus. There are many strains of HPV; some of them can cause genital warts in men and women, and other kinds can cause cervical dysplasia in women, which, if left untreated, can lead to cervical cancer.

Immune system: The body's natural defense system, which works to protect the body from pathogens.

Jaundice: A condition in which accumulation of the pigments in the blood produces a yellowing of the skins and eyes.

Opportunistic infections: Infections that seldom cause disease in people with normal immune function but "take the opportunity" to cause disease in people with a present illness or a lowered immune system, such as caused by HIV/AIDS.

Pelvic inflammatory disease (PID): A general term describing an infection of the internal female reproductive tract that can lead to infertility, chronic pain, or ectopic pregnancy. PID is usually caused by a sexually transmitted infection such as chlamydia or gonorrhea that spreads into the upper reproductive tract.

Prodrome: Period of infectiousness before the first signs of infection are present.

Pus: A substance composed of dead bacteria, dead white blood cells, and fluid that is most commonly the result of an infection process.

Retrovirus: A virus that has the ability to take over certain cells and interrupt their normal genetic function.

Sexually transmitted infections (STIs): Infections of the reproductive tract that are transmitted by sexual intimacy. Sexually transmitted infections include Chlamydia, gonorrhea, syphilis, herpes, genital warts, hepatitis, and human immunodeficiency virus (HIV) infections.

Sitz baths: A tub in which one bathes in a sitting position with hips and buttocks under water and legs out.

Syphilis: A sexually transmitted bacterial infection that causes small, painless sores in the genital area, a rash, flu-like symptoms, and, after many years, systemic damage.

Toxic shock syndrome (TSS): A rare but serious infection cause by strains of the bacteria *Staphylococcus aureus*. For reasons not fully understood, these bacteria release toxins (poisons) into the bloodstream after deep wounds, surgery, or tampon use (especially high-absorbency tampon use).

Trichomoniasis: A vaginal infection cause by *Trichomonas vaginalis*, a single-cell protozoan parasite with a whip-like tail that it uses to propel itself through vaginal and urethral mucus.

Viruses: Small pathogens incapable of independent metabolism; can only reproduce inside living cells.

Western blot test: Laboratory test used to detect antibodies; Western blots are performed after two positive ELISA tests to test for HIV.

Yeast infection: A vaginal infection caused most commonly by the fungal organism, *Candida albicans*. Symptoms of yeast infections include abnormal vaginal discharge, vaginal and labial itching and burning, redness and inflammation of the vulvar skin, pain with intercourse, and painful urination.

■■■■

Websites

AIDS Education Global Information System: http://www.aegis.com

American Social Health Association: http://www.ashastd.org

Centers for Disease Control and Prevention, Division of STIs: http://www.cdc.gov/STI

EngenderHealth: http://www.engenderhealth.org

Hepatitis Foundation International: http://www.hepfi.org

HIVandHepatitis.com: http://www.hepatitisandhiv.com

International Herpes Alliance: http://www.herpesalliance.org

Planned Parenthood: http://www.plannedparenthood.org

Sexuality Information and Education Council of the United States: http://www.siecus.org

The Body: The Complete HIV/AIDS Resource: http://www.thebody.com

UNAIDS: http://www.unaids.org

■■■■

References

1. Hanson, J., Ponser, S., Hassig, S., et al. (2005). Assessment of sexually transmitted diseases as risk factor for HIV seroconversion in a New Orleans sexually transmitted disease clinic, 1990–1998. *Annals of Epidemiology* 15(1): 13–20.

2. Centers for Disease Control and Prevention [CDC]. (2010). Sexually transmitted disease treatment guidelines. *Morbidity and Mortality Weekly Report* 59: 1–109.

3. Centers for Disease Control and Prevention [CDC]. (2008). National representative CDC study finds 1 in 4 teenage girls has a sexually transmitted disease. Available at: http://www.cdc.gov/stdconference/2008/media/release-11march2008.htm.

4. Centers for Disease Control and Prevention [CDC]. (2011). *Sexually transmitted disease surveillance 2010*. Atlanta, GA: U.S. Department of Health and Human Services.

5. Rietmejer, C., Van Bemmelen, R., Judson, F., et al. (2002). Incidence and repeat infection rates of Chlamydia trachomatis infections among male and female patients in an STD clinic: Implications for screening and rescreening. *Sexually Transmitted Diseases* 29: 65–72.

6. Chesson, H., Blandford, J., Thomas, L., et al. (2004). The estimated direct medical costs of sexually transmitted disease among American youth, 2000. *Perspectives on Sexual and Reproductive Health* 36(1): 11–19.

7. Joint U.N. Programme on HIV/AIDS (UNAIDS). (2010). *UNAIDS report on the global epidemic, 2010*. Geneva, Switerland: UNAIDS.

8. Adderley-Kelly, B., & Stephens, E. (2005). Chlamydia—A major threat to adolescents and young adults. *Association of Black Nursing Faculty* May/June: 52–55.

9. Rein, D., Kassler, W., Irwin, K., et al. (2000). Direct medical cost of pelvic inflammatory disease and its sequelae: Decreasing but still substantial. *Obstetrics and Gynecology* 95: 397–402.

10. Schwebke, J., & Desmond, R. (2005). Risk factors for bacterial vaginosis in women at high risk for sexually transmitted diseases. *Sexually Transmitted Diseases* 32(11): 654–658.

11. Myer, L., Kuhn, L., Stein, Z., et al. (2005). Intravaginal practices, bacterial vaginosis, and women's susceptibility to HIV infection: Epidemiological evidence and biological mechanisms. *Lancet Infectious Diseases* 5(12): 786–794.

12. Klebanoff, M., Schwebke, J., Zhang, J., et al. (2004). Vulvo-vaginal symptoms in women with bacterial vaginosis. *Obstetrics and Gynecology* 104: 267.

13. Zhang, J., Hatch, M., Zhang, D., et al. (2004). Frequency of douching and risk of bacterial vaginosis in African-American women. *Obstetrics and Gynecology* 104: 756–760.

14. Schiffman, M., & Castle, P. (2005). The promise of global cervical-cancer prevention. *New England Journal of Medicine* 353(20): 2101–2104.

15. Xu, F., Sternberg, M. R., Kottiri, B. J., et al. (2006). Trends in herpes simplex virus type 1 and type 2 seroprevalence in the United States. *JAMA* 296(8):964–973.

16. Corey, L., Wald, A., Patel, R., et al. (2004). Once-daily valacyclovir to reduce the risk of transmission of genital herpes. *New England Journal of Medicine* 350: 11–20.

17. Holmes, K., Levine, R., & Weaver, M. (2004). Effectiveness of condoms in preventing sexually transmitted diseases. *Bulletin of the World Health Organization* 82(6): 454–461.

18. Centers for Disease Control and Prevention. (2010). *Viral hepatitis surveillance, 2009*. Atlanta, GA: U.S. Department of Health and Human Services.

19. Prejean, J., Song, R., Hernandez, A., et al. (2011). Estimated HIV incidence in the United States, 2006–2009. *PLoS ONE* 6(8): e17502. doi:10.1371/journal.pone.0017502

20. HIV outbreak began decades earlier than thought. (October 1, 2008). *Washington Post*. Available at: http://www.washingtonpost.com/wp-dyn/content/article/2008/10/01/AR2008100101660.html.

21. Joint U.N. Programme on AIDS. (2010). 2008 report on the global AIDS epidemic. Geneva: UNAIDS.

22. Centers for Disease Control and Prevention [CDC]. (2011). HIV surveillance—United States, 1981–2008. *Morbidity and Mortality Weekly Report* 60(21): 689–693.

23. Bunders, M., Bekker, V., Scherpbier, H., et al. (2005). Haematological parameters of HIV-1 uninfected infants born to HIV-1 infected mothers. *Acta Paediatrica* 94(11): 1571–1577.

24. Centers for Disease Control and Prevention [CDC]. (2001). *Fact sheet for public health personnel: Male latex condoms*. Available at: http://www.cdc.gov/nchstp/od/condoms.pdf

Menopause and Hormone Therapy

Chapter Objectives

On completion of this chapter, the student should be able to discuss:

1. Demographic aging trends in the United States and social and cultural reflections on menopause.

2. Menopause and the different stages that women experience before, during, and after menopause.

3. The biology of natural menopause.

4. The biology, and reasons for, induced menopause.

5. Symptoms of menopause.

6. Complications of menopause.

7. The medicalization of menopause.

8. History of hormone use for menopause management.

9. The Women's Health Initiative and Million Women Study and their significance.

10. Medical and nonmedical options for managing menopause.

11. Concerns with "bio-identical" hormone products.

12. Informed decision-making strategies for women about menopause.

womenshealth.jbpub.com

Women's Health Online is a great source for supplementary women's health information for both students and instructors. Visit

http://womenshealth.jbpub.com

to find a variety of useful tools for learning, thinking, and teaching.

Introduction

Women, as they reach midlife, experience menopause, the end of their menstrual cycles. Menopause is not synonymous with midlife for a woman; it is a specific event that occurs during her midlife years that brings both physical and emotional changes. Menopause, a topic that was once not discussed in public, is now recognized as an important women's health issue. While women now are better informed about menopause than before, many women continue to lack basic information about menopause, such as its effects on the body, the potential benefits and drawbacks to menopausal hormone therapy, and other forms of menopause management.

This chapter reviews how cultural and social attitudes about aging and medicine have influenced attitudes about menopause, the negative and positive effects that menopause can have on a woman's life, the basic biology of menopause, and its health effects. In addition, the chapter will review the medicalization of menopause, the history of hormone use to manage menopause, and the two major studies about menopause and their results. The chapter concludes with informed decision-making guidance for women and the special caution to be exercised with popular "bio-identical" menopausal therapies.

Social and Cultural Reflections on Menopause

Menopause needs to be understood in the context of the demographic aging trends of the United States. Because menopause is a natural aging process, all women who live to enjoy their later years will experience it. However, it was not until the 20th century that the life expectancy of U.S. women reached a point where most women lived much beyond menopause. Today most women will live one-third or more of their lives postmenopausally. As the median age of the population continues to increase (see **Figure 8.1**), a growing proportion of women will have experienced, or will be experiencing, menopause. In 2010, nearly 23 million women were between the ages of 45 and 54, the age group at which menopause most often begins.[1]

Over the past century, the medical and public health communities have conducted major in-depth studies to better understand the clinical and demographical dimensions of menopause. Media coverage and public discussions of the emerging research, along with alternative menopause

Figure 8.1

Older population by age: 1900–2050.

Source: U.S. Census Bureau. (2000)

management options, have often been inaccurate, misunderstood, and exaggerated. As a result, many women remain unsure about how to best manage many of the natural symptoms associated with menopause.

In the United States, where society values and media emphasis is on youthful behaviors and appearance in women, menopause has often been viewed as a negative event. This trend is not universal. In many Asian countries, for example, women have traditionally gained respect and influence, often becoming the head of the household, as they reached middle age. In the United States, popular culture has portrayed menopause as a difficult time for women, during which they experience uncontrollable moodiness, irritability, and depression. In the 1800s and early 1900s, popular myths and stereotypes, often encouraged by the medical community, depicted menopause as a tragedy that caused hypochondria, hysteria, and irritability. This view implied that solace from these conditions could be found only in a physician's office with pharmacological remedies or surgical intervention. In the 1940s and 1950s, treatment for menopause often focused on psychiatric conditions of depression and melancholy.

Popular culture depicted menopausal women as burdens to themselves, to their families, and, if they were married, to their suffering husbands. In subsequent decades, menopause was examined as a "disease," with clinical concern focused on women reporting symptoms and seeking medical intervention for specific symptom relief. An explosion

■ Women today are more open in their discussions about all aspects of their sexual well-being, including menopause.

of commercial pharmacological options and the heavy marketing of them to clinicians and women made the situation even more complicated.

Now menopause is understood as a process of normal change. Open discussions about sexuality and life issues have allowed women to talk about menopause and aging without fear, embarrassment, or stigmatization. Many women either welcome menopause or do not fear it. The cessation of menses frees them from contraceptive concerns, in some cases leading to increased sexual satisfaction. Other women appreciate the freedom from menstrual periods, which may have been inconvenient or uncomfortable. Menopause may be a time of fewer family obligations, accompanied by increased opportunities in the workforce. For some, this life stage is more flexible in terms of leisure time and financial resources, increasing the opportunities for new forms of activity and self-expression. For others, it is merely the continuation of intense work, with many women taking on childcare responsibilities for grandchildren or caring for their own parents.

While the symptoms of menopause, as well as how those symptoms are perceived, vary from woman to woman, all women should understand the biological and psychological factors associated with this important and inevitable life change. A survey found significant information gaps remain about menopause in in all age groups. In fact, almost one in four women (24%) said they have more information about symptoms and treatments for erectile dysfunction for men than menopause for women.[2]

Menopause

Also known as the climacterium or "change of life," menopause marks the end of menstruation and childbearing capability. Menopause is the permanent end of menstruation and fertility, officially occurring 12 months after a woman's last menstrual period. Menopause is a natural, predictable biological process, not a medical illness or a disease. The transitional stage immediately before menopause is called **perimenopause**. During this period, physical changes begin to accelerate and women are most likely to experience perceptible physical changes due to drops in hormone production. These symptoms usually last about one year after a woman's last menstrual period. **Postmenopause** follows menopause and lasts the rest of a woman's life.

Like the onset of a girl's first period, the age of onset of menopause varies. Most women enter and complete menopause between the ages of 45 and 55, with the average age of natural menopause being 51.[3] Many factors influence the age at which a woman has her last period. These factors include family history, environmental factors, personal behaviors, and genetics.[4] Menopause is considered "late" when it occurs after age 55. One study found that late menopause was associated with a moderate protective effect for premature death.[5] Early menopause is defined as going through menopause before age 46, either naturally or surgically through removal of both ovaries. Early menopause is a potential risk factor for cardiovascular disease.[6] Women who smoke, who have not graduated from college, who are formerly married, who are unemployed, and who have had heart disease all reach natural menopause sooner than other women. Late menopausal women are more likely to have taken the pill, be ethnically Japanese, and to have given birth.[7]

Biology of Natural Menopause

Natural menopause occurs when the ovaries stop responding to the luteinizing and follicle-stimulating hormones that are produced in the anterior pituitary, which is under the control of the hypothalamus. As a woman approaches her late 30s, her ovaries produce less **estrogen** and **progesterone**, the hormones that regulate menstruation. As a result, ovulation becomes somewhat erratic. The mechanisms underlying these changes are not well understood. Whatever the reasons, a woman entering menopause will have more luteinizing and follicle-stimulating hormones present in the bloodstream and less estrogen and progesterone than she had during her regular menstrual cycling. Fertility begins to decline due to these hormonal effects. Pregnancy remains a possibility, however, because ovulation may occur in sporadic intervals during this time. In her 40s, the changes become more pronounced for a woman. Her menstrual periods may become longer or shorter, heavier or lighter, and more or less frequent until her ovaries cease to produce eggs and her periods end. Early in the transition process, many women experience 2-week cycles. Further into the process, women may skip periods for months at a time, and these skipped periods can be followed by a heavier period. The number of consecutively skipped periods increases as the time of the last period approaches. Based on population studies, scientists have classified the stages of menopause transition according to the woman's menstrual bleeding pattern and the changes in her FSH levels.[8] Natural menopause occurs when the ovaries fail to respond to the luteinizing and follicle-stimulating hormones produced in the anterior pituitary, which is under the control of the hypothalamus. Menopause is considered complete once monthly periods have ceased altogether for at least 12 months.

> *I guess that I was one of the lucky ones. My menopause was fairly short and easy. One of my friends had severe hot flashes and another friend was moody. Menopause has been different for each of us, but we all got through it in one piece.*
>
> **—55-year-old woman**

After menopause, women continue to produce estrogen, but the estrogen the ovaries produce drops sharply. Most postmenopausal estrogen is produced through the adrenal glands, which makes precursors of estrogen that stored fat converts to estrogen. Far less estrogen, however, is produced in this manner than was produced in the ovaries before menopause.

Smoking can also influence the biology of menopause. Women who smoke produce less estrogen and tend to experience menopause earlier than nonsmoking women. A woman who smokes in her youth or who is exposed to

secondhand smoke is also at increased risk for low bone mass. The number of cigarettes a woman smokes, as well as the length of her habit both increase her risk for fractures in later life. In addition, smokers with fractures take longer to heal than nonsmokers and may experience more complications during the healing process.[9]

Menopause Caused by Other Factors

In addition to the normal age-associated decline in hormones that leads to natural menopause, the condition can result from other causes. "Surgically induced menopause" happens with **hysterectomies**, the surgical removal of the uterus. It is the second most-frequently performed procedure, after cesarean sections, on women of reproductive age in the United States.[10] Hysterectomies are performed for certain reproductive cancers and for other conditions such as fibroids, which are benign growths that can develop on the uterus. Hysterectomy performed with the removal of both ovaries and the fallopian tubes, known as a **total hysterectomy** and **bilateral salpingo-oophorectomy**, has become increasingly common (**Figure 8.2**). When a woman's ovaries are surgically removed, a more abrupt and earlier menopause results. The pituitary gland continues to produce luteinizing and follicle-stimulating hormones, but the ovaries are not present to respond with ovulation. Estrogen and progesterone are no longer produced at the same level as they were before surgery because of the absence of the ovaries. Although the adrenal glands still produce these hormones, the levels are considerably lower without the ovarian production. Women who have had both ovaries removed before the onset of menopause experience more severe menopausal symptoms.[11] Hysterectomy in women aged 50 years or younger increases the risk for cardiovascular disease later in life; oophorectomy appears to increase the risk of both coronary heart disease and stroke.[12]

This high prevalence of surgical procedures continues to be controversial. Hysterectomies can have serious, lifelong consequences for women, yet women often either receive little information about these consequences or have little chance to consider them. Approximately 600,000 hysterectomies are performed annually in the United States, and approximately 20 million U.S. women have had a hysterectomy.[13] More than one-third (37%) of hysterectomies with oophorectomy are performed on women aged 15–44 years; the majority of these procedures are performed for benign (noncancerous) conditions.[10] The frequency of hysterectomy also varies greatly by geography (**Figure 8.3**). This variance suggests that access to care and the preferences

Figure 8.2

Four types of hysterectomy.

Partial hysterectomy: only the uterus is removed.

Total hysterectomy: both the uterus and cervix are removed.

Total hysterectomy with bilateral salpingo-oophorectomy: both ovaries, the fallopian tubes, the uterus, and the cervix are removed.

Radical hysterectomy: both ovaries, the fallopian tubes, the uterus, the cervix, and the lymph nodes are removed.

of doctors, rather than pure medical need, influence who undergoes this serious medical procedure.

In addition to hysterectomies, chemotherapy and/or radiation therapy, which are common cancer treatments, can induce menopause. Menopausal symptoms such as hot flashes often present during the course of treatment or within 3 to 6 months.

Primary ovarian insufficiency is another condition that results in early menopause. Approximately 1% of women experience menopause before the age of 40.[14] This condition may result from ovarian failure to produce normal levels of reproductive hormones. The condition may be due to genetic factors or autoimmune disorders but for many women, the primary cause is not known.

Menopause Symptoms

Hormonal changes during menopause affect women physically and emotionally (Figure 8.2). Studies examining menopause show considerable variance in the prevalence of symptoms, especially severe symptoms. The duration and severity of symptoms for any individual woman cannot be predicted in advance.

The most frequently reported physical symptom is the vascular response or instability, also known as **hot flashes** or hot flushes due to hormonal fluctuations. Hot flashes are generally described as uncomfortable sensations of internally generated heat, beginning in the chest and moving to the neck and head, or spreading throughout the body. Increased heart rate and temperature, shallow breathing,

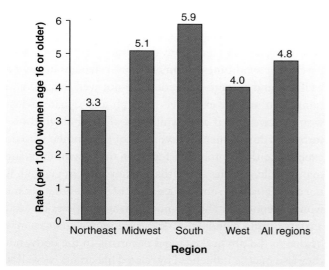

Figure 8.3

Hysterectomy rates by geographic region, United States.

Source: Wu, J., et al. (2007). Hysterectomy rates in the United States, 2003.

and sweating followed by chills are all common during hot flashes. In some women, hot flashes can be so intense as to raise the body temperature by a few degrees in a short period of time. Despite the discomfort to the woman, the hot flashes are not considered to be harmful. In addition, a significant number of women do not find them disturbing.[15] Hot flashes may begin before a woman has stopped menstruating, and they may continue for several years after menopause. Hot flashes can also be an early and acute sign of estrogen deficiency.

Besides hot flashes, common symptoms of menopause include:[16,17]

- Menstrual periods that occur less often and eventually stop
- Decreased fertility, progressing to infertility
- Heart pounding, racing, or irregular heartbeats (palpitations)
- Night sweats
- Skin flushing
- Sleep disturbances
- Decreased interest in sex and decreased response to sexual stimulation
- Forgetfulness
- Increased abdominal fat
- Thinning hair
- Loss of breast fullness
- Headaches
- Mood swings including irritability, depression, and anxiety
- Urine leakage
- Vaginal dryness and painful sexual intercourse
- Vaginal infections
- Joint aches and pains

Menopausal symptoms also vary depending on the woman's lifestyle, menstrual status, race/ethnicity, and socioeconomic status.[18] Cross-cultural differences suggest that symptom reporting is not consistent and that there are significant ethnic differences in the frequency and severity of the total physical, psychological, and psychosomatic symptoms.[19,20] African American women often present with menopausal symptoms earlier than White women of the same age, while Asian American women seem to have the fewest symptoms.[18] Symptoms such as mood changes, fatigue, and vaginal dryness tend to be more common and more severe for Hispanic women.[17,20]

It is often difficult for women to directly associate any or all of their symptoms with menopause. Other factors such as aging, family life, health issues, work, and home stresses can affect the process and how women interpret them. Symptoms such as hot flashes, can occur at night, disrupting sleep and contributing to much of the insomnia associated with menopause.

Thinning of the vaginal lining, known as **vaginal atrophy**, also sometimes occurs after menopause. As estrogen levels decline, layers of the vaginal surface become drier and more sensitive. The vaginal wall becomes thinner, less elastic, and more vulnerable to infection. Some women experience pain or burning during intercourse, vaginal discharge, and more frequent vaginal infections. Physiological changes that affect the vaginal tract may affect a woman's sexual response as well. For example, lack of vaginal lubricant may affect sexual arousal. A change in hormone levels—specifically androgen production—may diminish libido.

Other symptoms associated with menopause include breast changes, changes in hair growth, and changes in skin. As estrogen levels decrease during menopause, a rapid loss of collagen occurs, causing the skin to become thinner and less elastic. The cycling levels of hormones also may cause a change in the prevalence or intensity of headaches.[21]

The medical community has associated a variety of psychiatric and mental health conditions with menopause. Many of these associations have been based on myths, stereotypes, unwarranted assumptions, and methodically flawed studies. Conditions associated with menopause include postpartum psychosis and depression, premenstrual syndrome, post-hysterectomy depression, and menopausal psychiatric syndromes. Perimenopausal changes in mental wellness and cognitive function are not well defined and remain an area of extensive research and debate. Most women have few, if any, symptoms of psychological disturbances during menopause; most of the women who do experience these problems feel that these symptoms are manageable. Studies show that menopause, in general, is not associated with an increased risk of depression.[22] Some women report irritability, mood swings, depression, and anxiety during menopause. These emotional changes may be due to the physical changes occurring in the body, but they also may be influenced by related life events, as well as traditional, cultural, and social expectations of a woman's worth expressed in relation to her reproductive capabilities. Significant psychosocial changes often happen during the midlife transition. Grown children may leave home, eliminating some women's view of their primary role as mother and forcing them to reevaluate their positions in life and in the family unit. A menopausal woman's parents may die or need chronic care, forcing her to take physical and emotional care of her own parents.

Medication or counseling may help women who experience severe symptoms. Estrogen has been correlated with a positive effect on mood and overall sense of well-being, and appears to be important for memory and mental functioning. As with all hormone-related issues, sensitivity and validation by a woman's physician is an important component of any treatment.

Menopause Complications

Cardiovascular disease, osteoporosis, urinary incontinence, and weight gain are the four major complications of menopause. Cardiovascular disease is the leading cause of death in women and men (see Chapter 10). Its incidence in women, which begins to rise in the perimenopausal years, continues to increase after menopause. Studies have found that low levels of estrogen after menopause increase the risk for developing cardiovascular disease in the smaller blood vessels.[15,20]

Osteoporosis, the loss of bone mass or bone density that leads to brittle bones that are more likely to fracture, and **osteopenia**, a related but less severe condition (see Chapter 11), are also serious concerns for many postmenopausal women. Osteoporosis is far more prevalent in women than men, and smaller and thinner women are at more risk than larger women. Osteoporosis tends to present in individuals with a family history of the disease.[21] It is a serious problem for many elderly women; falls resulting from or leading to bone fractures are a major cause of death and disability in older women. Postmenopausal women are especially susceptible to fractures of their hips, wrists, and spine.[15] Bone loss is particularly rapid in the first few years following menopause. During this time, the spine may also lose flexibility and begin to curve. The prevalence of reduced bone density in older women varies by race and ethnicity. Low bone density and osteoporosis are most common among non-Hispanic White and Asian women.[22]

Urinary incontinence is another possible complication of menopause. As the vagina and urethra lose their elasticity, some women may also experience atrophy of the urinary tract. Diminished muscle tone may result in urinary incontinence. Some women also experience an increase in the frequency and duration of urinary tract infections.

Weight gain is a common complication for women after menopause. Estrogen appears to help regulate body weight; with lower estrogen levels, metabolic rates drop and it is easier to gain weight. However, other factors also influence weight gain associated with menopause. Some women become less active and exercise less as they age. Physical inactivity leads to lost muscle mass, which also decreases resting metabolism, making it easier to gain weight. In addition, aerobic capacity declines with age, so for women to use the same energy as in the past and lose weight, they need to increase the amount and intensity of their physical exercise.

Dementia is another complication hypothesized to be associated with menopause. Some researchers have speculated that the loss of estrogen in older women might affect the development of **Alzheimer's disease** because more women than men have the disease and almost two-thirds of all Americans living with Alzheimer's are women.[23] However, studies examining the association of hormones and menopause have often found conflicting results.[24] The most recent epidemiological data suggest that the larger portion of older women than men who have Alzheimer's disease or other dementia is due to the fact that women live longer than men. In addition, other studies have found no significant gender incidence differences in Alzheimer's or other dementias. Experts are now concluding that women are *not* more likely than men to develop dementia at any given age.[23]

Medicalization of Menopause

"Medicalization" is a process in which societies or individuals define and treat basic human conditions as medical conditions to be solved or cured. These conditions thus become the subjects of medical study, diagnosis, prevention, or treatment. Education to consumers and clinicians about the topic becomes framed in medical jargon and in "solutions" that typically earn profits for the medical community. Once a significant proportion of society accepts a condition as a medical condition, the medical model dominates other social models for management, understanding, and reimbursement. Many factors, some of them well-intentioned, can contribute to medicalization. Medicalization can occur as new scientific evidence or treatment emerges, as social attitudes change, or through the influence of medically oriented marketing and advertising.

In the United States, both childbirth and menopause have been heavily "medicalized." Many have suggested that menopause in the United States became medicalized when it was promoted as an estrogen-deficiency disease. For menopause, medicalization means that all dimensions of a woman's aging are inextricably linked to the shut down of her estrogen production; rather than being considered a natural part of the life span, menopause is managed as an estrogen-deficiency disease.

Hormone Therapy

For decades, **hormone** therapy has been the standard treatment for symptoms of menopause. The idea behind these therapies has been to replace or supplement the hormone levels that fall during menopause. Modern hormone therapy comes in two primary forms: estrogen alone, or estrogen and progesterone (or progestin, a synthetic form of progesterone). In 2002, the Women's Health Initiative (WHI), a major clinical trial, found increased risks for breast cancer and heart disease associated with hormone therapy. While millions of women stopped taking hormone therapy as a result, hormone therapy remains a common treatment today.

Estrogen alone is usually prescribed for women who do not have a uterus. If a woman's uterus is intact, her hormone therapy is typically a combination of estrogen and progesterone.[28] This combination lowers her risk of possible uterine cancer. The ideal regimen, if any, for a woman

Table 8.1	**Types of Menopause Treatments and Drugs**

Menopause is unique to each woman. These treatments and drugs are often used to address specific symptoms:

- Hot flashes:
  - Hormone therapy
    - Estrogen
    - Estrogen plus progesterone
  - Low-dose antidepressants
  - Other drugs
- Bone loss:
  - Bisphosphonates
  - SERMS
- Vaginal dryness:
  - Tablets, rings, and creams

will depend on her own symptoms, risks, and feelings; flexibility and discussion with a healthcare provider are key to determining the correct dose and form of hormone therapy for each individual.

Hormonal therapy to treat menopause carries potential risks and benefits. Hormone therapy appears to be a

Table 8.2	**Hormone Therapy Timeline**
1890s	Experiments of hormone therapy (HT) with testicular extracts for aged men
1920s	Estrogen distilled from urine of pregnant women
1930s	Pharmaceutical companies manufacture purified and synthesized hormones
1938	DES, a powerful synthetic, nonsteroidal estrogen formula published
1939	*Journal of the American Medical Association* (JAMA) publishes "Estrogen Therapy—A Warning" cautioning against use of DES, a possible carcinogen
1940	Thirteen drug companies apply to FDA to market DES but FDA does not approve their applications. The companies band together and form an aggressive campaign to gain approval.
1941	As a result of the campaign, FDA approves DES for use in menopausal symptoms and menstrual disorders. Physicians began to use it "off-label" for preventing miscarriages—later shown to be the most harmful use of DES.
1942	FDA approves Premarin, made from urine of pregnant horses
1950s	William Masters promotes expansion of short-term HT to long-term, describing "ovarian failure as the Achilles heel" for women
1960	FDA approves oral contraceptives, beginning long-term hormonal use by many women
1960s	Large scale manufacturing and marketing of psychotropic drugs and hormones
1966	Robert Wilson writes the best selling book *Feminine Forever*, promoting the prevention of menopause with HT
1970s	Premarin is one of top five prescribed medications in the United States
1971	Studies show DES use to prevent miscarriage during pregnancy causes vaginal cancer in their daughters
1971	NIH conference examines use of estrogen therapy for menopause; deplores lack of data and concerns
1975	Retrospective studies find that estrogen use caused endometrial cancer
1976	FDA mandates patient labeling for estrogen
1977	NIH Consensus Development Conference to assess estrogen use and provide guidance for clinicians

Table 8.2   Hormone Therapy Timeline *(Continued)*

1980	Synthetic progesterone, progestin, added to HT as "opposed therapy or combo"
1980s	Studies find protective effect of estrogen on bone loss and osteoporosis in women who had surgical menopause; hormones were promoted for osteoporosis protection for all women; some studies show small elevations of breast cancer risk in long-term hormone users
1984	NIH Consensus Conference warns against widespread use of hormone therapies but also notes estrogen to be effective against osteoporosis. Messaging to women begins to emphasize osteoporosis prevention and minimize cancer risk
1985	Nurses' Study shows estrogen users had reduced risk of CHD
1986	FDA approves estrogen as treatment for postmenopausal osteoporosis
1980–1990	Opposed therapy becomes one of the most prescribed drugs in America, being used by nearly 40% postmenopausal women
1987	PEPI (Postmenopausal Estrogen/Progestin Interventions) Trial started to assess HT on CVD risk factors
1990s	Studies find decreased risk of heart disease in women on HT
1991	WHI started. Four components to study were: (1) estrogen–progestin vs. placebo, (2) conjugated estrogen vs. placebo, (3) calcium and vitamin D vs. placebo, and (4) non-intervention cohort
1992	Premarin ranks #1 in prescribed U.S. drugs—promoted to prevent heart attacks and osteoporosis
1992	Nurses' Study shows increased risk of breast cancer among hormone therapy users; contradictory findings in Framingham study show increased risk but study participants were older and had received higher doses
1993	HERS study begins to see if combination hormone therapy alters the risk for CHD in women with established coronary disease
1995	PEPI Trial results find combination hormone therapy better than estrogen for protection against uterine cancer; progesterone found to interfere with the beneficial effect estrogen has on cholesterol
1996	PEPI Trial results find estrogen alone greater risk for hyperplasia than placebo
1997	Premarin sales reach $1 billion
1998	HERS study finds that hormone therapy does not protect women with heart disease against further progression of heart disease. The use of hormone therapy nearly triples the participant risk of having a blood clot.
1999	Studies confirm elevated risk of breast cancer in long-term hormone therapy users
2002	HERS II study finds no CVD prevention benefit to combination hormone therapy but does find an increased risk of stroke, clots, and need for gallbladder surgery
2002	WHI component (1) trial ended early due to greater incidence of CHD, breast cancer, stroke, and blood clots in treatment group vs. placebo. Findings also show decreased risk of colorectal cancer and fewer fractures in the treatment group.
2002	NAMES guidelines released saying estrogen–progestin should not be used for the prevention of heart disease
2003	Five articles in *JAMA* find: (1) Combination hormone therapy did not improve women's quality of life, vitality, mental health, depressive symptoms, or sexual satisfaction; (2) Hormone users had a two-fold increased risk of developing dementia; (3) An increased risk of stroke in the hormone therapy treatment group; (4) An increased risk of breast cancer with hormone therapy and cancers in hormone users are diagnosed at a more advanced stage than placebo users; and (5) The longer women used combined HT, the greater their risk of developing breast cancer.
2003	FDA strengthens warning label requirements for hormone products. Products have to highlight increased risks for heart disease, heart attacks, strokes, and breast cancer and have to state that products have not been approved for heart disease prevention or memory loss.
2003	Results of the Million Women Study show women taking hormones are at higher risk of breast cancer. Women taking estrogen alone had an increased risk of uterine and breast cancers.
2004	WHI component (2) terminated 1 year early because estrogen alone did not reduce risk of heart disease; however, it did decrease risk for colon cancer and hip fracture
2005	NIH State-of-the Science Conference changes "hormone replacement therapy" to its current name—menopausal hormone therapy—shifting emphasis away from the concept of "replacing" hormones
2003–present	FDA recommends hormone therapy for post-menopausal women be at the lowest doses for the shortest amount of time needed to reach treatment goals

Source: Data from: Rothenberg, C. J. (2005) *The rise and fall of estrogen therapy: The history of HRT.* Harvard Law School. Paper submitted in satisfaction of the Food and Drug Law course and the third year written work requirement. Available at: http://leda.law.harvard.edu; Watkins, E. S. (2007). *The estrogen elixir: A history of hormone replacement therapy in America.* Baltimore, MD: The Johns Hopkins University Press; *Project MUSE.* (2012). Available at: http://muse.jhu.edu/

higher health risk for some groups of women, such as older women and smokers. At the same time, used properly, and by women in low-risk groups, hormone therapy is usually a safe product that can provide relief for women with severe symptoms associated with menopause.

History of Hormone Use in the United States

For the latter half of the 20th century, millions of women received hormone therapy to treat symptoms of menopause and protect their long-term health (see **Table 8.2** for a timeline view of hormone therapy use over the past 100 years). Large pharmaceutical companies have used their influence to shape public policy and national education campaigns. Commercial emphasis on positive attributes of therapies has misled women and clinicians, while risks were minimized or ignored.[25] At the same time, many of the supposed negative effects of current hormonal products for menopause have been exaggerated, misunderstood, or falsely inferred.

The Food and Drug Administration (FDA) approved the first product for use in menopausal symptoms in 1941. Diethylstilbestrol (DES), a synthetic form of estrogen, became used for both symptoms of menopause and for the prevention of miscarriage. For the next 40 years, various hormonal combinations were positioned as a cure for many afflictions of aging. In addition, doctors often prescribed these products as preventative drugs for chronic conditions such as heart disease, osteoporosis, and dementia. Over the years many observational and case studies supported these positive attributes of hormones, and a billion-dollar business system evolved. The pathway to widespread adoption became more complicated in the 1970s. During this decade, studies found increased rates of vaginal cancers in women whose mothers used DES during pregnancy. In addition, research also found a link between estrogen and uterine cancer, with the suggestion of possible links with hormone therapies and other cancers. However, until large-scale studies provided clearer insight, American women continued to routinely receive hormones for menopausal symptom treatment and chronic disease prevention.

Major Studies

In 1991, the federal government embarked on an expansive, rigorous set of clinical studies to better understand life after menopause. The Women's Health Initiative (WHI) was a 15-year research program aimed at learning more about cardiovascular disease, cancer, and osteoporosis, the most frequent causes of death, disability, and low quality of life in postmenopausal women. The clinical trials also examined the effects of two major postmenopausal hormone therapies, estrogen alone and estrogen plus progestin, compared to placebo. Additional studies examined the effects of diet modification, calcium, and vitamin D supplements on heart disease, fractures, and breast and colorectal cancer. The WHI studies were the largest studies ever conducted in the United States. The trials and an observational study recruited more than 161,000 generally healthy postmenopausal women. The studies were complex, and the interpretation of the findings has been the subject of hundreds of professional papers and medical presentations.

In 2002, the estrogen plus progestin portion of the WHI was stopped early due to a lack of overall benefit and an increased risk of breast cancer and heart disease. Women in this group also had a slightly lower risk of developing hip fractures and colon cancers, but the increased risk for other diseases outweighed these benefits. The effects that estrogen plus progestin had on these conditions, while statistically significant, were still small for any individual woman. For example, the study found that for every 10,000 women taking estrogen pills:

- 38 developed breast cancer each year, compared to 30 breast cancers seen in every 10,000 women taking placebo.
- 37 had a heart attack, compared to 30 out of every 10,000 women taking placebo.
- 10 had hip fractures, compared to 15 out of every 10,000 women taking placebo.
- 10 developed colon cancer, compared to 16 out of every 10,000 women taking placebo.

Women in the estrogen-alone portion of the WHI continued taking pills until 2004, when researchers concluded that estrogen alone did not appear to decrease the risk for heart disease or stroke. **Table 8.3** presents the major findings from these two studies in greater detail.

In 2003, the Million Women Study, the largest observational study of all time, showed that women taking hormones had a higher risk of developing breast cancer than the women not taking hormones. The study, conducted in the United Kingdom, also confirmed the increased risk for uterine cancer in women who had their uterus and were taking estrogen alone. Consistent with other studies, the findings showed that prior use of hormones did not seem to affect the current risk of developing breast cancer, suggesting that the effects of the hormones on breast cancer risk diminished within 2 years of stopping them.[26]

Table 8.3	Results from the Estrogen Plus Progestin Study Compared to the Results from the Estrogen-Alone Study

Results from the Estrogen Plus Progestin Study	Results from the Estrogen-Alone Study
Compared with the placebo, the estrogen plus progestin resulted in:	Compared with the placebo, estrogen alone resulted in:
Increased risk of heart attack	No difference in risk for heart attack
Increased risk of stroke	Increased risk of stroke
Increased risk of blood clots	Increased risk of blood clots
Increased risk of breast cancer	Uncertain effect for breast cancer
Reduced risk of colorectal cancer	No difference in risk for colorectal cancer
Reduced risk of fractures	Reduced risk of fractures
No protection against mild cognitive impairment and increased risk of dementia (study included only women aged 65 and older)	

Source: Data from Heiss, G., Wallace, R., Anderson, G., Aragaki, A., Beresford, S., Brzyski, R., et al. (2008). Health risks and benefits 3 years after stopping randomized treatment with estrogen and progestin. *Journal of the American Medical Association, 299*(9), 1036–1045.

While the findings of the WHI and Million Women Study are important, they have still not answered all the questions about menopause and hormone therapy. Today experts continue to debate the merit of the studies and the interpretations of their data.[27]

Current Medical Menopause Management Options

Although millions of women stopped taking hormones after the studies, hormone therapy continues to be prescribed for women who want relief from menopausal symptoms. The absolute risk of heart disease or breast cancer to an individual woman taking hormones is low. For a woman who has severe symptoms such as intense hot flashes, the benefits of hormonal therapy may outweigh the risks. Many clinical studies have provided evidence that estrogen with or without progesterone effectively helps such conditions such as hot flashes, vaginal dryness, night sweats, and bone loss. These benefits can lead to improved sleep, sexual relations, and quality of life. Hormone therapy does not "cure" any disease; rather, hormone therapy helps to reduce symptoms associated with the hormone changes that result from menopause. Women most often take hormone therapy during menopause and perimenopause. The consensus guidance for hormones today is to take the lowest possible dose for the shortest amount of time possible for menopausal symptom relief. The FDA has approved many hormone products for use in hormone therapy; these products have received extensive testing, are manufactured under precise criteria for uniformity, and are only available with a medical prescription. The prescriptions are available as pills, patches (transdermally), creams, gels, or sprays. Vaginal creams, suppositories, tablets, or rings that release hormones within the vagina are also available. Oral preparations are prescribed most frequently. Women can take hormone therapy daily, or only on certain days of the month. Each of these methods has dose options that can be tailored to a woman's specific needs. Hormone therapy delivered through the skin and low-dose oral estrogen may have lower risks of blood clots and strokes than standard doses of oral estrogen. Vaginal creams containing estrogen can help women whose only symptom is vaginal dryness, but they do not appear to provide other benefits, such as relief from hot flashes. Transdermal application of hormone therapy can benefit women whose livers respond to oral doses of estrogen by deactivating it with enzymes that raise triglycerides, which contribute to heart disease, but oral doses of estrogen increase levels of HDL cholesterol, the "good" cholesterol, for some women. Long-term

■ Menopausal hormone therapy is available in a variety of preparations, routes of administration, and dosages.

studies are underway evaluating these newer hormone delivery options and their associated risks and benefits.[28] Despite recent controversy and negative study results, the hormone therapy market continues to grow and is estimated to reach $3.04 billion in 2017.[29]

Special populations that often depend upon hormone therapy are women who experience premature menopause (before age 40) or women who have lost normal ovarian function, called premature ovarian failure, before age 40. These women have a different set of health risks compared to women who reach menopause near the average age of 50, including a higher risk of coronary heart disease (CHD). In these special, younger populations, of women, hormone therapy appears to actually reduce their risk of CHD.[30]

Current Nonmedical Menopause Management Options

The question of whether menopause should be medically treated, and if so, how, remains a controversial and misunderstood topic. Some experts are concerned that menopause, a natural and normal life process, is often considered a condition to be cured with medical treatment. Many of these experts note that nonmedical lifestyle options can be at least as effective as medical procedures for reducing unwanted symptoms of menopause, while also improving overall health. Regular exercise; avoiding smoking; a balanced, healthful diet; a thorough, honest examination of one's position in life; and, if warranted, counseling, allow women to take an active role in maintaining health, rather than relying on prescribed medications that imply illness or disease. Women can also take actions to avoid specific symptoms: for example, wearing less restrictive clothing or lowering the temperature to deal with hot flashes, or reducing stress and eliminating caffeine to cope with insomnia.

Regular physical activity is critical in the menopausal years, a time when a woman is at increased risk for osteoporosis and osteoporosis-related fractures, heart disease, and chronic diseases such as diabetes. Weight-bearing exercise can increase bone density and improve balance and flexibility to decrease falls, thereby reducing fractures. Aerobic exercise can reduce a woman's risk for cardiovascular by improving cardiac function, decreasing high body weight, and lowering LDL cholesterol levels. In addition to its many other benefits (Chapter 9), exercise also may reduce the incidence and severity of hot flashes. Other symptoms associated with hormonal changes of menopause, such as insomnia, depression or other mood changes, weight gain, and headache, all may improve with exercise.[31]

"Bio-Identical" Hormones

In recent years, large marketing campaigns have promoted "bio-identical" hormones as alternative therapies to prescriptive medical hormones. Fueled by the controversy associated with hormone research studies and preying on the fears of women with menopausal symptoms, these products claim to be identical to natural female hormones. The FDA has expressed concern that these products pose a potentially serious risk to women. "Bio-identical" hormones are not sanctioned by the FDA. Sellers of these products often claim that they are safe, "all natural," and free of the risks that present with the FDA-approved drugs for hormone therapy. The "bio-identical" products have not been subjected to the rigorous testing required by the FDA for drugs. FDA-approved drugs for hormone therapy are sold by prescription only.

"Bio-identical drugs" are compounded in pharmacies where practices do not always conform to FDA standards, and these drugs have not been systematically evaluated to ensure safety and effectiveness. Often the manufacturers claim that their products that contain estriol, a weak form of estrogen, are safe. However, the FDA has not reviewed any data on these products. In addition, claims from companies to "create a personal drug" based on a saliva test have not been validated.

Millions of women have tried custom-compounded hormones or herbal supplements like black cohosh and red clover to cope with symptoms of menopause. Alternative remedies such as these often appeal to women who like to research and find their own solutions to medical problems. However, instead of a safer option, they are getting products of unknown risk that still contain the estrogen many of them fear.

In summary, the nonprescriptive option of a risk-free hormonal product is appealing to many women. However, products that have not been evaluated by the FDA have inherent risks. To date, the FDA is not aware of any credible scientific evidence to support claims made regarding the safety and effectiveness of compounded "bio-identical" products, and they urge women to consult with their healthcare provider before consuming them.[32]

I am approaching menopause and I feel very frustrated with the lack of clear information about menopause and hormone therapies. First, hormone therapy was supposed to be a cure-all; now, everyone seems to think you're risking your life if you choose to take it. Haven't we been using this stuff for decades? Why is there so much we still don't know?

—46-year-old woman

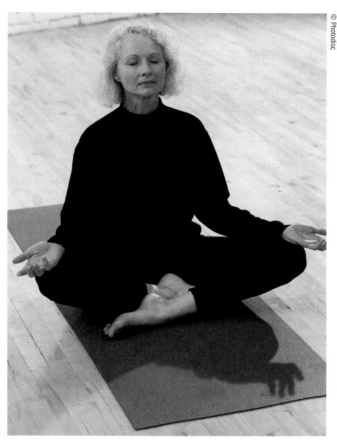

© Photodisc

■ Symptoms associated with hormonal changes of menopause, such as hot flashes, may improve with regular exercise.

I started exercising when menopause started and it has helped me in so many ways. I am glad that exercise is now a regular part of my daily routine.

57-year-old woman

Informed Decision Making

Learning about the advantages and disadvantages of hormone therapy from unbiased sources and one's own health-care provider are two key steps women can take to decide if and how hormone therapy is right for them. Family history, personal medical history, and the lifestyle choices made before menopause should also influence an individual's risk for hormone therapy. A person who stopped having periods before 40 or lost her normal ovarian function before 40 has a different set of health risks compared to women who reached menopause at age 50.

Limiting the risks with any hormone therapy is important. Three strategies have been proposed for limiting such risk:[30]

- Start hormone therapy early, because it does not appear to significantly increase the risk of heart disease in women under age 60. Some studies suggest that estrogen may protect against heart disease when taken early in the menopausal years.

- Minimize the amount of medication. Use the lowest effective dose for the shortest amount of time needed to alleviate symptoms.

- Try a form of hormone therapy with limited systemic effects, such as patches, gels, creams, or suppositories.

Although it is commonly believed that health problems are inevitable as women age, many can actually be prevented or controlled. Clearly, it is best to have a full lifetime of healthful behaviors, but changing unhealthful behaviors, even in later years, can improve both the quality and the quantity of life. Health-promoting behaviors include tobacco cessation, good nutrition, maintaining a healthy weight, and regular physical exercise. For some women, menopause is a time for reflection and renewed determination to engage in healthier living. Protecting the body from age-related diseases such as heart disease and osteoporosis means engaging in these healthful behaviors.

Staying informed about health research and new options is important for women. Unfortunately, many women are uninformed about their health and about the steps they can take to become and remain healthy. The confusing and complicated historical reality of hormone therapy, as well as the lack of in-depth, nuanced coverage of the subject, has not helped. One study found that most women discontinued hormone therapy after the WHI results were published. Given their experience with therapy, some women,

■ Seemingly contradictory findings about hormone therapy, as well as lack of nuanced media coverage of the subject, has made it difficult for many women to decide whether hormone therapy is right for them.

particularly nonwhites, are now less trusting of medical recommendations and less likely to take drugs for cardiovascular disease prevention.[30]

■■■■

I started hormone therapy but with all the contradictory news I decided that I preferred to not take 'medicine' to get through a normal transition. Yes, I did have hot flashes, but they were manageable. I got through it.

—**61-year-old woman**

The decision about whether to take hormone therapy is a personal one. No two women respond exactly the same way to the same therapy. Ethnic differences may influence perception of menopausal symptoms. Many women choose to live with symptoms because they consider them signs of normal developmental transition and aging. The presence of symptoms does not necessarily indicate the need for a medical intervention. If a therapy is selected, dosages, products, and regimens may require readjusting more than once to find an appropriate balance. Women with difficult menopause symptoms; who have thin bones, as measured by a bone density test; or who are at high risk of heart disease are possible candidates for hormone therapy. Women who have a history of liver disease, who are prone to blood clots, or who have had breast cancer are generally considered to be at too high a risk to begin hormone therapy (**Table 8.4**). As with other forms of treatment, the benefits must be carefully weighed and considered against the spectrum of associated risks before a decision is made (see **Self-Assessment 8.1**).

Improving women's access to accurate, relevant information in this regard will help them better make these important health decisions.

Table 8.4 **Conditions That May Preclude the Use of Hormone Therapy**

- Personal history of breast cancer
- History of blood clots in legs, lungs, or eyes
- Undiagnosed or abnormal vaginal bleeding
- Preexisting cardiovascular conditions, such as blood clots, stroke, or uncontrolled hypertension
- History of liver, gallbladder, or pancreatic disease; impaired liver function

■■■■

Summary

Once considered "the beginning of the end of life," menopause should instead be seen as the beginning of a new life phase, no longer confined or defined by procreative abilities. Fears about aging and the myths and misconceptions about the aging process should be replaced with better knowledge and insight into the myriad opportunities that exist in the second half of a woman's life. For some women, menopause brings physical symptoms; for others, it inspires questions about their roles and place in life. Menopause management—especially hormone therapy—remains a complex area that deserves continuing research and requires individual choices by women and their physicians. For some women, this therapy is a solution to distressing symptoms associated with menopause. For other women, hormone therapy may cause more health problems than it solves. Women should learn all they can about emerging options and consult with their providers to understand the best course of action for themselves as it relates to menopause and their individual process of aging.

Self-Assessment 8.1

Strategies for Hormone Therapy Decision Making

The decision to use hormone therapy is a personal and private one.

Women should consider several factors when making the decision:

1. Person and family medical history
   - History of breast cancer
   - Blood clots in the legs, lungs, or eyes
   - Abnormal vaginal bleeding
   - Preexisting cardiovascular conditions, such as blood clots, stroke, or uncontrolled high blood pressure
   - Liver, gallbladder, or pancreatic disease

2. Menopausal symptoms and their severity
   - Hot flashes
   - Vaginal irritation and discomfort
   - Urinary tract problems
   - Emotional and mood changes

3. Review risks and benefits

4. Reevaluate decision periodically

Profiles of Remarkable Women

Lynn Johnston (1947–)

Lynn Johnston is a cartoonist and the creator of the comic strip *For Better or For Worse*. The strip has been a staple in North American newspapers since its debut in 1979. Johnston grew up in British Columbia, where she studied art and began her career as an illustrator. She spent the early 1970s as a commercial artist. In 1975 she developed *For Better or For Worse*, a comic strip set in Canada and loosely based on her own family experiences. The strip is a perennial favorite and appears internationally in several languages. Johnston is the first woman to receive a Rueben Award for Cartoonist of the Year by the National Cartoonist Society, in 1985. She has also received the Order of Canada and claims a star on Canada's Walk of Fame. Her comic strip ended in 2007.

Johnston's characters, loosely based on her own family members and friends, aged together more than 30 years over during the course of the comic strip. She humorously depicted social, cultural, and physical realities of women, families, work, and relationships. While focusing on the daily life of a typical middle-class household, Johnston has not been afraid to tackle controversial issues, such as menopause, gay marriage, and child abuse. Johnston has been candid about her personal experiences with abuse and her own doubts about childrearing during her lifetime. Many of her strips captured real dimensions of her own thoughts and experiences during menopause. Her humor and honesty have been inspirational to her readers and she is a model for women around the world.

Additional information about Lynn and her work can be found at: http://www.fbofw.com/

Topics for Discussion

1. Why has medical research been slower to understand the physiological and psychological dimensions of menopause than those of other reproductive health matters?

2. What can be done to continue to change societal images of menopause, aging, and older women?

3. What can women do to better understand and appreciate menopause as an exciting stage of life?

4. What can a woman do to maximize the effectiveness of her decision making about menopausal symptom management?

5. What are some of the physical, emotional, and social dimensions of menopause?

6. What are some new areas that merit research in the arena of midlife and maturity for a woman?

7. If you were experiencing severe symptoms of menopause, what course of action would you take? How would you go about making this decision?

Key Terms

Alzheimer's disease: An irreversible, progressive brain disorder that occurs gradually and results in memory loss, behavior and personality changes, and a decline in cognitive abilities.

Bilateral salpingo-oophorectomy: Surgical excision of the fallopian tube and the ovary.

Estrogen: A class of hormones that produce female secondary sex characteristics and affect the menstrual cycle.

Hormone: A chemical produced by one part of the body that influences activity, growth, or metabolism in another part of the body.

Hot flash: An uncomfortable sensation of menopause consisting of internally generated heat beginning in the chest and moving to the neck and head or spreading through the body. Also known as hot flushes.

Hysterectomy: The surgical removal of the uterus, resulting in surgically induced menopause.

Natural menopause: The failure of the ovaries to respond to the luteinizing and follicle-stimulating hormones that are produced in the anterior pituitary, which is under the control of the hypothalamus. As a result of this failure, ovulation becomes somewhat erratic. The mechanisms for these changes are not well understood. Menopause is considered complete once monthly periods have ceased altogether.

Osteopenia: Decreased calcification or density of bone. This descriptive term is applicable to all skeletal systems in which such a condition is noted.

Osteoporosis: A age-related debilitating disorder characterized by a general decrease in bone mass and structural deterioration of bone tissue.

Perimenopause: Refers to the years immediately preceding and following the last menstrual period.

Postmenopause: Life after the final menstrual period.

Progesterone: The hormone produced by the corpus luteum of the ovary that causes the uterine lining to thicken.

Total hysterectomy: Surgical removal of the uterus performed in conjunction with the removal of both ovaries and fallopian tubes.

Vaginal atrophy: A condition often associated with menopause that refers to the thinning of the vaginal lining.

Websites

American College of Obstetricians and Gynecologists: Provides provider and consumer information from OB-GYN specialists: http://www.acog.org

American Heart Association Provides information about women and cardiovascular disease: http://www.goredforwomen.org

American Society for Reproductive Medicine National healthcare provider resource on all reproductive topics: http://www.asrm.org

Association of Reproductive Health Professionals Nonprofit organization of physicians and health care providers: http://www.arhp.org

Black Women's Health Imperative National nonprofit devoted to the health of black women and girls: http://www.blackwomenshealth.org

Global Library of Women's Medicine Provides library of women's medicine—over 40,000 references: http://www.glowm.com

The Hormone Foundation:
Offers information about all hormone therapies: http://www.hormone.org

National Institute on Aging Information Center:
National site with resources on aging for clinicians and consumers: http://www.nia.nih.gov

National Women's Health Information Center:
Offers comprehensive information for professionals and consumers: http://www.womenshealth.gov

National Women's Health Resource Center:
Comprehensive resource about all women's health issues: http://www.healthywomen.org

North American Menopause Society:
Comprehensive resource for women and clinicians on menopause: http://www.menopause.org

Office of Research on Women's Health
National Institutes of Health resource focused on issues regarding women's health: http://www.orwh.od.nih.gov

Power Surge:
An online community for menopausal women: http://www.power-surge.com

Society for Women's Health Research:
National non-profit promoting research on women's health: http://www.womenshealthresearch.org

Wise Woman
Hosted by the Centers for Disease Control and Prevention for underserved women to prevent disease: http://www.cdc.gov/wisewoman

Women's Voices for Change (WVFC)
Provides information and motivation for self discovery: http://womensvoicesforchange.org/

■■■■

References

1. U.S. Census Bureau. (2012). *Annual estimates of the resident population by sex and five year age groups for the United States. April 1, 2000–July 1, 2009.* (NC-EST2009-01). June 2010. Available at: http://www.cenus.gov/popest/national/asm/NC-EST2009-01.xls

2. OWL—The Voice of Midlife and Older Women. (2012). *OWL releases menopause survey findings.* Available at: http://www.owl-national.org/pages/press-releases

3. National Institute of Aging. (2012). *Health and aging—Age page: Menopause.* Available at: http://www.nia.nih.gov/health/publication/menopause

4. Stolk, L. Perry, J. R.B., Chasman, D. I., et al. (2011). Meta-analysis identifies 13 loci associated with age at menopause and highlight DNA repair and immune pathways. *Nature Genetics 44*: 260–268. Available at: http://www.nature.com/ng/journal/v44/h3/full/ng.1051.html

5. Jacobson, B. K., Heuch, I., & Kvale,G. (2002). Age at natural menopause and all-cause mortality: A 37-year follow-up of 19,731 Norwegian women. *American Journal of Epidemiology 157*(10): 923–929.

6. The Endocrine Society. (2010). Early menopause linked to higher risk of future cardiovascular disease, study finds. *ScienceDaily.* Available at: www.sciencedaily.com/releases/2010/08/100821133948.htm

7. Guttmacher Perspectives. (2001). *Multiple factors, including genetic and environmental components, influence when menopause begins 35*(5). Available at: http://www.guttmacher.org/pubs/journals/3323601.html

8. Burger, H. (2008). The menopause transition—endocrinology. *Journal of Sexual Medicine Oct 5*(10): 2266–2273.

9. NIH Osteoporosis and Related Bone Diseases National Resource Center. (2011). *Smoking and osteoporosis.* Available at: http://www.niams.nih.gov/health_info/bone/Osteoporosis/Conditions_Behaviors/bone_smoking.asp

10. Whiteman, M. K., Hillis, S. D., Jamieson, D. J., et al. (2008). Inpatient hysterectomy surveillance in the United States. *American Journal Obstetrics and Gynecology 198*(1): 34.e1–7.

11. Hunter, M. S., Gentry-Maharai, A. Burnell, M., et al. (2012). Prevalence, frequency and problem rating of hot flashes persist in older postmenopausal women: impact of age, body mass index, hysterectomy, hormone therapy use, lifestyle and mood in a cross-sectional cohort study of 10,418 British women aged 54–65. *British Journal of Gynecology 119*(1): 40–50.

12. Ingelsson, E., Lundholm, C., Johansson, A. L. V., et al. (2010). Hysterectomy and risk of cardiovascular disease: a population based cohort study. *European Heart Journal 32*(6): 745–750.

13. Centers for Disease Control and Prevention [CDC]. (2009). Women's reproductive health: Hysterectomy.

Available at: http://www.cdc.gov/reproductivehealth/womensrh/Hysterectomy.htm

14. Beck-Peccoz, P. & Persani, L. (2006). Premature ovarian failure. *Orphanet Journal of Rare Diseases 1*: 9. Available at: http://www.ojrd.com/content/1/1/9

15. Luoto, R. (2009). Hot flashes and quality of life during menopause. *BMC Women's Health 9*: 13. Available at: http://www.biomedcentral.com/1472-6874/9/13

16. National Institutes of Health, National Library of Medicine. (2011). Menopause. *MedlinePlus Medical Encyclopedia*. Available at: http://www.nlm.nih.gov/medlineplus/ency/article/000894.htm

17. Mayo Clinic. (2011). *Menopause*. Available at: http://www.mayoclinic.com/health/menopause/DS00119

18. Gold, E. B., Sternfeld, B., Kelsey, J. L., et al. (2000). Relation of demographic and lifestyle factors to symptoms in a multi-racial/ethnic population of women 40–55 years of age. *American Journal of Epidemiology 152*(5): 463–473.

19. National Institutes of Health [NIH]. (2005). *NIH State-of-the-Science Conference on Management of Menopause-Related Symptoms*. Available at: http://consensus.nih.gov/2005/menopausestatement.htm

20. Im, E., Lee, B., Chee, W., et al. (2010). Menopausal symptoms among four major ethnic groups in the U.S. *Western Journal of Nursing Research 32*(4): 540–565.

21. Geweke, L. O. (2007). Menopause and migrane. *Menopause Management*. Available at: www.menopausemgmt.com/issues/16-05/MM0910_feature.pdf

22. National Institute of Mental Health. (2007). *Women and depression*. Available at: http://psychcentral.com/lib/2007/women-and-depression/all/1

23. Alzheimer's Association. (2011). *Alzheimer's disease facts and figures*. Available at: http://www.alz.org/alzheimers_disease_facts_and_figures.asp

24. Shumaker, S. A., Legault, C., Rapp, S. R., et al. (2003). Estrogen plus progestin and the incidence of dementia and mild cognitive impairment in postmenopausal women. *Journal of the American Medical Association 289*(20): 2651–2662.

25. Rothenberg, C. J. (2005). *The rise and fall of estrogen therapy: The history of HRT*. Harvard Law School. Paper submitted in satisfaction of the Food and Drug Law course and the third year written work requirement. Available at: http://leda.law.harvard.edu

26. Narod, S. A. (2011). Hormone replacement therapy and the risk of breast cancer. *Nature Reviews Clinical Oncology 8*(11): 669–676.

27. Chlebowski, R. T., &Anderson, G. L. (2012). Changing concepts: Menopausal hormone therapy and breast cancer. *Journal of the National Cancer Institute 104*(7): 517–527.

28. The North American Menopause Society. (2012). *Hormone therapy for women in 2012*. Available at: www.menopause.org/psht12patient.pdf

29. Global Industry Analysts, Inc. (2011). Global hormone replacement therapy (HRT) market to reach US$3.04 billion by 2016. *PRWeb*. Available at: http://www.prweb.com/releases/hormone_replacement/therapy_HRT/prweb8853368.htm

30. Mayo Clinic. (2010) *Hormone replacement therapy and your heart*. Available at: http://www.mayoclinic.com/health/hormone-replacement-therapy/WO00131

31. National Cancer Institute. (2011). *Menopausal hormone therapy and cancer fact sheet*. Available at: http://www.cancer.gov/cancertopics/factsheet/Risk/menopausal-hormones

32. Food and Drug Administration [FDA]. (2008). *Consumer health information. Bio-identicals: Sorting myths from facts*. Available at: http://www.fda.gov/forconsumers/consumerupdates/ucm049311.htm

Physical and Lifespan Dimensions of Women's Health

Chapter Nine

Nutrition, Exercise, and Weight Management

Chapter Objectives

On completion of this chapter, the student should be able to discuss:

1. How a balanced diet and an active lifestyle improve health and lower the risk for disease.

2. The USDA food plate, as well as other dietary guidelines.

3. The six major nutrients and how they fit into a healthful diet.

4. The building blocks of nutrition.

5. Factors contributing toward unbalanced diets and sedentary lifestyles, as well as ways to overcome those challenges.

6. The physiological and psychological benefits of regular physical activity.

7. The complementary benefits of aerobic exercise and strength training.

8. How to calculate one's body mass index (BMI) and maximum and target-range heart rates.

9. Physical fitness concerns specific to women.

10. Myths and facts about exercise and fitness.

11. Reasons why women should maintain a healthy weight.

12. Biological, cultural, and economic factors contributing to weight gain.

13. The effects of obesity and overweight on health.

14. Effective ways that women can reach or maintain a healthful weight.

15. Sociocultural influences on body image.

16. Global and national perspectives on hunger.

womenshealth.jbpub.com

Women's Health Online is a great source for supplementary women's health information for both students and instructors. Visit

http://womenshealth.jbpub.com

to find a variety of useful tools for learning, thinking, and teaching.

Introduction

Healthful eating and regular exercise are two of the simplest, most effective ways that women (and men) can improve their health. These behaviors improve mental and physical health in the present; prevent disease; and help people live longer, healthier, happier lives in the future.

A balanced diet that is low in fat and high in fruits, vegetables, and fiber lowers the risk of cardiovascular disease, various cancers, diabetes, hypertension, and other chronic conditions. It also makes the body stronger and more capable in every aspect of life. Regular physical activity brings many of the same benefits. Additionally, regular physical activity improves the mood and quality of sleep; reduces stress, controls body fat and fat distribution; and builds healthy muscle, bones, and joints. Exercise also helps older adults maintain function and preserve independence.

Despite these findings, many women continue to follow unhealthful eating patterns and lead sedentary lives. These two behaviors are responsible for 400,000 deaths each year. Together, unhealthful diets and a sedentary lifestyle are the second-leading preventable cause of death in the United States, just behind tobacco use.[1]

It's Your Health

Food manufacturers use a variety of claims to get consumers to purchase their products. Many claims focus on nutritional aspects of their food, drawing attention to the fact that a product is low in calories, sugar, or fat. These terms can be useful, but women should evaluate them with a critical eye. Many candies, while high in sugar, are fat-free, while a bag of corn chips may have no sugar and be high in fat and sodium. Neither of these products is good for the body; both are high in calories while offering few or any nutrients.

Other food-related claims have developed as consumers have grown more concerned about the conditions under which the food is grown or raised. These claims may focus on the absence of antibiotics or harmful chemicals used during farming, the environmental impact of farming practices, whether the business model justly compensates farmers and workers, the living conditions of farmed animals, or a combination of these factors. In many cases, these conditions may work together naturally: A farm that operates without pesticides may add fewer toxins to nearby rivers and cause less harm to the environment and its laborers.

Being aware of the meaning of the following conditions will help women become more knowledgeable and responsible consumers.

Nutritional Claims:

- *Enriched:* The replacement of nutrients in a product that may have been lost during processing; for example, bread may be enriched with iron, niacin, thiamin, and riboflavin. The nutrients added during enrichment usually only partially replace the nutrients that processing takes away.

- *Fortified:* The addition of vitamins and minerals that were not originally present in a food product; for example, orange juice may be fortified with calcium.

- *Light:* A food that is labeled "light" typically meets the definition for "low calorie" or "low fat." "Light in sodium" means the sodium content has been reduced by at least 50%. In some cases, "light" may refer to the color or texture of a food rather than to low quantities of sodium, fat, or calories; in these cases, the food will be specifically labeled to this effect.

- *Low-calorie:* Food that has fewer than 40 calories per serving and less than 0.4 calorie per gram.

- *Low-fat:* Food that has 3 grams or fewer of fat per serving. Food manufacturers sometimes add large amounts of sugar to low-fat foods to compensate for the taste.

- *Low-sodium:* Food that has 140 mg or less of sodium per serving; food labeled as "very low sodium" has 35 mg or less per serving.

- *Natural:* Meat, poultry, and egg products labeled as "natural" have no artificial ingredients and are minimally processed. For other types of food, the term may be used without any specific requirements (and thus has little guaranteed meaning). "Natural" does not mean nutritious; many foods labeled as natural are highly processed, high in fat or sugar, or loaded with preservatives.

- *RDA:* Recommended Dietary Allowance, the estimated amount of various nutrients needed each day to maintain good health. The guidelines were developed to address dietary needs for large populations; individual needs may vary owing to genetic, personal, and demographic factors.

- *Reduced:* A food that has at least 25% less of a given characteristic (such as calories, fat, cholesterol, sodium, or sugar than a regular preparation of a given product). The product label must display the nutritional comparison.

- *Sugarless and sugar-free:* Contains less than 0.5 grams of sugar per serving.

Ethical/Responsibility Terms

- *Biodynamic:* a stricter method of organic farming that focuses on reducing environmental impact and using sustainable methods (see terms below).

- *Cage-Free:* Poultry and egg products with this label are farmed in a common area with unlimited access to food and water. Caged birds often live their lives in a small cage with several other birds; "cage-free" birds may still live in crowded conditions but at least have the freedom to move around.

- *Fair Trade:* Foods with the fair trade logo are grown on farms where farmers are equitably compensated and where safe, nonexploitative conditions exist for farm workers. Some products without this label, such as chocolate, coffee, or sugar, are often produced in conditions where laborers and farmers work in dangerous conditions and receive little of the products' net profit.

- *Free-Range:* Farmers may label poultry and egg products as "free range" if the birds have access to the outdoors. Because of the flexibility of this definition conditions from on different "free range" farms may vary widely, from a crowded pen where thousands of chickens share access to a single ledge, to an open farm where animals can roam freely.

- *Grass-Fed:* Beef, lamb, and other animal meat with this label comes from animals that get most of their nutrients from grass, rather than from grain. Grass-based diets are more natural and healthy for cows and sheep than grain-based diet. Many nutrition experts believe that grass-fed meat may also be more nutritious, environmentally friendly, and less likely to contain harmful bacteria than grain-fed meat.

- *Humane, or Humanely Raised:* This term implies that farm animals are raised within certain basic living standards. It may refer to an animal's shelter, access to food and water, or the absence of hormones and antibiotics used to raise animals. In the absence of a standard definition, what this label means often varies from company to company.

- *Locally grown or raised:* Food that is either grown or raised within a certain distance of where it is sold, often within the same or a neighboring state. Locally grown food supports local agriculture and reduces the greenhouse gases needed for transportation. Food referred to as regionally grown or raised may be produced at a slightly farther, but relatively moderate, distance.

- *Organic:* Food produced using renewable resources and without traditional pesticides or artificial fertilizers. Animals that produce organic products, meat, and eggs receive no antibiotics or growth hormones. Organically grown food may be more nutritious than conventionally grown food, but the extent of this difference is still being researched.

- *Pasture-raised:* Pasture-raised animals live and grow up on open grazing fields, with a diet focusing on grass, rather than grains.

- *Sustainable:* A method of raising food that does not cause lasting harm to the environment, provides just compensation for farmers and workers, and uses a variety of plant and animal species.

It's Your Health

Dietary Guidelines for Americans

The USDA makes the following recommendations for the five food groups as part of a healthful, 2,000-calorie per day diet:

Vegetables

- Vary the vegetables you eat. Try to eat at least two different colors of vegetables every day.
- Try to eat 2.5 cups of vegetables a day.
- Especially nutritious vegetables include:
  - Dark green vegetables like spinach and broccoli.
  - Orange vegetables like carrots and sweet potatoes.
  - Dry beans and peas like kidney beans, pinto beans, and lentils.

Fruits

- Eat a variety of fruit.
- Try to eat 2 cups of fruit every day.
- Get most of your fruit whole or cut up, rather than from juice.

Grains

Eat 6 ounces of grains every day (1 ounce equals one 1 cup of cereal, ½ cup of cooked rice or pasta, or 1 slice of bread).

- Make at least half of the grains you eat whole, rather than refined grains.

Dairy Products

- Consume about 3 cups of dairy products or other calcium-rich foods every day.
- Consume low-fat dairy products when possible.
- Calcium-fortified soy products are a healthful alternative to dairy foods.

Proteins

- Eat 5.5 ounces of protein-rich foods every day.
- Consume baked, broiled, or grilled meat products when possible.
- Eat seafood as a protein source twice a week (roughly 8 ounces per week).
- Make beans and peas a regular protein source.
- Limit consumption of processed meats such as sausage, luncheon meats, and hot dogs.

This chapter describes the basic nutritional components of a healthful diet, and discusses different types of physical activity and their importance. It also discusses ways to maintain a healthful weight, provides perspectives about body image, and discusses hunger from global and national perspectives.

Healthful Eating and Nutrition

Nutrition is the science that explores the need for food and the role of food in nourishing the body and fostering good health. To survive and stay healthy, the human body needs six basic **nutrients**, which fall into three types:

- *Macronutrients*, which include carbohydrates, proteins, and fats, are needed in large amounts.

- *Micronutrients*, which include vitamins and minerals, are needed in smaller amounts.

- *Water*, a substance often overlooked as a nutrient, is indispensable for virtually every bodily function.

Dietary Guidelines

The U.S. Department of Agriculture (USDA) has issued updated dietary guidelines for Americans every 5 years since 1980. These guidelines offer rough estimates of how much of each basic food group to eat to maintain a balanced, healthful diet. The 2010 guidelines use a plate as a basic visual metaphor (see **Figure 9.1**) Fruits and vegetables make up the left side of the plate, with vegetables taking up a slightly larger share than fruit. Grains and protein foods (meat, poultry, seafood, beans and peas, and nuts and seeds) make up the right half of the plate, with each taking up a roughly equal amount. Each of these plate "halves" corresponds to just under half of a healthful diet. Dairy products, represented by a cup next to the plate, make up the remaining portion of the diet. The USDA also has recommendations within each food group. **It's Your Health:** Dietary Guidelines for Americans summarizes these recommendations.

Unfortunately, the typical American diet includes too many foods high in fat (particularly saturated fats), sugar, salt, and "empty calories" as well as too few fruits, vegetables, and whole grains.[2] More than three-fourths (78%) of American high-school students do not get enough fruits and vegetables each day; a higher percentage drinks at least one can of soda or soft drinks on a daily basis.[3] Poor eating habits that begin during childhood and adolescence typically carry into adulthood and become harder to break.[4]

Other food guide pyramids challenge or complement the USDA's food guide. Food guides exist for special populations, such as people older than 70 years of age and vegetarians. Culture-specific food guidelines, including ones for Arabic, Chinese, Indian, Russian, and Mexican populations, also offer guidance for a balanced, healthful diet.

The Mediterranean food guide, based on the dietary traditions of Greece and southern Italy, has received much attention. In that region, rates of chronic disease such as heart disease and stroke are consistently lower than they are in many other regions, while life expectancy remains high. The food guide highlights the following characteristics of the Mediterranean diet:

■ Fruits and vegetables should make up roughly half of a balanced diet.

- An abundance of food from plant sources, including fruits and vegetables, bread and grains, beans, nuts, and seeds

- Emphasis on fresh, locally grown foods

- Olive oil as the principal fat

- Moderate amounts of fish, poultry, cheese, and yogurt

- Moderate consumption of wine

- Limited consumption of red meat, dairy products and sweets

Figure 9.1

MyPlate: The 2010 USDA food plate.

Source: Reproduced from U.S. Department of Agriculture. http://www.choosemyplate.gov/

Other food guides attempt to correct what some experts see as the excesses of a Western diet. Author and food expert Michael Pollan summarized one approach with seven words: "Eat food, not too much, mostly plants."[5] The first part, "Eat food," refers to avoiding processed foods—food with long ingredient lists, artificial ingredients, or ingredients that a person would not have recognized as food 100 years ago. The second part, "not too much," encourages people to keep snacks between meals to a minimum and to stop eating just before one feels full. The third part, "mostly plants," encourages people to make fruits, vegetables, and grains the bulk of their diet, with meat and dairy products acting as supplementary, not primary, sources of energy.

Nutrition Facts Label

The Nutrition Facts label is designed to help people make healthful food choices and compare the nutritional quality of foods. The food label lists information on serving size, calories, nutrients, and vitamins and minerals, as well as other important facts relevant to a balanced diet (**Figure 9.2**). The Daily Value (%DV) section indicates the amount of each of the major nutrients (expressed as a percentage of a person's daily requirement of that nutrient) in a serving of food. These values are based on recommendations for a 2,000-calorie diet. A woman under doctor's orders to eat a higher- or lower-calorie diet will need to recalculate these numbers to fit her own needs.[2]

Carbohydrates

Carbohydrates provide the basic fuel for the body and are available in two forms: simple carbohydrates (sugars) and complex carbohydrates (starches). Complex carbohydrates are almost always more nutritious than simple carbohydrates. Simple carbohydrates often provide little more than a quick burst of energy (fruit is a notable exception). Foods rich in complex carbohydrates are more likely to contain vitamins, minerals, and other nutrients than sugar-rich foods.

During digestion, the body breaks down all carbohydrates into sugar. The body breaks down simple

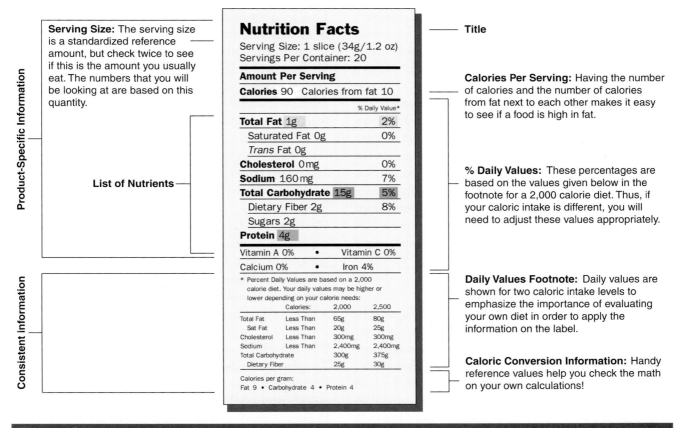

Figure 9.2

Example of the Nutrition Facts label.

carbohydrates quickly, making them little more than a quick energy source. Starches are broken down at a slower, steadier pace, providing a source of energy that lasts for a longer time. Whether it comes from simple or complex carbohydrates, sugar enters the blood, where cells throughout the body use it for energy. The pancreas makes a hormone called insulin, which allows cells to absorb sugar from the blood. A diet rich in complex carbohydrates allows the body to make insulin at a comparatively steady pace, while a diet rich in simple sugars creates rapid swings in blood sugar, forcing irregular insulin production that can overwork the pancreas and harm overall health.

Simple Carbohydrates

Simple carbohydrates, or sugars, have four virtually identical forms: sucrose, glucose, fructose, and lactose. They are present in many foods, from fruit to ice cream to ketchup. Processed foods often have much more sugar than their natural counterparts. A typical 12-ounce soft drink contains the equivalent of 8 teaspoons of sugar, and a chocolate bar contains about 3 teaspoons of sugar per ounce. Foods high in sugar are often high in fat, and a high-fat diet is a major culprit in cardiovascular disease, obesity, and other chronic diseases. Sugar provides "empty calories," or calories without significant nutritional value. In addition, consumption of a sugared product, such as a soft drink, usually occurs in lieu of something else that may be nutritious, such as a glass of skim milk or water.

Foods high in sugar are also harmful to dental health because sugar nourishes cavity-causing bacteria. The physical structure of the food can also affect its effect on dental health. Sugar in sticky foods, for example, clings to the teeth and encourages bacterial growth. High consumption of sugar promotes the growth of plaque, the toxin-producing film that forms on teeth; plaque can lead to periodontal (gum) disease, the leading cause of tooth loss among U.S. adults. In addition, research has linked periodontal disease with an increased risk of heart disease.[6]

Complex Carbohydrates

Complex carbohydrates are found in breads, cereals, legumes, rice, pastas, and "starchy" vegetables such as beans and potatoes. Digestion breaks down complex carbohydrates into simple sugars. Because complex carbohydrates take longer to digest than simple carbohydrates, they are a good long-term source of energy. According to USDA dietary guidelines, complex carbohydrates should provide the major supply of calories in diets, approximately 55% to 60% of total calories consumed.

© DUSAN ZIDAR/ShutterStock, Inc.

■ Complex carbohydrates are a good source of minerals, vitamins, and fiber.

Fiber is not a single substance, but rather a group of substances with varied physical properties. Fiber comes from the parts of plants that cannot be digested by enzymes in the human digestive tract. Although not considered a nutrient because it cannot be digested, it is an essential to digestion and helps improve overall health.

There are two kinds of fiber: soluble and insoluble. Both kinds benefit the body. Soluble fiber absorbs water in the digestive tract and is easily fermented by bacteria in the large intestine. Oats, for example, are rich in soluble fiber, which helps lower blood cholesterol and manage blood sugar levels. In contrast, most insoluble fiber remains essentially unchanged during digestion. Wheat bran, whole-grain breads and cereals, broccoli, carrots, and pears are all rich in insoluble fiber, which tends to increase stool bulk. A high-fiber diet lowers the risk for heart disease, high blood pressure, and diabetes.[7]

Women 50 and younger should aim for roughly 25–28 grams of fiber a day; women over 50 can aim for roughly 20–25 grams a day. Most women, however, do not get this amount. A woman adding fiber to her diet should do so gradually. Opting for less-processed food, such as an apple rather than applesauce or apple juice, is one way to increase fiber intake. The skins of fruits and vegetables are also rich sources of fiber (see **It's Your Health**).

Glycemic Index

The **glycemic index** measures how fast glucose enters the bloodstream after a carbohydrate is eaten and thus how quickly the carbohydrate increases a person's blood sugar. In general, foods that are mostly simple sugars, are highly processed, or contain refined sugars have a high glycemic index. This group includes refined breakfast cereals, white bread, white rice, white spaghetti, soft drinks, and sugar. Some complex carbohydrates, such as potatoes, behave just as simple carbohydrates do, elevating blood sugar to an excessive level. These complex carbohydrates have a high glycemic index, while complex carbohydrates that are high in fiber tend to have a lower glycemic index. Fiber slows digestion, so sugars in high-fiber foods take longer to be absorbed into the bloodstream. Interestingly, ice cream has a fairly low glycemic index because the fat in ice cream tends to slow blood sugar absorption.

The rationale for avoiding high-glycemic-index foods relates to the resulting production of insulin. Avoiding high-glycemic-index foods and eating only low glycemic-index foods may facilitate fat loss by reducing excess insulin. The weakness of this theory, however, is that obese and severely overweight individuals are already producing excess insulin, thus consuming a low-glycemic-index diet will not help them to achieve meaningful weight loss. A food's glycemic index is only one part of the larger picture. Many fruits, for example, have very high glycemic indexes but are high in desirable fiber and vitamins.[8]

Proteins

Protein provides the framework for muscles, bones, blood, hair, and fingernails. It is the main supply of amino acids— the building blocks that construct, repair, and maintain body tissues. There are nine "essential" amino acids that the body cannot manufacture itself and must receive from dietary sources. Complete sources of protein contain all of the essential amino acids in their required amounts; incomplete sources of protein lack one or more of the essential amino acids. Complete proteins include meat, fish, poultry, and dairy products. Incomplete sources include beans, peas, peanuts, grains, and potatoes. Complementary proteins are protein sources that, when eaten together, supply

© Robyn Mackenzie/ShutterStock, Inc.

■ With the exception of fish and shellfish, all animal-based sources of protein contain saturated fat.

the necessary amounts of all the essential amino acids. An example of complementary proteins is cooked dried or canned beans eaten with rice. One difficulty for vegetarians, vegans, or even people eating a diet low in animal proteins is that the body cannot store amino acids. To benefit the body, a person must consume all the essential amino acids at the same meal.

The Food and Drug Administration (FDA) recommends that women between the ages of 19 and 30 eat 5.5 ounces of protein-rich foods per day. For a healthful diet, women should vary their sources of protein to include beans, peas, fish, seafood, and other sources in addition to meat and poultry.

Some high-protein diets focus on obtaining a significant percentage of daily calories from protein. One problem with these diets is that they encourage consumption of proteins high in saturated fat, such as red meat and cheese, while discouraging consumption of healthy carbohydrates such as fruit, vegetables, and fiber. Diets high in saturated fat increase a person's risk for heart disease and certain types of cancer. In addition, the body receives no benefit for excessive amounts of protein; extra protein is simply converted into fat. Finally, high-protein diets also may increase a woman's risk for osteoporosis, as excess dietary protein increases calcium loss in the urine.

Soy is another vegetarian-based protein source. Soy-based products have no saturated fat, and they can be a low-fat source of calcium, protein, and other nutrients. Excessive consumption of soy isoflavones, a product found in soy, may be harmful to women because isoflavones can act like estrogen in the human body. However, when consumed in moderation, soy-based products are probably not a major health risk.[8]

It's Your Health

Ways to Eat More Fiber

1. Eat whole fresh fruit instead of just drinking juice.
2. Eat the skins of fruits and vegetables, such as apples and potatoes.
3. Eat fruits with edible seeds, such as berries and kiwis.
4. Eat whole-grain foods.
5. Eat more of the stems when having broccoli or asparagus.
6. Peel citrus fruits and eat the sections with their membranes.
7. Eat more beans and peas.

Fats

Fats perform many essential bodily functions. They store energy, maintain healthy hair and skin, carry **fat-soluble vitamins**, supply essential fatty acids, affect levels of blood cholesterol, and create a feeling of "fullness." **Cholesterol** is a type of fat produced by the liver. It is a vital constituent of cell membranes and nerve fibers and serves as a building block for estrogen, testosterone, vitamin D, and bile. Cholesterol is transported in the bloodstream in protein packages called lipoproteins, which are assembled in the intestinal tract and liver. **Low-density lipoproteins (LDLs)**—called the "bad" cholesterol—carry the cholesterol through the blood, dropping it off where it is needed for cell building and leaving any excess in arterial walls and other tissues. This excess accumulates in the arterial walls, causing blockage. **High-density lipoproteins (HDLs)**—known as the "good" cholesterol—pick up cholesterol deposits and bring them to the liver for reprocessing or excretion. Increased levels of LDLs are associated with an increased risk of heart disease. Increased levels of HDLs seem to have a protective effect against heart disease, though some studies suggest they may simply be a marker of other factors that lower the risk for heart disease. The body normally produces all of the cholesterol that it needs, so dietary cholesterol (found in foods from animal sources such as eggs, meats, and dairy products) is unnecessary.

There are three types of fats:

1. **Saturated fats** come primarily from animal sources such as meat, poultry, milk, cheese, and butter. Some vegetable oils, such as coconut, palm kernel, and palm oil, also are saturated fats. At the molecular level, saturated fats are "saturated" with hydrogen atoms; each molecule holds as many as it can possibly carry. Saturated fats are generally solid at room temperature. They raise both LDL and HDL cholesterol, thereby increasing the risk of heart disease.

2. **Unsaturated fats** come from plants and include most vegetable oils. Carbon atoms in unsaturated fats have multiple bonds with each other, which prevents them from carrying the maximum number of hydrogen atoms they can carry (hence the name "unsaturated"). In turn, this configuration gives the molecules "kinks" that prevent unsaturated fat molecules from solidifying. They include two types:

   ■ **Monounsaturated fats**, such as those in olive, peanut, grapeseed, and canola oil

   ■ **Polyunsaturated fats**, such as those in safflower, sunflower, corn, and flaxseed oil

Like saturated fats, unsaturated fats are high in calories. In all other respects, however, unsaturated fats are a much more healthful nutrient. Both types of unsaturated fats lower LDL cholesterol and raise HDL cholesterol, which has a positive effect on overall blood cholesterol levels and can therefore lower the risk of heart disease.

3. **Trans fats** form when vegetable oils are processed into margarine or shortening. They are found in snack foods such as potato chips, commercial baked goods with "partially hydrogenated vegetable oil" or "vegetable shortening," many types of fast foods (french fries and onion rings), stick margarine, and some dairy products. Trans fats are solid or semi-solid at room temperature. These fats are worse than saturated fats because they raise LDL cholesterol and lower HDL cholesterol. A report from the Institute of Medicine concluded that there is no safe level of

© Christian Jung/ShutterStock, Inc.

■ Monounsaturated fats like olive oil are more healthful choices than saturated fats (fats that are solid at room temperature).

trans fats in the diet, and the FDA now requires that trans fats be listed on the Nutrition Facts food label used in the United States. The Centers for Disease Control and Prevention (CDC) estimates that artificial trans fats are responsible for 10,000–20,000 heart attacks and 3,000–7,000 coronary heart disease deaths each year in the United States.[9]

Lowering one's intake of saturated fat, trans fat, and dietary cholesterol is one of the major modifiable risk factors for coronary heart disease. Lowering intake of dietary cholesterol has less effect on blood cholesterol levels than lowering intake of saturated fat.[10,11]

Most women should obtain 30% or less of their daily calories from fat, with unsaturated fats making up the majority of their fat intake. Only 10% or less of a woman's daily calories should come from saturated fat (**Table 9.1**). Women should also avoid trans fats, as any amount of these fats appears to be harmful. Additionally, diets should contain less than 300 mg of cholesterol per day.[10] How well these guidelines fit a person's diet as a whole is more important than how well they fit any given day. A two-egg omelet eaten once or twice per week may be a perfectly healthful breakfast, even if it contains 360 mg of cholesterol. These guidelines, which parallel the dietary guidelines endorsed by the USDA and the U.S. Department of Health and Human Services, emphasize careful eating patterns from early childhood to old age. Currently, few American women meet these standards. **Self-Assessment 9.1** reviews the method for calculating daily fat intake.

Vitamins

Vitamins are organic substances that perform a variety of functions and are needed by the body in very small amounts. Vitamins are essential for life. They help promote good vision, form normal blood cells, create strong bones and teeth, and ensure proper functioning of the heart and nervous system. Although vitamins do not provide energy, they do help the body efficiently convert foods into energy. Vitamin supplements are one tool women can use to get their daily requirements for vitamins, but supplements should not be used to replace a balanced diet. Vitamin supplements cannot turn a junk-food meal into a healthful one, and getting vitamins naturally through food provides greater benefits than taking them as supplements. Taking large doses of vitamins far beyond their **Recommended Daily Allowances (RDAs)** does not provide any benefit; in fact, overdosing on large amounts of vitamins can be harmful to one's health.

| **Table 9.1** | Differences in Saturated Fat and Calorie Content of Common Foods |

This table compares the saturated fat content of different forms of common foods. Even foods that are similar in nature (such as regular cheddar cheese and low-fat cheddar cheese), may have significantly different amounts of fat and saturated fat.

Food Category	Portion	Saturated Fat Content (grams)	Calories
Cheese			
Regular cheddar cheese	1 oz	6.0	114
Low-fat cheddar cheese	1 oz	1.2	49
Ground beef			
Regular ground beef (25% fat)	3 oz (cooked)	6.1	236
Extra lean ground beef (5% fat)	3 oz (cooked)	2.6	148
Milk			
Whole milk (3.24%)	1 cup	4.6	146
Low-fat (1%) milk	1 cup	1.5	102
Breads			
Croissant	1 medium	6.6	231
Bagel, oat bran	1 medium (4 inch)	0.2	227
Frozen desserts			
Regular ice cream	½ cup	4.9	145
Frozen yogurt, low-fat	½ cup	2.0	110
Table spreads			
Butter	1 tsp	2.4	34
Soft margarine with zero trans fat	1 tsp	0.7	25
Chicken			
Fried chicken (leg with skin)	3 oz (cooked)	3.3	212
Roasted chicken (breast, no skin)	3 oz (cooked)	0.9	140
Fish			
Fried fish	3 oz	2.8	195
Baked fish	3 oz	1.5	129

Source: U.S. Department of Agriculture, U.S. Department of Health and Human Services. (2010). *Dietary guidelines for Americans.*

There are 13 essential vitamins: A, C, D, E, K, and the eight vitamins of the B complex. The body stores fat-soluble vitamins (A, D, E, and K) in the liver for relatively long periods of time; **water-soluble vitamins** (B-complex vitamins and C) are stored for very short periods of time. Each vitamin carries out specific functions. The body generally cannot manufacture vitamins; instead, they must be ingested from food sources. Some diseases can result

Calculating Daily Fat Limits

To determine the maximum number of daily grams of fat:

1. Calculate approximately how many calories are consumed on a daily basis, then

2. Divide the answer above by 33.

Women who find that they are eating more grams of fat than the calculated number should work on achieving this desired amount. Women with an intake of greater than 30% of calories from fat are at greater risk for many chronic diseases as well as obesity.

---

if a person does not get enough of a particular vitamin. **Table 9.3** summarizes facts known for each of the essential vitamins.

Folic Acid

Folate is a B vitamin found in chickpeas, spinach, strawberries, kidney beans, and citrus fruits and juices. It is vital for cell growth and function and for the development of healthy neural tubes in fetuses. Folic acid, a form of folate, is used to fortify grain-based foods, such as bread, flour, rice, pasta, and cereal. Folic acid and folate are also present in prenatal vitamins. Neural tube defects, including spina bifida, are birth defects affecting the brain and spinal cord. Since fortification of cereal grains with folic acid

Table 9.2 **Typical American Diets Compared to Recommended Intake Levels**

Foods to Eat More of:	Average American Intake
Whole Grains	15% of recommended levels
Seafood	44% of recommended levels
Dairy Products	52% of recommended levels
Fruits	42% of recommended levels
Vegetables	59% of recommended levels
Healthful Oils	61% of recommended levels
Foods to Eat Less of:	
Refined Grains	200% of recommended levels
Sodium	149% of recommended levels
Saturated Fat	110% of recommended levels
Calories from added sugar and solid fats	280% of recommended levels

Source: Data from U.S. Department of Agriculture, U.S. Department of Health and Human Services. (2010). *Dietary guidelines for Americans.* Available at http://health.gov/dietaryguidelines/dga2010/DietaryGuidelines2010.pdf

began in the United States in 1998, the incidence of neural tube disorders has decreased by 20–30%. All women of childbearing age should include 400–600 micrograms (0.4–0.6 mg) of folate or folic acid in their daily diet. However, on average, women of childbearing age consume an average of 200 micrograms per day, only half of the recommended amount.[12] Folic acid also helps maintain levels of homocysteine, an amino acid that builds and maintains tissues, but it can increase the risk of cardiovascular disease if consumed at excessive levels. Folic acid fortification is a public health intervention that, like immunization, actually saves money; one economic analysis concluded that folic acid fortification in the United States saves $88 million to $145 million annually and is associated with an overall economic benefit of $312 million to $425 million per year.[13]

Antioxidants and Phytochemicals

Antioxidants, which include vitamins E and C, are substances that can neutralize oxidants, harmful molecules that can build up in the body. Antioxidants and **phytochemicals** (substances such as carotenoids and flavonoids that appear to act as antioxidants) have been widely studied for their roles in disease prevention and health promotion. Diets rich in fruits, vegetables, and grains—all of which are sources of antioxidants—are associated with a decreased risk of cardiovascular disease and cancer. Damage to cells from oxidation is associated with an increased risk of various diseases. Antioxidants appear to block some of the oxygen-induced cell damage by stabilizing and neutralizing the effects of free radicals (toxic particles) in the body.

Some studies show that vitamin E protects against damage in the artery lining, thereby decreasing the risk of coronary artery disease. Eating fruits and vegetables rich in vitamin C and beta-carotene (the carotenoid that is the precursor of vitamin A) may reduce the risk for many cancers. Carotenoids and flavonoids, which are found in foods such as onions, broccoli, red wine, green tea, and black tea, also reduce the risk for heart disease.

To stay healthy, nutritionists recommend that people eat foods high in carotenoids, such as red, orange, and deep yellow fruits and vegetables (e.g., tomatoes, carrots, sweet potatoes) and dark green leafy vegetables (e.g., spinach, broccoli); vitamin E (e.g., vegetable oils, salad dressings, margarine, whole grains, peanut butter); and vitamin C (e.g., citrus fruits, strawberries, broccoli). Eating a variety of fruits and vegetables supplies the body with vitamins, fiber, and antioxidants that may reduce the risk of heart disease and some kinds of cancer.[8] Getting these vitamins

Table 9.3   Facts About Vitamins

Vitamin	Women's RDA*	Sources	What It Does
Vitamin A	700 mg	Liver, eggs, dairy products, carrots, bell peppers, green leafy vegetables, squash	Promotes good vision; helps form and maintain healthy skin and mucous membranes; helps fight infections
Vitamin B$_1$ (thiamin)	1.1 mg	Whole grains, dried beans, lean red meats, fish, sunflower seeds	Helps release energy from carbohydrates; necessary for healthy brain and nerve cells and for functioning of heart
Vitamin B$_2$ (riboflavin)	1.1 mg	Dairy products, liver, whole grains, spinach, broccoli	Aids in the release of energy from food; helps form antibodies and red blood cells
Vitamin B$_3$ (niacin)	14 mg	Nuts, dairy products, liver, enriched grains, poultry	Aids in the release of energy from food; involved in the synthesis of DNA; maintains normal function of skin, nerves, and digestive system
Vitamin B$_5$ (pantothenic acid)	5 mg	Whole grains, dried beans, eggs, nuts	Aids in the release of energy from food; essential for synthesis of numerous body materials
Vitamin B$_6$ (pyridoxine)	1.3 mg	Fortified breakfast cereals, meat, nuts, beans	Important in chemical reactions of proteins and amino acids; involved in normal functioning of brain and formation of red blood cells
Vitamin B$_{12}$ (cobalamin)	2.4 mg	Liver, beef, eggs, milk, shellfish	Necessary for development of red blood cells; maintains normal functioning of nervous system
Biotin	30 mg	Yeast, liver, eggs, milk	Important in the formation of fatty acids; helps metabolize amino acids and carbohydrates
Vitamin C† (ascorbic acid)	75 mg	Citrus fruits and juices, bell peppers, tomatoes, spinach, broccoli	Promotes healthy gums, capillaries, and teeth; aids iron absorption; maintains normal connective tissue; aids in healing wounds
Choline	425 mg	Whole grains, egg yolks, legumes, liver, soybeans, green leafy vegetables	Manages cholesterol in body; important for brain function; involved in production of hormones; necessary for functioning of folic acid
Vitamin D (calciferol)	15 mg	Dairy products, mackerel, sardines, salmon and other cold-water fish	Promotes strong bones and teeth; necessary for absorption of calcium
Vitamin E (tocopherol)	15 mg	Nuts, vegetable oils, whole grains, margarine, dark green vegetables	Protects tissue against oxidation; important in formation of red blood cells; helps body use vitamin K
Folate (folic acid/folacin)	400 mg	Liver, fortified breakfast cereals, lentils, chickpeas, spinach, beans	Important in the synthesis of DNA; acts together with vitamin B$_{12}$ in the production of hemoglobin; vital to healthy fetal development
Vitamin K	90 mg	Leafy green vegetables, soybeans, broccoli, cauliflower	Aids in the clotting of blood

*Pregnant or breastfeeding women need additional levels of these vitamins.

†Smokers should consume an additional 35 mg daily of vitamin C.

Sources: U.S. Department of Agriculture, U.S. Department of Health and Human Services. (2010). *Dietary guidelines for Americans*; Willet, W. C. (2002). *Eat, drink and be healthy: The Harvard Medical School guide to healthy eating.* New York, NY: Simon and Schuster.

naturally from one's diet appears to provide substantially more health benefits than getting them from supplements.

Minerals

Minerals are inorganic substances essential to bone formation (calcium), enzyme synthesis (iron), blood pressure maintenance (sodium), and normal functioning of the digestive process (potassium). Minerals make up the earth's surface. Carried into the soil, groundwater, and sea by erosion, they are taken up by plants and subsequently consumed by animals and humans. As components of the body, minerals are present in small amounts. Six minerals (calcium, chloride, magnesium, phosphorus, potassium, and sodium) are generally designated as macrominerals, or major minerals; other nutrients, which are equally essential but needed in smaller amounts, are referred to as microminerals. **Table 9.4** summarizes facts about each of the essential minerals. Calcium and iron are especially important for women's health.

Because of the complex interactions between minerals and the dangers of overdosing, taking mineral supplements in doses greater than the RDAs should be avoided.

Table 9.4   Facts About Minerals

Mineral	Adult RDA*	Sources	What It Does
Calcium	1,000–1,200 mg*	Milk and milk products, sardines and salmon eaten with bones, dark green leafy vegetables, certain types of tofu and soy milk, fortified orange juice	Builds bones and teeth and maintains bone density and strength; helps prevent osteoporosis; helps regulate heartbeat, blood clotting, muscle contraction, and nerve conduction; helps prevent hypertension
Chloride	700 mg	Table salt, fish, pickled and smoked foods	Maintains normal fluid shifts; balances pH of the blood; forms hydrochloric acid to aid digestion
Magnesium	310–320 mg*	Whole grains, raw leafy green vegetables, nuts (especially almonds and cashews), soybeans, tofu, hard water	Aids in bone growth; assists function of nerves and muscles, including regulation of normal heart rhythm; important in energy metabolism
Phosphorus	700 mg*	Meats, poultry, fish, egg yolks, dried peas and beans, milk and milk products, nuts; present in almost all foods	Aids bone growth and strengthening of teeth; important in energy metabolism
Potassium	4,700 mg†	Oranges and orange juice, melons, bananas, dried fruits, dried peas and beans, potatoes	Promotes regular heartbeat; active in muscle contraction; regulates transfer of nutrients to cells; controls water balance in body tissues and cells; contributes to regulation of blood pressure
Sodium	500–2,300 mg (estimated safe amount for dietary intake)	All from salt and foods containing salt	Helps regulate water balance in body; helps maintain blood pressure; excess sodium may raise blood pressure to unhealthful levels
Chromium	50–200 mg†	Meat, cheese, mushrooms, oysters, peanuts, brewer's yeast, potatoes	Important for glucose metabolism; may be a cofactor for insulin; regulates cholesterol production in liver; aids in digestion of protein
Copper	900–1,000 mg†	Wheat, peanuts, shellfish (especially oysters), nuts, beef and pork liver, dried beans	Formation of red blood cells; cofactor in absorbing iron into blood cells; assists in production of several enzymes involved in respiration; interacts with zinc
Fluorine (fluoride)	3.1 mg†	Fluoridated water, foods cooked with or grown in fluoridated water, fish, tea, gelatin	Contributes to solid bone and tooth formation; prevents dental cavities; may help prevent osteoporosis
Iodine	0.15 mg*	Primarily from iodized salt, but also seafood, seaweed food products, vegetables grown in iodine-rich areas, eggs, certain cheeses, whole milk	Necessary for normal function of the thyroid gland; essential for normal cell function; keeps skin, hair, and nails healthy; prevents goiter
Iron	18 mg*	Liver (especially pork liver), kidneys, red meats, egg yolks, peas, beans, nuts, dried fruits, green leafy vegetables, enriched grain products, blackstrap molasses	Essential to formation of hemoglobin, the oxygen-carrying factor in the blood; part of several enzymes and proteins in the blood
Manganese	320–350 mg†	Nuts, whole grains, vegetables, fruits, instant coffee, tea, cocoa powder, beets, egg yolks	Required for normal bone growth; helps maintain healthy skin; important for metabolism of glucose and fatty acids
Molybdenum	75–250 mg	Peas, beans, cereal grains, organ meats, some dark green vegetables	Important for normal cell function
Selenium	50–55 mg	Fish, shellfish, red meat, egg yolks, chicken, legumes, whole grains	Protects cells against effects of free radicals that can damage cells; essential for normal functioning of the immune system and thyroid gland
Zinc	8 mg	Meat, liver, eggs, oysters, legumes, whole grain cereals, nuts	Essential for growth and skeletal development; important for immune system; assists in production of DNA and RNA

*These figures are not applicable to pregnant or breastfeeding women, who need additional minerals.

†Although there is no RDA for these minerals, the Food and Nutrition Board recommends this value as an average healthy intake.

Sources: U.S. Department of Agriculture, U.S. Department of Health and Human Services. (2010). *Dietary guidelines for Americans*. Willet, W. C. (2002). Eat, drink and be healthy: The Harvard Medical School Guide to healthy eating. New York, NY: Simon and Schuster.

Megadoses of certain minerals may do serious harm. The best way to ensure an adequate, but not excessive, supply of minerals is to eat a varied, balanced diet.

Calcium

Calcium is a mineral of special concern to women. It is an integral component of bones and teeth, and calcium deficiency is a major contributor to osteoporosis. Calcium helps regulate heartbeat, blood clotting, muscle contraction, and nerve conduction. This mineral also helps prevent high blood pressure, is essential in the development of the fetus during pregnancy, and may reduce the risk for colon cancer. When calcium levels in the blood fall too low, the body draws the mineral from the supply in the bones to meet its needs elsewhere. This process accelerates the gradual bone loss that occurs most dramatically in postmenopausal women.

The RDA's recommendation that women receive 1,000 mg of calcium per day is deceptive. Adolescents, young women (ages 11 to 24), and postmenopausal women are advised to consume 1,200 mg daily. Three to five cups of milk or servings of other calcium-rich foods such as collard greens, cheese, tofu, cornbread, or sardines can supply the daily recommended amount. (See **It's Your Health**.)

When possible, women should get calcium through their diets rather than through supplements. For years, healthcare providers have recommended that women take calcium and vitamin D supplements to improve their long-term bone health. However, recent research indicates that calcium and vitamin D supplements do not appear to prevent cancer or reduce the risk of bone fractures; in addition, women who take the equivalent of their RDA of calcium and vitamin D as supplements every day may have a slightly increased risk for kidney stones.[14] The risk for supplements appears to be the greatest when women take the equivalent of one or more RDA of calcium per day. The evidence is less clear about smaller doses of calcium (such as taking daily supplements to provide 50% or less of the RDA, or taking the RDA on an irregular basis to supplement dietary calcium). Getting calcium through the diet, however, is the better choice.

The 2010 "My Plate" food guide continues to emphasize dairy products as an important part of a healthy diet. Dairy foods are an excellent source of calcium as well as protein, vitamin D, and other nutrients; however, they often contain large amounts of saturated fat and calories, and they are not an option for lactose-intolerant individuals. Women do not have to rely on dairy products for their calcium. A cup of collard greens, for example, has virtually the same amount of calcium as a cup of skim milk (see **It's Your Health**).

Iron

Iron is necessary to produce **hemoglobin**, a key component of red blood cells and the oxygen-carrying protein that gives blood its red color. The body only needs small amounts of iron each day—about 18 mg each day for an average adult—but without iron the body becomes fatigued

It's Your Health

Calcium Sources

Food	Amount	mg Calcium	Percentage of RDA	
			1,000 mg/day	1,200 mg/day
Plain yogurt	1 cup	415	41%	35%
Sardines with bones	3 oz	372	37%	31%
Skim milk	1 cup	302	30%	25%
Collard greens	1 cup	290	29%	24%
Swiss cheese	1 oz	262	26%	22%
Cheddar cheese	1 oz	213	21%	18%
Canned salmon, with bones	3 oz	167	17%	14%
Low-fat cottage cheese	1 cup	154	15%	12%
Blackstrap molasses	1 tbsp	137	14%	12%
Cooked broccoli	1 cup	136	14%	12%
Dried and cooked beans	1 cup	90	9%	7%
Orange	1 (medium)	54	5%	4%

and weak. Reduced levels of hemoglobin result in anemia, a serious risk for women whose diets are chronically deficient in iron. Symptoms of iron-deficiency anemia include headaches, fatigue, general weakness, and pallor. In severe cases, anemia can lead to an irregular or increased heart rate. Iron-deficiency anemia is relatively common in the United States today, with 12% of women ages 12 to 49 experiencing some form of iron deficiency.[15] In addition to being found in hemoglobin, iron is stored in the liver, spleen, bone marrow, and other tissues.

Iron absorption is a complex process that varies with the types and combination of foods consumed and the body's needs. There are several healthful ways to increase iron intake. Eating lean red meats is one method. Liver is one of the best sources of iron, but it should not be eaten more than once a week owing to its high cholesterol content. Chicken and fish typically contain one-third to one-half the iron of red meat. Vegetarian sources of iron include chickpeas, soybeans, kidney beans, and lentils. Choosing breads, cereals, and pasta labeled "enriched" or "fortified" and unrefined whole grains, such as whole-wheat bread, supplies a fair amount of iron. In addition, eating foods high in vitamin C facilitates the body's absorption of iron. For vegetarians and vegans, consuming vitamin C with meals is a must. Cooking in cast-iron cookware also helps to increase the iron content of foods. The more acidic the food (such as spaghetti sauce) and the longer it cooks, the more iron will be absorbed. Other compounds, such as coffee, tea, and dietary fiber, block the body's ability to absorb iron.

Sodium

Sodium is another macromineral necessary for human health. Unlike other macrominerals, however, the main health concern in the United States (and other developed countries) is not too little sodium, but too much. The average American consumes about 3,400 mg of sodium per day—about 7 times what the body needs to function.[2] The Dietary Guidelines recommend that Americans reduce their sodium intake to a maximum of 2,300 mg a day (1,500 mg a day for people with hypertension or people who are at risk).

The main health concern regarding excessive sodium intake is sodium's effects on blood pressure. Sodium is a major risk factor for hypertension, which itself raises the risk for heart disease, stroke, and other conditions. About half of Americans appear to be "salt sensitive," meaning that their blood pressure rises in response to extra sodium intake. The blood pressure of people who are not salt sensitive is mostly unaffected by sodium intake. However, there is no easy way of distinguishing between people who are salt sensitive and people who are not.

Almost all dietary sodium comes from salt (baking soda, monosodium glutamate, and some other foods can also add sodium to the diet). This salt may be naturally present in foods, added during cooking or processing, or added at the table. However, processed and restaurant foods are the greatest contributors to salt in the American diet. Women can reduce their sodium consumption by cutting back on processed foods such as rolls, cold cuts and luncheon meats, and soups, eating less fast food and other high-sodium meals at restaurants, and paying attention to the sodium content of the nutrition facts label of foods purchased at the grocery store.

Water

The human body is approximately 50% to 70% water. Every system in the body depends on water to function: Water regulates body temperature and chemical actions, disposes of waste, lubricates joints, cushions the fetus during pregnancy, transports nutrients, prevents bowel problems, and helps enzymes function properly.

The average female requires 8 to 9 cups of fluid per day; pregnant women have a slightly higher requirement. Some of this fluid comes from the food a woman eats; the rest must come from what she drinks. Drinking water is one healthful option. Another is drinking milk, skim milk, or fruit juice, which can also supply the body with minerals, protein, and vitamins.

Water is so essential that the human body can survive only 3 days without it, even though the body can be denied food for a few weeks and still recover. As little as 2% to 5% loss of body weight from water loss results in symptoms of dehydration, including headache, fatigue, flushed skin, and excessive thirst. Greater need for fluids occurs during exercise and conditions of high temperature, high altitude, and low humidity, and when it is necessary to counter the effects of high intakes of caffeine and alcohol, which promote fluid loss.

Sugary sodas and sports drinks have become a daily part of life for millions of Americans. These drinks add sugar and calories to the diet while offering no additional nutritional benefit. While diet or unsweetened sodas typically contain almost no sugar or calories, water still appears to be a more healthful choice. Saving these drinks for special occasions, or eliminating them entirely, is a simple way to improve one's diet and improve one's overall health.

© Chuck Wagner/ShutterStock, Inc.

■ Sports and energy drinks may claim to "replenish" body fluids, but often contain large amounts of sugar. Water alone is usually a better (and cheaper) option.

Table 9.5	Percentage of U.S. Women Engaging in Adequate Physical Activity, 2007–2009
Total	**14.7%**
Age Groups	
18–24	17.4%
25–44	17.1%
45–64	14.8%
65 and older	7.9%
Race and Ethnicity	
White, non-Hispanic	16.9%
Black, non-Hispanic	9.4%
Hispanic	9.5%
Native American/Alaska Native	14.9%
Asian, non-Hispanic	10.3%
Multiple race, non-Hispanic	16.0%

Source: Modified from U.S. Department of Health and Human Services, Health Resources and Services Administration, Maternal and Child Health Bureau. *Women's health USA 2011.* Rockville, Maryland: U.S. Department of Health and Human Services, 2011.

Exercise and Fitness

Regular physical activity improves mental and physical health, lowers risk of early death, increases quality of life, and reduces the risk for disease and injury. This physical activity can come in the form of intense exercise sessions or from more moderate-intensity activities, such as walking, dancing, or yoga.

However, physical inactivity remains a serious national problem. Only about one out of six (14.7%) women in the United States get the government-recommended levels of physical activity of 2.5 hours per week of moderate physical activity.[16] More than one-half of U.S. adults do not get enough physical activity to provide even basic health benefits. Physical activity decreases with age and is less common among those with lower incomes, less education, and non-White ethnicity/race (see **Table 9.5**).[17]

Physical Fitness

"Physical fitness" means different things to different people. A dancer and a long-distance swimmer may both be physically fit even if they have different strengths, stretch different muscles, and have different workout goals. Fitness is also relative—a woman may be "more fit" this year than she was last year, and there is no clear endpoint at which fitness occurs. Defining fitness as the ability to perform specific tasks can also be problematic. A paraplegic woman may be unable to walk a mile even if she has strong upper body strength and her circulatory system is in excellent shape. From a broad perspective, however, fitness should include the ability to perform daily tasks without getting tired and the ability to perform additional physical tasks if needed.

I've made a real effort to incorporate exercise into my daily routine this semester. On Mondays, Wednesdays, and Fridays I go straight to the gym after class, and I go running Tuesdays, Thursdays, and Saturdays, taking Sunday off. It's funny, because I never really thought about exercise much until this year, but now it's a normal part of my life.

—20-year-old student

Benefits of Exercise

Regular exercise offers many physical and psychological benefits that improve quality and quantity of life (**Table 9.6**). Adults and children of all age groups and body types, including people with disabilities, benefit greatly from regular physical activity. Substantial health benefits occur if a person gets at least 150 minutes (2.5 hours) of moderate-intensity activity a week, or 75 minutes (1 hour and 15 minutes) of high-intensity exercise a week. Alternatively, a combination of both high- and moderate-intensity exercise can also be used to reach the total of 150 minutes, with every minute of high-intensity exercise counting for 2 minutes of moderate-intensity exercise. Greater health benefits occur if a person gets twice that amount or more (300 minutes a week of moderate-intensity activity, 150 minutes of high-intensity activity,

Table 9.6	Benefits of Regular Physical Activity

Long-term:

- Reduces the risk of early death
- Reduces the risk of developing coronary heart disease and stroke
- Lowers the risk of breast, lung, colon, and other cancers
- Reduces the risk of developing type 2 diabetes, osteoporosis, and depression; for people with these conditions, reduces the severity of symptoms
- Lowers high blood pressure and cholesterol
- For older adults, improves ability to complete day-to-day tasks, reduces the risk of falls, and improves mental cognition

Short-term:

- Improves aerobic capacity, muscle strength, and muscle endurance
- Helps maintain healthy muscles, joints, and bones
- Can improve mood
- Can reduce symptoms of depression and increase cognitive functioning
- Helps control weight, build muscle, and reduce body fat
- Can promote better sleep and increase energy

■ Organized sports are one form of exercise.

or a combination of both).[18] However, even small amounts of physical activity are better than none at all. Regular exercise reduces death and injury from heart disease, the leading cause of death in the United States. Physical activity improves overall cardiovascular status and affects other risk factors for heart disease. For example, regular physical activity lowers blood pressure, reduces body fat, builds lean body weight, improves blood cholesterol levels, and reduces stress. Exercise reduces the risk of developing colon cancer, type 2 diabetes, osteoporosis, obesity, and other diseases. Women who exercise just an hour per week or more are 33% less likely to die from cancer, 50% less likely to die from cardiovascular disease, and 66% less likely to die early than women who do not excercise.[19]

Regular physical activity also has many short-term benefits. People who get regular physical activity sleep better than people who are inactive. Regular physical activity keeps muscles, bones, and joints healthy and maintains a sense of balance and coordination, which reduces a woman's risk of fall-related fractures in later life.

Studies have confirmed the potential value of aerobic exercise, along with medication if necessary, as a complementary therapy for depression.[20] People who exercise regularly report being happier, feeling better about themselves, and in general experience a better quality of life than people who do not. Regular exercise may also reduce anxiety and depression that can appear during pregnancy.[21] Other psychological benefits from exercise include decreased stress, increased sense of well-being, and improvements in cognitive function and mood. Proper exercise during pregnancy also has many benefits, including improved psychological well-being, shorter labor, and speedier recovery after childbirth (see Chapter 6).

Components of Physical Fitness

Exercise physiologists usually define fitness in four major areas:

- Cardiovascular endurance
- Muscular strength
- Muscular endurance
- Flexibility

Modern lifestyles do not require much physical movement, and few U.S. women are naturally fit as a result of daily activities. Most women who wish to become fit in today's society will need to commit time and energy to exercise.

Cardiovascular endurance, the ability to carry on vigorous physical activity for an extended period of time, is the most vital element of fitness. It is a measure of the heart's ability to pump blood efficiently through the body. Developing cardiovascular endurance enhances the ability of the heart, blood vessels, and blood to deliver oxygen to the body's cells and then remove waste products. Although muscles are able to draw on quick sources of energy for short-term exertion, when exercise lasts more than a minute or two, the muscles require oxygen from the blood. Such physical activity is called aerobic exercise. With repeated regular exercise, the heart becomes able to pump blood and deliver oxygen with greater efficiency. The muscles' capacity to use this oxygen also improves. The coupled events are referred to as the "training effect." The heart rate, both at rest and exertion, decreases as a result of this regular exercise, and the heart acquires the ability to recover from the stress of exercise more quickly.

Muscular strength is the total force that muscle groups produce in one effort, such as a lift, jump, or heave. Strength training with free weights, weight machines, or other equipment is the best way to increase muscle strength. Strength gains come most quickly from heavy resistance and few repetitions.

Muscular endurance is the ability to perform repeated muscular contractions over time without tiring. Although muscle endurance requires strength, it is not a single, all-out effort. The keys to increasing endurance are repetition, working at a moderate level, and building up to a specified goal. Women can build both muscle strength and endurance by varying the amount of weight lifted and the number of repetitions per workout.

Flexibility is the ability of the joints to move through their full range of motion. Natural flexibility varies from person to person and from joint to joint. Women tend to be more flexible than men because of differences in their skeletons, muscle mass, and body composition. Good flexibility protects the muscles against pulls and tears because short, tight muscles may be more likely to be overstretched. Stretching the major body areas (legs, shoulders, arms, neck, and back) for 15–30 seconds at a time, at least 3 times a week, is the best way to improve and maintain flexibility.[22] Some women find that stretching certain muscle groups helps relieve or prevent pain. Stretching hamstring and lower back muscles may alleviate lower back pain, and calf stretches may help prevent leg cramps. To lower the chances of injury and receive the most benefit, stretch after, rather than before a workout.

Body composition refers to the ratio of lean body weight (muscle and bone) to fat weight. Exercise affects body composition in two major ways: by reducing excess body weight through energy expenditure and by increasing the body's overall metabolism rate. The body burns extra calories during both the period of physical exercise, and for several hours after exercise ends (known as afterburn). The longer and more intense the exercise, the longer the **basal metabolic rate (BMR)** remains elevated. Regular exercise improves overall muscle tone, contributing to a trimmer appearance.

■ Maintaining a strong back through strength training protects it from injury.

Exercise can also improve balance, coordination (the ability to skillfully use different body parts and the senses together), and agility (the ability to coordinate multiple movements and to react quickly and safely).

Exercise

Physical activity consists of any movement of moderate intensity that lasts a few minutes or more. Many day-to-day activities, such as climbing a flight of stairs, count as physical activity. **Exercise** refers to a deliberate session of physical activity for the purpose of improving health. Exercise tends to fall into two rough categories: aerobic training and strength training. Both types of exercise provide benefits. Aerobic training increases the body's ability to use oxygen, strengthens the heart and blood vessels, and improves the general health of the body. Strength training strengthens specific muscle groups, improves the health of bones, and helps with everyday living. Together, aerobic and strength training provide better benefits than either form of exercise alone. Coupled with a healthy diet, the combination program also may be the most efficient way to lose weight. In addition to burning calories while working out, the resultant muscle mass from strength training boosts the basal metabolic rate because muscle consumes more energy than does fat.

Aerobic Exercise

Aerobic exercise significantly raises the heart rate for a sustained period of time and is the form of physical activity most important for general health. Aerobic exercise seems to lower body cholesterol levels and blood pressure more than strength training. It also improves cardiovascular fitness, the ability of the heart and lungs to supply the muscles with oxygen; strength training generally does not provide such a benefit.

Components of Aerobic Exercise.

Health experts generally measure three important parts of an aerobic workout: intensity, duration, and frequency. Intensity, duration, and frequency all affect the amount of health benefits any exercise program provides; no one of these variables is more important than the others.

Exercise intensity is the work per unit of time. It can be monitored by measuring the target heart rate—the exercise heart rate needed to produce a training effect—for 20 to 30 minutes during each workout. See **Table 9.7** for examples of moderate- and high-intensity activities.

Exercise duration is the length of one exercise session. To benefit the heart, aerobic exercise must be intense enough to increase the heart rate and must continue for a minimum amount of time depending on the intensity of the workout. Aerobic activity provides the most benefit when performed for 30 minutes or more, but sessions as short as 10 minutes can still strengthen the heart and body.[18]

Exercise frequency measures the number of exercise sessions over the long term. Engaging in regular periods of exercise is essential for any exercise program. Exercising in three to five half-hour periods per week builds muscle and improves fitness faster and more safely than exercising for the same length of time in one long weekly workout.

Table 9.7	Examples of Moderate- and High-Intensity Activities

Moderate-Intensity Activities
Walking briskly (3 mph or more)
Ballroom dancing
Playing tennis, doubles
Bicycling 5 to 9 mph, level terrain
Weight-lifting
High-Intensity Activities
Swimming laps
Hiking with a heavy backpack or on hilly terrain
Aerobic dancing
Playing tennis, singles
Jumping rope

Source: Department of Health and Human Services. (2008). *2008 physical activity guidelines for Americans.*

Maximum and Target Range Heart Rates.

No aerobic exercise program will be beneficial unless it forces the heart to pump beyond its normal output. To determine this ideal pace, check whether the heart is beating within the target heart range—fast enough to ensure that the activity pushes the heart muscle to the point of improving fitness, but not so fast that it will become quickly exhausted or cause physical harm. (See **Figure 9.3** to determine maximum and target heart rates.) Checking the pulse during or immediately after exercise is one way to determine the intensity level of a workout (see **Self-Assessment 9.2**). An exercise program should keep the heart rate within

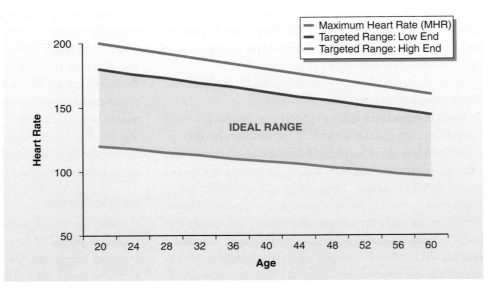

Figure 9.3

Maximum and targeted heart rates.

How to Check Your Pulse

Each "pulse" you feel when you put your fingers on an artery represents the blood pushed by one pump of a person's heart. The easiest way to measure your pulse is to place your fingers on the carotid artery on your neck or the radial artery on your wrist.

1. To find the radial artery, place your first two or three fingers on the thumb side of your inner wrist. To find the carotid artery, place your fingers just below the edge of the jaw bone. Apply gentle pressure. Do not use your thumb.

2. Using a stopwatch or clock with a second hand, count the number of pulses in 30 seconds. Multiply by 2 to get the number of beats per minute.

the target range. If the heart does not reach the lower limit of the target heart range during an exercise activity, increase the intensity by exercising more vigorously. If the heart rate exceeds the upper limit of the target heart range, particularly in the early phases of an exercise program, reduce the intensity to stay within the range.

Aerobic workouts should begin with a 5 to 10-minute warm-up period. Warming up prepares the body for exercise by gradually increasing the heart rate and blood flow, raising the temperature of the muscles, and improving muscle function. It may also decrease the chance of sports-related injury. There are many different ways to warm up, including walking; jogging in place; jumping jacks; or doing a few sets of push-ups, crunches, and squats. Stretching is not a wise way to begin a workout, because stretching cold muscles increases the risk of injury. Sudden exercise without a gradual warm-up can lead to an abnormal heart rate and blood flow and changes in blood pressure, which can be dangerous, especially for older exercisers. A cool-down is as important as a warm-up. A cool-down is a 5–10 minute period of exercising at a slow but steady rate. This less intense activity helps to prevent muscle stiffness and potentially dangerous sudden drops in blood pressure that occur when vigorous activities stop abruptly. Stretching after exercise can reduce the likelihood of injury.

Forms of Aerobic Exercise.

Regular exercise is important. The form it takes is of secondary importance. Some women enjoy sticking with a single form of exercise that works for them. Others keep their interest in exercise by changing their physical activity

on a regular basis. Seasonal variations, changes in schedules, and access to equipment and facilities also influence women's exercise habits.

The 2008 Physical Activity Guidelines for Americans distinguish between moderate and intense forms of aerobic exercise. Both forms raise the heart rate and improve overall health; however, intense aerobic activity provides roughly the same benefits as moderate aerobic activities in about half the time. A woman can reach the recommended guidelines by performing 2 hours and 30 minutes (150 minutes) of moderate aerobic activity a week, 1 hour and 15 minutes (75 minutes) of intense activities, or a combination of the two. Moderate forms of aerobic exercise include brisk walking, bicycling at a slow pace, dancing, water aerobics, gardening, doubles tennis, and using a manual wheelchair. Intense forms of aerobic exercise include aerobic dance or cardio-kickboxing classes, playing soccer or basketball, fast or hilly riding on a bicycle, singles tennis, and swimming laps.[17]

Moderate- to brisk-paced walking is an easy, safe, and enjoyable way to stay healthy. Walking for 30 to 45 minutes a day provides excellent health benefits and burns as many calories as running or jogging the same distance. Walking is also an activity that people of most abilities and body types can participate in. Most problems with walking can be avoided by simply wearing good walking shoes, warming up beforehand, and practicing good walking technique.

Jogging is aerobic exercise somewhere between a fast walk and a run, usually defined as moving at a pace slower than a 9-minute mile, with running defined as a 9-minute mile or faster. Both activities count as intense forms of aerobic exercise. While running and jogging are excellent forms of aerobic exercise, women (and men) should be careful not to put too much stress on their knees, ankles, and other joints. Ways to reduce joint stress while running or jogging include using good running shoes; running on grass, dirt, or asphalt rather than concrete; running or jogging no more than 12–15 miles per week; and alternating between running or jogging, and other forms of aerobic exercise.

Bicycling, whether on a stationary bike or outdoors, can be an excellent cardiovascular conditioner as well as an effective way to control weight. Stationary biking in aerobic settings, often referred to as "spinning," offers a variety of speed resistances to simulate biking a hilly course or race.

Stair climbing, either in buildings or on stair machines, is another excellent form of aerobic exercise. A major advantage of stair climbing, particularly with machines, is that it involves less impact on the joints and feet than other forms

■ Aerobic exercise can take many forms. It is not limited to running or exercise classes.

of aerobic exercise such as running or jogging. Step aerobics is another form of this exercise. Stair climbing and bicycling can each act as moderate or intense forms of aerobic exercise, depending on their pace.

Swimming is an excellent way to strengthen and tone muscles as well as promote aerobic fitness. It does not, however, appear to be as effective for losing weight as other forms of exercise. A major benefit of swimming is that it places no excess stress on the joints, as do many other forms of aerobic exercise.

Aerobic dance is exercise combining music with kicking, stretching, bending, and jumping, to deliver the same benefits as running, cycling, or swimming. Aerobic classes based on kickboxing or other martial arts are another form of exercise. These intense classes combine punches, kicks, and other activities with an aerobic workout to provide excellent benefits in strength, coordination, balance, speed, flexibility, and agility.

Tennis was a big part of my life when I was in high school. Our school's women's tennis team was one of the best in the state, but we were always a second priority to the men's team, which was pretty mediocre. The female players weren't even allowed to wear our letters on our school jackets. My younger daughter plays soccer, and I love seeing her play. It's nice to see the women's teams getting some recognition!

—55-year-old doctor

Strength Training

Strength training is another essential component of a well-balanced exercise program. Like aerobic exercise, strength training helps prevent or delay many of the declines associated with aging or inactivity. The 2008 Physical Activity Guidelines for Americans recommend that adult men and women do strength training two or more times a week. A good strength training workout should involve all the major muscle groups, and should use enough weight that a person can just barely do 8–12 repetitions in a row.

Strength training is not just a tool for bodybuilders and muscle enthusiasts. An equally valid term for strength training could be "body conditioning." Strength training helps to tone the body, build bone strength, and improve overall health in addition to increasing muscle mass. A woman can use free weights, dumbbells, barbells, resistance bands, weight machines, or her own body weight (as in push-ups, chin-ups, and pull-ups) for strength training.

Strength training offers many benefits:

■ Well-toned muscles help maintain good posture. Maintaining a strong back through strength training reduces the risk of injury. Lower back pain often results from weakness of back and abdominal muscles, both of which help support the back.

■ Muscle strength produces benefits in daily living, from lifting items to engaging in physical activity, by increasing stamina and self-confidence.

■ Strength training can help prevent or delay many of the declines associated with aging or inactivity.

■ Strength training increases bone density, thereby helping to delay or minimize osteoporosis and vulnerability to fractures.

■ Injury prevention is another important benefit of strength training, especially for musculoskeletal injuries induced by exercise, such as runner's knee or shin splints. These injuries are due in part to muscle weakness and imbalances as well as joint instability. Such conditions are often corrected with strength training.

Women tend to have less muscle mass than men, especially in the upper body. Gender differences in size, hormones, and normal activity levels contribute to this discrepancy. Women who work out, however, gain strength at the same rate as men. Many women have avoided strength training out of fear of becoming "muscle bound." A moderate program will not create obvious muscle bulk in men or women but will result in a firmer, trimmer physique.

Physical Fitness and Women

Psychological, social, historical, and cultural factors all affect how women think about fitness and exercise. Historically, women were labeled "the weaker sex" and were not encouraged to become as fit as their male counterparts. Prejudices have traditionally limited women's access to and full participation in sports. Self-esteem and self-confidence with physical activity are developmental tasks of childhood. Because young girls were not encouraged to excel or compete in the physical arena, they often lacked the self-esteem and confidence necessary to participate in sports as they grew older. It was not until 1978 that legislation known as **Title IX** mandated that public schools provide equal funding for girls' sports. Even since its passage, opportunities, resources, and, perhaps most importantly, encouragement for physical fitness have not been equally distributed to children, regardless of gender. Groups like the Women's National Basketball Association and a new generation of popular women's sports stars are revising the societal rule that says only male athletes can be admired.

Traditionally, men have excelled in physical competition against women. In general, men are able to run longer and faster, jump higher and farther, lift more and longer, and so forth. Over the past 30 years, however, women have become more competitive in all athletic arenas. Despite these advances, young girls and boys are still often raised with different levels of emphasis, encouragement, and training in physical fitness.

The fact that men are stronger than women reflects the larger absolute quantity of their muscle mass. Individual muscle fibers do not appear to be different, and women's bodies respond to training as quickly as do men's. Women appear to be about half as strong as men in the upper body areas of the shoulders, arms, and backs and two-thirds as strong in the legs and lower body, primarily because men have larger muscle fiber areas and greater lean body weight (total weight minus body fat). Women's naturally higher percentage of body fat, essential for reproduction and general health, may have more of an effect on their physical performance than any other factor. Typically about 25% of a woman's body weight is fat, compared with 15% for men. Women's extra body fat may be a hindrance in sports such as running, but an advantage in sports such as swimming. In general, women also have a lower blood volume, about 5% less hemoglobin, smaller hearts, and less lung capacity than men.

Women's performances in endurance sports have dramatically increased over the past 30 years. Over the same period, the gender gap in biking, swimming, and other sports has been gradually shrinking. Female professional athletes may not reach the same levels of absolute performance as their male counterparts for every sport, but women should not let prejudice or feelings of inferiority prevent them from reaching their own optimal fitness levels. Reaching the level of fitness that best fits a person's individual preference and goals is the responsibility of an adult of either gender.

Exercise Myths and Facts

Fear and misinformation about fitness, workouts, or muscles cause many women to avoid exercise or to exercise inappropriately. Current medical knowledge shows that these fears are usually unfounded and that their resultant behaviors are often harmful.

Myth: Exercise increases the appetite.

Fact: Many factors affect the appetite more than exercise. Depending on the circumstance, exercise may increase, decrease, or have no noticeable effect on the appetite. Women who do eat more when they exercise usually add fewer calories than they burn in their workouts. Exercise raises the basal metabolic rate, which remains elevated not only for the exercise period, but also for an extended time after the physical activity ends. Calories are thus burned at a higher rate for an extended period of time.

Myth: I am too out of shape or old to exercise.

Fact: People of all ages and body types benefit from physical activity. Exercise programs can begin with a few

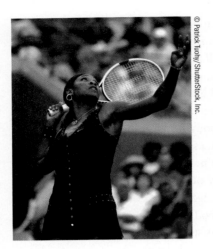

■ Women are increasingly being recognized as proficient athletes, whether in competition with one another or in mixed sports.

■ It is a myth that a woman will develop bulging muscles if she lifts weights.

minutes of activity per day, such as walking or climbing a flight of stairs, and gradually increasing the amount of activity. This will help a person get in better shape and prepare him or her for additional activity. Any amount of physical activity provides some health benefits.

Myth: Exercising special spots will reduce local fat.

Fact: There is no such thing as effective "spot reduction." Fat tissue cannot be converted into muscle. When a woman exercises, she uses energy produced by burning fat in all parts of the body—not just around the muscles that are doing the most work. Sit-ups will not take fat off the abdomen any faster than any other body area. Sit-ups can, however, strengthen the abdominal muscles, which may help hold the abdomen in more.

Myth: No pain, no gain.

Fact: Exercise does not have to hurt to provide benefits. If a person is beginning or intensifying an exercise program, some muscle discomfort is probable. However, this discomfort should not extend beyond the feeling of a slight ache into actual pain. It is best to avoid pain during and after exercise by intensifying workouts slowly and by beginning each session with a warm-up and ending it with a cooldown.

Myth: Lifting weights gives women a bulky, masculine physique.

Fact: Because most women have relatively low levels of the hormone testosterone, it is more difficult than it is for men to build the musculature associated with male bodybuilders. Strength training offers as many benefits to bone strength and general health as it does to major muscle groups.

Myth: The more sweat produced, the more fat lost.

Fact: Exercising in extreme heat or while wearing a plastic suit will, indeed, cause a person to sweat and lose weight, but sweat reflects the loss of water, not fat. Normal consumption of food and water will soon cause the weight to return. An individual who sweats too much during exercise without replenishing essential liquids runs the risk of developing heat exhaustion or dehydration. The amount of sweat produced is not a measure of energy expended. Sweating depends more on temperature, humidity, lack of conditioning, body weight, and individual variability.

Myth: Exercise is not good for weight loss because weight is gained in muscle.

Fact: Aerobic exercises burn more fat than they add muscle. With exercises such as weight-lifting, muscle gain may indeed weigh more than burned-off fat. Usually, however, this tradeoff results in increased trimness because the added muscle is less dense and bulky than the lost fat. One added benefit is that the few extra pounds of muscle do not carry the health risks of excess fat. Another is that the body burns 15 to 20 times the calories to maintain a pound of muscle than it burns to maintain the same amount of fat.

Myth: Women cannot perform well athletically while menstruating.

Fact: Most women can perform physical activities consistently throughout their menstrual cycles. Researchers have found no significant differences in physical capabilities, such as oxygen intake, throughout the menstrual cycle. In fact, exercising during menstruation helps relieve pain and discomfort associated with the menstrual cycle.

Exercise and Aging

Exercise becomes more important with age. Many problems commonly associated with aging, such as increased body fat, decreased lean body weight (muscle mass), decreased muscle strength and flexibility, loss of bone mass, lower metabolism, and slower reaction times, are often signs of inactivity that can be minimized or even prevented by exercise. Reduced muscle strength is a major cause of physical disability in the elderly. Maintaining muscle strength and flexibility are critical components of maintaining the ability to walk and remain independent. For people 65 years and older, falls account for 80% of injuries requiring a hospital visit.[23] In addition to improving physical fitness, exercise reduces the risk of developing type 2 diabetes and osteoporosis, and can reduce symptoms for people with these conditions (see Chapter 11). The combination of strength training and aerobic exercise seems to be the best method for preventing these chronic debilitating conditions. Exercise also promotes a sense of well-being and reduces symptoms of depression, a common problem among aging women.

Exercise Abuse

Pressure to be svelte and physically attractive bombards women from many directions. Being healthy and fit are desirable and noble goals, but occasionally individuals become so zealous in the pursuit of fitness or the desire to be attractive that injury or harm results. Exercise abuse occurs when exercise or fitness supplants family, friends, work, and education in importance; when the body is pushed beyond healthful limits; or when athletic injuries are ignored. A body part or the entire body is considered overused if it is exercised beyond its biological limit to the point of injury. Common overuse injuries affect the

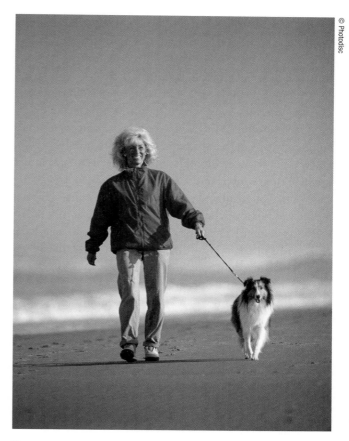

© Photodisc

■ Exercise throughout the life span can reduce or prevent many of the health problems associated with aging.

muscles, tendons, ligaments, joints, and skin. Excessive exercise, faulty technique, and poor equipment are all common causes of overuse injuries. Pushing beyond discomfort into pain is dangerous because the pain of overexertion is the body's message indicating that something is wrong; such a problem should be addressed, not ignored.

Some women may exercise so much that they stop menstruating. This condition, known as athletic amenorrhea, usually is the direct result of excessive exercise and an abnormally low ratio of body fat to body weight. The long-term consequences of prolonged athletic amenorrhea include the early onset of osteoporosis and its resultant risk for injury and debilitation. Athletic amenorrhea often affects adolescent female athletes who train in sports that emphasize slenderness, such as long-distance running, gymnastics, figure skating, and ballet, or women who are endurance athletes, such as distance swimmers and runners.[24] The **female athlete triad** is the relationship among disordered eating, amenorrhea, and osteoporosis. This problem usually begins with disordered eating. The combination of poor nutrition and intense athletic training causes weight loss and a decrease in or shutdown of estrogen production. Consequently, amenorrhea occurs. The final condition in the triad, osteoporosis, may follow if estrogen levels remain low and the woman's diet continues to lack calcium and vitamin D.

Anabolic steroid use is another form of exercise abuse. Anabolic steroids are synthetic derivatives of the male hormone testosterone. Although steroid use is most common among teenage males, women use these drugs as well. Men and women who take steroids with heavy resistance training increase their muscle and lean body mass, but also experience severe physical and psychological side effects. Documented adverse physical effects of steroid use in women include enlargement of the clitoris, growth of facial hair, changes in or cessation of the menstrual cycle, deepened voice, and breast diminution. Other potential side effects include increased risk of heart disease and stroke, increased aggression, liver tumors and jaundice, aching joints, bad breath, and acne.

In adolescents, steroid use can halt growth prematurely. The AIDS epidemic has introduced another liability from steroid use: increased risk of human immunodeficiency virus (HIV) transmission from sharing needles. The psychological effects of long-term, high-dose anabolic steroid use may lead to addiction, drug cravings, and withdrawal symptoms when use of the drugs is stopped.[25] Hepatitis B and C, two diseases that can seriously damage the liver, are also easily spread by needle sharing. Clearly, anabolic steroids should be totally avoided.

Maintaining a Healthy Weight

To maintain a healthful weight, a woman should balance calories she consumes as part of a balanced diet with the calories she burns through daily physical activities. Weight loss should occur at the level of no more than 0.5 to 1 pound per week. For a rough estimate of their ideal weight, adults can evaluate their weight-for-height ratio, or **body mass index (BMI)**. (See **It's Your Health** and **Self-Assessment 9.3**.) A BMI of between 25 and 29.9 indicates overweight and a BMI of 30 or higher indicates obesity in adults. While it is a useful tool, the BMI is only effective for certain body types. A person who has a lot of muscle, a large body frame, and little fat may have a BMI above the healthy range but may still be healthy; similarly, a person who has a lot of fat and little muscle may have a BMI in the healthy range, but may not be at their ideal weight. Another way to define overweight is to measure the proportion of fat in the body, though it is a difficult measurement to perform accurately, even with professional training.

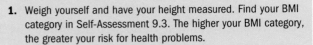

It's Your Health

Evaluate Your Weight (Adults)

1. Weigh yourself and have your height measured. Find your BMI category in Self-Assessment 9.3. The higher your BMI category, the greater your risk for health problems.

2. Measure around your waist while standing, just above your hip bones. If it is greater than 35 inches for women or 40 inches for men, you probably have excess abdominal fat. This excess fat may place you at greater risk of health problems, even if your BMI is about right.

3. The higher your BMI and waist measurement, the more you are likely to benefit from weight loss.

In addition to total weight, weight distribution is an important consideration. Women whose body-fat distribution favors the upper body ("apples") rather than the hips and thighs ("pears") are at higher risk of developing type 2 diabetes, coronary artery disease, hypertension, gallbladder disease, and polycystic ovarian syndrome.[26] Consequently, waist measurement has been used as a loose measure of one's chance of developing heart disease, cancer, or other chronic diseases. A waist larger than 35 inches for a woman and 40 inches for a man is considered to be a risk factor for the aforementioned diseases.

What Causes Weight Gain

Many factors influence weight loss and gain. In most cases, overweight and obesity result from excess calorie consumption and/or inadequate physical activity. A small percentage of people may have a genetic predisposition to gain weight or a genetic need to eat more than they need for energy; a larger percentage may simply have a body that tends to store extra fat, making it harder for them to lose weight (and keep weight off).

When a woman takes in more calories than she burns, she will gain weight. Burning calories through physical activity can offset calories consumed and can help a person maintain or lose weight. Beneath this simple truth, however, lies a more complex reality. Today, most Americans work, study, and relax in environments that require little physical activity and have easy access to widely advertised processed foods that are cheap; high in calories, fats, and sugars; and low in nutrients. Women still have ultimate responsibility for taking care of their health, but these cultural, social, and economic factors make getting adequate physical activity and eating a balanced diet difficult for millions of women.

Self-Assessment 9.3

Are You at a Healthy Weight?

Body Mass Index Table

Height (inches)	Normal						Overweight					Obese										Extreme Obesity															
BMI	19	20	21	22	23	24	25	26	27	28	29	30	31	32	33	34	35	36	37	38	39	40	41	42	43	44	45	46	47	48	49	50	51	52	53	54
															Body Weight (pounds)																					
58	91	96	100	105	110	115	119	124	129	134	138	143	148	153	158	162	167	172	177	181	186	191	196	201	205	210	215	220	224	229	234	239	244	248	253	258
59	94	99	104	109	114	119	124	128	133	138	143	148	153	158	163	168	173	178	183	188	193	198	203	208	212	217	222	227	232	237	242	247	252	257	262	267
60	97	102	107	112	118	123	128	133	138	143	148	153	158	163	168	174	179	184	189	194	199	204	209	215	220	225	230	235	240	245	250	255	261	266	271	276
61	100	106	111	116	122	127	132	137	143	148	153	158	164	169	174	180	185	190	195	201	206	211	217	222	227	232	238	243	248	254	259	264	269	275	280	285
62	104	109	115	120	126	131	136	142	147	153	158	164	169	175	180	186	191	196	202	207	213	218	224	229	235	240	246	251	256	262	267	273	278	284	289	295
63	107	113	118	124	130	135	141	146	152	158	163	169	175	180	186	191	197	203	208	214	220	225	231	237	242	248	254	259	265	270	278	282	287	293	299	304
64	110	116	122	128	134	140	145	151	157	163	169	174	180	186	192	197	204	209	215	221	227	232	238	244	250	256	262	267	273	279	285	291	296	302	308	314
65	114	120	126	132	138	144	150	156	162	168	174	180	186	192	198	204	210	216	222	228	234	240	246	252	258	264	270	276	282	288	294	300	306	312	318	324
66	118	124	130	136	142	148	155	161	167	173	179	186	192	198	204	210	216	223	229	235	241	247	253	260	266	272	278	284	291	297	303	309	315	322	328	334
67	121	127	134	140	146	153	159	166	172	178	185	191	198	204	211	217	223	230	236	242	249	255	261	268	274	280	287	293	299	306	312	319	325	331	338	344
68	125	131	138	144	151	158	164	171	177	184	190	197	203	210	216	223	230	236	243	249	256	262	269	276	282	289	295	302	308	315	322	328	335	341	348	354
69	128	135	142	149	155	162	169	176	182	189	196	203	209	216	223	230	236	243	250	257	263	270	277	284	291	297	304	311	318	324	331	338	345	351	358	365
70	132	139	146	153	160	167	174	181	188	195	202	209	216	222	229	236	243	250	257	264	271	278	285	292	299	306	313	320	327	334	341	348	355	362	369	376
71	136	143	150	157	165	172	179	186	193	200	208	215	222	229	236	243	250	257	265	272	279	286	293	301	308	315	322	329	338	343	351	358	365	372	379	386
72	140	147	154	162	169	177	184	191	199	206	213	221	228	235	242	250	258	265	272	279	287	294	302	309	316	324	331	338	346	353	361	368	375	383	390	397
73	144	151	159	166	174	182	189	197	204	212	219	227	235	242	250	257	265	272	280	288	295	302	310	318	325	333	340	348	355	363	371	378	386	393	401	408
74	148	155	163	171	179	186	194	202	210	218	225	233	241	249	256	264	272	280	287	295	303	311	319	326	334	342	350	358	365	373	381	389	396	404	412	420
75	152	160	168	176	184	192	200	208	216	224	232	240	248	256	264	272	279	287	295	303	311	319	327	335	343	351	359	367	375	383	391	399	407	415	423	431
76	156	164	172	180	189	197	205	213	221	230	238	246	254	263	271	279	287	295	304	312	320	328	336	344	353	361	369	377	385	394	402	410	418	426	435	443

Source: Adapted from Clinical Guidelines on the Identification, Evaluation, and Treatment of Overweight and Obesity in Adults: The Evidence Report.

BMI measures weight in relation to height. The BMI ranges shown above are for adults. They are not exact ranges of healthy and unhealthy weights, but rather show that health risk increases at higher levels of overweight and obesity. Even within the healthy BMI range, weight gains can carry health risks for adults.

Directions: Find your weight on the bottom of the graph. Go straight up from that point until you come to the line that matches your height. Then look to find your weight group.

Healthy Weight: BMI from 18.5 to 24. **Overweight:** BMI from 25 to 29. **Obese:** BMI 30 or higher.

People who are overweight or obese are often assigned responsibility for overindulging or overeating, while people who lose weight or stay at a healthy weight are praised for their discipline. Although this perspective does sometimes have elements of truth, taking a population-based perspective can also yield insights into the problems of obesity, overweight, and difficulty maintaining weight. It is not only discipline and a desire to be fit that influence whether a person chooses to exercise—it is also how much free time a woman has; whether she lives in a neighborhood with safe and satisfying places to walk, run, or play sports; and whether her work schedule allows her to visit a health club while it is open.

Similarly, if a woman lives in an area where healthful foods are unavailable, inconvenient, or considerably more expensive than processed foods high in fats and sugars, she is less likely to eat a well-balanced diet than if she lives in an area where those foods are easily accessible. The processed food industry uses a variety of tactics to sell its products, many of which are unhealthy. Companies use deceptive advertising methods to portray their products as healthy, such as emphasizing that a product is low in sugar even as it is high in fat and salt (or vice-versa).

Another tactic has been to increase portion sizes to market the idea of customers getting a "better deal." These tactics have earned hundreds of millions of dollars for the fast-food and carbonated-beverage industries in particular. Unfortunately, these same tactics have also resulted in millions of people eating extra, unneeded calories without adding nutrients to their diet. **Table 9.8** provides examples of changes in portion size over the past 20 years.

Overweight and Obesity

Although the word "overweight" is often used subjectively or with judgmental overtones, the word also has a medical definition, meaning that a person weighs more than is generally healthy for a certain height. A person is considered to be **overweight** if he or she has BMI of 25 to 29.9. **Obesity** defines people with additional unhealthful weight beyond the overweight range, with a BMI of 30 or greater. Obesity is a complex, multifactorial chronic disease. Overweight and obesity are increasing in both genders and among all population groups. Today, more than one-third of U.S. adults are obese.[25] There are more than twice as many overweight children and three times as many overweight adolescents as there were in 1980.[27] Overweight children and adolescents are more likely to become overweight or obese adults. More than two-thirds of adults in the United States are overweight or obese, and more than 1 out of 20 are extremely obese (see **Figure 9.4**).

Approximately one out of five U.S. children are overweight, and one-third of those who are at a healthy weight are at risk of soon becoming overweight.[28] The prevalence of obesity is higher among African American women and Hispanic women than among White and Asian American women. Obesity and overweight also more common among people with low incomes and low education, in part because these people have less access to healthful foods and opportunities to exercise.[27]

One important factor behind this increase in rates of obesity appears to be the jump in average calorie intake over the past 30 years. Today, the average daily calorie consumption is over 300 calories more than the average

Table 9.8	**Portion Distortion**		
Food Item	Size and Calories		Ways to Burn the Extra
	20 Years Ago	Today	
Bagel	3-inch diameter/ 140 calories	6-inch diameter/ 350 calories	Rake leaves for 50 minutes to burn extra 210 calories
French fries	2.4 ounces/ 210 calories	6.9 ounces/ 610 calories	Walk 2 hours, 20 minutes to burn extra 400 calories
Soda	6.5 ounces/ 85 calories	20 ounces/ 250 calories	Garden for 35 minutes to burn extra 165 calories
Turkey sandwich	320 calories	820 calories	Bike for 1 hour, 25 minutes to burn extra 500 calories

Source: National Heart, Lung and Blood Institute. *Stay young at heart.*

■ Food portions have become noticeably larger in the past 20 years. Single portions now often provide enough food for at least two people.

consumption in 1980. Refined grains, added fats, and added sugars account for most of this increase.[29]

Overweight and obesity are the second-leading preventable causes of death in the United States, just behind tobacco use. Obesity increases the risk for heart disease, stroke, many forms of cancer, hypertension, diabetes, and other conditions. Every year, about 50,500 cases of cancer among women (about 7% of total cancers in women) occur as a direct result of obesity.[30] Cancers of the thyroid, esophagus, colon, endometrium (uterine lining), kidney, pancreas, gallbladder, and other areas are more likely to develop in people who are overweight or obese. Being 30 pounds overweight can increase a woman's risk of endometrial cancer threefold and being 50 pounds overweight can increase

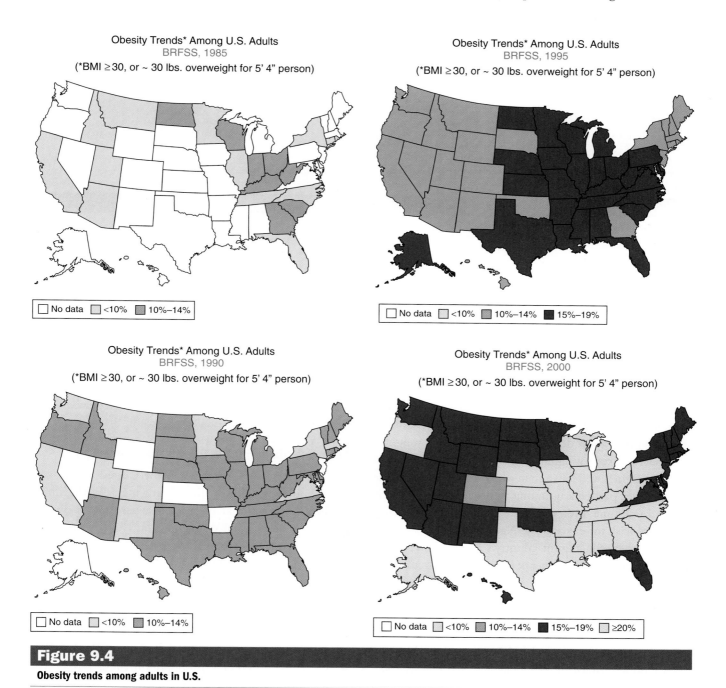

Figure 9.4

Obesity trends among adults in U.S.

Source: Reproduced from the Centers for Disease Control and Prevention. Obesity Trends Among U.S. Adults, BRFSS, 1985, 1990, 1995, 2000, 2005, 2010

(continues)

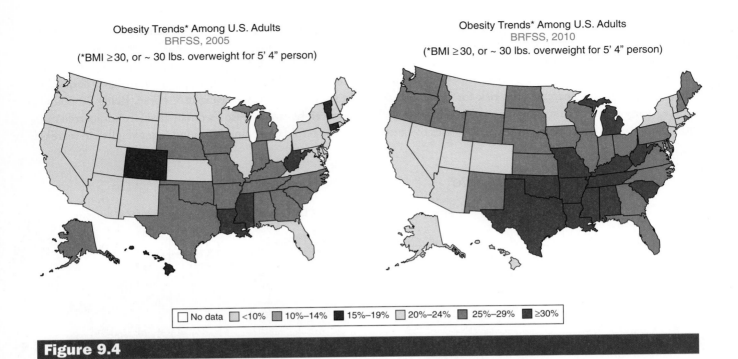

Figure 9.4

Obesity trends among adults in U.S. *(Continued)*

her risk tenfold.[30] People who are obese also are subject to discrimination and social stigmatization, and consequently they may suffer from low self-esteem and depression.

Being overweight or obese can lead to many health problems, including adult-onset diabetes, hypertension, coronary heart disease, gout, gallbladder disease, and arthritic conditions. Women suffer from additional obesity-related problems, including irregular menstrual cycles, amenorrhea, infertility, and polycystic ovarian syndrome. Studies show that the risk of death rises with increasing weight.

Moderate excess weight (10 to 20 pounds for a person of average height), even for women who exercise, increases the risk of death, particularly among adults age 30 to 64 years. At the same time, even moderate weight loss can reduce a woman's risk for cancer: The National Cancer Institute estimates that reducing the country's average BMI by 1% (about 2 lbs of weight loss per person) would prevent about 100,000 cases of cancer.[32]

Obesity was only recognized as a major health issue in the latter half of the 20th century. Discussions of obesity as a potential public health concern began in the 1970s, but it was not until 1985 at the NIH Consensus Development Conference was it acknowledged that obesity leads to increased morbidity and mortality. Concern over the subject has increased as the proportion of people who are obese or overweight has grown.

Although the development of obesity is complex, the benefits of treatment are certain. The ideal goal is to return a person to a healthful weight. However, even a small loss of weight (such as 5–10% of a person's body weight), if maintained, has significant health benefits. Obesity treatments often begin with weight loss, employing reduced-calorie diets along with physical activity, behavior therapy, medications, and weight-loss surgery for people who are severely obese (BMIs equal to or greater than 40).

Economic Dimensions of Obesity and Overweight

The medical costs for obesity in the United States were $148 billion in 2008.[33] This figure includes the direct medical costs to treat diseases associated with obesity such as diabetes, joint problems, and heart disease, and the indirect costs of injuries associated with the condition. In addition, overweight and obesity carry indirect costs from lost productivity, premature disability, and early death. Healthcare costs and the likelihood of complications from surgery for obese and overweight people are higher than those for people of healthful weight. Individuals and families face additional costs, such as specially designed chairs and beds to support an obese frame, specialty clothes, and higher-than-average numbers of medications. Together these items can create a significant cost burden to families.

How Women Can Lose Weight

To lose weight, it is necessary to burn more calories than are ingested. However, this simple claim is more difficult than it sounds. For millions of Americans, opportunities to exercise are limited. Cities and suburbs are often designed with cars, not pedestrians, in mind, making walking unpleasant or dangerous; for people living in some neighborhoods, being outside for an extended period can be a safety risk. The profits of the multibillion-dollar weight-loss, fast-food, and soft-drink industries all depend on continued growth: These industries spend hundreds of millions of dollars to advertise their products. Advertisements and commercials constantly tout ways that their methods or products can help people lose weight, but their claims are often biased, exaggerated, or inaccurate.

Americans spend more than $60 billion every year, most of it unsuccessfully, addressing weight concerns. This money includes health-club memberships, home gym equipment, diet books, and participation in weight-loss programs. About 70 million people—almost one out of four people in the United States—attempt to lose weight every year. Only about 5% of these people are ultimately successful.[34]

These statements are not intended to cause anyone to lose hope. Achieving and maintaining a healthful weight can be done and is a worthwhile goal. For millions of Americans, however, reaching this goal will require acknowledging the obstacles in one's path and making significant lifestyle changes.

The most important way that the body burns calories is through one's resting metabolism, or basal metabolic rate (BMR), the process that maintains body heat and controls automatic activities such as breathing and heartbeat. Nearly 75% of calorie use is devoted to these functions. When a woman attempts to lose weight by drastically cutting calories, her body responds as it would to starvation, by burning fewer calories. Shifting from an intake of about 2,000 calories per day to a 1,200-calorie diet reduces resting metabolism by 5% to 10%, and a more stringent 800-calorie diet lowers it by 10% to 20%. Even after resuming a more normal calorie consumption, other changes keep the metabolic rate low. Much of the weight lost on a low-calorie, low-activity diet can come from lost muscle tissue and water, and the muscles may shrink further as the woman stays at the lower weight because they do not have to work as hard to carry the body around. Less muscle tissue means a lower metabolic rate. The net effect is simple: The more weight that is lost through strict dieting, the more the metabolic

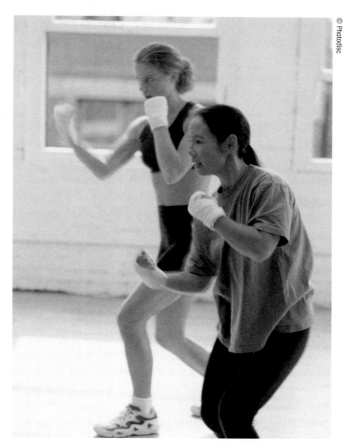

■ Regular exercise is an essential component of any weight-control program.

rate will decline—and the greater the tendency to regain the weight that was lost.

The key to successful weight loss is to combine regular exercise with calorie control while maintaining a healthful diet. The most effective way to safely reduce calories in one's diet is to eliminate (or greatly reduce) intake of "empty calorie" foods. Whether or not a woman is attempting to lose weight a diet should include be based on fruits, vegetables and whole grains. Lean, varied sources of protein should be present, as well as limited (but not eliminated) sources of fat. The main difference in a diet geared toward weight loss should be in portion size. A modest, sustained reduction in total calories consumed is generally more effective than a dramatic, but unsustainable reduction in calories.

Regular exercise should also be a part of any weight-control program. A vigorous 20- to 30-minute workout can easily burn 200 to 300 calories, and even brisk walking can have significant benefits. Equally important, exercise increases the metabolic rate by building muscle and by keeping muscle from shrinking as a result of weight loss. Adding exercise to a diet program helps steady the metabolic rate, making it easier to keep the weight off. After exercise, a person's metabolism remains higher for several hours afterward, so calories are burned at a higher rate, even during inactivity.

Aerobic exercise burns calories faster than weight training, but weight training builds muscle, which an important part of weight loss. A pound of muscle needs 30 to 50 calories per day for maintenance, whereas fat needs only 2 maintenance calories per day. Substituting muscle for fat will therefore result in an increased daily caloric expenditure. Rather than simply promoting weight loss, exercise appears to affect the body in a more complex, integrated way, bringing appetite and energy expenditure into balance. In addition, exercise trims a physical profile even without weight loss. Muscle is denser than fat, so it is possible to appear thinner while the weight holds steady if a larger amount of fat is replaced with a smaller amount of muscle. Bathroom scales do not measure these changes. Regardless of its direct effects on weight and body fat, exercise improves overall health by lowering blood pressure, improving cholesterol levels, strengthening the cardiovascular system, helping prevent type 2 diabetes and other conditions, and reducing stress.

Keeping a food and exercise diary may help some women identify their eating and exercising patterns. Meals, snacks, drinks, and all forms of physical activity should all be recorded in the diary. After a review of a few days of diary notes, a woman can objectively examine her own eating habits and set realistic goals that rely on a diet based on healthy foods and regular exercise. Women can monitor their progress through the food diary and weekly (not daily) checks with the scale. Once the reasonable desired weight loss is achieved, the focus should be on maintenance through sensible eating and exercise.

Ways Not to Lose Weight

Women (and, increasingly, men) spend countless hours worrying, thinking, and obsessing over weight loss. Diet books, programs, and plans make enormous profits by preying on women's insecurities about their weight, and then offering their new product as an easy solution to this "problem." When women do not lose weight, or lose weight but gain it back, they often blame themselves, even if the diets themselves are flawed, ineffective, or unrealistic.

Starvation, hunger, or completely eliminating fats (or another food group) is not the solution to any weight-loss effort. Food substitution, in which a woman consumes twice as many calories from carbohydrates as she does from fat, is far better than food restriction. Foods such as pasta made from whole grains are nutritious, filling, and low in calories when they are not smothered in high-fat products,

It's Your Health

Helpful and Unhelpful Weight-Loss Strategies

Helpful

Allow occasional treats or servings of favorite foods.

Develop realistic, long-term goals that can be maintained.

Reduce but do not eliminate fat from the diet.

Use monounsaturated oils like olive oil more than other sources of fat.

Stick with the program even if there are lapses.

Plan meals and snacks to include more complex carbohydrates, fruits, and vegetables.

Limit intake of fatty foods, oils, and dressings.

Avoid packaged snack foods.

Develop new interests that do not involve food.

Vary sources of protein to include fish and seafood and peas and beans in addition to meat and poultry.

Eat foods slowly.

Exercise regularly.

Drink water rather than carbonated beverages or sports drinks.

Reduce sugar intake—look for levels of simple carbohydrates.

Join a support group or share the process with a friend.

Clean the pantry—give away foods that are not part of the new healthy eating plan.

Try a new low-fat recipe each week.

Eat small meals throughout the day to keep from getting too hungry.

Unhelpful

Setting unrealistically high expectations.

Focusing solely on short-term goals.

Choosing a program that makes eating unpleasant.

Unconventional theories to explain how food combinations add or decrease body weight.

Following a diet that omits any one food group, or focuses on one particular food, such as grapefruit or yogurt.

Daily caloric intake less than 1,200 calories unless under medical supervision.

Any diet that promotes megadoses of vitamins to make up for nutritional deficits.

Fasting or starvation diets.

Any pill or potion that "melts fat."

Appetite-suppressant drugs.

Giving up all sweets or breads.

Using muscle stimulators or body wraps.

such as butter, mayonnaise, and margarine. Alcohol should also be considered contraindicated in a weight-loss effort. Alcohol provides empty calories that contribute to weight gain without providing any nutritional benefit. Furthermore, alcohol affects the BMR because the body burns fat more slowly in the presence of alcohol, thus alcohol promotes the storage of body fat.

Dieting without exercise is the least effective way to lose weight. **Yo-yo dieting** is a term characterizing the repeated, chronic pattern of dieting that describes most dieters' behavior. In addition to being frustrating, yo-yo dieting may be hazardous to health, as it may increase the risk for coronary heart disease, although separating the direct physiological effects of the behavior and the resulting stress that comes with trying and failing to lose weight is difficult.[35] Yo-yo dieting may also weaken the immune system, making dieters more likely to become and stay sick.[36] Yo-yo dieters may store more and more fat in the abdominal area with each failed diet; abdominal fat is more harmful to one's health than fat in other places.

Diet supplements are another unhealthful way to lose weight. Weight-loss supplements often contain stimulants, which in high amounts may lead to an increased heart rate, heart attacks, nervousness, insomnia, headaches, seizures, or death. Many women have begun to use supplements such as Ephedra, which has been linked to adverse health outcomes and even death. Because the products are not subjected to the same testing standards as substances regulated by the FDA, supplements may have a higher rate of contamination or contraindications not stated on warning labels. Other weight-loss products may also be harmful or simply ineffective.

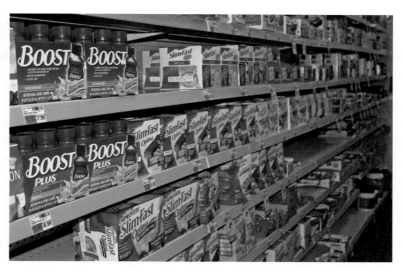

■ Weight-loss products should be used only when prescribed by a healthcare provider; in these seleted patients, the products should be used in combination with lifestyle changes to increase the success of long-term weight loss.

I have tried every diet in the book. I have had times where I have eaten only grapefruit, only rice, or only salads. I have also tried all the gimmicks—pills, liquids, body wraps. You name it, I've tried it. But nothing has really worked. I quickly gain the weight back, sometimes more, within a short time after I lose it. I always swear I won't try another stupid method, but as soon as I read an ad or see a new product, I feel that I have to give it a try.

—22-year-old woman

Other Weight-Loss Strategies

Many popular diets encourage specific eating regimens to attain maximum weight loss. In the 1990s, diets typically focused on high-carbohydrate/very-low-fat daily regimens. Later, the high-protein, high-fat, low-carbohydrate (Atkins) diet reemerged as a popular weight-loss strategy. Many people were not able to lose weight on these diets because they mistakenly believed that they could eat unlimited amounts of certain foods. In reality, excessive calories from any food source cause weight gain. Low-fat foods are often packed with sugar to make up for the loss of flavor when fat is removed. Several high-profile diets, including the Atkins diet and the Zone diet, identify high-protein/low-carbohydrate meals as being optimal. These diets have become financial empires, with books, snacks, prepared meals, and energy drinks all being sold to the millions of people who are subscribing to them. A Consumer Reports analysis found that people in Atkins and the Zone weight-loss programs were at least as likely as people in other top-rated weight-loss programs to lose weight in the short term but were more likely to drop out in less than a year. They were also more likely to eat too much saturated fat and not enough fruits and vegetables.[36]

Weight-loss surgery has gained attention as a tool for people who are severely overweight or obese. Gastrointestinal surgery for obesity, also called **bariatric surgery**, alters the digestive process. The operation promotes weight loss by closing off parts of the stomach to make it smaller. Operations that only reduce stomach size are known as "restrictive operations" because they restrict the amount of food the stomach can hold. Other operations, known as malabsorptive operations, combine stomach restriction with a partial bypass of the small intestine. These procedures create a direct connection from the stomach to the lower segment of the small intestine, bypassing portions of the digestive tract that absorb calories and nutrients. These operations often make eating and swallowing food extremely painful. These procedures are typically appropriate only for severely obese individuals who have not been able to control their weight with diet, exercise, and appropriate pharmaceutical interventions.

Body Image and Shape

Body image is a result of a complex interrelationship among self-perception, family attitudes toward bodies and food, social norms, and individual experiences. Standards for beauty and desirability are not absolute; they vary over time and from culture to culture. The ideal promoted by Madison Avenue and Hollywood often includes women who are either severely underweight or women whose images have retouched and digitally reshaped with computer design software. In Greek and Roman representations of Aphrodite and Venus as, well as in paintings by Titian, Rubens, and Rembrandt, "ideal" women often had ample thighs, hips, waists, and abdomens. The Venus de Milo, one of the most beautiful of the classical female torsos, is muscular and rounded. Contemporary society is weight conscious, fashion conscious, exercise conscious, diet conscious, and not very tolerant of perceived physical imperfection.

Modern Western society trains women to believe that their physical attractiveness determines their social value.

■ Women have been socialized to believe that an ultra-thin body shape is desirable.

Advertisements, magazines, television shows, and movies have further distorted this message by airbrushing images to produce flawless complexions, whitening and brightening of teeth and eyes, digital enhancement to increase breast size and decrease fat, and celebration of models and movie stars who are not representative of the average woman. These images, which appear on commercials, Internet advertisements, magazines, movies, and other locations, have serious unconscious psychological effects. A study examining physical measurements of Miss America contestants, models, and Playboy Playmates over the course of the 20th century found that women in all three groups were likely to be underweight and were often thin enough to meet the World Health Organization's [WHO's] definition of anorexic. The weight and BMI of all three groups of women have also fallen even as the weight of the average American woman has increased over the past 50 years.[37]

The gulf between what women see in the media and what they see in the mirror results in excessive dieting, eating disorders, a perceived need for plastic or cosmetic surgery, and feelings of self-loathing and inadequacy in many women, as seen in the following statistics:

- A national poll found that 24% of the people who said they would try any diet to lose weight were obese women, whereas only 9% were obese men. Obese women were also much more likely than men to feel guilty about eating.[38]

- Females account for 90% of the estimated 8 million sufferers of eating disorders.[39]

- Nearly 10 million cosmetic surgical and nonsurgical procedures were performed in the United States in 2011, according to the American Society for Aesthetic Plastic Surgery (ASAPS). This represents an increase of more than 400% compared to the number of procedures performed in 1997. Although the number of surgical procedures, such as liposuction, breast augmentation, and eyelid surgery, also grew, the biggest increase has been in procedures that do not require actual surgery, such as Botox injections and laser hair removals.[40]

In the early 1990s, studies found that compared with women in other countries, girls and women in the United States dieted more and were less satisfied and more self-conscious about their bodies.[41] However, later international studies of body language showed increased discontent with bodies, appearance, and weight by women across Western nations, suggesting a more global problem.[42] This phenomenon begins early, with inappropriate eating habits and high anxiety about being overweight prevalent among adolescent girls. A large U.S. school-based study found that more than one-third of adolescent girls believed they were overweight, and more than 60% of female adolescents were trying to lose weight.[3] High school girls use starvation, fad diets, and purging methods, which can result in disordered eating behaviors, to lose weight. This finding is especially disturbing given the importance of high calcium intake for building healthy bones and developing critical bone mass, as well as the need for dietary fat to ensure healthy breast development in adolescents. Another concern is that a girl's preoccupation with body image and discontent with body shape during adolescence may persist for life.

Excessive dieting and bodily preoccupation increase the likelihood that a person will have or will develop an eating disorder. New research findings and growing numbers of activists are seeking to influence the women and girls who are alienated from their bodies and obsessed with dieting (**Table 9.9**).

| **Table 9.9** | Comparison of the Average Woman with Unrealistic Models |

	Average Woman	Barbie	Store Mannequin
Height	5' 4"	6' 0"	6' 0"
Weight	145 lb	101 lb	Not available
Dress size	11–14	4	6
Bust	36–37"	39"	34"
Waist	29–31"	19"	23"
Hips	40–42"	33"	34"

Sources: Health magazine, September 1997; NEDIC, a Canadian eating disorders advocacy group; Anorexia Nervosa and Related Eating Disorders, Inc., 2003.

I guess when I look in the mirror I see only the things that I feel are wrong. I wish I was thinner and taller, with a flatter stomach and a bigger chest. When I think about it, I realize that there are many things I actually like about myself but I can't seem to focus on them. When I look at other women, I notice their attributes. I wonder why I can't do that with myself.

—26-year-old woman

It's taken me most of my life, but I've finally gotten comfortable with my body. I'm not skinny. But you know what? I'm not overweight or out of shape, either. I exercise, I eat a good diet, and I don't smoke. And guess what? I can stay out dancing at a club hours after most of the skinny girls are wiped out.

—24-year-old librarian

Sociocultural Perspectives on Body Image

Women who grew up in largely African American communities often have a very different perspective on body ideals than women who grow up in White-dominated communities. Similarly, girls who grow up in families where their mothers had their own disordered eating habits or poor body images are more likely to internalize those signals and adopt similar attitudes. Religion also can influence a girl's or woman's concept of her body, through doctrines of self-restraint, hard work, negative viewpoints on sloth, or in other ways. Even when these attitudes are not specifically directed toward body size, these messages can translate into feelings of blame for girls and women who struggle to control their weight. Cultural norms significantly influence weight management. A woman who wishes to change

her eating habits may have to rebel against the traditions of her family or community.

Millions of women suffer from eating disorders, illnesses that develop around harmful, unusual eating habits. Eating disorders are most common among young, educated

Photographed by Kimberly Potvin.

■ Women's perceptions about their bodies often are inaccurate.

White and Hispanic females from middle to upper social classes, with new cases peaking at age 18. Eating disorders can have roots in social, emotional, and even biological factors in women's lives; pressure to "fit in" with popular cliques or peers; a desire to avoid consumption as a way of dealing with strong emotions or maintaining control over one's life; and even feelings of euphoria that can occur when a person skips meals can all encourage a woman (or man) to adopt or continue an eating disorder. At the same time, these behaviors undermine one's health, self-esteem, and sense of competency. (For more on eating disorders, see Chapter 12.)

Hunger

Hunger is the painful or uneasy feeling and biological harm caused by the continuous, unwanted lack of food. Hunger continues to be the world's greatest health risk, affecting one in seven people around the world.[43] Chronic hunger results when a person's daily calorie intake is not enough for the individual to lead an active, healthy life. **Malnutrition** refers to an imbalance between the body's nutritional needs and the intake or digestion of nutrients. Malnutrition may result in disease or death, and can be caused by an unbalanced diet or from problems in digesting or absorbing food.

Millions of people die each year from chronic hunger and malnutrition; millions more are permanently or seriously sickened or injured. Although most people think of malnutrition as **undernutrition**, this term also includes **overnutrition**, which results from overeating, insufficient exercise, or excessive intake of vitamins and minerals. Overnutrition can lead to overweight and obesity, epidemics that are growing around the world.

Almost 1 billion people around the world regularly do not get enough food to eat.[43] Most of these people live in the developing world. For people living in hunger, finding and preparing food typically takes more time, resources,

Gender Dimensions: Health Differences Between Men and Women

Extreme Dieting

Many women who try restrictive or long-term diets experience troublesome changes in the way they think, feel, and act. These women may feel cold, listless, and tired; have recurring, obsessive thoughts about food; grow anxious or afraid; and feel a reduced sex drive. Society has often designated these feelings as somehow feminine in nature. But the results of a landmark study conducted more than 50 years ago found that these symptoms are not unique to either gender, but instead reflect the body's reaction to starvation. This same study also found that diets that severely restrict calorie intake are ultimately unproductive in producing lasting weight loss.

In 1944, researcher Ancel Keys enrolled 36 male volunteers in what would be known as the Minnesota starvation experiment. This experiment was designed to examine the effects of a "semi-starvation diet" that many Europeans had been forced to adopt during World War II, with the goal of learning how to best help such people. The study results of the experiment, first published in 1950, are still cited by scientists studying the thought and behavioral patterns of people with eating disorders.

All of the participating men were young, healthy, tested to be emotionally stable, and of normal weight. The requirements of the semi-starvation diet were actually less restrictive than the diets many women put themselves through today. Participants received a low-fat, low-protein diet of 1,800 calories a day over a 6-month period, with the goal of losing about 25% of their body weight. The men also were required to walk about 3 miles a day.

Physical symptoms appeared soon after the men started the diet and increased as time progressed. They became gaunt, lost hair, and broke out in rashes. The men reported feeling dizzy, tired, slow, clumsy, and cold. Participants slept under layers of blankets during the warm summer weather, and their sex drive plummeted.

But the researchers were even more surprised by the psychological changes that occurred. The men became withdrawn and irritable. Several men who were taking classes at the university had to withdraw because they couldn't concentrate. The men also became increasingly obsessed with food: They developed rituals, such as chewing food slowly, watering down meals, or drinking cup after cup of tea, that today are associated with eating disorders.

Even after the 6-month period of food restriction was over, the men's metabolism continued to be affected by the diet restrictions. Symptoms continued for weeks after the restrictions were lifted. Many men did not feel full, no matter how much they ate; several men gorged themselves in attempts to do so. Most of the weight they gained back returned as fat, not muscle. Although the men eventually made full recoveries, the process was painful, difficult, and slow. The study found that vitamins and minerals weren't enough—participants also needed to consume a diet containing 4,000 calories a day for weeks to fully recover.

Interviewed more than 50 years later, the surviving study participants said they would do the experiment again because of the beneficial research it produced. Nevertheless, they all cited the study as the most difficult part of their lives.

Now that the risks of severely limiting calorie intake are known, the Minnesota starvation experiment would never be allowed today. The participants of the study enrolled because they believed their results could help victims of war. Women (or men) who are considering a similar diet plan today may want to ask themselves if their sacrifice is worth the effort.

Source: Kalm, L., & Semba, R. (2005). They starved so that others might be better fed: Remembering Ancel Keys and the Minnesota experiment. *Journal of Nutrition 135*: 1347-1352.

and effort than for people who do not live in hunger. Many factors contribute to hunger: artificially low food prices that make it hard for local farmers to compete with large farms in the developed world, global warming, increased demands for energy, and the recent global financial crisis.[44]

Poverty is also a major contributing factor to hunger. Today, one out of five people in the world lives on less than $1 a day; twice that population lives on less than $2 a day. One out of every five people around the world has no regular access to clean water, and two out of every five people lack access to sanitation.[45] Providing these simple services could save millions of lives per year and prevent much pain and suffering.

Populations at risk of malnutrition include infants and children, women who are pregnant or breastfeeding, the elderly, vegetarians, fad dieters, alcoholics or substance abusers, and people with certain chronic diseases. Malnourishment magnifies the effects of every disease, causing malnourished children to be ill nearly 160 days each year, almost half of their daily lives. The most destructive form of malnutrition, which mainly affects infants and young children, is **protein-energy malnutrition (PEM)**. Children have high energy and protein needs, and therefore they suffer most when protein is lacking in their diets. Protein-energy malnutrition affects more than one-fourth of the world's children. More than 70% of PEM-afflicted children live in Asia, 26% in Africa, and 4% in Latin America and the Caribbean.[46]

Other nutrients that are extremely important for health include the following:

- *Vitamin A.* Vitamin A deficiency (VAD) is the leading cause of preventable blindness, reduces the body's resistance to disease and infection, and can cause growth retardation in children. An estimated 250,000 to 500,000 children lose their sight every year due to VAD, and half of these children die within 12 months after becoming blind. This deficiency also poses a risk to pregnant women and their fetuses, causing night blindness, increased risk of maternal mortality, premature birth, low birthweight, and infection. Breastfeeding is the best way to protect babies from VAD, because breast milk is a natural source of vitamin A.

- *Iron.* Iron deficiency is the principal cause of anemia, which affects more than 30% of the world's population. Iron deficiency and anemia impose a heavy economic burden on society, because affected individuals are less able to work and be productive members of a community. In many developing countries, malaria and worm infections consume iron from the body, making problems caused by iron deficiency even worse. Health consequences for pregnant women and their fetuses include premature birth, low birthweight, and increased risk of maternal death. Twenty percent of all maternal deaths have been attributed to anemia.

- *Iodine.* Iodine deficiency is primarily known for causing goiters (enlarged thyroid glands), a condition that can be dramatically disfiguring. Iodine deficiency disorders (IDDs) threaten the mental health of children, representing the world's most prevalent cause of brain damage. Iodine deficiency during pregnancy may result in stillbirth, miscarriage, congenital abnormalities, and mental impairment in the baby. More than 13% of the world's population (740 million people) is affected by this problem. Salt iodization has improved iodine status in many countries.

Hunger is also a serious concern in the United States. Along with poverty, hunger increased in the United States as a result of the global financial crisis. In 2010, 49 million people in the United States, or almost one in seven Americans, did not have consistent access to a varied diet throughout the year, compared to 36 million in 2006. Considerable variety existed within these households. About one-third of households (about 5 million households) had very low food security; people in these homes not only went hungry from time to time, but had to make serious changes to their eating habits at some point during the year. People in other households faced some shortages but were often able to cope by reducing the variety in their diets, obtaining food from emergency kitchens, or participating in federal food programs.[47] People at greatest risk of food insecurity live in households with the following characteristics:

- Having children and headed by a single woman
- Hispanic or Black
- Located in the South
- Located in large cities or rural areas[47]

Informed Decision Making

Nutrition

Healthful eating is essential to health promotion and disease prevention. To develop sensible eating habits, women should eat balanced meals containing carbohydrates, fats, and proteins, as well as the essential vitamins and minerals. A healthful diet should focus on fruits and vegetables, whole grains, and varied sources of protein while limiting processed foods and other sources of empty calories. The USDA's dietary guidelines and the nutrition facts labels on foods can help women choose foods based on their nutrient content. Women should also be aware of the dangers of nutrient deficiencies as well as nutritional excesses.

Maintaining a Personal Exercise Program

Exercise provides enormous benefits to health and disease prevention. Exercise should be not just a means to an end, such as "losing another 5 pounds," but a permanent part of a person's life. The most health benefits come from at least 150 minutes (2.5 hours) of exercise per week of moderate-intensity physical activity. High-intensity physical activity (activity that, when you are performing it, works you hard enough that conversation is difficult) can be included in this total, with every 1 minute of high-intensity activity counting for 2 minutes of moderate-intensity activity. The ideal exercise program should include both aerobic and strength training activity. Additional exercise beyond 150 minutes per week provides additional benefits, and any amount of exercise is better than none at all.

Common perceived barriers to exercise for women include lack of time to exercise, lack of encouragement from family and friends, not wanting to exercise alone, the desire to avoid exertion or soreness, and a fear of looking silly.[48] Staying committed to exercise can also be a challenge: About 50% of people who start structured exercise programs drop out in 6 to 12 months. Habits that can make sticking with an exercise program easier include:

- Keeping an exercise log
- Recording total calories burned in a workout, distance traveled, or improvements in performance
- Exercising with a friend or in a class
- Choosing activities that are personally enjoyable
- Switching to new programs or rotating between programs to maintain interest
- Giving oneself periodic rewards for continuing to exercise

Imagining exercise as a normal part of one's routine maintenance (like brushing one's teeth) can also help a woman stay on a program: A woman who misses an exercise session or who forgets to brush her teeth before going to bed one night should not give up on either activity, but should continue both habits the next day as if nothing unusual had happened.

Body Image and Weight Management

A woman who decides to lose weight should begin by examining her diet and activity level, as well as her motives for doing so. Some women want to lose weight to improve their health; others to improve their physical appearance. Many women feel a combination of both desires. However, women who feel an especially powerful desire to lose weight may want to reflect on their own body image. Society places enormous pressure on women to be thin and to conform to artificial body types that may be unhealthy or impossible to achieve. Developing a healthy body image, with the help of a medical professional if necessary, may benefit some women more than an Olympian-level fitness program.

Extra weight neither accumulates nor disappears overnight. Weight-loss programs that focus on slow but steady weight loss are healthier and more likely to keep weight off than programs that focus on dramatic short-term results. An average weekly loss of 1 pound is a realistic, safe goal for weight loss. Joining a group or making a serious arrangement for support with a friend can help sustain a long-term commitment.

A woman who adopts a healthful diet or starts an exercise program should not stop either activity once she reaches her initial weight-loss goal. A balanced diet and exercise continue to provide benefits only for as long as they are practiced. Reverting to unhealthy habits not only harms the body, but also is likely to result in the return of lost weight.

■■■■

Summary

The human body needs six nutrients to function and stay healthy:

- Carbohydrates, which can be simple (sugars) or complex (starches), provide fuel for the body.
- Proteins supply amino acids, which construct, repair, and maintain body tissues.
- Fats store energy and perform many other functions. Many Americans consume too much fat; however, no diet should eliminate this vital nutrient.
- Vitamins, which the body uses for nearly all aspects of function, are needed in small but regular amounts.
- Minerals are inorganic substances that help with bone formation, enzyme synthesis, maintaining blood

Profiles of Remarkable Women

Michelle Obama (1964–)

Michelle Obama is a lawyer, community activist, a mother of two, and the husband of the 44th U.S. President, Barack Obama. Since becoming the First Lady of the United States in 2008, she has been a strong advocate for a balanced diet and physical fitness. In 2010, she launched a national initiative, *Let's Move!*, to reduce and prevent childhood obesity and improve the health of American children. *Let's Move* takes a multipronged approach by working to improve access to healthful, affordable foods; increase children's physical activity; provide healthful foods in school;, and educate and empower parents and guardians.

Mrs. Obama was born and raised in Chicago as the second of two children of Marian and Fraser Robinson. She was an excellent student and went on to study sociology in Princeton, and then law at Harvard Law School. She joined Sidley Austin, a Chicago law firm and met her future husband when she was assigned to be his mentor. Mrs. Obama left Sidley Austin in 1991 to work for the government of Chicago and to direct a Chicago nonprofit that encouraged young people to become socially active and participate in public service. Mr. and Mrs. Obama were married in 1992.

From 1996 to 2002, Mrs. Obama worked for the University of Chicago, where she helped build the University's Community Service Center. She later worked for the University of Chicago hospitals and the University of Chicago Medical Center. Mrs. Obama continued to work part-time while she raised their two daughters, Sasha and Malia, and to help with her husband's Senate, and later, Presidential campaigns.

In addition to working to improve children's physical fitness, Mrs. Obama works to help support military families, promote national service, help women balance career goals and family aspirations, and encourage education in the arts.

© spirit of america/ShutterStock, Inc.

pressure, and digestive function. Calcium and iron are especially important minerals for young women.

- The body needs water for all its actions. Women should consume 8 to 9 cups of water per day.

Women in the United States spend most of their waking hours in sedentary activity. By incorporating physical activity into their daily routine, women can become more fit, improve their quality of life, and reduce their risk of chronic disease and premature death. These dramatic benefits to activity can also be pleasurable.

Around the world and in the United States, both obesity and overweight, and hunger are serious public health concerns. Obesity and overweight cause a variety of health problems and raise the risk of developing cancer, heart disease, and other conditions. Hunger affects about one in seven people in the United States and around the world, causing a variety of health problems.

Topics for Discussion

1. How well do your eating habits compare to those outlined in the *2010 Dietary Guidelines for Americans*? What patterns are healthful, and what patterns could use improvement?

2. How does the modern American lifestyle make getting regular physical activity and a balanced diet difficult? What are some ways to overcome these challenges?

3. Women who are physically active are healthier and therefore at lower risk of chronic disease and early mortality than those who are inactive. Should they have to pay the same insurance rates as those women whose lifestyles place them at greater risk for illness? If so, how should insurance policies be implemented to be fair and accurate?

4. Some believe that the physical fitness craze has been detrimental to the women's movement because it has added another layer of pressure to conform to an "ideal" body shape or size. How valid is this argument? How can efforts to improve physical fitness avoid alienating and discouraging women?

5. What can be done to improve women's attitudes toward exercise and physical fitness?

6. In an effort to curb obesity, the government of New York City recently proposed banning the sale of sodas and soft drinks of more than 16 ounces at restaurants and stadiums. Is this concern about public health, personal freedom, or both? Is the ability to purchase soft drinks of a certain serving side comparable to freedom of speech?

7. What are the biggest challenges to regular exercise and a healthy diet that you face? How are these challenges going to change over the next five years? How do they differ from the challenges your female friends have in these areas?

■■■■

Key Terms

Anabolic steroids: Synthetic derivatives of the male hormone testosterone usually taken to increase muscle mass. Their use often results in serious physiological and psychological side effects.

Antioxidants: Substances that prevent cells called "free radicals" from harming the body's tissues. Antioxidants are present in many fruits and vegetables. They work to neutralize free radicals and protect genes from damage, possibly decreasing the risk of cancer and heart disease and delaying the effects of aging.

Bariatric surgery: Gastrointestinal surgery for obesity that alters the digestive process. The operation promotes weight loss by closing off parts of the stomach to make it smaller.

Basal metabolic rate (BMR): The amount of energy needed to maintain essential body functions under resting conditions, usually expressed in terms of calories per hour per kilogram of body weight.

Body composition: Proportions of fat, muscle, and bone making up the body. Body composition is usually expressed as percentage of body fat and percentage of lean muscle mass.

Body mass index (BMI): Weight (in kilograms) divided by height squared (in meters). A value or 25 or greater indicates obesity-related health risks.

Calcium: A mineral found mainly in the bones and the teeth. Calcium is important for bone health throughout life. Sources include dairy products, canned fish, seeds and nuts, some green vegetables such as broccoli and kale, and calcium-fortified foods.

Carbohydrate: An organic compound such as starch, sugar, or glycogen, composed of carbon, hydrogen, and oxygen. Carbohydrates are a source of bodily energy.

Cardiovascular endurance: The ability of the body to perform aerobic activities for extended periods of time.

Cholesterol: One of the steroids or fat-like chemical substances manufactured by the body and also consumed in foods of animal origin. It is essential for the manufacture and maintenance of cells, sex hormones, and nerves throughout the body.

Complex carbohydrates: One of the main sources of fuel for the muscles. Complex carbohydrates are found in breads, cereals, pasta, rice, and vegetables such as potatoes and corn.

Exercise: Routine or structured physical activity that a person performs with the goal of improving his or her health.

Fat: A lipid with one, two, or three fatty acids, which is responsible for multiple body functions.

Fat-soluble vitamins: Vitamins absorbed with the aid of fats in the diet or bile from the liver through the intestinal membrane and stored in the body.

Female athlete triad: The interrelationship among disordered eating, amenorrhea, and osteoporosis. Beginning with disordered eating, the combination of poor nutrition and intense athletic training causes weight loss and a decrease in or shutdown of estrogen production. Consequently, amenorrhea occurs. The final condition in the triad, osteoporosis, may follow if estrogen levels remain low and the woman's diet continues to lack calcium and vitamin D.

Fiber: Plant parts that cannot be digested in the human digestive tract. High-fiber diets protect against certain cancers and heart disease.

Flexibility: The range of motion permitted by joints.

Folate: A B vitamin found in foods such as chickpeas, spinach, strawberries, kidney beans, and citrus fruits and juices.

Glycemic index: A measure of how fast glucose enters the bloodstream after a carbohydrate is eaten and thus how quickly the carbohydrate increases a person's blood sugar.

Hemoglobin: The iron-containing protein in the red blood cell that carries oxygen from the lungs to the cells and carbon dioxide away from the cells to the lungs. It also is responsible for the red color of blood.

High-density lipoproteins (HDL): A type of lipoprotein in the blood that carries cholesterol and fats out of the body. It is often referred to as the "good" cholesterol.

Hunger: The painful or uneasy feeling caused by the continuous and involuntary lack of food.

Iron: A mineral that is needed to make hemoglobin (a compound in the blood).

Low-density lipoprotein (LDL): A type of lipoprotein that contains cholesterol and triglycerides and is considered harmful because it promotes fatty deposits on the inner lining of arteries. Also called "bad" cholesterol.

Malnutrition: An imbalance between the body's nutritional needs and the intake or digestion of nutrients, which may result in disease or death. Malnutrition can be caused by an unbalanced diet, digestive problems, or absorption problems.

Mineral: A naturally occurring inorganic substance. These nutrients are essential in small amounts for regulating body functions.

Monounsaturated fat: A type of fat that comes from both plant and animal sources and is liquid at room temperature and solid or semi-solid when refrigerated. Monounsaturated fats help to lower blood cholesterol.

Muscular endurance: The ability to withstand the stress of physical exertion.

Muscular strength: Physical power, such as the amount of weight one can lift, push, or press in a single effort.

Nutrient: A substance essential to life that the body cannot produce on its own. Nutrients are provided by food and assist in the growth and development of the body.

Nutrition: The science of studying the need for and the effects of food on an organism.

Obesity: The excessive accumulation of fat in the body; a condition of being 20% or more above ideal weight.

Overnutrition: A form of malnutrition caused by overeating, insufficient exercise, and excessive intake of vitamins and minerals. Overnutrition can lead to overweight and obesity.

Overweight: Having a body mass index (BMI) of 25 to 29.9.

Phytochemicals: Plant chemicals found in fruits and vegetables that protect the body from cancer by blocking the carcinogenic activities of certain substances in the human body.

Polyunsaturated fat: A type of fat that is liquid at room temperature and when refrigerated. Such fats help lower both LDL and HDL cholesterol.

Protein: A substance that is basically a compound of amino acids; one of the essential nutrients.

Protein-energy malnutrition (PEM): A deficiency syndrome caused by the inadequate intake of protein and/or energy. PEM, the most destructive form of malnutrition, main affects infants and young children.

Recommended Daily Allowance (RDA): Daily nutrient allowance recommended for healthy adults by the National Research Council.

Saturated fats: Fats that come primarily from animal sources.

Simple carbohydrates: A sugar. It provides the boy with glucose and a quick spurt of energy.

Sodium: A macromineral and major component of salt. Most Americans get too much sodium in their diets.

Title IX: The portion of the Education Amendments of 1972 that prohibits gender discrimination in educational institutions that receive any federal funds. If educational institutions are found to violate Title IX, their federal funding can be withdrawn.

Trans fats: Fats that are formed when vegetable oils are processed into margarine or shortening. Trans fats are found in snack foods such as potato chips, commercial baked good with "partially hydrogenated vegetable oil" or "vegetable shortening," many types of fast food (e.g., French fries and onion rings), stick margarine, and some dairy products. These fats are solid or semi-solid at room temperature and raise levels of LDL cholesterol.

Undernutrition: Poor health resulting from the depletion of nutrients due to inadequate nutrient intake over time.

Unsaturated fats: Fats that come from plants and include most vegetable oils.

Vitamin: An organic substance needed by the body in a very small amount. The various vitamins have many different functions in metabolism and nutrition.

Water-soluble vitamins: Vitamins used up or excreted in urine and sweat; must be replaced daily.

Yo-yo dieting: The practice of losing weight and then regaining it, only to lose it and regain it again. This practice makes it more difficult to succeed in future attempts to lose weight because thyroid hormone levels may drop very low in subsequent dieting, thereby significantly slowly basal metabolism.

■■■■
Websites

American Council on Exercise: http://www.acefitness.org

American Dietetic Association: http://www.eatright.org

American Society of Bariatric Physicians: http://www.asbp.org

Center for Nutrition Policy and Promotion: http://www.usda.gov/cnpp

Dietary Guidelines for Americans: http://www.health.gov/dietaryguidelines

International Food Information Council Foundation: http://www.ific.org

National Eating Disorders Association: http://www.nationaleatingdisorders.org

National Institute of Mental Health Center on Eating Disorders: http://www.nimh.nih.gov/publicat/eatingdisorders.cfm

Nutrition.gov: http://www.nutrition.gov

The Obesity Society: http://www.obesity.org

The President's Council on Physical Fitness and Sports: http://www.fitness.gov

USDA: Center for Food Safety and Applied Nutrition: http://www.cfsan.fda.gov

■■■■
References

1. Mokdad, A. H., Marks, J. S., Stroup, D. F., et al. (2004). Actual causes of death in the United States, 2000. *Journal of the American Medical Association 291*: 1238–1245.

2. U.S. Department of Health and Human Services & U.S. Department of Agriculture. (2010). Dietary guidelines for Americans. Available at: www.dietaryguidelines.gov

3. Eaton, D., Kann, L., Kinchen, S., et al. (2011). *Youth Risk Behavior Surveillance—United States, 2009*. Atlanta, GA: Centers for Disease Control and Prevention.

4. Lowry, R., Galuska, D. A., Fulton, J. E., et al. (2002). Weight management goals and practices among U.S. high school students: associations with physical activity, diet, and smoking. *Journal of Adolescent Health 31*(2): 133–144.

5. Pollan, M. (2009). *Food rules: An eater's manual*. New York, NY: Penguin Books.

6. Rufail, M. L., Schenkein, H. A., Barbour, S. E., et al. (2005). Altered lipoprotein subclass distribution and PAF-AH activity in subjects with generalized aggressive periodontitis. *Journal of Lipid Research 46*: 2752–2760.

7. James, S. L., Muir, J. G., Curtis, S. L., et al. (2003). Dietary fibre: A roughage guide. *Internal Medicine Journal 33*(7): 291–296.

8. Willet, W. C. (2005). *Eat, drink and be healthy: The Harvard Medical School guide to healthy eating*. New York, NY: Simon and Schuster.

9. Centers for Disease Control and Prevention [CDC]. (2010). *Trans fat: The facts*. Available at: http://www.cdc.gov/nutrition/everyone/basics/fat/transfat.html

10. Mensink, R. P., Zock, P. L., Kester, A. D., et al. (2003). Effects of dietary fatty acids and carbohydrates on the ratio of serum total to HDL cholesterol and on serum lipids and apolipoproteins: A meta-analysis of 60 controlled trials. *American Journal of Clinical Nutrition 77*(5): 1146–1155.

11. Caro, J., Huybrechts, K. F., Klittich, W. S., et al. (2003). Allocating funds for cardiovascular disease prevention in light of the NCEP ATP III guidelines. *American Journal of Managed Care 9*(7): 477–489.

12. Egen, V., & Hasford, J. (2003). Prevention of neural tube defects: Effect of an intervention aimed at implementing the official recommendations. *Soz Praventivmed 48*(1): 24–32.

13. Grosse, S. D., Waitzman, N. J., Romano, P. S., et al. (2005). Reevaluating the benefits of folic acid fortification in the United States: Economic analysis, regulation, and public health. *American Journal of Public Health 95*: 1917–1922.

14. U.S. Preventive Services Task Force. (2012). *Vitamin D and calcium supplementation to prevent cancer and osteoporotic fractures in adults: U.S. Preventive Services Task Force recommendation statement.* Available at: http://www.uspreventiveservicestaskforce.org/draftrec3.htm

15. Centers for Disease Control and Prevention [CDC]. (2002). Iron deficiency—United States, 1999–2000. *Morbidity and Mortality Weekly Report 51*(40): 897–899.

16. U.S. Department of Health and Human Services, Health Resources and Services Administration, Maternal and Child Health Bureau. (2011). *Women's Health USA 2011*. Rockville, Maryland: U.S. Department of Health and Human Services.

17. Centers for Disease Control and Prevention [CDC], National Center for Health Statistics. (2008). *National Health Interview Survey.* Analysis conducted by the Maternal and Child Health Information Resource Center.

18. U. S. Department of Health and Human Services. (2008). *2008 physical activity guidelines for Americans.* Available at: http://www.health.gov/PAGuidelines/

19. Hu, F. B., Willet, W. C., Li, T., et al. (2004). Adiposity as compared with physical activity in predicting mortality among women. *New England Journal of Medicine 351*(26): 2694–2703.

20. Elavsky, S., McAuley, E., Motl, R. W., et al. (2005). Physical activity enhances long-term quality of life in older adults: Efficacy, esteem, and affective influences. *Annals of Behavioral Medicine 30*(2): 138–145.

21. Da Costa, D., Rippen, N., Drista, M., et al. (2003). Self-reported leisure-time physical activity during pregnancy and relationship to psychological well-being. *Journal of Psychosomatic Obstetrics and Gynaecology 24*(2): 111–119.

22. Page, P. (2012). Current concepts in muscle stretching for exercise and rehabilitation. *International Journal of Sports Physical Therapy 7*(1):109–119.

23. Kannus, P., Sievanen, H., Palvenen, M., et al. (2005). Prevention of falls and injuries in elderly people. *Lancet 366*(9500): 1885–1893.

24. Warren, M. P., & Goodman, L. R. (2003). Exercise-induced endocrine pathologies. *Journal of Endocrinological Investigation 26*(9): 873–878.

25. Hall, R. C., Hall, R. C. W., & Chapman, M. J. (2005). Psychiatric complications of anabolic steroid use. *Psychosomatics 46*(4): 285–290.

26. Savard, M. & Svec, C. (2005). The body shape solution to weight loss and wellness. New York, NY: Atria.

27. Centers for Disease Control and Prevention [CDC]. (2008). *Obesity and overweight: U.S. obesity trends.* Available at: http://www.cdc.gov/nccdphp/dnpa/obesity/trend/maps/.

28. Hedley, A. A., Ogden, C. L., Johnson, C. L., et al. (2004). Prevalence of overweight and obesity among U.S. children, adolescents, and adults, 1999–2002. *Journal of the American Medical Association 291*: 2847–2850.

29. Food and Agriculture Organization of the United Nations [FAO]. (2006). *Country profile: United States, 2004*. Rome, Italy: FAO.

30. Polednak, A. (2008). Estimating the number of U.S. incident cancers attributable to obesity and the impact on temporal trends in incidence rates for obesity-related cancers. *Cancer Detection and Prevention 32*(3): 190–199.

31. Calle, D., Rodriguez, C., Walker-Thurmond, K., et al. (2003). Overweight, obesity, and mortality from cancer in a prospectively studied cohort of U.S. adults. *New England Journal of Medicine 348*: 1625–1638.

32. National Cancer Institute. (2012). *Obesity and cancer risk*. Available at: http://www.cancer.gov/cancertopics/factsheet/Risk/obesity

33. Finkelstein, E., Trogdon, J., Cohen, J., et al. (2009). Annual medical spending attributable to obesity: Payer and service-specific estimates. *Health Affairs 28*(5): 822–831.

34. Palmer, H. (May 30, 2007). *Our loss, diet industry's gain*. American Public Media radio broadcast. Available at: http://marketplace.publicradio.org/display/web/2007/05/30/our_loss_diet_industrys_gain/.

35. Ward, E. M. (1994). Researchers disagree on the dangers of yo-yo dieting. *Environmental Nutrition 17*(6): 2.

36. Rating the diets from A to Z. (June 2005). *Consumer Reports 70*(6): 18–22.

37. Byrd-Bredbenner, C., Murray, J., & Schlussel, Y. (2005). Temporal changes in anthropometric measurements of idealized females and young women in general. *Women and Health 41*(2): 13–20.

38. Yin, S. (2004). Size and gender. *American Demographics 26*(2): 14.

39. National Institute of Mental Health. (2011). *Eating disorders*. Available at: http://www.nimh.nih.gov/health/publications/eating-disorders/eating-disorders.pdf

40. American Society for Aesthetic Plastic Surgery. (2012). *15th Annual Cosmetic Surgery National Databank Statistics*. Available at: http://www.surgery.org/sites/default/files/ASAPS-2011-Stats.pdf

41. Rothblum, E. (1990). Women and weight: Fad and fiction. *Journal of Psychology 124*: 5–24.

42. Garner, D. M. (January–February 1997). The 1997 body image survey results. *Psychology Today*. Available at: http://www.psychologytoday.com/articles/pto-19970201-000023.htm

43. Food and Agriculture Organization of the United Nations [FAO]. (2010). *Global hunger declining, but still unacceptably high*. Available at: http://www.fao.org/docrep/012/al390e/al390e00.pdf

44. Food and Agriculture Organization of the United Nations [FAO]. (2008). *Clinton at UN: Food, energy, financial woes linked*. Available at: http://www.fao.org/newsroom/en/news/2008/1000945/index.html

45. UNICEF. (2007). *State of the world's children, 2008*. New York, NY: United Nations.

46. World Health Organization [WHO]. (2003). *Nutrition*. Available at: http://www.who.int/nutrition/index.htm

47. Feeding America. (2012). *Hunger & poverty statistics*. Available at: http://feedingamerica.org/hunger-in-america/hunger-facts/hunger-and-poverty-statistics.aspx

48. Harne, A. J., & Bixby, W. R. (2005). The benefits and barriers of strength training among college-age women. *Journal of Sport Behavior 28*(2): 151–166.

Chapter Ten

Understanding and Preventing Cardiovascular Disease and Cancer

Chapter Objectives

On completion of this chapter, the student should be able to discuss:

1. The main components and functions of the circulatory system and blood.

2. The processes leading to atherosclerosis and myocardial infarction.

3. The conditions that contribute to congestive heart failure.

4. Types of congenital heart disease and its associated prevalence and mortality rates.

5. The cause and effects of rheumatic heart disease.

6. The significance of angina pectoris.

7. Conditions that lead to peripheral artery disease.

8. The major causes of cerebrovascular accidents.

9. The major modifiable risk factors for cardiovascular disease.

10. Cardiovascular disease (CVD) from an epidemiological perspective including sex/gender, race/ethnicity, and socioeconomics.

11. The process of cancer development and metastasis.

12. Cancer from an epidemiological perspective including sex/gender, race/ethnicity, and socioeconomics.

13. Types of benign conditions of the breast, cervix, uterus, and ovaries.

14. Risk factors, screening methods, and treatment modalities for breast, cervical, uterine, and ovarian cancer.

15. Pap smears and HPV tests and how they relate to benign cervical conditions as well as cervical cancer.

16. Risk factors, screening methods, and treatment modalities for lung cancer, colorectal cancer, and skin cancer.

17. Prevention of cardiovascular disease and cancer through lifestyle changes and health screening.

womenshealth.jbpub.com

Women's Health Online is a great source for supplementary women's health information for both students and instructors. Visit

http://womenshealth.jbpub.com

to find a variety of useful tools for learning, thinking, and teaching.

Introduction

Cardiovascular disease and cancer are, by far, the biggest causes of death in the United States. In almost every case, these chronic conditions are caused not by infectious disease. Instead, a combination of genetics and lifestyle factors affect who gets, and who dies from, these conditions. Genetics clearly influences who is at highest risk for cardiovascular disease and cancer. Lifestyle alone cannot totally counter a heavy genetic loading for either condition; however, behaviors can greatly reduce the risk of developing the disease and help limit the effects of diseases that develop. This chapter reviews cardiovascular disease and cancer, and discusses them in terms of epidemiology, risk factors, screening, treatment, and personal decision making to reduce the risk of disease.

Cardiovascular Disease

Cardiovascular disease (CVD) comprises a group of diseases that affect the heart and blood vessels, including stroke, a condition that affects the brain's blood vessels. **Figure 10.1** presents the major cardiovascular diseases.

Cardiovascular disease is the leading cause of death worldwide, with over 17.3 million people dying in 2009.[1] In the United States, more than 82 million people are living with CVD; of those, 42 million are women. Every year, about 420,000 U.S. women die of CVD, equaling a rate of about 1 death less than every 37 seconds. Stroke accounts for approximately 1 in 18 deaths. Cardiovascular disease costs the United States about $300 billion in a year, with women accounting for 38% of the cost (more than $100 billion).[2]

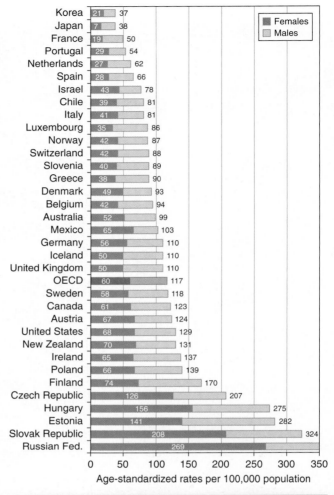

Figure 10.2

Ischemic Heart Disease Mortality by Country and Sex

Source: Adapted from OECD (2011), Health at a Glance 2011: OECD Indicators, OECD Publishing. Available at http://dx.doi.org/10.1787/health_glance-2011-en

Figure 10.1

Major Cardiovascular Diseases

Source: Reproduced from Miniño AM, Klein RJ. (2010). Health mortality from major cardiovascular diseases: United States, 2007. Health E-Stats. National Center for Health Statistics.

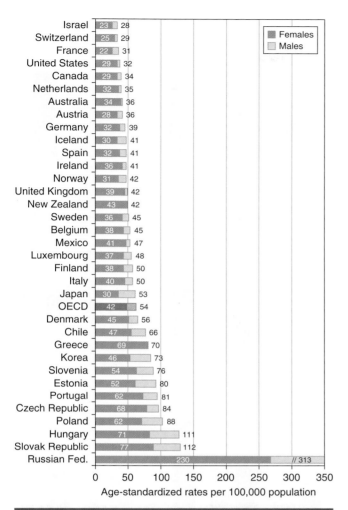

Figure 10.3

Stroke Mortality Rates for Males and Females Internationally

Source: Adapted from OECD (2011), Health at a Glance 2011: OECD Indicators, OECD Publishing. Available at http://dx.doi.org/10.1787/health_glance-2011-en

Cardiovascular deaths usually occur in later years when women are beset with a variety of comorbid conditions, such as high blood pressure, high blood cholesterol, osteoporosis, and diabetes. **Figures 10.4** and **10.5** illustrate the death rates from cardiovascular diseases among women of different races.

Cardiovascular disease is a leading cause of disability in women. Heart disease can be severely disabling, reducing the kinds of activities a person can enjoy and requiring major lifestyle changes. Stroke can lead to paralysis, incontinence, language impairments, and loss of memory. Heart conditions and stroke are not an inevitable consequence of aging, but are often related to behaviors such as cigarette smoking, poor nutrition, lack of exercise, and insufficient attention to CVD risk factors such as high blood pressure, high blood cholesterol, diabetes, and overweight and obesity.

Perspectives on Cardiovascular Disease

Epidemiology

Cardiovascular disease is the leading cause of death for women, regardless of racial or ethnic group. Of the various forms of CVD, coronary heart disease (CHD), or diseases in which the coronary arteries that supply blood to the heart become narrowed or blocked, is the leading cause of death. Every year, about 190,000 women die from CHD, slightly less than the number of deaths of men (216,000). Among these women, 64% died suddenly with no warning symptoms. Stroke, the third leading cause of death among women (after heart disease and cancer), kills about 82,000 (60%) women a year, compared with about 54,000 (40%) men.[2]

Although some cardiovascular diseases occur among children and adolescents, they typically occur among men

Figure 10.4

Age-adjusted Death Rates for Coronary Heart Disease by Female Sex and Race/Ethnicity, US, 2008

Source: Data from NHLBI. (2012). Morbidity & Mortality Chartbook on Cardiovascular, Lung, and Blood Diseases. Available at: http://www.nhlbi.nih.gov/resources/docs/2012_ChartBook_508.pdf

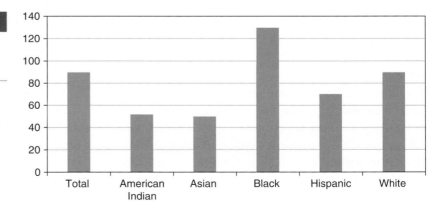

Figure 10.5

Age-adjusted Death Rates for Stroke by Female Sex and Race/Ethnicity, 2008

Source: Data from NHLBI. (2012). Morbidity & Mortality Chartbook on Cardiovascular, Lung, and Blood Diseases. Available at: http://www.nhlbi.nih.gov/resources/docs/2012_ChartBook_508.pdf

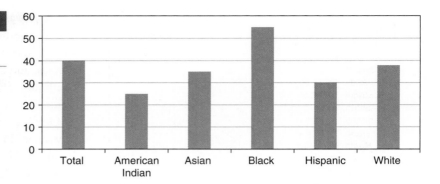

Figure 10.6

Age-adjusted Death Rates for Coronary Heart Disease for Coronary Heart Disease by Sex and Race/Ethnicity, 2008

Source: Data from NHLBI. (2012). Morbidity & Mortality Chartbook on Cardiovascular, Lung, and Blood Diseases. Available at: http://www.nhlbi.nih.gov/resources/docs/2012_ChartBook_508.pdf

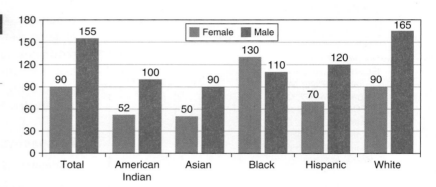

Figure 10.7

Age-adjusted Death Rates for Stroke by Sex and Race/Ethnicity 2009

Source: Data from NHLBI. (2012). Morbidity & Mortality Chartbook on Cardiovascular, Lung, and Blood Diseases. Available at: http://www.nhlbi.nih.gov/resources/docs/2012_ChartBook_508.pdf

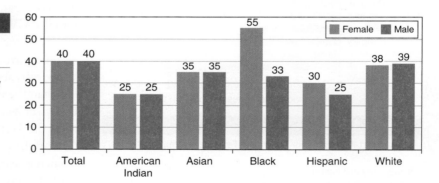

who are at least 50 years old. The incidence of CHD begins to rise for women between the ages of 55 and 60, about 10 years later than it does for men. The incidence of stroke begins to sharply rise in both women and men after the age of 60.[2]

Economic Dimensions

Cardiovascular disease imposes a heavy burden on the healthcare system in the United States, particularly on emergency medical departments and hospitals. Clinical care of CVD patients is costly and often prolonged. The estimated cost of cardiovascular disease and stroke in the United States in 2007 was $286 billion.[1] This figure includes both direct and indirect costs.

- Direct costs ($167 billion): health expenditures including those for physicians and other professionals, hospital and nursing home services, medications, home health care, and other medical durables
- Indirect costs ($119 billion): lost productivity resulting from morbidity and mortality

Cardiovascular disease often affects individuals during their peak productive years at work, causing significant disruption to families who depend on the person's income. The high rate of CVD also influences the national economy by killing or disabling otherwise productive workers. In addition, the emotional cost to women and their families and friends from such disease is incalculable.

Global Dimensions

Over the past century, cardiovascular disease has surpassed infectious diseases to become the leading cause of death and disability. With an ever-increasing life expectancy, countries that once were overwhelmed with infectious and communicable diseases, maternal and infant deaths, and malnutrition are now besieged with CVD. Cardiovascular disease is a leading cause of death among women worldwide.[3]

The growing convenience and lower price of high-fat, high-calorie processed foods, a decrease in physical exercise, and high rates of cigarette smoking have all contributed to this problem. According to the World Health Organization (WHO), American women rank 18th in the world in levels of obesity. More than 20% of women are obese in the Middle East, the United States, and some South American countries (see **Figure 10.8**).[3] Heart disease death rates vary widely among women across the continents (see Figure 10.2). The Russian Federation leads in death rates, whereas rates in Japan and France are much lower.

In the United States, smoking rates among women have begun to plateau or decline, in part because of strong and widespread public health education and intervention. Yet, marketing that targets women, especially young women, remains quite successful and many continue to smoke or to use smokeless tobacco. In some countries, predominantly in Asia, women may use smokeless forms such as chewing tobacco.[2] In addition, women often have a more difficult time quitting. Some interventions may not be as successful in women as in men, in part because many programs were initially designed for a male audience. On average, women smokers die about 14.5 years earlier than women nonsmokers.[4] **Table 10.1** presents examples of smoking trends among women and men in different world regions.

Cultural attitudes affect lifestyle habits. Women in many countries have moved from rural areas to urban areas—from physically active lifestyles such as farming to more sedentary work in offices and industry. Another concern is the "migration" effect that occurs among women who migrate from developing to developed countries. As with migration from farm to city, women who migrate to more developed countries are exposed to different cultures and styles of living. Unhealthful foods may be convenient, cheap, and present in greater quantities, while nutritious foods and opportunities for physical activity may be more rare. These lifestyle changes put immigrant women at particularly high risk for obesity, high blood pressure, high blood cholesterol, and diabetes—all risk factors for CVD. Unfortunately, in many countries and for many women immigrants to the United States, disease prevention and health care remain fragmented.

The Heart

Cardiovascular disease cannot be understood without an appreciation of the heart as a vital organ. The heart relentlessly pumps blood throughout the body 24 hours a day, without stopping, throughout a person's life.

The heart is located in the chest behind the **sternum**, also known as the breastbone. The **cardiovascular system** consists of the heart, arteries, veins, and capillaries (Figure

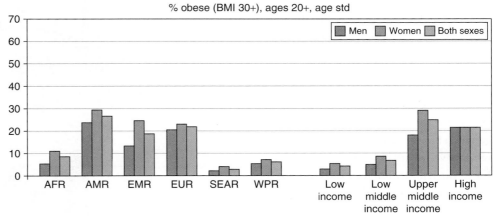

Figure 10.8

Percent Obesity Among Men and Women, Age 20 and Above, 2008

Source: Adapted from World Health Organization. (2010) Obesity: Situation and trends. Available at: http://www.who.int/gho/ncd/risk_factors/obesity_text/en/index.html

% obese (BMI 30+), ages 20+, age std

Men Women Both sexes

AFR : African Region
AMR : Americas
EMR : Eastern Mediterranean
EUR : Europe
SEAR : South East Asia
WPR : Western Pacific

Table 10.1 Smoking Prevalence and Number of Smokers Among Adults (Age 15 and Older), by WHO Region and Gender, 2006

WHO Region	Smoking Prevalence %			Total Smokers (millions)	% of all Smokers
	Male	Female	Overall		
African Region (AFR)	16	2	9	41	4
Regions of Americas (AMR)	27	17	22	145	12
Eastern Mediterranean (EMR)	30	4	17	60	5
European (EUR)	44	22	32	238	21
South-East Asia (SEAR)	37	4	21	248	21
Western Pacific (WPR)	57	5	31	430	37
World Total	40	9	24	1,164	100

Source: Reproduced from *Tobacco Use and Its Impact on Health*. WHO. Available at http://www.who.int/tobacco/publications/gender/en_tfi_gender_women_prevalence_tobacco_use.pdf. Based on *WHO Report on the Global Tobacco Epidemic, 2009: Implementing Smoke-Free Environments*. Geneva, World Health Organization, 2009.

10.5). The heart has four major chambers: the **right atrium**, **right ventricle**, **left atrium**, and **left ventricle**. The right and left atria are the upper blood-receiving chambers, and the right and left ventricles are the lower blood-pumping chambers. The right atrium and ventricle and the left atrium and ventricle are each separated by a valve. The right atrium and ventricle are separated by the **tricuspid valve**; the left atrium and ventricle are separated by the **bicuspid** or **mitral valve**. Blood flows from the atrium through the valve to the ventricle below. A thick muscular wall known as the **septum** separates the right and left sides of the heart.

Oxygen-poor blood from throughout the body travels to the heart so that it can be pumped to the lungs for oxygenation. The oxygen-poor blood enters the right atrium of the heart from the **inferior** and **superior vena cava** (major veins). From the right atrium, blood flows through the tricuspid valve into the right ventricle, where it is pumped to the lungs via the **pulmonary arteries**.

In the lungs, carbon dioxide and waste products are removed from the blood and exchanged for fresh oxygen. The newly oxygen-rich blood leaves the lungs via the **pulmonary veins** and flows into the left atrium. From the left atrium, it passes through the mitral valve into the left ventricle. The left ventricle contracts and forces the oxygen-rich blood through the **aortic valve** into the **aorta** (the main artery) and from there throughout the major **arteries**, flowing gradually into smaller and smaller arteries,

arterioles, and finally **capillaries** throughout the body. The capillaries—microscopic vessels with thin walls—are the sites where the nutrients and oxygen in the blood are exchanged for waste and carbon dioxide at the cellular level. From the capillaries, the oxygen-poor but carbon dioxide–rich blood flows into the **venules** and veins as it makes its way back to the heart. The cycle then begins again.[4]

For this system to function properly, the pump—the heart—must remain strong and forceful. It must contract forcefully and quickly when a woman runs a marathon, yet it must slow for rest during sleep. The heart is activated to perform its pumping function by electrical stimuli pulsed

Ascending aorta

Right atrium

Right coronary artery

Right ventricle

Aortic arch

Left pulmonary artery

Auricle of left atrium

Left coronary artery

Left ventricle

Descending aorta

Figure 10.9

Illustration of a Heart

■ An electrocardiograph (ECG) can detect a normal heart rhythm or abnormalities such as a heart attack or a congenitally damaged tricuspid valve.

from specialized tissues called nodes buried in the cardiac muscle. This electrical stimulation can be detected by a special device known as an **electrocardiograph (ECG)**, sometimes known as an EKG. An ECG can detect a normal heart rhythm or abnormalities such as a heart attack or a congenitally damaged tricuspid valve.

Similar to the heart, the arteries have muscles and must expand and contract vigorously to meet the demands placed on the body, yet remain supple and open. Veins, although they must also remain supple and open, do not have muscles and must therefore rely on surrounding muscles to move the blood along through the venous system to its destination.

Blood is the vehicle for transporting food and waste throughout the body. An average woman circulates about six quarts of blood per day. Blood consists of many critical components, which are all suspended in plasma, the liquid in which the different components of the blood travel. The primary components are as follows:

■ The **red blood cells (erythrocytes)** carry oxygen and carbon dioxide. Hemoglobin is an important protein in the red blood cells that carries oxygen from the lungs throughout the body; it also gives blood its red color.

■ The **white blood cells (leukocytes)** act as scavengers to rid the blood and body of bacteria and waste. Several types of white blood cells exist, each of which has a role in fighting bacterial, viral, fungal, and parasitic infections.

■ The **platelets (thrombocytes)** cause the blood to clot.

If the heart's electrical signal loses its regular pattern, the heart can begin to beat irregularly and less effectively, a condition called **arrhythmia**. Arrhythmias are very common and can occur in an otherwise healthy heart; in some cases, however, they may indicate a serious problem and can lead to heart disease.

When the atria emit uncoordinated electrical signals, the condition is called **atrial fibrillation** (AF); when disordered electrical activity causes rapid, uncoordinated contractions of the ventricle, the condition is called **ventricular fibrillation** (VF). Atrial fibrillation is not usually life threatening in itself, but it can lead to other, more serious conditions. For example, when the atrium doesn't pump blood evenly, some blood may remain in the atrium and form a clot. If this clot enters the bloodstream, it can travel to the brain and cause a stroke. In VF, little or no blood may be pumped from the heart, which can result in collapse and sudden death. Physicians can detect heart abnormalities and will first determine the origination of the arrhythmia and its severity before considering treatment.[5]

Pathophysiology of the Heart

Cardiovascular disease encompasses both heart disease (coronary heart disease, congestive heart failure, rheumatic heart disease, angina pectoris, peripheral artery disease, hypertension) and cerebrovascular disease (stroke). Many of these diseases can be prevented or controlled with lifestyle modifications or medications (see "Risk Factors for Cardiovascular Disease").

Heart conditions can typically be diagnosed by a variety of tests. Which test (or tests) is used often depends on a woman's risk factors, her history of heart problems, and her current symptoms. Tests include noninvasive tests such as electrocardiograms and magnetic resonance imaging (MRI), nuclear imaging tests that require a needle puncture, and possibly invasive imaging tests such as cardiac catheterization. (For more information on diagnostic tests, visit the websites listed at the end of this chapter.)

Treatment also varies greatly for each patient depending on the severity of the condition. This chapter describes the many medications, surgical interventions, and lifestyle changes that can help prevent and treat heart disease.

Coronary Heart Disease

Coronary heart disease (CHD) is a result of narrowed or clogged arteries. **Arteriosclerosis** is a generic term that describes any disease of the arteries that leads to thickening and hardening of the artery walls. **Atherosclerosis**, a form of arteriosclerosis, is the major culprit in CHD. It causes the heart vessels to become clogged, thereby impairing a woman's heart's ability to function. This can happen in a variety of ways:

- The arteries can become clogged with waste, usually fat deposits (**plaques**). Low density lipoproteins (LDL), or "bad" cholesterol, and other waste deposits penetrate the inner lining of the arteries. There, they build up over years, impeding the flow of blood.

- The arteries can become stiff with age or disease, rendering them less able to respond to the demands placed on them. If the blood flow is compromised, the area being fed by that particular artery or arteries does not receive proper nutrients and can become damaged or die.

When arteries surrounding the heart become twisted and tortuous, they are particularly prone to developing atherosclerosis. When that occurs, a woman is at increased risk of suffering a **heart attack** (**myocardial infarction**).[6] A heart attack, or death of a portion of the heart, occurs when one or more of the coronary arteries in the heart become damaged or clogged and, consequently, the arteries close off (Figure 10.6). Such blockages can occur from a circulating blood clot called an **embolus**. As an embolus moves through the bloodstream, it can become lodged in an artery, blocking any further blood from getting through. The resulting blockage is called a **thrombus** (stationary blood clot). A clot can also form as a result of plaque (cholesterol) buildup within the inner arterial wall. Whatever the cause, blood cannot flow downstream from the blockage. As a result, the part of the body fed by the blocked artery does not receive blood carrying oxygen and nutrients and becomes severely impaired or dies. Blockages within different coronary arteries create different problems. For example, if the blockage occurs within the major artery feeding the left ventricle (the main pump of the heart),

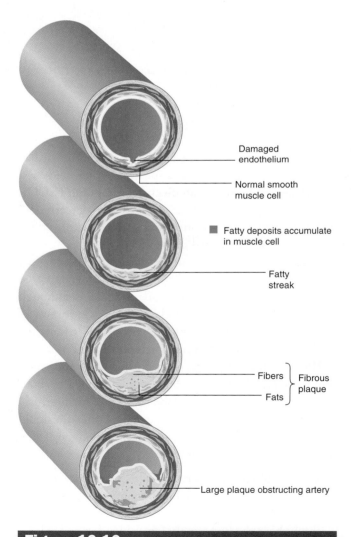

Damaged endothelium

Normal smooth muscle cell

■ Fatty deposits accumulate in muscle cell

Fatty streak

Fibers ⎱ Fibrous
Fats ⎰ plaque

Large plaque obstructing artery

Figure 10.10

Picture of Clogged Arteries

the entire ventricle can cease to pump. This stops blood flow to the rest of the body; if this situation is not reversed immediately, a woman can die or suffer irreversible brain damage within a matter of minutes from lack of oxygen to the brain. The heart also can become damaged from other diseases or conditions, such as rheumatic heart disease, or from injury, such as a heart attack, which can lead to congestive heart failure, a condition in which the heart is impaired and cannot pump effectively.[6]

Atherosclerosis cannot be cured, but its progression can be slowed. Treatment often depends on which organs are involved.

For heart conditions, cholesterol-lowering medications, which can control high cholesterol levels, are a critical factor in treatment. Surgical procedures are often common. In **balloon angioplasty**, a procedure used to open narrowed or blocked coronary arteries, a surgeon inserts a small, hollow tube called a catheter into an artery near the blockage, and then inflates a balloon near the end of the catheter. This action widens the vessel and allows blood to flow more freely. The surgeon usually places a wire mesh stent at the site of the original narrowing to keep the artery open. In contrast, **coronary artery bypass graft (CABG) surgery** creates a new passage around the blocked part of the coronary artery to restore blood flow to the heart muscle. When the brain is affected, antiplatelet medications, including aspirin, and anticoagulant medications, such as warfarin and heparin, may help prevent strokes. When atherosclerosis narrows arteries that supply the bowel, balloon angioplasty may be used or a bypass arterial graft may be performed.[7]

Some of these treatments also may be useful in treating a patient after a heart attack. The ultimate goal of such treatment is to minimize damage by restoring blood flow to the heart muscle.

People with heart disease are more likely to suffer from depression than otherwise healthy people. People with depression also are at greater risk for developing heart disease. Furthermore, depression and low perceived social support after a heart attack are associated with higher morbidity and mortality. While treating depression in recent heart attack patients does not appear to reduce the risk of death or second heart attack, it may help the symptoms of depression and improve quality of life.[8]

Acute Coronary Syndrome

Acute coronary syndrome (ACS) describes individuals who present with specific cardiac symptoms: myocardial infarction (heart attack) or unstable angina (chest pain that is unexpected or unusual and may be more severe than usual).[9] This important diagnostic category identifies individuals when they are moving toward a heart attack (unstable angina) or are in the early stages of a heart attack. The goal is to intervene before serious damage occurs.

Congestive Heart Failure

Congestive heart failure (CHF) occurs when heart muscles are weak and cannot pump with proper vigor. In such a case, the heart loses its ability to contract properly or sufficiently to meet the demands placed on it. Even if the arteries remain open, without a strong pumping action from the heart, the nutrient-rich and oxygen-rich blood may not be able to reach cells, and the cells may suffer damage or die. Additionally, the heart muscle itself depends on a rich blood supply from the coronary arteries, which must remain open and supple if the heart is to function with vigor. As a result, circulation suffers and fluids begin to accumulate in veins, causing breathing problems, kidney problems, and swelling in the extremities, particularly the legs. Congestive heart failure may have many causes, but it is often a disease of older women who have suffered heart damage from high blood pressure, atherosclerosis, arteriosclerosis, or heart attack. In some cases, CHF occurs because of a congenital defect or damage to the heart from a bacterial disease, such as rheumatic heart disease.[2]

Congestive heart failure can often be prevented or minimized by controlling high blood pressure, treating underlying bacterial infections, and following lifestyle modifications that prevent other forms of CVD. Medication, salt reduction, and possibly surgery to alleviate blockages in coronary arteries may help to improve heart function once CHF has been diagnosed. Women are about 50% more likely to die from CHF than are men.[2]

Congenital Heart Disease

Congenital heart disease is an abnormality of the heart that is present at birth. It can include one or more of the following:

- A hole in the septum
- Imperfectly formed blood vessels
- Valvular damage
- Left ventricular imperfections

Patent ductus arteriosus is a congenital condition in which the ductus arteriosus (passageway between the pulmonary artery and aorta) does not close. It is a common condition in premature babies. Another congenital heart disease, called **pulmonary stenosis**, occurs when the valve between the ventricle and the pulmonary artery is defective and does not open properly. Atrial or ventricular septal defects occur when an opening appears between the two upper or lower chambers of the heart. Most of these imperfections can be corrected with surgery.

Nearly 36,000 babies are born each year with congenital heart defects.[2] Mortality associated with congenital heart defects declined, however, due to advances in diagnosis and surgical treatments. From 1997 to 2007, for example, death rates declined 33% for congenital cardiovascular defects.[2] However, the majority of congenital heart defect deaths occur in children less than 1 year old. Congenital heart defects or imperfections often can be corrected with surgery.

Rheumatic Heart Disease

Rheumatic heart disease results from a bacterial infection (Streptococcus) that has been inadequately treated and causes damage to the heart valves. Rheumatic heart disease is a complication from an inadequately treated strep throat, which progresses to rheumatic fever and affects the entire body. The brain, heart, and joints can be permanently damaged. In the heart, rheumatic heart disease can damage the valves by closing them off either completely or partially. This condition may require surgery and valve replacement. The best treatment is prevention—for example, treatment of the initial infection, which precludes further damage. Modern antibiotic therapy has sharply reduced mortality from rheumatic heart disease. In 1950, approximately 15,000 Americans died of this disease; in 2007, there were 3,200 deaths, an 80% decline. The highest death rates were in women, especially White women.[11]

Angina Pectoris

Angina pectoris (or just angina) is chest pain resulting from an insufficient supply of blood, and thus oxygen, to the heart muscle. The symptoms can range in severity from a mild cramping ache to a crushing pain in the chest. The impairment of blood flow can result from atherosclerosis or a spasm of a normal artery. Angina is as common in women as it is in men.[12] Angina is also a symptom of CVD and may be a predictor of future myocardial infarction; however, angina symptoms precede only 18% of coronary attacks.[1] Depending on the cause of the impairment, the pain can be relieved by medication, often nitroglycerin, a strong vasodilator (opening the closed blood vessel), which reduces the heart's need for more oxygen.

Peripheral Artery Disease

Peripheral artery disease (PAD) is a disease of the extremities (hands, arms, or, most commonly, legs and feet) in which the blood supply is diminished, sufficient oxygen and nutrients do not reach these areas properly, and waste products accumulate. A woman with PAD can experience symptoms ranging from cramping and numbness to gangrene (tissue death), which may require amputation of the extremity. The cause of PAD is related to atherosclerosis and arteriosclerosis and is particularly associated with diabetes, smoking, and hypertension. Of all the known risk factors, smoking and diabetes are the most strongly related to PAD. Treatment options include lifestyle modifications, such as smoking cessation, increased exercise, anticoagulant or antiplatelet medications, angioplasty, or bypass surgery. While women may know about PAD, many do not understand the risk factors for it, especially smoking and diabetes.[2]

Metabolic Syndrome

Metabolic syndrome is a group of diseases that can occur together and increase risk for CVD. The National Heart, Lung, and Blood Institute and the American Heart Association note that the presence of three or more of the following diseases predisposes a person to an increased risk for metabolic syndrome.

- Elevated waist circumference
    - Men: Equal to or greater than 40 inches (102 cm)
    - Women: Equal to or greater than 35 inches (88 cm)
- Elevated triglycerides
    - Equal to or greater than 150 mg/dL
- Reduced HDL ("good") cholesterol
    - Men: Less than 40 mg/dL
    - Women: Less than 50 mg/dL
- Elevated blood pressure
    - Equal to or greater than 130/85 mmHg
- Elevated fasting glucose
    - Equal to or greater than 100 mg/dL

The principal factors contributing to metabolic syndrome appear to be central obesity and insulin resistance—factors that are increasingly common among women. One in three women (33%) have this condition, with prevalence varying among women of different racial/ethnic groups (White 32%, Black 39%, and Mexican American 41%).[2] Preventive actions to address metabolic syndrome

Table 10.2	Warning Signs of a Heart Attack in Women

- Pain or discomfort in the chest: Heart attacks often involve pain or discomfort in the chest. The pain can be intense, mild, or in-between. Discomfort can feel like a sense of squeezing, pressure, or fullness.
- Pain or aching in other parts of the upper body. A heart attack can cause pain or uncomfortable feelings in the back, neck, jaw, one or both arms, or stomach.
- Unexplained feelings of nausea, dizziness, or shortness of breath, or feeling lightheaded, that last a few minutes or more.

are weight loss and control, healthy eating, and increased physical activity.

Cerebrovascular Accident (Stroke)

Cerebrovascular accident, commonly called **stroke**, is a condition in which blood vessels leading to and within the brain become damaged. The process of blood flow blockage that occurs in the coronary vessels of the heart is similar to that which occurs in the brain. The other major process involved in stroke is vessel rupture, often resulting from atherosclerotic vessels. When the blood vessel is blocked or bursts, part of the brain cannot get blood, and therefore oxygen, which it needs to survive. The most common type of stroke, **ischemic stroke**, is caused by blockage; the clot in such cases is called a cerebral thrombus or cerebral **embolism**. **Hemorrhagic strokes** are caused by ruptured blood vessels.[13]

An **aneurysm** is one type of weakened blood vessel that can cause a stroke. It involves a ballooning of a weakened region of a blood vessel resulting from several factors including a congenital defect, chronic high blood pressure, or an injury to the brain. If left untreated, the aneurysm will continue to weaken until it ruptures and bleeds in the brain[2] (**Figure 10.11**).

Warning signs (**Table 10.3**) may precede a stroke in the form of a **transient ischemic attack (TIA)**. In a TIA, the artery may close momentarily in a spasm, and the woman may have a brief memory lapse or garbled speech. Such an event often occurs very quickly, and the woman may have little memory of it. Recognition of stroke warning signs and subsequent action varies. About 42% of women recognize the symptoms, considerably more than men (35%). In addition, individuals with a higher education also appear to respond more quickly and to seek intervention.[2]

Thrombus

Embolism

Aneurysm (ruptured)

Figure 10.11
Cerebrovascular Accident (Stroke)

A variety of tests can diagnose a stroke by examining the brain and outlining the injured brain area:

- Imaging tests, such as a CT (computed tomography) or CAT (computerized axial tomography) scan, produce a picture of the brain similar to X-rays.
- Electrical tests, such as an EEG (electroencephalogram) or an evoked response test, record the electrical impulses of the brain.

Table 10.3	Warning Signs of Stroke

- Sudden numbness or weakness of the face, arm, or leg, especially on one side of the body
- Sudden confusion, or trouble speaking or understanding
- Sudden trouble seeing in one or both eyes
- Sudden trouble walking, dizziness, loss of balance or coordination
- Sudden, severe headache with no known cause

In the event of a stroke, immediate action is required. Call 911 or the local emergency system and get medical treatment immediately.

Source: American Heart Association. *Stroke warning signs.* Available at: http://www.americanheart.org/presenter.jhtml?identifier=4742

- Blood flow tests, such as B-mode imaging, Doppler testing, duplex scanning, and angiography (arteriography or arteriogram), show any problem that may cause changes in blood flow to the brain.

Stroke therapies include surgery, drugs, acute hospital care, and rehabilitation. Treatment of an ischemic stroke focuses on removing the obstruction and restoring blood flow.[15] The most promising medication for ischemic stroke is the clot-busting drug, tissue plasminogen activator (tPA). For maximum benefit, tPA therapy must be started within 3 hours of the onset of stroke symptoms. Unfortunately, only 3% to 5% of people who suffer a stroke reach the hospital in time to be considered for this treatment. Although tPA carries a risk of bleeding in the brain, its benefits generally outweigh the risks when an experienced doctor uses it properly.[17]

Doctors sometimes use balloon angioplasty and the implantable steel screens called stents to restore blood flow to a clogged artery. When the carotid artery (a major artery in the neck) is partially blocked by a fat buildup (plaque), a technique called carotid endarterectomy might be performed to remove the plaque. Antiplatelet agents, such as aspirin, and anticoagulants, such as warfarin, interfere with the blood's ability to clot and can reduce the likelihood of ischemic stroke.

To treat a hemorrhagic stroke, an obstruction needs to be introduced to prevent rupture and bleeding of the affected blood vessel. Surgical treatment may involve placing a metal clip at the base of the aneurysm (rupture) or to removing the abnormal vessels. Endovascular procedures are less invasive and involve the introduction of a catheter through a major artery in the leg or arm; a surgeon then guides the catheter to the aneurysm, where it deposits a mechanical agent, such as a coil, to prevent rupture.

After a stroke, rehabilitation is often necessary to help survivors relearn skills that are lost when part of the brain is damaged and learn new ways of performing tasks to compensate for any disabilities. Therapy begins in the acute-care hospital after the patient's medical condition has been stabilized, often within 24 to 48 hours after the stroke. Poststroke rehabilitation requires the services of physicians; rehabilitation nurses; physical, occupational, recreational, speech-language, and vocational therapists; and mental health professionals.

The types and degrees of disability that follow a stroke depend on which area of the brain is damaged. Generally, stroke can cause five types of disabilities:

- Paralysis is one of the most common disabilities resulting from stroke. It usually appears on the side of the body opposite the side of the brain damaged by stroke,

© Shaywitz, et al., 1995 NMR Research/Yale Medical School

■ Functional MRI scans show that male subjects predominantly rely on areas of the left hemisphere of the brain, while females activate both the left and right regions for certain aspects of language.

and may affect the face, an arm, a leg, or the entire side of the body.

- Stroke patients may lose the ability to feel touch, pain, temperature, or position. Some experience pain, numbness, or odd sensations of tingling or prickling in paralyzed or weakened limbs. The loss of urinary continence and/or bowel control is fairly common immediately after a stroke and often results from a combination of sensory and motor deficits. Permanent incontinence after a stroke, however, is uncommon.

- At least one-fourth of all stroke survivors experience language impairments, involving the ability to speak, write, and understand spoken and written language. There are sex-related differences in language impairments, depending on which portion of the brain is affected. Functional MRI scans have shown that males predominantly rely on areas of the left hemisphere of the brain, whereas females activate both the left and right regions for certain aspects of language. A stroke that occurs in the left hemisphere can therefore have disastrous results for men in terms of speech, whereas women can use the other, unaffected side to regain speech. This knowledge helps to explain why women are more resilient to the effects of such injury and are more likely than males to recover language ability after suffering a left-hemisphere stroke.

- Stroke can damage parts of the brain responsible for memory, learning, and awareness. Stroke survivors may have dramatically shortened attention spans or may lose their ability to make plans, comprehend meaning, learn new tasks, or engage in other complex mental activities.[17]

- Survivors of stroke often feel fear, anxiety, frustration, anger, sadness, and a sense of grief for their physical and mental losses. The physical effects of brain damage are responsible for some of these emotional disturbances and personality changes. Clinical depression appears to be the emotional disorder most commonly experienced by stroke survivors.

Whatever the cause of the stroke, the damage to the artery prevents oxygen and nutrients from reaching a particular area of the brain. As a result, that portion of the brain dies. Depending on where the stroke occurs in the brain, speech, memory, thought, and movement can be diminished or lost. Stroke is a leading cause of severe, long-term disability. Recovery depends on many factors, many of which stem from the individual's pre-stroke status: age, mental status, physical abilities, economic support, and cultural perceptions. Often women are older when they experience a stroke and frequently do less well compared to men in recovering physical and mental functioning.[18]

Although a stroke can happen at any time to anyone, it generally occurs in older individuals. The risk of a stroke substantially increases for people older than 55. Women are more prone to die of stroke than are men. About 60% of stroke deaths are in women, with the highest rates in Black and White women.[2]

Rates of stroke, as well as deaths from stroke, vary within the United States. This area at highest risk, which includes eight southern states—North Carolina, South Carolina, Georgia, Mississippi, Tennessee, Louisiana, Alabama, and Arkansas—is called the "stroke belt" (**Figure 10.12**). The average mortality from strokes in this region is approximately 20% greater than the rest of the country.[2]

© Photodisc

- Recovery from a stroke can be very difficult.

**Stroke death rates, 2000–2006
women ages 35+, by county**

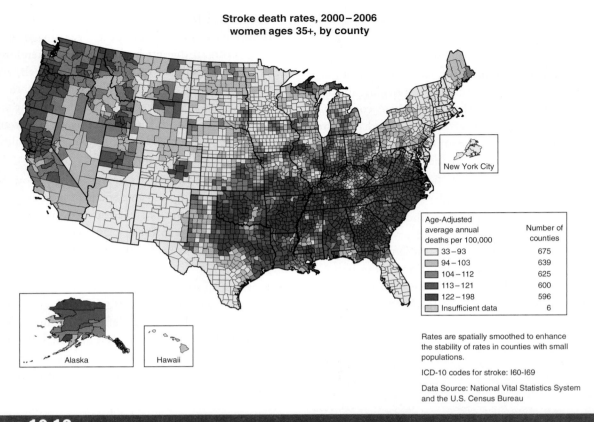

Age-Adjusted average annual deaths per 100,000	Number of counties
33–93	675
94–103	639
104–112	625
113–121	600
122–198	596
Insufficient data	6

Rates are spatially smoothed to enhance the stability of rates in counties with small populations.

ICD-10 codes for stroke: I60-I69

Data Source: National Vital Statistics System and the U.S. Census Bureau

Figure 10.12

US Map of the "Stroke Belt"

Source: Reproduced from CDC. (2010). Stroke Death Rates for Women. Available at: http://www.cdc.gov/dhdsp/maps/national_maps/stroke_women.htm

Risk Factors for Cardiovascular Disease

Cardiovascular diseases result from a complex interaction of genetics, lifestyle, and environmental factors that lead to different pathological conditions of the cardiovascular system. The major risk factors for CHD that can be modified or controlled include tobacco use, high blood pressure, high blood cholesterol, diabetes, obesity, and sedentary lifestyle (see **Self-Assessment 10.1**). Risk factors that cannot be changed or controlled include increasing age, family history of CVD, and race. Although these factors can contribute to a person's risk of disease, they are not perfect predictors of disease. A woman with normal cholesterol levels, for example, may have heart disease. Conversely, a woman with high cholesterol may not have heart disease even though she does have one of the factors that put her at risk.

Tobacco Use

Tobacco use is the greatest preventable cause of death in the United States. Tobacco use increases the risk of several kinds of cancers, and also sharply increases the risk of heart attack (especially sudden death from heart attack), stroke, and PAD. Although smoking rates have declined sharply since 1960, about 19% of women still smoke. Smoking rates vary by age, race, and income.[2]

- In 2009, an estimated 19% of girls in grades 9–12 smoked—a substantial decline since the 1990s.
- More female than male students in grades 9–12 tried to quit.
- Smokers by race and gender
  - Asian men vs women: 16.9% vs 7.5%
  - Hispanic men vs women: 19% vs 9.8%
  - American Indian/Alaskan Native men vs women: 29.7% vs 17.5%
  - Black men vs women: 24.1% vs 19%
  - White men vs women: 24.6% vs 22.2%

Furthermore, smoking is highest among women with little education and lowest among women with a bachelor's degree or higher.[19]

Self Assessment 10.1

Heart Disease

The first step toward heart health is becoming aware of your own personal risk for heart disease. Some risks, such as smoking cigarettes, are obvious: Every woman knows whether or not she smokes. But other risk factors, such as high blood pressure or high blood cholesterol, generally don't have obvious signs or symptoms. So you'll need to gather some information to create your personal "heart profile."

You and Your Doctor: A Heart Healthy Partnership

A crucial step in determining your risk is to see your doctor for a thorough checkup. Your doctor can be an important partner in helping you set and reach goals for heart health. But don't wait for your doctor to mention heart disease or its risk factors: Many doctors don't routinely bring up the subject with women patients. Here are some tips for establishing good, clear communication between you and your doctor:

- Speak up. Tell your doctor you want to keep your heart healthy and would like help in achieving that goal. Ask questions about your chances of developing heart disease and how you can lower your risk.

- Keep tabs on treatment. If you already are being treated for heart disease or heart disease risk factors, ask your doctor to review your treatment plan with you. Ask: Is what I'm doing

in line with the latest recommendations? Are my treatments working? Are my risk factors under control? If your doctor recommends a medical procedure, ask about its benefits and risks. Find out if you will need to be hospitalized and for how long, and what to expect during the recovery period.

- Be open. When your doctor asks you questions, answer as honestly and fully as you can. While certain topics may seem quite personal, discussing them openly can help your doctor find out your chances of developing heart disease. It can also help your doctor work with you to reduce your risk. If you already have heart disease, briefly describe each of your symptoms. Include when each symptom started, how often it happens, and whether it has been getting worse.

- Keep it simple. If you don't understand something your doctor says, ask for an explanation in simple language. Be especially sure you understand how to take any medication you are given. If you are worried about understanding what the doctor says, or if you have trouble hearing, bring a friend or relative with you to your appointment. You may want to ask that person to write down the doctor's instructions for you.

Source: Reproduced from National Heart, Lung, and Blood Institute. (2010). The healthy heart handbook for women. Available at: http://www.nhlbi.nih.gov/educational/hearttruth/lower-risk/find-out.htm

---

I started smoking last year. It's helped me lose weight, and gives us something cool to do before school. I'm not worried about getting cancer—that takes years to develop, and I can quit any time I want.
15-year-old female student

Pregnant women are less likely to smoke than were non-pregnant women,[2] yet from 2000 to 2004 an estimated 776 infants died as a result of maternal smoking during pregnancy.[14] In addition, smoking during pregnancy can result in low birthweight babies and preterm birth.[20]

Certain components in cigarette smoke act as **vasoconstrictors**, meaning they narrow the blood vessels. One such compound is carbon monoxide, a gas that reduces the amount of oxygen that red blood cells can carry. This poor oxygen-carrying ability reduces the amount of oxygen available to the heart, brain, muscles, and every organ in the body. Nicotine is another vasoconstrictor. By narrowing the blood vessels, it increases the likelihood of a blood clot forming. Over time, vasoconstriction contributes to the increased fragility and brittleness of arteries, which in turn contributes to atherosclerosis.

The good news is that when a woman stops smoking, her risk for heart disease begins to decline within months. According to data from the Nurses' Health Study, the risk

from death from any cause went down by 13% in the first 5 years of quitting. Twenty years after quitting, the risk of death declined to the same as that of people who have never smoked. The most rapid lowering of risk occurred among the cardiovascular diseases.[21]

Secondhand smoke, also known as **environmental tobacco smoke (ETS)**, comes from nearby tobacco products that are burning. The toxins contained in secondhand smoke include more than 60 cancer-causing agents, nicotine, and carbon monoxide. Secondhand smoke is associated with a number of potentially lethal conditions: lung cancer, sinus cancer, lung conditions (such as asthma, or impaired lung function, especially in young children), heart disease, low birthweight in babies (especially when mothers smoke during pregnancy), and others. Repeated exposure to secondhand smoke almost doubles the risk of heart disease.[22]

Hypertension

Blood pressure is the pressure exerted against the walls of the arteries when the heart pumps, specifically when the left ventricle contracts. This pressure is crucial in maintaining equilibrium throughout the vascular system as different forces affect this system. For example, when an athlete runs

■ All women should know their personal risk for hypertension and regularly monitor their blood pressure.

a race, the heart must pump faster and harder to meet the demands of the cells for oxygen. As part of this process, the arteries must constrict to keep the pressure constant to accomplish the task of running.

Blood pressure is measured with a **sphygmomanometer**. This cuff device is connected to a hose, which is in turn connected to a measuring device. The cuff is wrapped around the woman's upper arm (or in rare instances the leg) and inflated, thereby constricting the underlying artery and stopping the blood flow—and with it the sound of the heartbeat. Gradually the pressure in the cuff is released, and the blood begins to flow back through the artery and the sound of the heartbeat returns.[23] The first number, which expresses the **systolic** pressure, represents the amount of force the blood exerts against the wall of the artery when the heart contracts. The second number, which expresses the **diastolic** pressure, represents the amount of pressure the blood exerts against the wall of the artery when the heart rests between beats.

Hypertension, also known as high blood pressure, is a blood pressure that remains elevated above what is considered a safe level. Hypertension is not the same as excessive stress or tension, as some individuals mistakenly imagine. Although numbers such as 120/80 mmHg have been noted over the years as "normal" blood pressure, blood pressure varies throughout the day and during different activities. A young woman may have a blood pressure of 90/70 mmHg during a visit to the doctor, whereas an older woman may have a blood pressure of 138/80 mmHg during her

doctor's visit; both may be deemed appropriate. The numbers used by the National Heart, Lung, and Blood Institute's National High Blood Pressure Education Program and by the American Heart Association to indicate high blood pressure are 140 mmHg systolic and 90 mmHg diastolic. Although blood pressure can reach heights such as 140/90 mmHg or greater in a healthy adult during exercise, these levels return to a lower level after exercise. Continuing levels of blood pressure at 140/90 mmHg or higher, however, are considered high blood pressure and, as such, increase an individual's risk for heart disease and stroke (see **Table 10.4**). The percentage of the U.S. population with high blood pressure rises with age:[2]

- 18–28: 5%
- 30–39: 15%
- 40–49: 25%
- 50–59: 38%
- 60–69: 58%
- 70–79: 65%
- 80+: 68%

Over time, high blood pressure damages small arteries, known as arterioles. Arterioles become thicker and less elastic, resulting in arteriosclerosis. This condition, coupled with the effects from atherosclerosis, greatly increases a person's risk. When faced with the demands of heavy exertion (such as running or shoveling snow), arterioles, particularly in the brain, heart, or kidneys, can close, rupture, or leak, causing a stroke, heart attack, or renal accident (in kidneys). About 69% of the people who have a first heart attack and 77% of people who have a first stroke have blood pressures greater than 140/90 mmHg.[2]

Table 10.4 Categories for Blood Pressure Levels in Adults (Ages 18 and Older)

Category	Blood Pressure Level		
	Systolic		Diastolic
Normal	Less than 120	and	Less than 80
Prehypertension	120–139	or	80–89
High Blood Pressure			
Stage 1	140–159	or	90–99
Stage 2	Greater than 160	or	Greater than 100

Source: National Heart, Lung, and Blood Institute. *Categories for blood pressure levels in adults.* http://www.nhlbi.nih.gov/hbp/detect/categ.htm

The highest rates of high blood pressure occur among African American and Hispanic women; those who are older, overweight, or obese; and those who are poor or near poor.[25] The risk of high blood pressure increases with age. More than half of women older than age 55 have elevated or high blood pressure, an with the rise in blood pressure comes a higher risk of heart disease and death.

In many cases, high blood pressure can be controlled by diet, weight loss, and weight control. In some women, especially African American women, salt sensitivity appears to affect the development and control of high blood pressure. People who are salt-sensitive have blood pressure that rises in response to the amount of salt they eat. For these people, consistently eating a low-salt diet can help lower their blood pressure. When necessary, medication can also lower elevated blood pressure. A woman with high blood pressure should be under the supervision of a healthcare provider. Blood pressure should be checked periodically, especially as a woman ages.

High Blood Cholesterol

Cholesterol is a waxy substance that is essential for cell manufacture and maintenance, as well as the production of sex hormones and nerves throughout the body. While cholesterol may be obtained through the diet, the body on its own manufactures enough cholesterol to serve its needs. In some individuals, however, blood cholesterol levels may be excessively high because of obesity, poor diet, or genetic abnormalities. High blood levels of cholesterol (greater than 240 mg/dL) are associated with an increased risk of mortality and morbidity from CHD.[26]

When excessive cholesterol is present, the body can become overwhelmed, and the body deposits unused cholesterol on the inner walls of the arteries. Over time (usually decades), these deposits penetrate the inner lining of the artery and accumulate, slowly narrowing the space for blood to flow (Figure 10.6). The inner walls become clogged and brittle, and pieces of the artery tear, leaving jagged edges. These jagged edges stick up and catch material that flows by in the bloodstream, thereby adding more waste deposits to the wall. The artery is gradually closed off either by a fatty plaque, a clot, or some other blockage, which may become lodged in the narrowed artery. Another type of smaller plaque, called an unstable plaque, also may cause blood to clot. If the plaque bursts within the artery wall, its contents are released into the bloodstream and can trigger a blockage. In any case, the blood does not reach a part of the body, and that part will die unless the artery is

once again opened. If this blockage happens in a coronary artery, a heart attack occurs.

The liver and small intestine manufacture cholesterol, which moves throughout the body in a **lipoprotein**. Lipoproteins consist of fats and protein bound together in a chemical structure that enables them to be transported in the blood. They are made up of the following key elements: low-density lipoproteins (LDL), high-density lipoproteins (HDL), very-low-density lipoproteins (VLDL), and triglycerides. Everyone has each of these substances in varying amounts in each lipoprotein molecule.

- LDL cholesterol is often referred to as "bad" cholesterol because of its affinity for sticking to the wall of the artery and lodging there.
- HDL cholesterol has often been referred to as "good" cholesterol because it appears to function somewhat like a trash collector, taking the LDL cholesterol out of the body. Recent studies, however, have questioned whether HDL cholesterol actively helps the body or is merely an indicator of other factors that lower risk.
- **VLDL** is associated with the transport of fats known as triglycerides.
- **Triglycerides** are a form of fat that comes from food and is also made in the body. High triglycerides are often a sign of high total cholesterol.[27]

When speaking of cholesterol levels in the blood, healthcare professionals generally refer either to the total blood cholesterol level, or to the LDL cholesterol and HDL cholesterol levels. Cholesterol levels are measured from a small amount of blood (about one teaspoonful) drawn from a vein. If the physician wishes to obtain an accurate measurement of the LDL cholesterol and the HDL cholesterol, the person must fast for 12 hours before the sample is drawn. The measurement is shown in milligrams per deciliter (mg/dL). As with blood pressure measurements, there is no one "normal" level for blood cholesterol.[28] **Table 10.5** summarizes the National Heart, Lung, and Blood Institute's recommendations for cholesterol and triglyceride levels.

Low levels of HDL ("good cholesterol") are a predictor of mortality from CHD in both young and older women, and are a stronger predictor in women than in men. Women, particularly those who are fit and slender and who have not experienced menopause, tend to have slightly elevated HDL cholesterol levels compared with men or with postmenopausal women. Elevated HDL cholesterol levels either protect against heart disease or indicate the presence of other factors that reduce the risk of

Table 10.5 Categories for Blood Cholesterol and Triglyceride Levels

Cholesterol	Status
Total Cholesterol	
Less than 200 mg/dL	Ideal
200–239 mg/dL	Borderline High
240 or more	High
LDL (Bad) Cholesterol	
Less than 100 mg/dL	Ideal
100–129 md/dL	Near optimal/above optimal
130–159 mg/dL	Borderline High
160–189 mg/dL	High
190 mg/dL and higher	Very High
HDL (Good) Cholesterol	
Less than 40 mg/dL	Major risk factor
40–59 mg/dL	The higher, the better
60 mg/dL and higher	Considered protective
Triglyceride Levels	
Less than 150 mg/dL	Normal
150–199 md/dL	Borderline
200–499 mg/dL	High
500 mg/dl or above	Very high

Source: Modified from National Heart, Lung, and Blood Institute. http://www.nhlbi.nih.gov/health/health-topics/topics/hbc/printall-index. html; Data from U.S. National Library of Medicine. National Institutes of Health. Available at http://www.nlm.nih.gov/medlineplus/ency/article/003493.htm

heart disease. Around menopause, a woman's hormone levels begin to change, and so do her cholesterol levels. Total cholesterol, especially LDL cholesterol and triglyceride levels, increase a woman's chance of experiencing or dying from a heart attack.[28,29] **Figure 10.13** demonstrates the differences in high blood cholesterol by sex.

A person's diet influences his or her cholesterol levels. A diet low in cholesterol and saturated fat is crucial in maintaining a low overall total cholesterol level. Saturated fats

eaten in food actually have a greater effect on blood cholesterol than cholesterol eaten in food. Eating saturated fats increases the total blood cholesterol, particularly LDL cholesterol. This means that a woman should to limit both the dietary cholesterol and the dietary saturated fat she eats. Daily consumption of essential nutrients remains crucial.

Even though cholesterol acts as a strong predictor of potential heart attack or stroke, almost half of people who have heart attacks have normal levels of cholesterol. Studies have shown that levels of **C-reactive protein** (CRP), a protein found in the blood when inflammation is present, may actually be a stronger predictor of potential cardiovascular disease than cholesterol levels. CRP levels can be measured by a simple blood test. The American Heart Association and the Centers for Disease Control and Prevention guidelines recommend that CRP screening should be reserved for people with moderate cardiovascular risk and that it should not replace assessment for major risk factors.[31] If CRP levels are high, treatments to lower cholesterol—such as exercise, aspirin, and **statins**—can also be used to lower CRP. Although CRP can be useful as a predictor, high levels of this protein can indicate other acute and chronic conditions, including arthritis, tuberculosis, cancer, pneumonia, or the common cold. Positive CRP also can occur during the last half of pregnancy or with the use of oral contraceptives.

Whether C-reactive protein should be used as a screening mechanism in women remains unclear. Even when controlling for other risk factors, CRP levels are generally higher in women of all racial and ethnic groups compared with men.

Another substance found in the blood is **homocysteine**, an essential amino acid. Increased levels harm the arterial lining and increase the risk for heart disease. Folic acid and vitamins B_6 and B_{12} can lower homocysteine levels, though whether such efforts reduce the rates of heart disease is not yet clear. Until the evidence is stronger, women at high risk for heart disease should make certain that their diet is

Figure 10.13

Prevalence of High Blood Cholesterol According to BMI in Men and Women

Source: Adapted from Rogers, VL et al. 2011. Risk Factors: High Blood Cholesterol and Other Lipids, Heart Disease and Stroke Statistics—2011 Update: A Report from the American Heart Association, e117, http://circ.ahajournals.org/content/1234/4/e18

*Defined as ≥240 mg/dL.

rich in folic acid and vitamins B_6 and B_{12} (fruits and green leafy vegetables).[31]

Diabetes

Diabetes is a disorder of the pancreas in which naturally occurring insulin (a hormone that is used to convert sugar, starches, and other types of food—mainly glucose—into energy) is not properly manufactured or used. The most common form of diabetes is type 2 diabetes (see Chapter 11 for more information). Diabetes causes many serious problems and can lead to life-threatening situations. Yet, the number of women with diabetes is rising, most often in those who are overweight or obese. Women who develop diabetes during pregnancy (gestational diabetes) are at higher risk of developing the disease again later in life.[2,33,34]

The presence of diabetes increases risk for heart disease and stroke. The reasons for this greater prevalence are not entirely clear, although higher rates of overweight and obesity certainly contribute to the risk. High levels of glucose in the blood may also accelerate damage to the blood vessels, increasing the rate of plaque development. The role of genetic predisposition to the disease among certain racial and ethnic groups is being explored. The critical issue for anyone with diabetes is to understand the disease and its effects on their health and well-being, and to assure that they maintain proper nutrition, exercise habits, and medication.

Overweight and Obesity

Overweight and obesity are major risk factors for many chronic diseases, especially for heart disease. Overweight is defined as having a body mass index (BMI) of 25 or greater; obesity is defined as having a BMI of 30 or greater. More than 64% of U.S. women are considered overweight or obese.[2] The highest rates of both are among African American and Hispanic women.

Perhaps one of the most troubling issues is the number of children who are overweight and obese: 16.8% of girls 12 to 19 years of age are obese.[35] This condition a major risk factor for the development of CHD through the heightened risk of developing high blood pressure, high blood cholesterol, and diabetes. Overweight and obesity are also correlated with poor nutrition and sedentary lifestyles—other CHD risk factors. Eating a diet rich in saturated fats and cholesterol can lead to clogged arteries. This compromises blood flow, especially to the heart, and can lead to a heart attack or stroke.

I know I've gotten overweight. In fact, our whole family could probably stand to lose a few pounds. But after work, I'm usually too tired to cook healthy meals or to get out to the health club. The thought of getting back into shape seems like so much work that I just want to give up.

35-year-old mother

Figure 10.14

Calculate BMI

BMI = weight (in pounds) divided by height (in inches) times height (in inches × 703)

$$\frac{\text{Weight}}{\text{Height} \times \text{Height}} \times 703 =$$

Example: For a 5' 5" woman weighing 146 lbs

$$\frac{146 \text{ lbs}}{65 \times 65} = \frac{146}{4,225} = 0.034 \times 703 = 24.9$$

Alternately, you can go to one of many websites and have it calculated for you. One such website is the National Institutes of Health's National Heart, Lung, and Blood Institute: www.nhlbisupport.com/**bmi/**

Figure 10.15

Children, 2–19 Years of Age, Either Overweight or Obese in the United States

Source: Data from American Heart Association. (2011). Overweight in children. Available at: http://www.heart.org/HEARTORG/GettingHealthy/Overweight-in-Children_UCM_304054_Article.jsp

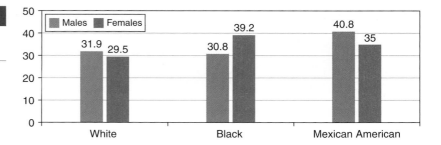

The way that fat is distributed on a woman's body may also affect her risk for heart disease. Truncal distribution of fat (around the stomach and upper body), as opposed to hip and thigh distribution, appears more risky. The truncal distribution pattern has been referred to as an "apple" shape, and the hip and thigh distribution a "pear" shape. More information on obesity appears in Chapter 9.

Physical Inactivity

Physical inactivity or a sedentary lifestyle is another important modifiable risk factor for cardiovascular disease. Physical inactivity simply means that a woman is not getting enough regular aerobic exercise—any movement that raises the heart rate significantly for an extended period of time. Overall, more than 34% of women do not participate in the recommended amount of physical activity and those percentages increase with age.[2] For all races, women are less physically active than men on average. Aerobic exercise is a critical factor in keeping the heart and other muscles strong and in good working condition. Regular exercise also aids in controlling weight, helping to raise HDL cholesterol levels, and both controlling and reducing the risk of developing diabetes. The Nurses' Health Study, a large, ongoing study observing female nurses, showed similar protective effects against coronary heart disease for brisk walking and vigorous exercise.[36,37] See Chapter 9 for more information.

Other Factors Affecting CVD Risk

Intrauterine Environment

This is a critically important factor in a child's development both in the womb (uterus) and in his or her subsequent development throughout life. If the mother does not have a healthy and sufficient lifestyle and diet while

■ The lifestyle choices a woman makes during pregnancy affect not only her health, but also the health of her developing fetus.

she is pregnant, the metabolic and endocrine status of the offspring may be severely compromised throughout life.[38]

This is particularly challenging if the child develops intrauterine growth restriction (IUGR), a condition in which the fetus grows more slowly than usual. As a result, when the child is born many exhibit a "catch-up" period in which excess consumption leads to increased fat (adipose tissue) and low adiponectin levels.[39] Adiponectin is a hormone produced by fat cells. This hormone regulates the metabolism of glucose and lipids.[40] This disregulation can lead to obesity, type 2 diabetes, and, ultimately cardiovascular disease. Thus, it is critically important for women to maintain a healthy lifestyle before and during pregnancy such that their babies have the best environment in which to develop.[41]

Menopause

After menopause (the cessation of menses), the risk for heart disease and stroke increases significantly for women. Coronary heart disease rates in women after menopause are two to three times higher than those in women of the same age who have not yet reached menopause. One reason appears to be related to the loss of natural estrogen. Scientists believe that during and after menopause, women experience a decrease in HDL cholesterol and an increase in LDL cholesterol and triglycerides. Increased plaque appears in the arteries, and heart attacks and strokes begin to occur. The decrease in estrogen as a result of natural and surgical menopause is associated with these changes in serum lipid profiles (blood cholesterol levels).[42]

Estrogen loss during menopause and the use of hormone therapy (HT) have inspired tremendous debate in the last several years. Observational studies in both animals and humans, carried out largely in the 1970s and 1980s, showed that HT could be beneficial in slowing the onset of heart disease. More recent clinical trials, carried out in the 1990s and early 2000s, however, showed that HT had no effect or was even dangerous. Recent examination of some of those clinical trials has shown where some of the differences in findings may lie. The increased risk appears to be greatest for women who started HT after they had been menopausal for several years or more, and those with established heart disease, especially for women on a particular regimen of HT. Women who started HT during or immediately after cessation of menstrual periods generally did not show an increased risk (see Chapter 8 for more information).[42,44] In addition, different types of medication, dosage, and routes of administration clearly affect how a woman responds.

Oral Contraceptives

Oral contraceptives (the "pill") were officially introduced in the 1960s.[45] With them came better birth control and some beneficial side effects: decreased risk of ovarian and endometrial cancers, pelvic inflammatory disease, and dysmenorrhea (painful periods). However, birth control pills also increased the risk for cardiovascular disease, especially in women who had risk factors for CVD, such as smoking and high blood pressure. Over time, scientists and drug manufacturers changed the formulation of oral contraceptives, significantly lowering dosages of estrogen and progestin, key hormonal agents. The question remained, however, as to whether the changed dosage would change the CVD risk. Studies examining the risks associated with oral contraceptives, especially the lower dosages, and CVD have shown that changing the dosage did reduce the risks for CVD, especially heart attack and stroke, but did not eliminate them. The risk of heart attack and stroke are uncommon in women of childbearing age. However, for women who are at risk for CVD, such as women who smoke and have high blood pressure, taking oral contraceptives can pose a risk.[46,47]

People who smoke, especially women on higher dose pills, may have an increase in blood pressure from oral contraceptives. Older women and obese women have the highest risk of increased blood pressure from oral contraceptives.

Concerns also have been raised regarding thromboembolism, also known as deep vein thrombosis (VTE), with oral contraceptive use. The estimated risk of VTE is low with all modern low-dose oral contraceptives; however, it is very important for the woman to check with her physician regarding her potential risk factors. Only then can the decision be made to proceed with the medication.[48]

Oral contraceptive users with a history of migraine are two to four times more likely to have an ischemic stroke than women with a history of migraine who do not use this form of birth control.[49] Studies suggest the risk is greater among women who have severe migraine headaches with "aura"—focal neurologic symptoms such as blurred vision, temporary loss of vision, seeing flashing lights or zigzag lines, or trouble speaking or moving. Experts now recommend that a woman who has migraine headaches with focal neurologic symptoms should not start combined oral contraceptives and a woman age 35 or older should choose another method if possible if she has migraine headaches even without focal neurologic symptoms. Mild or severe headaches that are not migraine-related do not rule out use of birth control pills.[50,51,52]

Because the risk of cardiovascular disease increases in oral contraceptive users with other risk factors, women should have a complete medical checkup before choosing oral contraceptives as their method of birth control.

Alcohol and Illicit Drugs

Consuming modest levels of wine or other alcohol (no more than one drink per day) can reduce the risk of coronary heart disease in women. There is, however, an increase in risk of stroke and other causes of morbidity and mortality with moderate to heavy consumption of alcohol.[53] Therefore, nondrinkers should not take this as a recommendation to begin drinking, and those who are drinking more than the recommended amount should cut back. One "drink" equals

- 1 to 1.5 fluid ounce (fl oz) of 80–100 proof alcohol,
- 5 fl oz wine, or
- 12 fl oz beer.[54]

Illicit drugs, such as cocaine, LSD (acid), and heroin, may cause short-term cardiovascular effects as well as long-term cardiovascular complications. Cocaine and LSD both increase heart rate and blood pressure while constricting the blood vessels. Cocaine can lead to medical complications such as heart attacks, strokes, heart failure, and irregular heart beats. Cocaine-related deaths are often a result of cardiac arrest.[55] Heroin slows down cardiac function during use. Its long-term effects include scarring and collapsing of the veins and bacterial infections of the blood vessels and heart valves, often leading to death. These drugs also are associated with many other short- and long-term negative effects. See Chapter 13 for more details.

Stress

Stress is a normal part of everyday life and, in fact, is essential to proper functioning of the body. External stimulation can push a person to study for a test, or to sprint the final lap in a race. A kiss from a loved one can also create stress, but most would not want to do without it. Stress also has negative side effects. The extent to which these negative side effects influence a person's sense of self and well-being differs greatly. However, continual exposure to psychological stress can damage the cardiovascular system.[56] Studies have associated heart disease with work-related stress, defined as low job control and high job demands.[57] Researchers are also investigating the link between anger in stressful conditions and increased risk of premature cardiovascular

© DWaschnig/ShutterStock, in

■ Chronic stress increases a woman's chances of heart disease, stroke and other conditions.

disease. Whether women manifest stress differently from men requires additional study.[58] What does seem clear is that stress makes both men and women more susceptible to heart disease and stroke.[59]

Compounding Risk Factors

Many risk factors affect a person's likelihood of developing CVD. Together, multiple risk factors have a cumulative effect. For example, consumption of a diet high in cholesterol and saturated fats leads to high blood cholesterol and deposition of fatty plaques in the arteries. That same diet, which is often also high in calories, leads to overweight and obesity, which strains the heart and arteries and contributes to high blood pressure and diabetes. These factors place additional strain on arteries already carrying increasing amounts of plaques. The addition of cigarette smoking compounds the problem, making the arteries fragile and more constrictive. Arteries become clogged with waste, and the supreme pump—the heart—becomes sluggish and weak. In short, the combination of these risk factors produces a scenario for disaster: heart attack, stroke, CHF, and peripheral vascular disease.

Such disaster events are not always fatal. If a woman survives the heart attack or stroke, she may be severely limited by a damaged heart or the effects of the stroke, such as impaired vision, memory, speech, or movement. Thus, even though she may be alive, the quality of her life and that of her family may be seriously diminished. Although no one can predict what will happen, establishing and maintaining good health habits early in life reduces the likelihood of cardiovascular disease and limits the effects of disease if it occurs.

Sex/Gender Differences in Cardiovascular Disease

Cardiovascular disease, particularly heart attack, is sometimes not considered a disease of women by women, their families, and even some healthcare professionals. Part of the reason may be that women present with signs and symptoms of the disease some 10 to 15 years later than men: Between the ages of 20 and 39, CVD is more prevalent in men, but by age 45, the rates of diseases of the heart in women begin to rise.[60] These differences may in part stem from estrogen loss as women age. Estrogen appears to have a positive effect on the cardiovascular system.[61] As women approach menopause, their rates of CVD begin to rise.

Overall, more women than men die from CVD. In 2007, 302,000 women died of diseases of the heart and 82,000 of cerebrovascular disease (see Figures 10.6 and 10.7).[62] Heart disease and stroke are the first and third leading causes of death for women, respectively; in contrast, heart disease is the leading cause for men, and stroke is the fifth leading cause for men. That does not imply that men are in better cardiovascular health than women—it simply means that other diseases, conditions, and behaviors affect men and their health differently than they do women. For example, the third leading cause of death in men is unintentional injuries (traffic and other accidents), while it is the sixth leading cause in women (**Table 10.6**). The signs and symptoms of a myocardial infarction (heart

Table 10.6	Top 10 Leading Causes of Death in Men and Women, 2007	

MALE	RANK	FEMALE
Diseases of the heart	1	Diseases of the heart
Malignant neoplasms	2	Malignant neoplasms
Unintentional injuries	3	Cerebrovascular diseases
Chronic lower respiratory disease	4	Chronic lower respiratory disease
Cerebrovascular disease	5	Alzheimer's disease
Diabetes mellitus	6	Unintentional injuries
Suicide	7	Diabetes mellitus
Influenza and pneumonia	8	Influenza and pneumonia
Nephritis, nephrotic syndrome and nephrosis	9	Nephritis, nephrotic syndrome and nephrosis
Alzheimer's disease	10	Septicemia

Source: Reproduced from Centers for Disease Control and Prevention, *Health United States, 2010,* www.cdc.gov/nchs/data/hus/hus10.pdf

attack) also underscore gender differences. Both men and women may experience the following symptoms:

- pain or discomfort in the chest region,
- pain or discomfort in the upper torso (trunk and arms),
- shortness of breath, and/or
- cold sweats, nausea, or dizziness.

However, women appear more prone to other symptoms, especially shortness of breath, nausea/vomiting, back or jaw pain, or unusual fatigue.[63]

Symptoms of a heart attack are sometimes milder in women than they are in men. Some women may not even be aware they are having a heart attack. These differences in symptoms present a challenge not only to the woman and her family, friends, and co-workers, but also to healthcare professionals. Cultural beliefs can play a critical role in the understanding of heart signs and symptoms.[64] Rather than a heart attack, some women may suspect gastrointestinal symptoms (gas, upset stomach) and thus not act quickly.[65]

Immediate action is essential at the first signs and symptoms of a heart attack. The sooner the person gets to treatment, preferably within the first 3 hours of symptom onset, the less heart damage may occur. Further complicating the issue is that women often experience a "silent" heart attack in which there are no signs or symptoms. This lack of symptoms puts them at great risk: 64% percent of women who experienced sudden death from CHD had no symptoms. Within 5 years of a heart attack, 47% of women 40 or older will die; among women who have had an heart attack, 6% will have a stroke within the next five years.[2] Women are 55% less likely than men to use rehabilitation, a key factor in post-heart-attack recovery.[66]

I started having chest pains, but I thought they were just due to stress. I didn't want to make a big deal of it. My doctor didn't suspect anything either—I guess I look pretty healthy. But when they did the tests, they found that I had had a "silent heart attack." I wish I had paid closer attention to the pain, and I wish that my doctor had been more sensitive about the possibility of my having a heart attack.

60-year-old woman

The reasons for these sex-related differences are not entirely clear. One key factor may be the age difference between women and men at the time of the event—women are generally older and have more compromising risk factors. Scientists are exploring these differences, but such studies take time because it is important to follow groups of individuals over decades to obtain accurate, reliable data. Such long-term studies, which have already provided important CVD data on women and men, include the Framingham Heart Study, the Nurses' Health Study, the Bogalusa Heart Study, the Rancho Bernardo Study, and many others.

Racial Differences in Cardiovascular Disease

The age-adjusted death rates for heart disease and stroke vary significantly among women in the five major U.S. designated racial and ethnic groups. Rates are highest among African American women, followed by White and Hispanic women. The lowest rates are among Asian American women.[62] The reasons for these disparities are not fully understood, though Mexican American and African American women have higher rates of obesity, high blood pressure, and diabetes than white women.

- Among Mexican American women:
  - 77% are overweight or obese and 45% are obese
  - 11% are diabetic
  - 19% have high blood pressure or are taking antihypertensive medication
  - 25% have a total cholesterol greater than 240 mg/dL or are taking cholesterol-lowering medication
  - 8% smoke
- Among African American women:
  - 78% are overweight or obese and 50% are obese
  - 23% are prediabetic and 13% have physician-diagnosed diabetes
  - 44% have high blood pressure or are taking antihypertensive medication
  - 25% have a total cholesterol greater than 240 mg/dL or are taking cholesterol-lowering medication
  - 17% smoke
- Among White women
  - 61% are overweight or obese and 33% are obese
  - 22% are prediabetic and 6% have physician-diagnosed diabetes
  - 28% have high blood pressure or are taking antihypertensive medication
  - 28% have a total cholesterol greater than 240 mg/dL or are taking cholesterol-lowering medication
  - 19% smoke
- Among Asian-American women:
  - 5.4% smoke

- Among Native American/Alaskan Native women:
  - 20% smoke[60,66–68]

Of particular concern is the number of children and youth who are also at elevated risk for CVD earlier in life because of these risk factors. Overweight is increasing among girls ages 6–11 and 12–19 years,[66] and among young women ages 18–44, only 19% met recommended aerobic activity and muscle-strengthening guidelines.[66]

Diabetes rates are rising along with obesity and high blood pressure rates. The prevalence of diabetes among women in the United States rose substantially from 8.7% in 1994 to 10.2% in 2010, and the prevalence of hypertension among women rose from 24.4% in 1988–1994 to 29.8% in 2005–2008.[66] The presence of two or more CVD risk factors compounds this risk. For example, women can lose from 3 to 5 years of life depending on the amount smoked and the level of obesity.[105]

Social Determinants

Social factors also play a critical role in the development of cardiovascular disease. Numerous factors play into these determinants: the environment in which an individual lives, the economy, resources, the healthcare system, health inequities, discrimination, as well as other local issues.

A woman living under challenging economic conditions in a location that does not have easily accessible health care, limited resources (healthy food sources, safe drinking water, safe air quality), and who has not been educated about health and staying healthy is at greatly increased risk for cardiovascular disease and its risk factors.[71] Furthermore, the force of a community or culture can have an important effect on how a woman sees herself—fat, thin, just right—what she eats, and how she maintains her health.

Cancer

Cancer is a disease characterized by uncontrolled cellular growth and reproduction. It is not new to science. Hippocrates, in the fourth century B.C., coined the term **carcinoma**, meaning a cancerous growth. More than 100 different diseases are categorized as "cancer." **Figure 10.16** summarizes the major types of cancer in women. Many distinctions may be made among these types of cancer, although they all follow similar basic processes.[72]

A **tumor**, also referred to as a neoplasm or "new growth," is any abnormal growth of cells. Some tumors are solid, whereas others known as cysts consist of a thin-walled sac filled with fluid. A **benign tumor** is one that remains localized and confined in its original growth site—that is, it does not invade the surrounding tissue or spread to distant body sites. Examples of benign tumors include skin warts or cysts. Because benign tumors are confined and localized, they often are left alone, drained, or surgically removed. Usually benign tumors are not life threatening unless they are located in a surgically inaccessible location.

In contrast to benign tumors, **malignant tumors**, also called malignant neoplasms, are capable of spreading to other tissues and organs and invading adjacent tissue, the definition of a cancerous growth.[72]

The process of cancer cell invasion and spreading is known as **metastasis**. Cancer cells circulate through the

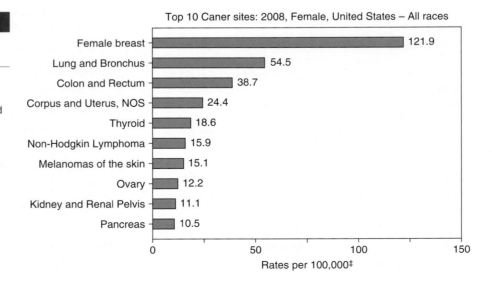

Figure 10.16

Leading Causes of Cancer Death in Women

Source: Reproduced from U.S. Cancer Statistics Working Group. (2012) United States Cancer Statistics: 1999–2008 Incidence and Mortality Web-based Report. Atlanta: U.S. Department of Health and Human Services, Centers for Disease Control and Prevention and National Cancer Institute. Available at: www.cdc.gov/uscs.

Top 10 Caner sites: 2008, Female, United States – All races

Cancer site	Rate per 100,000
Female breast	121.9
Lung and Bronchus	54.5
Colon and Rectum	38.7
Corpus and Uterus, NOS	24.4
Thyroid	18.6
Non-Hodgkin Lymphoma	15.9
Melanomas of the skin	15.1
Ovary	12.2
Kidney and Renal Pelvis	11.1
Pancreas	10.5

Rates per 100,000‡

blood or lymphatic system and can invade healthy cells in other parts of the body. These circulating cells often become trapped in the first network of capillaries that they encounter, usually the lungs. Blood leaving every organ other than the intestines travels to the lungs to get oxygenated, so the lungs are the most common site for metastasis. Blood leaving the intestines goes to the liver, the second most common site of metastasis.[73] Some cancer cells have an affinity for other receptors and, therefore, may metastasize to certain types of tissues. Once metastasis has occurred, localized surgical treatment is usually impossible.

There are two main types of **carcinogens**: those that damage genes that control cell reproduction and migration and those that enhance the growth of tumor cells. Many agents, including chemical substances, viral or bacterial carcinogens, physical agents, and natural substances in the blood can cause **carcinogenesis**. However, as noted by the American Cancer Society,

> Carcinogens do not cause cancer in every case, all the time. Substances labeled as carcinogens may have different levels of cancer-causing potential. Some may cause cancer only after prolonged, high levels of exposure. And for any particular person, the risk of developing cancer depends on many factors, including how they are exposed to a carcinogen, the length and intensity of the exposure, and the person's genetic makeup.[74]

Tobacco use is one of the major causes of carcinogenesis. Smoking cigarettes is associated with increased risk for cancers of the lung, mouth, nasal cavities, pharynx, larynx, esophagus, stomach, pancreas, liver, cervix, kidney, and bladder. The frequency of smoking, tar content, and duration of the habit all influence the initiation and promotion of cancer-cell growth.

Factors in the diet also affect the development of cancer. What a woman consumes as part of her diet is just as important as what she avoids. Saturated fat; non-nutrient food additives such as salt, nitrates, and nitrites; and alcohol all have been associated with increased risk of cancer. In contrast, vegetables and fruits containing phytochemicals (see Chapter 9) may reduce the risk for cancer.[74,75]

Radiation, occupational carcinogens such as asbestos, and even certain drugs or medications can cause cancer. Viral carcinogens also have been recognized as contributors to cancer: For example, the human papillomavirus (HPV) causes all cases of cervical cancer, and some cases of ano-genital cancer.[76]

Perspectives on Cancer

Epidemiological Overview

Cancer is the second leading cause of death for women in the United States, with an estimated 275,000 women dying from this disease in 2012.[77] Cancer is the second leading cause of death for Black, White, and Hispanic women, but is the leading cause for American Indian/Alaskan Native and Asian women.[66] Although anyone can develop cancer, most cases affect adults beginning in middle age. Most cancers are diagnosed in women age 65 and older.[78]

The most common type of cancer in new cancer cases among women in the United States is breast cancer. Breast cancer killed more than 39,000 women in 2011.[79] Death rates from breast cancer, however, have declined at about 2% a year since 1999, with the greatest decline among women younger than 50 years of age.[79] White and Black women have higher rates of new cases and deaths than other racial and ethnic groups.[80]

Lung cancer is the second most commonly diagnosed cancer among both men and women. While breast cancer is the most common cancer among women, lung cancer is the most deadly. Less than one out of every five women who develop breast cancer will die from it, but lung cancer kills most of the women who have it.

Since 1999 the incidence rates for lung cancer in women have been fairly level.[81] This decline in both sexes reflects, to a large extent, a decline in smoking rates. However, 21% of adult men and 17% of adult women still smoke.[82] The 5-year survival rate for lung cancer is low (16%), and early detection of the disease is difficult because symptoms often do not appear until the disease has reached an advanced stage.[83]

Men and women differ in their reasons for smoking. For example, men appear to find the nicotine in cigarettes makes them more assertive, while women apparently find cigarettes calming and they also enjoy "cigarette breaks" with others. Women have greater difficulties quitting smoking and are more vulnerable to relapses.[84]

Regional variations also exist. For example, new cases of lung and bronchial cancers in women ranged from 39.4 cases per 100,000 population in New Mexico to 79.5 per 100,000 in Kentucky[85] (**Figure 10.17**).

Colorectal cancer is the third leading cancer diagnosed in women, though the number of cases has declined sharply since the 1990s. Nevertheless, an estimated 25,000 women died from colorectal cancer in 2012, with the death rates rising as a woman ages.[85] When diagnosed at an early

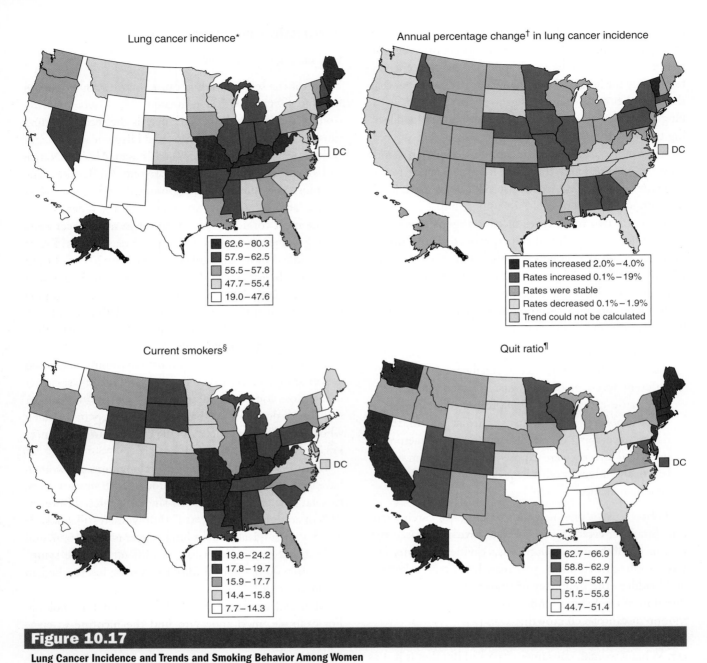

Figure 10.17

Lung Cancer Incidence and Trends and Smoking Behavior Among Women

Source: Reproduced from CDC. (2011). State-Specific Trends in Lung Cancer Incidence and Smoking–United States, 1999–2008. Available at: http://www.cdc.gov/mmwr/preview/mmwrhtml/mm6036a3.htm

stage, the death rates from this type of cancer are low. The 5-year survival rates are as high as 74% if diagnosed at a localized stage and as low as 6% if diagnosed at a distant stage.[86] Some of the major risk factors for colorectal cancer include obesity, smoking, alcoholic beverages, and a substantial consumption of meats, especially red meats.[87]

Endometrial cancer, or cancer of the uterine lining, is the fourth most common cancer in women with 46,000 cases diagnosed in 2011. In 2012, an estimated 8,000 women died from this disease. If diagnosed and treated early, there is a 96% survival rate for endometrial cancer, but only a 16% survival rate if diagnosed at a late stage. A major risk factor for endometrial cancer is estrogen exposure. This exposure comes in several ways: obesity (estrogen is contained in fat cells), estrogen therapy for postmenopausal women, late menopause, or a history of polycystic ovary syndrome.[90]

Ovarian cancer causes more deaths than any other cancer affecting the female reproductive system. Although ovarian cancer only accounts for 3% of all female cancers, nearly twice as many deaths are attributable to this cause than to endometrial cancer. A family history of ovarian or breast cancer or those with a BRCA1 or BRCA2 gene are at increased risk for developing the disease.[91]

Cervical cancer is another important form of cancer for women. This form of cancer is caused by certain "high-risk" strains of a sexually transmitted virus called human papillomavirus. Approximately 12,000 cases of cervical cancer occur every year, with an estimated 4,000 deaths—despite the fact that cervical cancer is nearly 100% preventable. Death rates from cervical cancer have declined over the past 40 years, largely due to widespread cervical cancer screening programs using the Papanicolaou (Pap) test. Other techniques and prevention methods may reduce this number even further (see Chapter 7).

Skin cancer is one of the 10 most common cancers in women, but unfortunately, this is not a reportable disease to cancer registries. However, approximately 3 million cases of basal cell and squamous cell carcinomas are diagnosed every year. Melanoma incidence cases in women are estimated at 32,000 in 2012, with an estimated 9,000 deaths. If detected at a localized stage, the 5-year survival rate for melanoma is 93%. This cancer is 10 times more prevalent in Whites than in those of African descent. Risk factors include excessive sun exposure (sun burns, sun tans, especially tanning beds), sun sensitivity, and a history of skin cancers.[92]

Racial/Ethnic and Socioeconomic Dimensions

The rates of death and disease from cancer vary by race/ethnicity as well as geography (see **Figure 10.18**). Although White women have higher rates of breast cancer, African American women are most likely to die from the disease. These racial differences in breast cancer mortality rates are due to a combination of factors, including the lower likelihood of African American women with breast cancer being diagnosed in the early disease stages and a lower survival rate in women whose disease has advanced.[93]

Because cancer risk is strongly associated with lifestyle and behavior, differences in key factors can play a critical role in an individual's health and well-being. Cultural values and belief systems can affect a person's willingness and ability to understand the need for preventive action or to seek medical care. Poor health knowledge and literacy can also make a person less likely to be aware of a problem or to seek medical care, leading to late diagnosis and poor survival. For example, some African American women believe that treatment for cancer is far worse than the disease. "Fatalismo," a belief among some Hispanic/Latina women, that "cancer is a death sentence" discourages women from seeking screening and treatment. Some Native American and Alaskan Native women believe that

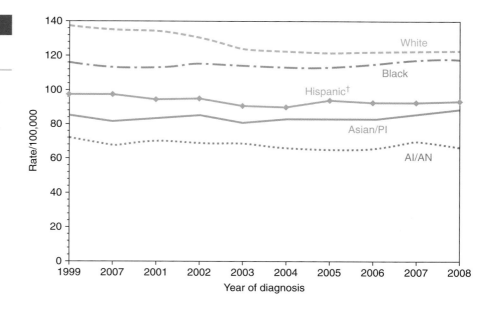

Figure 10.18

Breast Cancer Incidence in Women by Racial/Ethnic Group

Source: Reproduced from Centers for Disease Control and Prevention. (2012) Breast cancer rates by race and ethnicity. Available at: http://www.cdc.gov/cancer/breast/statistics/race.htm

speaking about an issue (breast cancer, for example), can cause it to happen. For some women of all racial and ethnic backgrounds, modesty is an issue and thus they may be reluctant to submit to a mammogram.[94–98] Individuals who are in the United States illegally have a particularly challenging time seeking and obtaining preventive screening and appropriate medical care.

Socioeconomic factors, such as lack of health insurance and/or transportation, type of job, busy work schedule, low income, or need for childcare, can impede women's access to care. These factors affect a woman's home and family and can produce high levels of stress that, over time, can have negative effects on health. Wealthier and more educated individuals of any racial or ethnic group tend to have better health than those less fortunate. Compared to people living in poverty, individuals of higher incomes smoke less, eat a healthier diet, have less overweight/obesity, and are more likely to exercise regularly. And, as pointed out by Cutler and colleagues, "education improves health." This begins in childhood. The healthier a woman is, the greater her chances of being able to advance intellectually and economically.[99]

To be effective, screening programs must be culturally sensitive and readily available. Language barriers, lack of health insurance, lack of availability and access to health care, and mistrust of the medical profession must be addressed if women are to advance and protect their health.

Economic Dimensions

The National Institutes of Health (NIH) estimates that cancer costs more than $227 billion a year, with $104 billion for direct medical costs and more than $123 billion in lost productivity.[99] Cancer patients and their families also face burdens in terms of time, reduced employment opportunities, payments for cancer treatments not covered by insurance, and emotional costs of pain and suffering.

Global Perspective

Cancer knows no boundaries and is estimated to be responsible for one in eight global deaths. Furthermore, the majority of cancer deaths, 60%, are to be found in low and middle-income countries, due, in part, to later stage diagnosis that has a negative effect on treatment options and survival rates. Limited access to the latest and most effective treatments is also a major issue.[100]

Better prevention, early detection, and improved treatment have helped many nations lower cancer incidence and mortality rates. Yet, in many developing countries, cancer rates continue to rise, especially in those where Western lifestyles—cigarette smoking, high-fat diets, and less physical activity—have been adopted.[101]

Breast Conditions

More than half of all women go through the frightening experience of finding a lump in a breast. In the majority of cases, the lump is benign and needs no treatment, but being able to understand the issues and concerns about breast conditions is an important dimension of women's health.

Benign Breast Diseases

Most breast lumps are not cancer. **Fibrocystic breast disease**, also called **cystic mastitis**, is the most common breast disorder and the most frequent cause of a breast lump in women younger than age 25. This disease is most prevalent in women between the ages of 30 and 50.[102] Typical symptoms of this condition include lumpy, tender breasts, particularly during the week before menses. Fibrocystic changes also may cause pain and swelling. In such cases, the doctor may recommend wearing a supportive bra and taking over-the-counter pain medications.[103] Although fibrocystic breast changes are not a medical problem, affected women may find it more difficult to detect lumps during breast self-exams.

Only a small subgroup of women with fibrocystic breast disease is at increased risk for breast cancer. These women have an atypical cell condition known as **hyperplasia**, which can be diagnosed by a breast **biopsy**, a procedure in which a small sample of breast tissue is removed and examined under a microscope.

Another nonmalignant form of breast tumor is **fibroadenoma**, which is common in women in their 20s and 30. This type of tumor produces a firm, movable, nontender lump. Fibroadenomas are usually removed both to confirm the diagnosis and to prevent further damage to breast tissue from continued localized tumor growth.[104]

Breast Cancer

Breast cancer is a frightening, conflicting, and sometimes misleading condition for women. Understanding breast cancer is important for all women, because this disease is one of the most treatable cancers if it is detected early.

The classification system for breast cancer consists of five levels:

- In situ stage breast cancer can be diagnosed by mammogram, but the tumors are usually too small to be felt. The five-year survival rate for in situ tumors is nearly 100%.

- Stage I breast cancer remains localized to the breast, generally is smaller than 2 cm in size, and has not spread to the lymph nodes.

- Stage II breast cancer tumors generally are larger—2 to 5 cm in size—and have not spread to the lymph nodes. Stage II tumors also may be smaller than 2 to 5 cm but have spread to nearby lymph nodes.

- Stage III tumors are growths that are larger than 5 cm in size or that have grown into the chest wall, skin, or distant lymph nodes.

- Stage IV tumors are classified as growths that have spread to other parts of the body.

Five-year breast cancer survival rates decline with increasing size and invasiveness of the tumor.[105]

Risk Factors

Several factors can increase a woman's chance of getting breast cancer.

- *Genetics:* Women with mothers or sisters (first-degree relatives) who have had breast cancer are generally at double the risk of developing the disease. Approximately 5–10% of breast cancer cases are believed to be inherited. Most of the hereditary cases result from mutations in two breast cancer genes: BRCA1 and BRCA2. These genes reduce the risk for breast cancer by manufacturing a protein that prevents abnormal cell growth. However, if the gene is mutated, it increases a woman's risk for breast cancer, ovarian cancer, and pancreatic cancer.

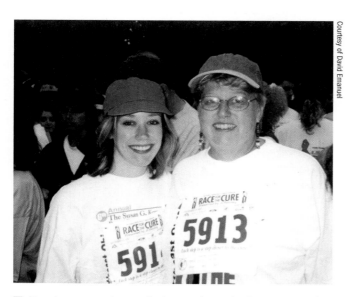

Courtesy of David Emanuel

■ Breast cancer survivors and advocates have raised awareness and billions of dollars for research.

Mutated BRCA1 or BRCA2 account for up to 10% of all breast cancer cases. Although BRCA1 and BRCA2 are generally the most common gene defects leading to breast cancer in women, other mutations also exist.

Although any woman can have such mutated genes, they are most common in women of Ashkenazi Jewish (generally of Eastern European origin), Norwegian, Icelandic, or Dutch ancestry. The increased frequency of mutated genes may be more common in these groups because of shared ancestry over many years.[106]

However, genetics are not the only factor. While White women are more likely to develop breast cancer, African American women are more likely to die of it. Genetic differences may play a part—it is possible that African American women are more likely have more aggressive tumors—but disparities in access to health care likely play a larger part. African American women may be less likely than White women to have cancers identified or obtain treatment in the early stages of the disease.

- *Hormones:* Exposure to two hormones, estrogen and progesterone, influence a woman's development and her ability to become pregnant and bear children. These hormones can also create some increased risk depending on a woman's lifetime exposure, the type of medication used, and how it is administered. Some examples follow:

  - Women who have early onset of menstruation (less than 12 years of age) or later menopause (after 50 years of age) have a somewhat greater risk. Part of the reason may be the longer exposure to the naturally occurring hormones estrogen and progesterone.

  - Never having had a child or having a child later in life (after age 30) may present an increased risk. These hormones play a crucial role in pregnancy.

  - Overweight and obesity: Estrogen is made largely in the ovaries; however, it is also manufactured in fat cells. After menopause, the estrogen in a woman's body comes largely from fat cells. The heavier the woman, the greater the exposure.[107]

  - Hormone replacement therapy (HT): Studies from the late 1990s have suggested that the use of estrogen alone or estrogen and progesterone together increase the risk of breast cancer.[147] However, more recent meta-analyses do not support those findings. Short-term use does not appear to pose a threat in most women. The threat of breast cancer development with the long-term use of estrogen plus progesterone is not absolutely clear. Furthermore, some women, especially those who drink alcohol, may be more susceptible to negative effects of HT.[109,110]

■ Oral contraceptives: While oral contraceptives are safe for most women, some women at risk for breast cancer and should not take oral contraceptives. They include women over 35 who smoke and/or have high blood pressure, women who have had or are at risk for heart disease or stroke, women who have migraines, women who have breast or estrogen-dependent cancers, and women who have liver disease. On the positive side, oral contraceptives can reduce risks for the following diseases: pelvic inflammatory disease, ovarian and endometrial cancers, colorectal cancer, and bone loss (osteopenia).[111,112,113]

My aunt was diagnosed with breast cancer when I was in high school. I couldn't believe it—she's only 10 years older than me, and has always been more like a big sister than an aunt. She had to have a lumpectomy and was really worried for a while. But almost four years later there's no sign of the cancer returning, and she just completed a marathon!

18-year-old woman

Screening and Diagnosis

Many risk factors for breast cancer cannot be modified by lifestyle behaviors. Early detection of breast cancer, however, can be lifesaving. Indeed, the prognosis for breast cancer strongly depends on the stage at which it is detected. There are three basic methods for early detection of breast cancer, all of which are important prevention behaviors:

■ **Breast self-examination** (BSE) consists of the systematic palpation of the breast tissue of each breast while lying on one's back. The most common sign of breast cancer is a new lump or mass in the breast, although other signs, such as swelling of the breast, skin dimpling, or nipple changes, may be present as well. The American Cancer Society recommends that women over the age of 20 years examine their breasts monthly after menses and at the same time each month. For women who have reached menopause, regular BSE should be done on a scheduled monthly basis. In addition to examining for lumps, women should check for breast discharge. **Figure 10.19** provides detailed guidance on the BSE procedure.[112]

■ Clinical breast examinations (CBE) are conducted by a woman's healthcare provider and should be performed every 3 years for women ages 20–39 and every year for women age 40 or older. The exam consists of observing the breasts for signs such as dimpling, feeling the breast and underarm for abnormal areas or swollen lymph nodes, and squeezing the nipples to check for discharge.[113]

■ **Mammography**, a low-dose radiograph of the breast tissue, can detect smaller breast lesions that cannot be felt through BSE or CBE. This technology has the potential to detect breast cancer at its earliest stages of development. Mammography involves compressing the breast between two flat disks. Two radiographs are taken of each breast, and one is taken from above the breast. Although mammograms can detect some breast cancers before they can be felt, other tumors may be felt through BSE or CBE that could not be detected by a mammogram. For this reason, it is extremely important to perform regular BSEs and have regular CBEs.

The National Cancer Institute and the American Cancer Society recommend screening mammograms for women age 40 years or older every 1 to 2 years. Women with a family history of breast cancer should discuss when to begin mammograms with their healthcare provider.[116]

Although a breast tumor may be suspected with an examination or mammography, the ultimate diagnosis is made by biopsy. The biopsy removes a sample of tissue, which is then examined for abnormal cell growth.

Magnetic resonance imaging (MRI) has been in use for years, but until recently has not been used for breast

Table 10.7   Breast Cancer Survival Rates

Stage At Diagnosis	Stage Distribution (%)	5-Year Relative Survival (%)
Localized (confined to primary site)	60	98.4
Regional (spread to regional lymph nodes)	30	83.9
Distant (cancer has metastasized)	5	23.8
Unknown (unstaged)	2	50.7

Source: Reproduced from Centers for Disease Control and Prevention. (2012). *Breast cancer rates by race and ethnicity.* Available at: http://www.cdc.gov/cancer/breast/statistics/race.htm

Breast Self–Examination

Breast self–examination should be done once a month so you become familiar with the usual appearance and feel of your breasts. Familiarity makes it easier to notice any changes in the breast from month to month. Early discovery of a change from what is "normal" is the main idea behind BSE. The outlook is much better if you detect cancer in an early stage.

If you menstruate, the best time to do BSE is 2 or 3 days after your period ends, when your breasts are least likely to be tender or swollen. If you no longer menstruate, pick a day such as the first day of the month, to remind yourself it is time to do BSE.

Here is one way to do BSE:

1. Stand before a mirror. Inspect both breasts for anything unusual, such as any discharge from the nipples or puckering, dimpling, or scaling of the skin.

The next two steps are designed to emphasize any change in the shape or contour of your breasts. As you do them, you should be able to feel your chest muscles tighten.

2. Watching closely in the mirror, clasp your hands behind your head and press your hands forward.

3. Next, press your hands firmly on your hips and bow slightly toward your mirror as you pull your shoulders and elbows forward.

Some women do the next part of the exam in the shower because fingers glide over soapy skin, making it easy to concentrate on the texture underneath.

4. Raise your left arm. Use three or four fingers of your right hand to explore your left breast firmly, carefully, and thoroughly. Beginning at the outer edge, press the flat part of your fingers in small circles, moving the circles slowly around the breast. Gradually work toward the nipple. Be sure to cover the entire breast. Pay special attention to the area between the breast and the underarm, including the underarm itself. Feel for any unusual lump or mass under the skin.

5. Gently squeeze the nipple and look for discharge. (If you have any discharge during the month— whether or not it is during BSE—see your doctor.) Repeat steps 4 and 5 on your right breast.

6. Steps 4 and 5 should be repeated lying down. Lie flat on your back with your left arm over your head and a pillow or folded towel under your left shoulder. This position flattens the breast and makes it easier to examine. Use the same circular motion described earlier. Repeat the exam on your right breast.

Figure 10.19

Breast self-exam.

cancer screening. The scans appear to be especially usefully in pre- and perimenopausal women, especially those who have dense breast tissue. For women who are at increased risk for breast cancer, MRI scans appear to be better at detecting tumors at an earlier stage. However, sometimes the test can show abnormalities when none exist. Therefore, this screening test is still being studied in a series of clinical trials.[117,118,119]

Treatment and Reconstruction

Surgery is the primary treatment for breast cancer, although it may be combined with radiation therapy or hormone therapy. There are several types of breast cancer surgery.

- A **lumpectomy** is often used for early-stage localized tumors when it is possible to remove only the tumor and some surrounding tissue. A separate incision may be made to remove the axillary lymph nodes (lymph nodes in the armpit area). In women with early cancer, a lumpectomy with subsequent radiation therapy has become the primary alternative to modified radical mastectomy. Lumpectomies are usually limited to those breast tumors that are well defined and less than 1 to 2 inches in total diameter.

- A **partial or segmental mastectomy** involves the removal of some breast tissue and some of the lymph nodes.

- A **simple mastectomy** involves the complete removal of the breast but not the lymph nodes under the arm or the chest wall muscles.

- A **radical mastectomy** is the removal of the entire affected breast, the underlying chest muscles, and the lymph nodes under the arm. Although once a very common surgery, this procedure is used less often today because of the disfigurement and the side effects it causes.

- A **modified radical mastectomy** has become the standard surgical procedure for most breast cancers that require removal of the entire breast. It involves removing the breast, some of the lymph nodes, and the lining over the chest muscles. This procedure has survival rates comparable to those with the radical mastectomy, but it is more conducive to breast reconstruction and results in greater mobility and reduced swelling.[121]

Adjuvant therapies—treatments that enhance surgical effectiveness—include **chemotherapy**, hormone therapy, and **radiation therapy**. Chemotherapy and hormone therapy may be used to treat localized tumors, as well as to control metastatic conditions. Hormone therapy may block the effects of certain hormones that promote the growth of some breast cancers. Tamoxifen is the most commonly used anti-estrogen drug. It is also being studied as a chemopreventive agent to reduce the risk of breast cancer in high-risk women. Although studies from the Breast Cancer Prevention Trial have shown that tamoxifen can prevent some cases of breast cancer, some users have reported serious side effects including endometrial cancer and blood clots in the lungs. Raloxifene, a drug used to reduce osteroporosis

in women, can also be effective in treating breast cancer. Like tamoxifen, raloxifene reduced invasive breast cancer by about 50%, but it was more effective in reducing uterine cancer and had a lower risk of causing blood clots. However, both drugs still increase the risk of blood clots.[122,123]

Targeted therapy can also be used. In this type of therapy, special substances such as monoclonal antibodies or tyrosine kinase inhibitors, such as Herceptin, attack specific cancer cells without killing normal cells.[123] In addition, other, even more advanced therapies are currently under investigation. However, they are in clinical trial stage—a period in which new drugs are thoroughly examined and compared to standard therapies to determine which is more effective.

After mastectomy, a woman faces the decision of whether to undergo breast reconstruction. Reconstruction of breast tissue may be an important part of breast cancer recovery for some women. The degree of difficulty associated with reconstruction varies with the extent of breast cancer surgery.

In addition, emotional support and social support are important components of recovery. Support groups may provide valuable information and assistance with physical and psychological breast cancer recovery issues.

Gynecological Conditions

A variety of malignant and benign conditions can develop in a woman's upper or lower reproductive tract. This section reviews major benign and malignant conditions of the cervix, uterus, and ovaries; it also discusses the risk factors, screening, and treatment of these conditions.

Benign Cervical Changes

Polyps are small benign growths that develop in the endocervical canal, often after the onset of menstruation. Polyps usually produce mild symptoms such as abnormal vaginal bleeding or discharge. Although they are rarely cancerous, the growths should still be examined. Treatment of a cervical polyp consists of removing the polyp and examining the tissue to rule out malignancy.

Cervical dysplasia, which involves abnormal changes in the cells of the cervix, is usually benign condition. It is considered precancerous, however, because severe, untreated **dysplasia** can result in invasive cervical cancer. Low-grade or mild dysplasia usually occurs in women from the ages of 25 to 35 years and often can be detected with a Pap smear. High-grade or moderate to severe dysplasia refers to the presence of a large number of precancerous cells covering the surface of the cervix. Also referred to as **carcinoma-in-situ**, severe dysplasia is more likely to become cancerous but can be successfully cured if detected and treated rapidly. Treatment varies depending on the severity of the dysplasia.[132]

Cervical Cancer*

It's Your Health

The cervix is technically part of the uterus, but because characteristics and risk factors for uterine and cervical cancer are distinctive, they are discussed separately.

Cervical cancer is a type of uterine cancer affecting the lower part of the uterus, which is referred to as the cervical canal. Most cancers of the cervix originate on the cells lining the surface of the cervix. Cervical cancer is classified into five stages, 0 through IV:[133,134]

- In its localized first stage, or carcinoma in situ (stage 0), cervical cancer involves only the cervix's innermost lining.

- Stage I cancer remains in the cervix only. There are two stages of this level: Stage IA and IB; in stage IB, the cancer is advanced slightly farther than in IA.

- Stage II cancer has spread beyond the cervix but not to the pelvic wall. Stage II cancer is defined either as Stage IIA or Stage II B. In Stage IIB, the cancer has spread into the tissue around uterus.

- Stage III cancer has spread to the pelvic wall and the vagina, and may affect the kidney. Again, it is presented in two sub stages: Stage IIIA and Stage IIIB.

- Stage IV cancer has spread past the pelvic wall and may be found in the bladder or rectum. It has two sub stages: Stage IVA and Stage IVB. In Stage IVB the cancer has spread to other body parts—liver, lungs, or distant lymph nodes.[135]

As with other forms of cancer, survival rates decline as the condition becomes more invasive.

Risk Factors

Cervical cancer is primarily caused by persistent infection with certain high-risk strains of the human papillomavirus (HPV). Some strains of HPV can cause genital warts, while others can (in some cases) lead to cervical cancer. HPV is a sexually transmitted infection that most sexually active women contract during their 20s. In fact, nearly 80% of women will have HPV at some point in their lives. Most women who become infected with HPV will clear the virus on their own, through their body's natural immune response. A few women will not clear the virus, however, and instead develop a long-term persistent infection. These women are at higher risk for developing cervical cancer.

Other factors that may contribute to the development of cervical cancer include: lower immune system suppression (often from taking immunosuppressant drugs), having HIV/AIDS, having multiple sexual partners, having other sexually transmitted diseases, smoking cigarettes, having a mother who took the drug diethylstilbestrol (DES), and having a family history of cervical cancer.[126] Women age 30 or older can now be tested for HPV when they get their Pap smear.

Invasive cervical cancer rarely occurs in women who have regular gynecological examinations. When it does, however, symptoms may include bleeding between menstrual periods, spotting after intercourse, and increased vaginal discharge. By the time symptoms of cervical cancer appear, a tumor is usually quite large and may have already invaded nearby tissue.

Screening and Diagnosis

Cervical cancer is one of the few cancers that is effectively preventable through regular screening. The Pap test, which is also known as a **Pap smear**, provides a method of screening for the cellular changes before cancer develops and to detect cancer at its earliest stages.

A newer screening method, the HPV test, looks for the DNA of cancer-causing types of HPV. The HPV test was first approved in the United States by the Food and Drug Administration (FDA) for follow-up evaluation in women whose Pap results are uncertain—typically referred to as ASC-US (atypical squamous cells of undetermined significance).

The American Cancer Society (ACS), the American College of Obstetrics and Gynecology (ACOG), and the U.S. Preventive Services Task Force have released new guidelines for cervical cancer screening.[130] There are slight variations among the three groups in regard to screening guidelines. In general, however, all three groups recommend that women begin cervical cancer screening at age 21. Note that ACOG does not recommend screening prior to the age of 21, while the other two groups recommend that screening commence 3 years after the onset of sexual activity. The details of screening recommendations are delineated in Table X: Cancer Screening Guidelines.

Women age 30 or older can have a Pap test with an HPV test; if both are normal, she can safely wait to have a repeat test in three years. Having a positive HPV test does not mean that a woman will get cervical cancer; it just means that she should be followed more closely by her healthcare provider. If a Pap smear is abnormal, regardless of the results of the HPV test, the clinician will want to perform a colposcopy and possibly a biopsy to view the cervical cells more closely. If Pap test results are inconclusive (also referred to as ASC-US), the HPV test can help the clinician clarify a woman's risk of cervical cancer. A negative HPV test means a woman is not at risk of developing cervical cancer in the next few years. Even when results are negative, all women should still continue to visit their healthcare provider for an annual exam. For more information on HPV, see Chapter 7.

Treatment

Treatment following an abnormal Pap smear depends on the results of the cervical biopsy. Inflammation of the cervix, known as **cervicitis**, may be associated with a vaginal infection or discharge that requires only local treatment with specific vaginal creams or suppositories. Treatment for dysplasia depends on its severity and usually consists of cryosurgery, cone biopsy, or laser cone biopsy.[131]

Cryosurgery destroys tissue by a freezing process. It is most often used to treat mild or moderate dysplasia. As a procedure, cryosurgery has the advantage of producing little or no discomfort. It also presents few risks for complications, such as bleeding, further infection, or infertility from scarring. A watery vaginal discharge is common for about 2 weeks after cryosurgery. It is generally recommended that women avoid intercourse, douching, or tampons during this recovery time.

A cone biopsy (or **conization**) is considered to be both a diagnostic and a therapeutic procedure because it provides tissue for an accurate diagnosis while removing the abnormal tissue. Cone biopsy procedures are less common today than they were a few years ago because of the widespread use of colposcopy. **Colposcopy** is performed in the physician's office using a **colposcope**, a special microscope that permits close examination of the cervix and vagina as well as biopsy.

Treatment of cervical cancer depends on the tumor's stage when diagnosed. Carcinoma-in-situ may be treated with cone biopsy in a woman who wishes to have more children. Surgery to remove abnormal tissue in or near the cervix will remove the tumor but leave the uterus and the ovaries intact. Definitive treatment of carcinoma-in-situ, however, may require a hysterectomy, surgical removal of the uterus, to ensure complete removal of the cancerous cells. Lymph nodes, as well as the fallopian tubes and ovaries, may also need to be removed. Depending on the stage of the cancer, radiation therapy or chemotherapy may be used as adjuvant therapy. Even after hysterectomy, a small percentage of women experience a recurrence of cancer in the vagina, so lifelong gynecological follow-up is important.[131]

Benign Uterine Conditions

Fibroids are benign tumors composed of muscular and fibrous tissue in the uterus (see **Figure 10.20**) and have different names depending of the type of fibroid: fibromyomas, leiomyomas, or myomas. The cause of uterine fibroids is not entirely understood. Hormones (estrogen and progesterone), other bodily chemicals such as insulin-growth factor, and, perhaps, genes may contribute to their development.[132] Risk factors for uterine fibroids also vary. Heredity and race appear to play a role. Fibroids are more common in Black women than in any other race. Clinical studies are also investigating whether obesity affects their development and whether oral contraceptives may be a deterrent.[132]

Fibroids often begin developing in women between the ages of 25 and 35. They are the primary cause of an abnormally enlarged uterus and one of the most common reasons for hysterectomy. Although single fibroid tumors occur, multiple tumors are more common. Symptoms depend

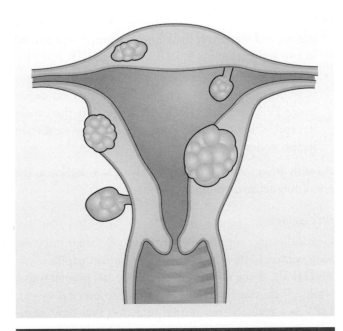

Figure 10.20

Uterine Fibroids.

on the size and location of the tumors and may include the following:

- Irregular vaginal bleeding
- Vaginal discharge
- Pain in the lower back
- Pain during sexual intercourse
- Frequent urination

Fibroids may grow under the influence of estrogen produced during pregnancy, from oral contraceptives, or from HT. They often shrink and disappear with menopause. These tumors are usually detected during routine pelvic examinations because they create an enlarged and irregular uterus.

Hormone-based treatments can temporarily reduce the size of the fibroid and relieve symptoms. A gonadotropin-releasing hormone (GnRH) agonist may be used to block the production of hormones, particularly estrogen, by the ovary. The most commonly used GnRH agonist in the United States is Lupron, which is given by an injection either once a month or every 3 months. Fibroids usually regrow, however, once treatment stops.

Surgery may be indicated for fibroids if they cause severe pain or bleeding. Surgery involves removing either the fibroid alone (**myomectomy**) or the entire uterus (hysterectomy). A hysteroscopic resection may be used for certain types of fibroids; in this procedure, a fiber-optic scope is inserted through the vagina while a dilation and curettage is used to remove the fibroid.

Nonsurgical procedures are another option to remove fibroids. In uterine artery embolization, a surgeon injects small particles of plastic or gelatin sponge through a catheter placed in the uterine artery. The particles block the blood supply to the fibroid, resulting in the death of the fibroid tissue. The fibroid shrinks and symptoms are usually relieved without the need for surgery. Focused ultrasound surgery is a surgery that uses an MRI scanner to locate the fibroids and then uses high-frequency and high-energy sound waves to destroy the fibroids.

Endometriosis is another benign condition of the uterus. In this condition, tissue that looks and acts like endometrial tissue begins to grow outside the uterine lining. This progressive condition is most common in women ages 30 to 40 years. Because endometrial tissue responds to hormonal influences during the menstrual cycle, women who have this disorder often feel pain just before or during menstruation. Endometriosis also may cause abdominal upset during menstruation and abnormal vaginal bleeding.

Many women, however, have advanced lesions without any symptoms.

For those with minimal or no symptoms or those women who do not want to have children, regular gynecological check-ups (every 6 to 12 months), exercise/relaxation efforts, and the use of anti-inflammatory medications such as ibuprophen (Advil) or naproxen (Aleve) may be sufficient to manage any symptoms of discomfort.

For others, the options include pain medications, hormonal medications, or surgery. Hormones can prevent ovulation and associated discomfort. However, hormonal therapy does not reverse damage that has already occurred or prevent scarring. When hormonal drugs fail to relieve symptoms of pain or when the endometriosis has progressed to the point of forming large cysts, surgery may be indicated. Through operative **laparoscopy**, deposits of endometriosis as well as more extensive disease involving cysts and adhesions can be removed using either electrocautery (burning of tissue) or a laser. The most radical surgery, as well as a more definitive cure for endometriosis, involves a complete hysterectomy that includes removal of the uterus, the fallopian tubes, and ovaries.[133]

Endometrial hyperplasia is an increase in the number of normal cells lining the uterus. Although the condition is not cancer, it may develop into cancer in some women if left untreated. Hyperplasia is caused by a constant production of estrogen and a lack of progesterone, which results in an abnormal thickening of the endometrium. Its most common symptoms are heavy menstrual periods and bleeding between periods. Treatment depends on the extent of the condition, and on the age of the woman. Young women are usually treated with progesterone, and the endometrial tissue is checked often. Hyperplasia in women near or after menopause may be treated with hormones if the condition is not severe. Hysterectomy is the usual treatment for severe cases.[134]

Malignant Uterine Tumors

Uterine cancer typically begins in the tissue lining of the uterus, the **endometrium**. Endometrial cancer is most common in women age 55 or older. Carcinoma-in-situ is found only on the surface layer of the endometrium. As the cancer progresses to stage I, it spreads to the muscle wall of the uterus. Stage II cancer spreads to the cervix and, possibly, the tissue supporting the cervix. By stage III, cancer has spread to the vagina, pelvic lymph nodes, and other membranes or organs in the pelvic cavity. The final stage of cancer involves the bladder, rectum, and possibly the abdominal lymph nodes.[135,136]

Risk Factors

Endometrial cancer accounts for most uterine cancers. The greatest risk factor for endometrial cancer is being older than 55 years of age. Risk factors of uterine cancer appear to involve excess stimulation of endometrial cell proliferation by estrogen in the absence of progesterone. Obesity increases endometrial cancer risk, perhaps owing to estrogen production in fat cells. Other risk factors include high blood pressure, diabetes, early menarche (before age 12), late menopause (after age 55), and never being pregnant. Failure to ovulate and a history of infertility also increase risk and may be associated with an estrogen imbalance. Other risk factors include postmenopausal long-term, high-dose estrogen replacement therapy.

Family history of endometrial cancer and personal history of breast, ovarian, or colon cancer increase a woman's risk as well. Finally, women using tamoxifen treatment for breast cancer are also at higher risk. Further research is needed to ascertain the mechanisms and roles of all these risk factors for endometrial cancer.[137]

Screening and Diagnosis

Because endometrial cancer affects the inside of the uterus, the tumor initially cannot be seen or felt during a pelvic examination. Unfortunately, a pelvic exam and Pap smear are only partially effective in the diagnosis of endometrial cancer and the disease is not usually detected until symptoms appear. The most common symptom of endometrial cancer after menopause is vaginal bleeding. Other symptoms include pain in the pelvic area, difficult or painful urination, pain during intercourse, and change in bowel patterns.

The American Cancer Society recommends that women at increased risk for endometrial cancer (i.e., those with a history of infertility or obesity) have an endometrial biopsy at menopause. Women on unopposed estrogen replacement therapy should have such biopsies repeated on a regular basis. A **transvaginal ultrasound** also has proven useful as a screening tool for endometrial cancer.

Diagnosis of endometrial cancer is made by biopsy, ultrasound, dilation and curettage (D&C), or **hysteroscopy**. These procedures permit the evaluation of the tissue and cells lining the uterine cavity.

Treatment

Treatment of endometrial cancer depends on several factors, including the stage of the disease. Because uterine cancer may spread rapidly, treatment of early-stage disease involves removal of the uterus as well as the fallopian tubes and ovaries. A combination of surgery and radiotherapy is effective in the treatment of localized disease. Regional spread of the cancer outside of the uterus is treatable by radiation. Advanced, metastatic endometrial cancer is generally treated by the administration of progesterone, which results in prolonged survival but not cure. Treatment for later-stage disease includes removal of not only the uterus, fallopian tubes, and ovaries, but also the cervix, part of the vagina, and lymph nodes.[138,139]

Benign Ovarian Growths

Cysts are fluid-filled growths that are extremely common. Ovarian cysts are usually benign and rarely cause discomfort or pain. If symptoms do occur, they often include pain or pressure in the pelvic cavity, irregular periods, and pain during intercourse.

Different types of cysts exist, depending on the tissue that makes up the cyst. The most common type results from the follicle that surrounds a mature egg. If the follicle does not rupture to release the egg during ovulation, it becomes a cyst. Many of these cysts go away without treatment within a few months.

Several treatments are available. Birth control pills are a common treatment for women who have recurrent cysts. If the cyst does not resolve, then surgery may be required. Laparoscopy, which is only mildly invasive, is often used for small cysts. Laparotomy, which involves an abdominal incision, is preferred for larger cysts and tumors.[140]

Polycystic ovarian syndrome, a condition that affects women of reproductive age, causes the formation of numerous cysts in the ovaries. The disorder results from increased levels and, often, an imbalance of hormones, including estrogen and testosterone. Women with polycystic ovarian syndrome are often obese (a probable effect of excess estrogen) and may have obesity-related risk factors: diabetes, high blood pressure, and high cholesterol levels. In addition, because of the effects of testosterone, some women may experience excess body or facial hair. The treatment for this condition may includes losing weight and hormonal medications, such as birth control pills to regularize the menstrual cycle, and anti-testosterone medication. Sometimes, medications used for diabetes may also be used.[141]

Ovarian Cancer

Ovarian cancer, the fifth leading cancer death in women, causes more deaths than any other cancer of the female reproductive system. This cancer usually affects women around the time of menopause or later (ages 50 to 70).

There are four stages considered in the diagnosis of ovarian cancer:

- Stage I: Cancer cells are limited to the ovaries.
- Stage II: Cancer cells have migrated from the ovaries to other parts of the pelvis.
- Stage III: Cancer cells have spread to the lymph nodes or other areas inside the abdominal cavity.
- Stage IV: Cancer cells have moved outside the abdomen and pelvis to other organ systems such as the lungs, liver, or other organs.[142]

Risk Factors

The risk factors for ovarian cancer are not fully understood and do not mean that a woman will get the disease. However, several risk factors are associated with the disease:

- A family or personal history of cancer, especially breast, uterine, colon, or rectal
- Age greater than 55 years
- Never been pregnant
- Possibly the use of hormone replacement therapy, especially estrogen

Other potential risk factors include obesity, hormone replacement therapy, and certain fertility drugs. However, it is not yet clear whether they are strong predictive risk factors.[193]

Screening and Diagnosis

Ovarian cancer, often called the "silent cancer," usually remains asymptomatic until it is relatively advanced, and cannot be detected by Pap smears. Early detection is best accomplished through regular pelvic examinations, transvaginal ultrasound, and a laboratory test for an ovarian tumor marker in the blood, called CA-125. Elevated levels of CA-125 are associated with ovarian cancer, but also may indicate other conditions.

Early symptoms of ovarian cancer include pelvic pressure, abdominal swelling, gas pains, indigestion, and vague abdominal discomfort. These symptoms are rarely attributed to ovarian cancer because they are also symptoms of other common benign conditions. Diagnosis of ovarian cancer is confirmed through ultrasound and/or biopsy.

Treatment

Definitive treatment for ovarian cancer consists of surgery, radiation, and chemotherapy. Surgical treatment involves removal of the uterus, fallopian tubes, and ovaries. If a woman desires to have children and has a slow-growing tumor, her doctor may remove only the affected ovary. Chemotherapy and radiation therapies are used after surgery to destroy remaining cancer cells and improve survival.[93]

Other Cancers of Special Concern to Women

Women are susceptible to cancer anywhere in their bodies. Lung cancer, colorectal cancer, and skin cancer, however, all deserve special consideration. The following section discusses the risk factors, screening guidelines, and treatment for each of these cancers.

Lung Cancer

Lung cancer is the leading cause of death among White, Black, Asian/Pacific Islander, and American Indian/Alaskan Native women and the second leading cause of death among Hispanic women.[93] Lung cancer is almost twice as deadly as breast cancer, although breast cancer is twice as common in women: 227,000 estimated new cases of breast cancer compared to 110,000 new cases of lung cancer in 2012. Although overall death rates from lung cancer declined during the 1990s, they have remained relatively stable for women since then. New lung cancer cases and deaths in women vary considerably by state. Some of the lowest rates of new cases in women are in the West while some of the highest are in the Northeast and Midwest. Death rates also vary, with the highest female death rates in Kentucky, West Virginia, Nevada, and Delaware.[93]

Most cases of lung cancer start in the lining of the bronchi, but the disease can originate anywhere in the lungs. Lung cancer develops over many years, and it often spreads before it can be detected radiographically. Causes of lung cancer vary, but most cases share a common factor—a persistent exposure to lung irritants, particularly those that are inhaled, such as cigarette smoke.

Risk Factors

Although exposure to radon, asbestos, radioactive materials, and some industrial compounds has been associated with lung cancer, cigarette smoking is clearly the most significant risk factor. This risk factor is responsible for more than 90% of lung cancer cases and almost 80% of lung cancer deaths.[143] A diagnosis of cancer usually reflects the cumulative effect of many years of smoking. Lung cancer in women appears to be different than lung cancer in men. Women who develop lung cancer typically have better survival rates that do men, possibly because women may metabolize chemicals in cigarettes differently than men. Furthermore, female hormones may also affect cancer growth.[144]

Secondhand smoke is also a risk factor. An individual living with a smoker has a 30% greater risk of developing lung cancer. Each year, over 3,000 nonsmoking adults die of lung cancer as a result of breathing secondhand smoke. A family history of lung cancer may increase a person's risk, although this increase may be associated with exposure to secondhand tobacco smoke from smoking family members as opposed to being a hereditary factor.[145]

> *My mom died of lung cancer at the age of 50. She never smoked a day in her life. But my dad smoked, my uncle who lived with us smoked, all her friends smoked, and many of her co-workers smoked in her office before her workplace became smoke-free. It makes me so angry when I see people smoking. Don't they realize that they're not just killing themselves but they're also killing their family and friends?*
>
> **32-year-old woman**

Workplace exposure to asbestos has been, especially in the past, a substantial risk factor for specific type of lung cancer called mesothelioma. Today, with much more stringent workplace regulations, asbestos exposure is much less common. Most women have not been exposed to work-related asbestos commonly found in plants, mills, mines, and other related work places. However, women may have been exposed via indirect means. This is especially true for women married to or living with men who work or have worked in workplaces where asbestos was used. The exposure for women comes largely from the dust from the worker's clothing or workplace equipment brought home.[146] Exposure to asbestos substantially increases a person's risk of developing lung cancer. Furthermore, workers exposed to asbestos and who smoke have a greatly increased risk for lung cancer than people in general.[147]

Other cancer-causing environmental agents exist, such as radon, radioactive ores, mineral exposures, and, potentially, air pollution.

Diagnosis

Early detection of lung cancer is difficult because symptoms often do not appear until the disease has reached an advanced stage. A persistent cough may then present as a predominant symptom. Along with cough, common symptoms of lung cancer include weight loss, bloody **sputum**, recurring bronchitis or pneumonia, chest pain, and/or voice changes. There are no specific screening techniques or guidelines for the early detection of lung cancer, but clinical studies are underway to determine the best methods for early detection of the disease. Newer tests, such as low-dose helical CT scans and molecular markers in sputum, have the potential to detect early lung cancer. A person with symptoms may have a chest radiograph, sputum tests, and fiber-optic examination of the bronchial passages for a more definitive diagnosis.[148] However, care must be given in administering too many high radiation tests for they, themselves, may present a risk.

Treatment

Because most lung cancers are not diagnosed until they are in advanced stages, treatment options are usually limited. Treatment typically includes surgical removal of the affected regions, followed by radiation and chemotherapy. A **lobectomy** removes a lobe of the lung; a **pneumonectomy** removes an entire lung; and a **segmentectomy** removes a section of a lobe of a lung.[149]

Colorectal Cancer

Colorectal cancer is the third most common cancer in men and women. This disease develops in a gradual, progressive manner and may present anywhere in the colon and rectal areas. Cancer affecting different areas of this anatomical region often presents with different symptoms. By far the most common colon cancer is **adenocarcinoma**, which begins in the glandular structure lining the colon. This is a slow-growing cancer, and it may not manifest symptoms for years.[150] The stages of colorectal cancer are:

- Stage 0 (Carcinoma-in-situ): Found in the lining of the colon or rectum
- Stage I: Cancer has moved from the lining of the colon to the muscles
- Stage II: Cancer has spread through the muscle layers into the serosa (outer layer of the colon wall)
- Stage III: Cancer has spread through the muscle wall and on to the lymph nodes
- Stage IV: Cancer has spread, via the blood and lymph nodes, to other organ systems such as ovaries, abdominal wall, liver, or lungs[151]

Risk Factors

Increasing age is the primary risk factor for colorectal cancer. Ninety percent of people with colorectal cancer are older than 50 years of age. The risk of developing colon and rectal cancers is about twice as high for individuals with an immediate family member who has had colorectal cancer or certain conditions such as **familial adenomatous polyposis**

Figure 10.21

Colon polyps.

(FAP). FAP is characterized by the presence of hundreds of polyps in the colon and rectum (see **Figure 10.21**). Likewise, a history of inflammatory bowel disease is associated with a high risk of developing colon cancer. An individual who has developed a polyp or carcinoma in the past is also at increased risk of developing a second carcinoma.

Dietary factors are important determinants of colon and rectal cancer risk. An increased incidence of these cancers is associated with diets that are high in fat and low in fiber or other components of fruits and vegetables. In particular, the most definitive dietary risk for colorectal cancer is a high-fat diet.[152,153]

Screening and Diagnosis

In its early stages, colorectal cancer usually causes no symptoms. Warning signs for advanced colorectal cancer include rectal bleeding, blood in the stool, a change in bowel habits, and cramping in the lower abdomen.

Similar to other forms of cancer, early detection of colorectal cancer greatly improves the likelihood of complete recovery. Approaches to the detection of colorectal cancer include fecal occult blood test, sigmoidoscopy, colonoscopy, and double contrast barium enema. In addition, clinical studies are investigating new and more efficient methods to screen for this disease.

- **Digital rectal examination** is a simple part of a routine physical examination; however, it is relatively insensitive as a screening test because very few colorectal lesions develop within the range of the examining finger.
- **Fecal occult blood test** tests an individual's stool (feces) for blood. This test, when done every 1 to 2 years, in individuals over 50, appears to reduce colorectal cancer death rates by as much as 33%.
- **Sigmoidoscopy** entails examination of the rectum and lower part of the colon with a thin, lighted tube. More tumors can be detected with this procedure than with the two previous tests. This test requires that the patient thoroughly cleanse his or her lower colon prior to the procedure.
- **Colonoscopies** are often used when a sigmoidoscopy detects a polyp or abnormality, or the person is at high risk for colorectal cancer. While sigmoidoscopies screen only the rectum and lower portion of the colon, a colonoscopy examines the entire colon. If a healthcare provider detects an abnormality, he or she can use the colonoscope to remove all or part of the polyp or inflamed tissue by passing tiny instruments through the scope. Medicines, lasers, and heat probes also can be passed through the scope to stop any bleeding.
- Double contrast barium enema requires that the individual have an enema with barium solution, followed by X-rays. The pictures from these X-rays provide an outline of both the rectum and colon. This procedure, while useful, may not discover small polyps.[152]

The U.S. Preventive Services Task Force and the American Cancer Society recommend that all individuals beginning at age 50 receive fecal occult blood tests annually, sigmoidoscopy every 3 to 5 years, and a colonoscopy every 10 years. Screening should begin earlier if there is a strong family or personal history of polyps, colorectal cancer, or chronic inflammatory bowel disease.[153,154]

Treatment

Treatment depends on several factors: the cancer stage, whether this is the first time discovery or a recurrence, and the patient's health. In general, there are four standard treatment options: surgery, chemotherapy, radiation therapy, or targeted therapy.

- Surgery can be done in several ways:
  - An incision into the abdomen to remove the tumor
  - Removal of part of the diseased colon and then sewing the healthy parts of the colon back together
  - Removal of the diseased portion of the colon and, if unable to connect the healthy parts back together, then creating a "stoma" (an opening) to the outside of the abdomen. A bag is attached to the stoma to collect the fecal material produced

- Targeted therapy: Radiofrequency ablation (a special probe using electrodes that can destroy cancer cells) or cryosurgery, a method that freezes the cancerous tissue

- Chemotherapy employs anticancer medications that destroy the tumor.

- Radiation therapy uses powerful "high energy" X-rays to destroy the cells.[155]

The death rates in colorectal cancer have declined during the past several decades. While rates are declining among most female racial and ethnic groups, the highest death rates are among African American women.[199] In addition, the decline is not even across the United States. Death rates are highest in some Southern and Midwestern states and lowest in Western and some East coast states (**Figure 10.22**).[157]

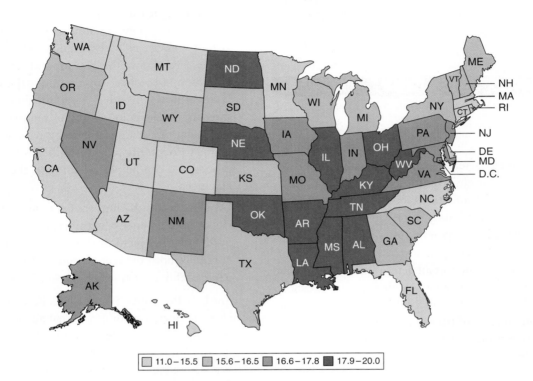

Color on Map	Interval	States
Light green	11.0 to 15.5	Arizona, California, Colorado, Connecticut, Florida, Hawaii, Idaho, Massachusetts, Minnesota, Montana, North Carolina, Rhode Island, Utah, and Washington
Medium green	15.6 to 16.5	Delaware, Georgia, Kansas, Maine, Michigan, New Hampshire, New York, Oregon, South Carolina, South Dakota, Texas, Vermont, Wisconsin, and Wyoming
Medium blue	16.6 to 17.8	Alaska, District of Columbia, Indiana, Iowa, Maryland, Missouri, Nevada, New Jersey, New Mexico, Pennsylvania, and Virginia
Dark blue	17.9 to 20.0	Alabama, Arkansas, Illinois, Kentucky, Louisiana, Mississippi, Nebraska, North Dakota, Ohio, Oklahoma, Tennessee, and West Virginia

*Rates are per 100,000 and are age-adjusted to the 2000 U.S. standard population.

Figure 10.22

Deaths from Colorectal Cancer, 2008

Source: Reproduced from U.S. Cancer Statistics Working Group. *United States Cancer Statistics: 1999–2008 Incidence and Mortality Web-based Report.* Atlanta (GA): Department of Health and Human Services, Centers for Disease Control and Prevention, and National Cancer Institute; 2012. Available at: http://www.cdc.gov/uscs.

Skin Cancer

Cancer of the skin, the most common of all cancers, comes in a number of different forms.

- Melanoma: The **melanocyte** cells in the skin, which are responsible for making pigment (coloring), can form a cancer known as melanoma. While it can occur on any skin area, it's usually found between the shoulders and hips. However, some sex differences are noted: Men tend to develop melanomas on the head, while women often develop them on their legs. This skin cancer is unusual in individuals with dark skin but it can occur, usually on the soles of the feet or palm of the hands. Occupational exposure to coal tar, pitch, creosote, arsenic compounds, or radium is also a risk factor.

- Basal Cell Carcinoma: This cancer is formed in the outer layer of the skin (epidermis). This is the most common cancer in individuals who are fair-skinned. The skin sites most vulnerable are those most often exposed to the sun.

- Squamous Cell Carcinoma: This cancer is formed on the skin surface in the squamous cells. In individuals who have dark skin, this tends to be the most common skin cancer. The most common sites are the feet and legs: areas less commonly exposed to the sun.[158,159]

I am a 65-year-old woman who for years was terrified of getting a colorectal screening. I went for mammograms, monitored my blood pressure and cholesterol, and exercised regularly. But the thought of a colorectal exam seemed so uncomfortable and painful. When my daughter showed me the statistics, I realized that I needed to take care of myself. Now, both my husband and I have gone for screening and it's so good to know we're healthy.

65-year-old grandmother of two

Risk Factors

A major risk factor is ultraviolet radiation from sunlight. Lifetime exposure, severe sunburn, and tanning each enhance the risk. People with lighter skin are especially vulnerable, as darker skin appears to provide some protection from the negative effect of the sun's rays. In addition, an individual's family history of skin cancer can play a role.

The presence of benign growths, such as moles, is not generally dangerous. Although they are benign, certain types of moles, such as **dysplastic nevi**, can increase a person's risk. Dysplastic nevi is the term for irregular moles (nevi is the medical term for multiple moles), and this condition often runs in families. Moles are considered irregular when they have an uneven border or color. A family history of melanoma is another important risk factor; individuals

■ The American Cancer Society emphasizes four warnings of melanoma: Asymmetry; Border irregularities; Color irregularities; and Diameter.

with a first-degree relative who has had melanoma are eight times more likely to develop melanoma themselves.[160]

Preventive measures for skin cancer include limiting or avoiding sun exposure during midday hours (10 A.M. to 4 P.M.), using sun lotion with a sun protective factor (SPF) of 15 or greater, and avoiding tanning beds and sun lamps. Unfortunately, not everyone uses protective measures against sun damage. Just over half (56%) of adults use sun-protective devices. Adolescents are even less likely to use protection, and many have had a least one sunburn in the past year.[161]

Screening and Diagnosis

Early detection of all skin cancers is critical and is essential to the outcome of melanoma. Recognizing changes in skin growths or the appearance of new growths is the best way to find early skin cancer.

Screening is best accomplished by skin examination. Basal cell carcinomas often appear as flat, scaly red areas or small, raised, translucent areas. Squamous cell carcinomas are growing lumps or flat, reddish patches. Melanomas may develop within a mole or as a new mole-like growth. They are characterized by increasing size and changes in color. The American Cancer Society emphasizes five warnings of melanoma (the ABCDE system):

- Asymmetry—the shape of one-half of a lesion or mole is different from the other.

- Border irregularities—the edge may be uneven, ragged, or blotched.

- Color irregularities—different colors (tan, brown, black, red, blue, or sometimes white) may be present in the mole or lesion.

- Diameter—the mole or lesion is usually greater than 6 mm (about 1/4 inch) in diameter.
- Evolution—the mole or lesion modifies appearance over time.[162]

I had so many sunburns as a child. My mom has had basal cells removed from her face and my grandfather had melanoma, so I know I'm at high risk for skin cancer. I get checked regularly by a dermatologist, but so far, the moles that she has removed from my back have been normal. I finally understand how important it is to protect myself from the sun.

30-year-old fair-skinned woman

If a skin growth looks suspicious, diagnosis will be performed through a skin biopsy (sample of the growth). A woman should check her own body on a monthly basis for new skin growths or changes. A cancer check by a dermatologist is recommended every three years for women ages 20 to 40 years, and every year for those older than age 40.

Treatment

There are five primary treatments for nonmelanoma skin cancer. Surgery is used in the majority of the cases. Radiation therapy, electrodesiccation, cryosurgery, and laser therapy are also employed for early forms of nonmelanoma skin cancer. Advances in treatment are increasingly available as studies produce valuable information. One such emerging treatment is biologic therapy, which uses the patient's immune system to attack the cancer.

Treatment for melanoma usually consists of surgical removal of the mole or lesion and possibly regional lymph nodes. Advanced cases of disease are treated with chemotherapy, radiation therapy, or immunotherapy. Survival rates are high for localized lesions, but metastatic disease is not responsive to therapy. Because melanomas are able to metastasize quickly, early detection is the major determinant of survival.[161]

Informed Decision Making

Women can reduce their risk of CVD and cancer in several ways. For most women, prevention and taking good care of one's long-term health are the most important steps. The old adage, "An ounce of prevention is worth a pound of cure," is still correct: It is much more effective to reduce your risk of suffering a life-threatening or disabling heart attack at 55 by never smoking, eating a prudent diet, and exercising—all behaviors that should begin in childhood. Although it is better to begin these behaviors

earlier in life rather than later, changing at any point can reduce one's risk.

Prevention Through Lifestyle

Lifestyle is a critical part of maintaining a woman's health and preventing disease. Such efforts also help to minimize problems when a woman is affected by a disease. Prevention and health enhancement include quitting smoking (or never starting), limiting alcohol intake, avoiding illegal and dangerous substances, practicing safe sex, being physically active, using sunblock and proper covering while in the sun, maintaining an appropriate weight, and eating a suitable diet. Enjoying life and maintaining a positive mental outlook are other important factors. These activities should be put in place as children and maintained throughout life. Another important part of maintaining health and preventing disease is for each woman to work with her physician or other healthcare provider.

Prevention Through Health Screening

Cardiovascular disease prevention involves getting screened and knowing one's family history of heart disease and stroke. When a woman visits her doctor, she should be ready to discuss her health and health concerns and to present her lifestyle habits: smoking, alcohol, dietary status, and any other issues that might influence her health. Her blood pressure, height, and weight should be measured. In addition, she should have regular blood tests to check for heart disease and risk factors: blood cholesterol and triglycerides, and fasting blood glucose.

Mammography is the best way to detect breast cancer in its earliest, most treatable stage—an average of 1.7 years before a woman can feel the lump. Clinical breast exams and monthly breast self-exams are recommended for women younger than age 40 and should supplement mammograms for women older than age 40. Any breast lumps; skin changes, such as flaking or crusting, or weeping eruptions around the nipple; discharge from the nipple; or dimpling or retraction of the skin should be evaluated by a physician.

I had a lump in my breast, and it had been there for some time. It didn't hurt. I guess that I was hoping it was nothing and would go away. I waited too long. This has been a rough year, but I am trying to tell other women not to make the same mistake. If you feel a lump, regardless of the size, have it checked right away.

42-year-old woman

Pap smears and HPV testing are screening methods that can greatly reduce invasive cervical cancer morbidity and mortality rates. Because cervical cancer is a slow-growing disease, screening programs started at age 21 dramatically decrease the risk of developing advanced disease. In fact, when cervical cancer is detected at its earliest stage, the 5-year survival rate is more than 90%. Pelvic exams are also essential for women to detect any abnormal changes of the reproductive system.

Self-examination of one's skin enables a woman to detect early forms of skin cancer. Women should become familiar with their bodies to be able to recognize any of the warning signs of cancer.

Table 10.8 summarizes the current cancer screening recommendations.

Table 10.8 | **Cancer Screening Guidelines (Centers for Disease Prevention and Control)**

Breast Cancer

Currently, mammograms are the best way to find breast cancer early, when it is easier to treat.

Cervical Cancer

The Pap test can find abnormal cells in the cervix that may turn into cancer. Pap tests also can find cervical cancer early, when the chance of being cured is very high.

Colorectal (Colon) Cancer

Colorectal cancer almost always develops from precancerous polyps (abnormal growths) in the colon or rectum. Screening tests can find precancerous polyps, so they can be removed before they turn into cancer. Screening tests also can find colorectal cancer early, when treatment works best.

Lung Cancer

Scientists have studied several types of screening tests for lung cancer. A review of these studies by experts shows that more information is needed. It is not known if these tests can help prevent deaths from lung cancer.

Ovarian Cancer

There is no evidence that any screening test reduces deaths from ovarian cancer.

Prostate Cancer

Because there is not enough evidence to decide if the potential benefits of prostate cancer screening outweigh the potential risks, not all medical experts agree that screening for prostate cancer will save lives.

Skin Cancer

The U.S. Preventive Services Task Force has concluded that there is not enough evidence to recommend for or against routine screening (total-body examination by a clinician) to detect skin cancers early.

Source: Reproduced from Centers for Disease Control and Prevention. (2012). *Cancer prevention and control.* Available at: http://www.cdc.gov/cancer/dcpc/prevention/screening.htm

---

It's Your Health

Quitting Tobacco

The positive effects of quitting begin very soon after you stop using tobacco and continue long after you've quit.

Short-Term Benefits

- Your blood pressure, pulse, and body temperature, which were abnormally elevated by nicotine, return to normal. Persons taking blood pressure medication should continue doing so until told otherwise by their physician.

- Your body starts to heal itself. Carbon monoxide and oxygen levels in your blood return to normal.

- Your chance of having a heart attack goes down.

- Nerve endings start to regrow. Your ability to taste and smell improves.

- Your breathing passages (bronchial tubes) relax, lung capacity goes up, and your breathing becomes easier.

- Your circulation improves.

- Your lungs become stronger, making it easier to walk.

- In your lungs, the cilia (hairlike structures on the lining) begin to regrow, increasing the ability of your lungs to handle mucus, to clean themselves, and to reduce infection.

- Coughing, sinus congestion, fatigue, and shortness of breath decrease. Your overall energy level increases.

Long-Term Benefits

- As a former smoker, your chance of dying from lung cancer is less than it would be if you continued to smoke. Your chance of getting cancer of the throat, bladder, kidney, or pancreas also decreases.

Source: National Cancer Institute, U.S. National Institutes of Health. Available at http://www.cancer.gov/cancertopics/factsheet/Tobacco/quitting-benefits.

Summary

Cardiovascular disease and cancer together represent the greatest risks to women's health. The underpinnings of disease causality and progression have been shown to be a complex interrelationship among an individual's family history, environment, lifestyle, and comorbid conditions. Though family history is not the only risk factor, women with genetic predispositions to cardiovascular disease and certain types of cancers are at increased risk for developing disease. Recognizing that these diseases affect women of all ages should be an incentive for women to begin making lifestyle changes in diet, physical activity, tobacco use, and health screening as early as possible.

Gender Dimensions: Health Differences Between Men and Women

Sex/Gender Differences in Breast Cancer

Breast cancer is well known and feared among women. Unfortunately, because it is far less common, breast cancer is not usually thought of as a threat to men's health, often with disastrous consequences. In 2008, an estimated 1,990 breast cancer cases were diagnosed in men—about 100 times less than among women—and about 450 men died from the disease.[83]

Men and women both have breast tissue. Both sexes also have "male" and "female" hormones, such as testosterone and estrogen, just in different amounts. The major difference in females and males is the amount of breast tissue and the hormonal influence on it. Females have more breast tissue than men and make far more female hormones than men do. These female hormones cause the breasts to develop and grow. In men, male hormones, made largely in the testicles, inhibit breast growth spurred by female hormones. Yet breast tissue, in both males and females, can become cancerous.

Several risk factors are associated with breast cancer in men:

- Radiation exposure in the chest area, as in radiation treatment for a disease
- Diseases that produce high levels of estrogen (female hormone) in the body, such as cirrhosis of the liver or Kleinfelter's syndrome (a genetic disorder in which men have more than one X chromosome, e.g., XXY)
- Female relatives who have alternations of the BRCA1 or BRCA2 genes
- Obesity, as fat cells produce estrogen

Known mutations in breast-cancer susceptibility genes—BRCA1, BRCA2, and CHEK2—pose a heightened breast cancer risk in women. BRCA1 and BRCA2 are also associated with breast cancer in men, and CHEK2 may also prove a risk. BRCA2 is the genetic mutation that appears most commonly in men and accounts for an estimated 5–10% risk. BRCA1 is less common and seems to appear more often in men of Jewish heritage.[84,85]

A study on the incidence of male and female breast cancer in a Veteran's Affairs population showed that men appeared to develop the disease later than women, and the median overall survival was 7 years for men and 9.8 years for women. The following were some of the important differences noted between the sexes in the study:

- Men presented with a greater disease stage.
- Men had greater lymph node involvement.
- Hormone treatment was less successful in men.
- Men were less likely to receive chemotherapy.[86]

This is a disease that deserves attention in both sexes. Yet, for many reasons men are more reluctant to acknowledge or be tested for the disease. Fortunately, men are becoming more aware and making efforts to educate both men and women about the disease in men. Websites are more prevalent and men are becoming more comfortable discussing it. However, much work remains to be done to promote public awareness of breast cancer in men.

Profiles of Remarkable Women

Elizabeth Barrett-Connor, M.D. (1935–)

Dr. Elizabeth Barrett-Connor is a world-renowned epidemiologist who has greatly increased the knowledge base regarding cardiovascular disease, diabetes, cancer, and osteoporosis, and the relationships of these diseases to lifestyle and behavior. Among her many accomplishments, she is widely recognized for conducting the Rancho Bernardo study, a long-term observational study of a group of largely middle-class women and their lifestyles and behaviors. This study has provided substantial knowledge about women as they age, particularly in the area of menopause.

She has been honored many times and has been the recipient of grants from organizations for her research in areas ranging from heart disease to diabetes to aging. Barrett-Connor is a member of numerous professional societies, a reviewer of 14 journals, and has been on the editorial boards of more than 10 journals.

Long an advocate for studies that bring exacting science to women's health issues, Barrett-Connor is noted for her work in chronic diseases that are common in older women. Her studies and her advocacy have advanced women's health knowledge substantially. For example, her studies on the role of hormone replacement therapy in the possible prevention of heart disease are internationally recognized. Barrett-Connor entered medicine at a time when few women had followed this path. She persevered and became a leader in the field. Over the years, Barrett-Connor has established herself as a role model through her leadership in medicine and her dedication to mentoring other women physicians and healthcare professionals.

Profiles of Remarkable Women

Nanette K. Wenger, M.D. (1930–)

Dr. Nanette Wenger is a Professor of Medicine (Cardiology) at Emory University School of Medicine. She is now also the Director of Cardiac Clinics, Chief of Cardiology, and Director of the Ambulatory Electrocardiography Laboratory at Grady Memorial Hospital in Atlanta, and a consultant at the Emory Heart Center.

Wenger has been honored and recognized numerous times, including being the recipient of the Atlanta Woman of the Year in Medicine award, the American College of Sports Medicine 1994 citation, the Best Doctor in America award for 1994–1998, and the Physician of the Year award from the American Heart Association in 1998. She has also been cited in Time magazine's "Women of the Year" issue for her accomplishments in cardiac rehabilitation and international medical teaching.

Wenger has been appointed as a member and chair on numerous boards and committees. At present, some of her appointments include member of the review board for the National Heart, Lung, and Blood Institute's Cardiovascular Health Study; a member of the Expert Advisory Panel in Cardiovascular Disease for the World Health Organization; Editor-in-Chief of the American Journal of Geriatric Cardiology; and consultant, editor, or reviewer for numerous journals.

Much of Wenger's work has highlighted gender and age differences in clinical outcomes. She has been involved in cardiac rehabilitation and education of heart disease in women for many years.

Profiles of Remarkable Women

Mary-Claire King (1946–)

Mary-Claire King is an American Cancer Society Professor in the Departments of Medicine and Genetics at the University of Washington in Seattle. King has received many honors, including election to the American Epidemiological Society, fellow in the American Association for the Advancement of Science, and election to the American Academy of Arts and Sciences. She has participated in numerous public advisory committees, including the Breast Cancer Program Review Group with the National Cancer Institute, the Board of Scientific Consultants at Memorial Sloan Kettering Cancer Center, the National Institutes of Health Office of Women's Health Scientific Advisory Committee, and the United Nations War Crimes Tribunal. King has been politically active since the Vietnam War, working with Ralph Nader's consumer-interest group, and consulting on a project to reunite kidnapped children from the Argentinean civil war with their grandparents.

King was the first person to suggest the idea that familial breast cancer could be traced to a particular gene. In 1990, she proved the existence of the gene for hereditary breast cancer, now known as BRCA1. She later found that the same gene could stop and in some cases reverse breast and ovarian cancers. King is also working on genetic research focused on AIDS and inherited deafness.

Adopting healthy lifestyle choices can greatly reduce a woman's risk. Women should become familiar with the risk factors for cardiovascular disease and cancer, and their changing risk status as they age. Women should follow prevention recommendations and screening guidelines for disease. By working cooperatively with healthcare providers, women can diminish their risk of developing disease and most effectively deal with treatment should the need arise. Knowledge, personal preventive measures, and lifestyle modifications are the best ways for a woman to reduce her chances of morbidity and mortality associated with these diseases.

Topics for Discussion

1. What factors influence women of different ages and cultures to adopt healthier lifestyles and engage in preventive action to reduce their risks of cardiovascular

disease and cancer? Discuss factors for different age groups beginning with the teen years.

2. How can women increase their awareness of cardiovascular and cancer threats? Discuss for different cultures and age groups beginning with the teen years.

3. What can public health agencies and community organizations do to increase women's awareness for cardiovascular and cancer risk factors?

4. Substantial differences exist in the incidence and prevalence of cancer and cardiovascular diseases across racial and ethnic groups. Discuss which factors influence these differences and why.

5. How can academic institutions take a more active role in disease prevention for young women?

■■■■

Key Terms

Adenocarcinoma: A cancer that originates from cells of the endocrine glands.

Adjuvant therapies: Methods such as chemotherapy and radiation therapy that enhance the effectiveness of surgery in cancer treatment.

Aneurysm: A type of weakened blood vessel that can cause a stroke. This ballooning of a weakened region of a blood vessel may result from several factors, including a congenital defect, chronic blood pressure, or an injury to the brain. If left untreated, the aneurysm continues to weaken until it ruptures and bleeds in the brain.

Angina pectoris: Chest pain resulting from insufficient supply of blood (oxygen) to the heart muscle.

Aorta: The great artery arising from the left ventricle of the heart; the largest artery.

Aortic valve: A valve located between the left ventricle and the aorta.

Arrhythmia: Erratic heartbeat.

Arteries: Vessels in the body that supply oxygenated blood to the tissues.

Arterioles: Small arteries.

Arteriosclerosis: Any arterial disease that leads to the thickening and hardening of the arterial walls, slowing the flow of blood.

Atherosclerosis: A type of arteriosclerosis characterized by deposits of fatty substances or plaques on inner walls of arteries that narrow blood vessels.

Atrial fibrillation: A disorder in which the heart's two small upper chambers (the atria) quiver instead of beating effectively. Because blood is not pumped completely out of them, it may pool and clot. If a piece of a blood clot in the atria leaves the heart and becomes lodged in an artery in the brain, a stroke results.

Balloon angioplasty: A procedure used to open narrowed or blocked coronary arteries. A surgeon inserts a small, hollow tube called a catheter in an artery and guides it to the blockage. The surgeon then inflates a balloon near the end of the catheter, widening the vessel and allowing blood to flow. A wire mesh stent is usually placed at the site of the narrowing to keep the artery open.

Benign tumor: A noncancerous growth that does not spread to other parts of the body.

Bicuspid valve: A valve that separates the left atrium and the left ventricle of the heart; also known as the mitral valve.

Biopsy: The removal and microscopic examination of a tissue sample to determine whether cancer cells are present.

Blood: Liquid medium of the circulatory system composed of plasma (fluid), erythrocytes (red blood cells), leukocytes (white blood cells), and platelets.

Breast self-examination: The systematic palpation of the breast tissue of each breast while lying on one's back.

C-reactive protein: A protein produced by the liver during periods of inflammation that is detectable in blood in various disease conditions. The C-reactive protein blood test is used as an indicator of acute inflammation.

Cancer: A general term for more than 100 diseases that are characterized by uncontrolled, abnormal growth of cells. Cancer cells can spread through the bloodstream and lymphatic system to other parts of the body.

Capillaries: Minute, hair-like vessels connecting arterioles and venules.

Carcinogenesis: The overall staging process by which normal cells become malignant. Chemical, physical, or viral agents may induce carcinogenesis.

Carcinogens: Substances or agents that is known to cause cancer. Examples of carcinogens include nicotine, asbestos, and ultraviolet radiation.

Carcinoma: A cancer that is the most common of all tumors, accounting for approximately 85% of all cancers.

This term generally refers to cancer that begins in tissues that line or cover an organ.

Carcinoma-in-situ: Cancer that involves only the top layer of the organ without invading deeper tissues.

Cardiovascular disease: A group of diseases that includes two major categories: diseases of the heart and cerebrovascular disease (primarily stroke).

Cardiovascular system: The network of structures that pump and carry blood through the body, including the heart, arteries, veins, and capillaries.

Cerebrovascular accident (stroke): A condition in which blood vessel damage occurs in the brain.

Cervical dysplasia: Abnormal changes in the cells of the cervix. This benign condition is considered precancerous but can develop into cancer if left untreated.

Cervicitis: An inflamation of the cervix.

Chemotherapy: The treatment of disease with anticancer drugs or chemicals.

Colonoscopy: An examination of the colon using a flexible lighted instrument called a colonoscope.

Colposcope: A lighted magnifying instrument used to examine the vagina and cervix.

Colposcopy: A procedure in which a colposcope is used to examine the vagina and cervix.

Congenital heart disease: A heart condition present when a baby is born. It may include many different conditions, most of which can be surgically corrected.

Congestive heart failure (CHF): A condition in which the heart loses its ability to contract properly of sufficiently to meet the demands placed on it.

Conization: The surgical removal of a cone-shaped piece of tissue intended to determine whether abnormal cells have invaded tissue beneath surface cells or to treat a precancerous lesion. Also called cone biopsy.

Coronary artery bypass graft (CABG) surgery: A type of surgery that creates a "bypass" around the blocked part of the coronary artery to restore the blood supply to the heart muscle.

Cryosurgery: Freezing of an infected area.

Cystic mastitis: The most common breast disorder in women, resulting in tender and lumpy breast tissues. Also known and fibrocystic breast disease.

Cysts: Abnormal growths of cells consisting of a thin-walled sac filled with fluid.

Diastolic: The second reading of blood pressure that represents the amount of pressure the blood exerts against the wall of the artery when the heart rests between beats.

Digital rectal examination: An examination intended to detect colorectal cancer in which the physician inserts a lubricated gloved finger into a rectum to feel for abnormal areas.

Dysplasia: Abnormal cells that are not cancerous; classified as mild, moderate, or severe.

Dysplastic nevi: Atypical moles.

Electrocardiograph (ECG): A device used to record the electric activity of the heart so as to diagnose heart problems.

Embolism: A condition in which an embolus (clot) traveling in the bloodstream suddenly becomes lodged in a blood vessel.

Embolus: A clot circulating in the bloodstream.

Endometriosis: A benign condition in which tissue that looks like endometrial tissue grows in abnormal places outside the uterus.

Endometrium: The tissue that lines the insides of the uterine walls.

Environmental tobacco smoke (ETS): Smoke resulting from others who are smoking cigarettes or cigars. Also referred to as passive or secondhand smoke.

Erythrocytes: Red blood cells. Erythrocytes carry oxygen and carbon dioxide.

Familial adenomatous polyposis (FAP): A condition in which polyps are inherited and affect the gastrointestinal tract. Individuals with FAP develop hundreds to thousands of polyps throughout the colon at young age.

Fecal occult blood test: A simple procedure of smearing a small sample of stool on a slide containing a chemical that changes color in the presence of hemoglobin. Developing tumors cause minor bleeding, which results in the presence of occult blood (small amounts of blood in the stool).

Fibroadenoma: A nonmalignant form of breast tumor.

Fibrocystic breast disease: The most common breast disorder in women, resulting in tender and lumpy breast tissues. Also known as cystic mastitis.

Fibroids: Benign uterine tumor composed of muscular and fibrous tissue.

Heart attack: Death of a certain portion of the heart.

Hemorrhagic stroke: A condition in which blood vessels leading to and within the brain rupture, causing the brain to no longer receive blood and oxygen.

Homocysteine: An essential amino acid found in the blood. Increased levels of homocysteine can harm the artery lining and increase risk for coronary artery disease.

Hyperplasia: A precancerous condition characterized by an increase in the number of normal cells.

Hypertension: A blood pressure that remains elevated above what is considered a safe level. Also known as high blood pressure.

Hysteroscopy: A procedure used to view the inside of the uterus through a telescope-like device called a hysteroscope.

Inferior vena cava: The major vein that carries oxygen-poor blood into the right atrium of the heart.

Ischemic stroke: A condition in which blood vessels leading to and within the brain become blocked, causing the brain to no longer receive blood and oxygen.

Laparoscopy: Examination of a woman's abdominal cavity to view the ovaries, fallopian tubes, and other structures.

Left atrium: One of the two upper chambers of the heart. It receives blood with oxygen from the lungs.

Left ventricle: One of the two lower chambers of the heart. It pumps blood from the heart to the body tissues.

Leukocytes: White blood cells. Leukocytes act as scavengers to rid the blood and body of bacteria and waster. Several types of white blood cells exist, each of which has its own role in fighting bacterial, viral, fungal, and parasitic infections.

Lipoprotein: A compound found in the bloodstream containing a core of lipids with a shell of protein, phospholipid, and cholesterol.

Lobectomy: Removal of the lobe of a lung.

Lumpectomy: A procedure in which only the cancerous lump and a small amount of surrounding tissue are removed from the breast.

Magnetic resonance imaging (MRI): A medical test used to provide a visual image of the body's internal structures. MRI scans may be used to examine the heart, brain, or other organs for signs of disease.

Malignant tumor: A tumor that is cancerous and capable of spreading to other tissues and invading adjacent areas.

Mammography: A procedure in which a low-dose X-ray of the breast is taken so as to detect tumors.

Melanocyte: A cell in the skin that produces pigment.

Metastasis: The spread of cancer from one part of the body to another. Cells in the metastatic tumor (the second tumor) are like those in the original tumor.

Mitral valve: The valve separating the left atrium and ventricle.

Modified radical mastectomy: Removal of the breast. Modified radical mastectomy is a less extensive procedure than radical mastectomy because the underlying chest wall muscles and some of the nearby lymph nodes are not removed. Also known as a total mastectomy.

Myocardial infarction: Heart attack.

Myomectomy: Surgical removal of a uterine fibroid.

Pap smear: A gynecological procedure in which a sample of cervical cells is examined for the presence of precancerous or cancerous cells.

Partial or segmental mastectomy: Surgery to treat breast cancer that involves the removal of some breast tissue and some of the surrounding lymph nodes.

Patent ductus arteriosus: A congenital condition common in premature babies in which the passageway between the pulmonary artery and aorta does not close.

Peripheral artery disease: A disease of the extremities (hands and arms but mainly in the legs and feet) in which the blood supply is diminished, and sufficient oxygen and nutrients do not reach these areas properly. Because waste is not removed from these areas effectively, the affected person may experience symptoms that range from cramping and numbness to gangrene (tissue death), which may require amputation of the extremity.

Plaques: Fatty deposits that develop inside the lining of the arteries that reduce blood flow and can eventually lead to a heart attack or stroke.

Platelets: Disk-shaped structures in the blood needed for blood coagulation. Also called thrombocytes.

Pneumonectomy: Removal of the lung.

Polycystic ovarian syndrome: A condition associated with the overproduction of male hormones, failure to ovulate, formation of cysts on the surface of the ovaries, inability to become pregnant, and abnormal hair growth on the body. Polycystic ovary syndrome occurs most often in women who are obese, and it generally can be reversed with weight loss. Also called polycystic ovarian disease (PCOD).

Polyps: Small benign growths that develop in the endocervical canal or colorectal region.

Pulmonary arteries: Vessels that receive blood from the right ventricle to carry to the lungs for oxygenation.

Pulmonary stenosis: A condition in which the valve between the ventricle and pulmonary artery is defective and does not open properly.

Pulmonary veins: Vessels that return oxygenated blood from the lungs to the left atrium.

Radiation therapy: Treatment with high-energy radiation from X-rays and other sources.

Radical mastectomy: Removal of the entire breast, underlying chest muscles, and underarm lymph nodes following a diagnosis of breast cancer.

Red blood cells: One of the formed elements in circulating blood. Red blood cells contain hemoglobin and transport oxygen. Also called erythrocytes.

Rheumatic heart disease: A heart condition resulting from a bacterial infection (*Streptococcus*) that has been inadequately treated. The infection can develop into rheumatic fever and damage the heart valves.

Right atrium: One of the two upper chambers of the heart. It collects the deoxygenated blood from the body.

Right ventricle: One of the two lower chambers of the heart. It pumps blood from the heart to the lungs to collect oxygen.

Segmentectomy: Surgery to remove a section of a lobe of a lung.

Septum: A dividing wall, such as that between the right and left sides of the heart.

Sigmoidoscopy: A procedure that uses a thin, lighted tube to examine the rectum and lower colon.

Simple mastectomy: Complete removal of the breast but not the lymph nodes under the arm or chest muscles following a diagnosis of breast cancer.

Sphygmomanometer: A cuff device connected to a hose an measuring device to ascertain blood pressure.

Sputum: A secretion that is produced in the lungs and the bronchi (tubes that carry air to the lung). This mucus-like secretion may become infected, become bloodstained, or contain abnormal cells that may lead to a diagnosis. Sputum is what comes up with deep coughing.

Statins: A class of cholesterol-lowering drugs.

Sternum: The breastbone.

Stroke: A condition in which blood vessel damage occurs in the brain.

Superior vena cava: The venous trunk draining blood from the head, neck, upper limbs, and thorax to the heart.

Systolic: First reading of blood pressure that represents the amount of pressure the blood exerts against the wall of the artery when the heart contracts.

Thrombocytes: Disk-shaped structures in the blood needed for blood coagulation. Also called platelets.

Thrombus: A blood clot that blocks an artery.

Transient ischemic attack (TIA): An event in which an artery closes momentarily in a spasm and may result in a brief memory lapse or garbled speech.

Transvaginal ultrasound: A method of imaging the genital tract in women. The ultrasound machine sends out high-frequency sound waves, which bounce off body structures and thereby create a picture. With the transvaginal technique, the ultrasound transducer (a hand-held probe) is inserted directly into the vagina.

Tricuspid valve: A heart valve that has three points or cusps and is situated between the right atrium and the right ventricle.

Triglycerides: Fatty substances found in the body's fatty tissues. High levels of triglycerides are associated with an elevated risks of heart disease.

Tumor: An abnormal mass of tissue that results from excessive cell division. It may be either benign or malignant.

Vasocontrictors: Compounds that result in narrowing of blood vessels.

Ventricular fibrillation: A disturbance in heart rhythm.

Venules: Small veins.

Very-low-density lipoprotein: A type of lipoprotein made up mostly of triglycerides. As with LDL, high levels of VLDL increase the risk atherosclerosis.

White blood cells: Elements in circulating blood that protect the body against pathogenic microorganisms. Also called leukocytes.

Websites

American Cancer Society: http://www.cancer.org

American Heart Association: http://www.heart.org

Breast Cancer Network of Strength: http://www.networkofstrength.org

CDC: Cancer Prevention and Control: http://www.cdc.gov/cancer/

Gynecological Cancer Foundation: http://www.thegcf.org

LungCancer.org: http://www.lungcancer.org

Lung Cancer Online: http://www.lungcanceronline.org

National Cancer Institute: http://www.cancer.gov

National Cervical Cancer Coalition: http://www.nccc-online.org

National Heart, Lung and Blood Institute: http://www.nhlbi.nih.gov

National Ovarian Cancer Coalition: http://www.ovarian.org

Ovarian Cancer National Alliance: http://www.ovariancancer.com

Skin Cancer Foundation: http://www.skincancer.org

Susan G. Komen for the Cure: http://www.komen.org

Women's Cancer Network: http://www.wcn.org

■■■■

References

1. World Health Organization. (2009). *Women's health.* Available at: http://www.who.int/mediacentre/factsheets/fs334/en/index.html

2. Rogers, V. L., Go, A. S., Lloyd-Jones, D. M., et al. (2011). Cardiovascular Diseases (Table 3-1), Heart Disease and Stroke Statistics—2011 Update: A Report from the American Heart Association. Available at: http://circ.ahajournals.org/content/1234/4/e18

3. World Health Organization, *Obesity: Situation and trends.* Available at: http://www.who.int/gho/ncd/risk_factors/obesity_text/en/index.html

4. National Heart, Lung, and Blood Institute. *What is the heart?* Available at: http://www.nhlbi.nih.gov/health/health-topics/topics/hhw/

5. National Library of Medicine, PubMed. *Coronary heart disease.* Available at: http://www.ncbi.nlm.nih.gov/pubmedhealth/PMH0004449/

6. National Library of Medicine, PubMed. *Heart attack.* Available at: http://www.ncbi.nlm.nih.gov/pubmedhealth/PMH0001246/

7. National Heart, Lung, and Blood Institute, People Science Health. *How is a heart attack treated?* Available at: http://www.nhlbi.nih.gov/health/health-topics/topics/heartattack/treatment.html

8. The Harvard Medical School Family Health Guide. *Different shades of gray for postheart attack depression.* Available at: http://www.health.harvard.edu/fhg/updates/Different-shades-of-gray-for-post-heart-attack-depression.shtml

9. Medscape Reference, Drugs, Diseases & Procedures. *Acute coronary syndrome.* Available at: http://emedicine.medscape.com/article/1910735-overview

10. National Library of Medicine, PubMed. *Heart failure.* Available at: http://www.ncbi.nlm.nih.gov/pubmedhealth/PMH0001211

11. National Heart, Lung, and Blood Institute. *What is angina?* Available at: http://www.nhlbi.nih.gov/health/health-topics/topics/angina/

12. Medscape, Emedicine. *Angina pectoris.* Available at: http://emedicine.medscape.com/article/150215-overview#showall

13. National Library of Medicine, PubMed Health. *Stroke.* Available at: http://www.ncbi.nlm.nih.gov/pubmedhealth/PMH0001740/

14. National Library of Medicine, PubMed Health. *Aneurysm.* Available at: http://www.ncbi.nlm.nih.gov/pubmedhealth/PMH0002387/

15. National Stroke Association. *Rehabilitation therapy after stroke.* Available at: http://www.stroke.org/site/PageServer?pagename=REHABT

16. Saver, J. L., & Yafeh, B. (2007). Confirmation of tPA treatment effect by baseline severity end [pomt reanalysis of the NINDS stroke trials. *Stroke*, 38: 414–416.

17. National Institute of Neurological Disorders and Stroke. Post-stroke rehabilitation fact sheet. Available at: http://www.ninds.nih.gov/disorders/stroke/poststrokerehab.htm#disabilities

18. Gargano, J. W., Reeves, M. J., & Coverdell, P. (2007). Sex differences in stroke recovery and stroke-specific quality of life: results from a statewide stroke registry. *Stroke* 38(9): 2541–2548.

19. Centers for Disease Control and Prevention. Vital signs: Current cigarette smoking among adults > 18 years—United States 2005–2010. *Morbidity and Mortality Weekly Report.* Available at: http://www. cdc.gov/mmwr/preview/mmwrhtml/mm6035a5.htm

20. Surgeon General. The health consequences of involuntary exposure to tobacco: A report of the Surgeon General, US, Department of Health and Human Services: Children are hurt by secondhand smoke. Available at: http://www.surgeongeneral.gov/library/ reports/secondhandsmoke/factsheet2.html

21. Kenfield, S. A., Stampfer, M. J., Rosner, B. A. et al. (2008). Smoking and smoking cessation is relation to mortality, *JAMA* 299(17): 2037–2047.

22. Centers for Disease Control and Prevention. Smoking and tobacco use, secondhand smoke. Available at: http://www.cdc.gov/tobacco/data_statistics/fact_ sheets/secondhand_smoke/general_facts/index.htm

23. National Heart, Lung, and Blood Institute, What is high blood pressure? Available at: http://www.nhlbi .nih.gov/health/health-topics/topics/hbp/

24. National Heart, Lung, and Blood Institute. (2012). Morbidity and mortality 2012 chart book on cardiovascular, lung, and blood diseases, Chart 3-67: Prevalence of hypertension and prehypertension by age, U.S., 1999–2008.

25. American Heart Association. Good versus bad cholesterol. Available at: http://www.heart.org/ HEARTORG/Conditions/Cholesterol/AboutCholesterol/Good-vs-Bad-Cholesterol_UCM_305561_ Article.jsp

26. McBride, P. (2008). Triglycerides and risk for coronary artery disease. *Current Atherosclerosis Reports* 10(5): 386–390.

27. Careurheart. No time for hesitation—Test your cholesterol levels. Available at: http://www.careurheart .com/heart-care-articles/cholesterol-blood-test.htm

28. Matthews, K. A., Crawford, S. L., Chase, C. U., et al. (2009). Are changes in cardiovascular disease risk factors in midlife women due to chronological aging or to the menopause transition? *Journal of the American College of Cardiology* 54(25): 2366–2372.

29. Pearson, T. A., Mensah, G. A., Alexander, R. W., et al. (2003). Markers of inflammation and cardiovascular disease: application to clinical and public health practice: a statement for healthcare professionals from the Centers for Disease Control and Prevention and the American Heart Association. *Circulation* 107: 499–511.

30. Smith, G. D., Timpson, N., & Lawler, D. A. (2006). C-reactive protein and cardiovascular risk: Still an unknown quantity? *Annals of Internal Medicine* 145(1): 70–73.

31. Wald, D. S., Law, M., & Morris, J. K. (2002). Homocysteine and cardiovascular disease: evidence on causality from a meta-analysis. *British Medical Journal* 325: 1202.

32. Malcolm, J. (2012). Through the looking glass: Gestational diabetes as a predictor of maternal and offspring long-term health. *Diabetes Metabolism Research Review* 28(4): 307–311.

33. Therani, T., Hashemi, S., Hasheminia, M., et al. (2012). Follow-up of women with gestational diabetes in the Tehran Lipid and Glucose Study (TLGS): A population based cohort study. *Journal of Obstetrical and Gynecological Research* 38(4): 698–704.

34. Verier-Mine, O. (2010). Outcomes in women with a history of gestational diabetes. Screening and prevention of Type2 Diabetes. Literature Review. *Diabetes Metabolism* 36(6 Pt 2): 595–616.

35. Centers for Disease Control and Prevention, NCHS Health E-State. Prevalence of obesity among children and adolescents: United States Trends 1963– 1965 through 2007–2008 Available at: http://www .cdc.gov/nchs/data/hestat/obesity_child_07_08/obesity_child_07_08.htm

36. Hu, F. B., Willett, W. C., Li, T., et al. (2004). Adiposity as compared with physical activity in predicting mortality among women. *New England Journal of Medicine* 351(26): 2694–2703.

37. Irwin, M. L., Yasui, Y., Ulrich, C. M., et al. (2008). Effect of exercise on total and intra-abdominal body fat in postmenopausal women. *Journal of the American Medical Association* 289(3): 323–330.

38. Rao, K. R., Pabmavathi, I. J., & Raghunath, M. (2012). Maternal micronutirent restriction programs the body adiposity, adipocyte function and lipid metabolism in offspring: A review. *Review of Endocrine Metabolism Disorders* 13(2): 103–108.

39. Varvarigou, A. A. (2010). Intrauterine growth restriction as a potential risk factor for disease onset in

adulthood. *Journal of Pediatric Endocrinology Metabolism* 23(3): 215–224.

40. Definition of Adiponectin. Available at: http://www.medterms.com/script/main/art.asp?articlekey=17982

41. DeBoo, H. A., & Harding, J. E. (2006). The developmental origins of adult disease (Barker) hypothesis. *Australian and New Zealand Journal of Obstetrics and Gynaecology* 46: 4–14.

42. Rosano, G. M., Vitale, C., Marazzi, G., et al. (2007). Menopause and cardiovascular disease: The evidence. *Climacteric* 10(Suppl 1): 19–24.

43. Koledova, V. V., & Khalil, R. A. (2007). Sex hormone replacement therapy and modulation of vascular function in cardiovascular disease. *Expert Review of Cardiovascular Therapy* 5(4): 777–789.

44. Qiao, X., McConnell, K. R., & Khalil, R. A. (2008). Sex steroids and vascular responses in hypertension and aging. *Gender Medicine* 5(Suppl A): S46–S64.

45. Dhont, M. (2010). History of oral contraception. *The European Journal of Contraception and Reproductive Health Care* 15(Supplement 2): S12–S18.

46. Baillargeon, J. P., McClish, D. K., Essah, P. A., et al. (2005). Association between the current use of low-dose oral contraceptives and cardiovascular arterial disease: a meta-analysis. *Journal of Clinical Endocrinology and Metabolism* 90(7): 3863–3870.

47. Beller, J. P., & McCarthy, C. R. (2012). Cardiovascular risk and combined oral contraceptives: Clinical decisions in settings of uncertainty. *American Journal of Obstetrics and Gynecology* [Epub ahead of print].

48. Manzoli, L., De Vito, C., Marzuillo, C., et al. (2012). Oral contraceptives and venous thromboembolism: A systematic review and meta-analysis. *Drug Safety* 35(3): 191–205.

49. Gillum, L. A., Mamidipudi, A. K., & Johnston, S. C. (2007). Ischemic stroke risk with oral contraceptives. *JAMA* 284(1): 72–78.

50. MacClellan, L. R., Giles, W., Cole, J., et al. (2007). Probable migraine with visual aura and risk of ischemic stroke: The stroke prevention in young women study. *Stroke* 38(9): 2438–2445.

51. Lampl, C., & Marecek, S. (2006). Migraine and stroke—why do we talk about it? *European Journal of Neurology* 13(3): 215–219.

52. Sacco, S., Ricci, S., Degan, D., et al. (2012). Migraine in women: The role of hormones and their impact on vascular diseases. *Journal of Headache Pain* 13(3): 177–189.

53. Movva, R., & Figueredo, V. M. (2012). Alcohol and the heart: To abstain or not to abstain? *International Journal of Cardiology* [Epub ahead of print].

54. Centers for Disease Control and Prevention. (2012). *Alcohol and public health*. Available at: http://www.cdc.gov/alcohol/faqs.htm

55. American Heart Association. (2012). *Cocaine, marijuana and other drugs and heart disease*. Available at: http://www.heart.org/HEARTORG/Conditions/More/MyHeartandStrokeNews/Cocaine-Marijuana-and-Other-Drugs-and-Heart-Disease_UCM_428537_Article.jsp#.T3YYIY7Y1sw

56. Ellins, E., Halcox, J., Donald, A., et al. (2008). Arterial stiffness and inflammatory response to psycho-physiological stress. *Brain, Behavior, and Immunity* 22(6): 941–948.

57. O'Donovan, A., Ndeylan, T. C., Metzler, T., et al. (2012). Lifetime exposure to traumatic psychological stress is associated with elevated inflammation in the Heart and Soul Study. *Brain, Behavior and Immunity* [Epub ahead of print].

58. Yoo, H., & Franke, W. D. (2011). Stress and cardiovascular disease in female law enforcement officers. *International Archives of Occupational and Environmental Health* 84(3): 279–286

59. Stansfield, S. A., Fuhrer, R., Shipley, M. J., et al. (2002). Psychological distress as a risk factor for coronary heart disease in the Whitehall II Study. *International Journal of Epidemiology* 31: 248–255.

60. Centers for Disease Control and Prevention. Health—United States, *Table 30, Death rates for diseases of heart, by sex, race, Hispanic origin, and age: United States, selected years 1950–2007.*

61. Stice, J. P., Lee, J. S., Pechenino, A. S. et al. (2009). Estrogen, aging, and the cardiovascular system. *Future Cardiology* 5(1): 93–103

62. Centers for Disease Control and Prevention. Health—United States, *Table 26: Leading causes of death and numbers of deaths, by sex, race, and Hispanic origin: United States, 1980 and 2007*

63. Cleveland Clinic. *Heart and vascular symptoms*. Available at: http://my.clevelandclinic.org/heart/disorders/cad/mi_symptoms.aspx

64. McSweeney, J. C., O'Sullivan, P., Cleves, M. A., et al. (2010). Racial differences in women's prodromal and acute symptoms of myocardial infarction, *American Journal of Critical Care* 19(1): 63–73.

65. Rosenfeld, A. G. (2004). Treatment-seeking delay among women with acute myocardial infarction: Decision trajectories and their predictors. *Nursing Research* 53(4): 225–236.

66. Witt, B. J., Jacobsen, S. J., Weston, S. A., et al. (2004). Cardiac rehabilitation after myocardial infarction in the community. *Journal of the American College of Cardiology* 44: 988–996.

67. Centers for Disease Control and Prevention. (2012). *Facts on women and heart disease*. Available at: http://www.cdc.gov/dhdsp/data_statistics/fact_sheets/fs_women_heart.htm

68. Centers for Disease Control and Prevention. *Diabetes among adults 20 years of age and over by sex, age, and race and Hispanic origin, Table 50, Health United States, 2010*.

69. Finkelstein, E. A., Brown, D. S., Wrage, L. A., et al. (2010). Individual and aggregate years of life lost associate with overweight and obesity. *Obesity 18*(2) 333–339.

70. Kreatsoulas, K., & Anand, S. S. (2010). The impact of social determinants on cardiovascular disease. *Canadian Journal of Cardiology* 26(supplement), 8C–13C.

71. National Cancer Institute. *What is cancer?* Available at: http://www.cancer.gov/cancertopics/cancerlibrary/what-is-cancer

72. National Cancer Institute. *Metastatic cancer*. Available at: http://www.cancer.gov/cancertopics/factsheet/Sites-Types/metastatic

73. American Cancer Society. *Known and probable human carcinogens*. Available at: http://www.cancer.org/Cancer/CancerCauses/OtherCarcinogens/GeneralInformationaboutCarcinogens/known-and-probable-human-carcinogens

74. American Cancer Society. *Find support and treatment*. Available at: http://www.cancer.org/Treatment/TreatmentsandSideEffects/Complementaryand AlternativeMedicine/HerbsVitaminsandMinerals/phytochemicals

75. National Cancer Institute. *Treatment for specific cancers*. Available at: http://www.cancer.gov/cancertopics/pdq/treatment/oropharyngeal/Patient

76. Centers for Disease Control and Prevention. *SEER stat fact sheets: Estimated new cancer cases and death for 2012*. Available at: http://seer.cancer.gov/statfacts/html/all.html

77. National Cancer Institute. *Surveillance epidemiology and end result*. Available at: http://seer.cancer.gov/csr/1975_2009_pops09/browse_csr.php?section=2&page=sect_02_table.07.html

78. American Cancer Society. *Breast cancer overview*. Available at: http://www.cancer.org/Cancer/BreastCancer/OverviewGuide/breast-cancer-overview-key-statistics

79. Breastcancer.org. *U.S. breast cancer statistics*. Available at: http://www.breastcancer.org/symptoms/understand_bc/statistics.jsp

80. Centers for Disease Control and Prevention. Breast cancer rates by race and ethnicity. Available at: http://www.cdc.gov/cancer/breast/statistics/race.htm

81. Centers for Disease Control and Prevention. *Lung cancer rates by race and ethnicity, 1999–2008*. Available at: http://www.cdc.gov/cancer/lung/statistics/race.htm

82. Centers for Disease Control and Prevention. *Number of smokers and number of smokers who have quit*. Available at: http://www.cdc.gov/tobacco/quit_smoking/how_to_quit/you_can_quit/alone/

83. National Cancer Institute. *SEER survival statistics, cancer of lung and bronchus (invasive) Table 15.12, 5-year survival*. Available at: http://surveillance.cancer.gov/statistics/types/survival.html

84. *Men, women, and the dangers of smoking: When it comes to smoking, there are clear differences between how men and women think about it and react to it*. Available at: http://www.everydayhealth.com/smoking-cessation/understanding/smoking-and-gender-differences.aspx

85. American Cancer Society. *Facts and figures, incidence rates for selected cancers by state, 2004–2008*. Available at: http://www.cancer.org/Research/CancerFactsFigures/CancerFactsFigures/cancer-facts-figures-2012

86. American Cancer Society. *Colorectal cancer*. Available at: http://www.cancer.org/Cancer/ColonandRectum

Cancer/DetailedGuide/colorectal-cancer-survival-rates

87. American Cancer Society. *What are the risk factors for colorectal cancer?* Available at: http://www.cancer.org/Cancer/ColonandRectumCancer/DetailedGuide/colorectal-cancer-risk-factors

88. US National Library of Medicine, PubMed Health. *Endometrial cancer.* Available at: http://www.ncbi.nlm.nih.gov/pubmedhealth/PMH0001908/

89. US National Library of Medicine, PubMed Health. *Ovarian cancer.* Available at: http://www.ncbi.nlm.nih.gov/pubmedhealth/PMH0001891/

90. US National Library of Medicine, PubMed Health. *Cervical cancer.* Available at: http://www.ncbi.nlm.nih.gov/pubmedhealth/PMH0001895/

91. American Cancer Society. *What are the key statistics about melanoma?* Available at: http://www.cancer.org/Cancer/SkinCancer-Melanoma/DetailedGuide/melanoma-skin-cancer-key-statistics

92. Siegel, R., Naishadham, D., Jemal, A. (2012). Table 9: Incidence and death rates by site, race, and ethnicity, United States, 2004–2008. *Cancer Statistics.* Available at: http://cacancerjournal.com

93. Simon, C. S. (2006). Breast cancer screening: Cultural beliefs and diverse populations, *National Association of Social Workers* 36–43.

94. Brown, D. R., Wilson, R. M., Booth, M. A. et al. (2011). Cervical cancer screening among ethically diverse black women: knowledge, attitudes, beliefs, and practices. *Journal of the National Medical Association* 103(8): 719–728.

95. Ackerson, K., & Gretebeck, L. (2007). Factors influencing cancer screening practices of underserved women. *Journal of the American Academic Nurse Practitioner* 19(11): 591–601.

96. Perdue, D. G., Henderson, J. A., Garoutte, E., et al. (2011). Culture and colorectal cancer screening on three American Indian reservations. *Ethnic Disparities* 21(3): 342–348.

97. Shelton, R. C., Goldman, R. E., Emmons, K. M., et al. (2011). An investigation into the social context of low-income, urban Black and Latina women: Implications for adherence to recommended health behaviors, *Health Education and Behavior* 38(5): 471–481.

98. Cutler, D. M., Lleras-Muney, A., & Vogl, T. (2008). Socioeconomic status and health: immersions and mechanisms. Available at: http://www.nber.org/papers/w14333

99. American Cancer Society. *Economic impact of cancer.* Available at: http://www.cancer.org/Cancer/CancerBasics/economic-impact-of-cancer

100. Jemal, A., Bray, F., Center, M. M., et al. (2011). *Global cancer statistics. CA: A Cancer Journal for Clinicians.* 61(2): 69–90.

101. American Cancer Society. *The global economic cost of cancer.* Available at: http://www.cancer.org/acs/groups/content/.../document/acspc-026203.pdf

102. American Cancer Society. *Non-cancerous breast conditions.* Available at: http://www.cancer.org/Healthy/FindCancerEarly/WomensHealth/Non-CancerousBreastConditions/non-cancerous-breast-conditions-fibroadenomas

103. National Library of Medicine, PubMed Health. *Fibrocystic breast disease.* Available at: http://www.ncbi.nlm.nih.gov/pubmedhealth/PMH0001910/

104. National Library of Medicine, PubMed Health. *Fibroadenoma—breast.* Available at: http://www.ncbi.nlm.nih.gov/pubmedhealth/PMH0004482/

105. National Cancer Institute. *Stages of breast cancer.* Available at: http://www.cancer.gov/cancertopics/pdq/treatment/breast/Patient/page2#Keypoint11

106. Genetic Home Reference. *Breast cancer.* Available at: http://ghr.nlm.nih.gov/condition/breast-cancer

107. National Cancer Institute. *General information about breast cancer.* Available at: http://www.cancer.gov/cancertopics/pdq/treatment/breast/Patient/page1

108. Porch, J. V., Lee, I. M., Cook, N. R., et al. (2002). Estrogen-progestin replacement therapy and breast cancer risk: The Women's Health Study (United States). *Cancer Causes Control* 13(9): 847–854.

109. Prentice, R. L., Chlebowski, R. T., Stefanick, M. L., et al. (2008). Conjugated equine estrogens and breast cancer risk in the Women's Health Initiative Clinical Trial and Observational Study. *American Journal of Epidemiology* 167(12): 1407–1415.

110. Humphrey, L. L. (2002). Hormone replacement therapy and breast cancer. *Systematic Evidence Reviews* No. 14 Available at: http://www.ncbi.nlm.nih.gov/books/NBK42718/?report=printable

111. Casey, P. M., Cehran, J. R., & Pruthi, S. (2008). Oral contraceptive use and risk of breast cancer. *Mayo Clinic Proceedings* 83(1): 86–91.

112. Borgelt-Hansen, L. *Oral contraceptives: An update on health benefits and risks: Menstrual cycle control.* Available at: http://www.medscape.com/viewarticle/421497_6

113. Medline Plus. *Breast self-exam.* Available at: http://www.nlm.nih.gov/medlineplus/ency/article/001993.htm

114. American Cancer Society. *Breast cancer.* Available at: http://www.cancer.org/Cancer/BreastCancer/DetailedGuide/breast-cancer-detection

115. National Cancer Institute. *Mammograms.* Available at: http://www.cancer.gov/cancertopics/factsheet/detection/mammograms

116. Berg, W. A., Zhang, Z., Lehrer, D., et al. (2012). Detection of breast cancer with addition of annual screening ultrasound or a single screening MRI to mammography in women with elevated breast cancer risk. *Journal of the American Medical Association* 307(13): 1394–1404.

117. About.com. *Breast MRI—Using MRI for breast cancer diagnosis and screening.* Available at: http://breastcancer.about.com/od/newlydiagnosed/a/mri_decisions.htm

118. National Cancer Institute, accessed 2012, Treatment Option Overview. Available at: http://www.cancer.gov/cancertopics/pdq/treatment/breast/Patient/page5

119. National Cancer Institute. *Breast cancer treatment.* Available at: http://www.cancer.gov/cancertopics/pdq/treatment/breast/Patient/page5

120. National Cancer Institute. (2006). *Results of the study of tamoxifen and raloxifene (STAR) released: Osteoporosis drug raloxifene shown to be as effective as tamoxifen in preventing invasive breast cancer.* Available at: http://www.cancer.gov/newscenter/pressreleases/

121. National Cancer Institute. *Hormone therapy.* Available at: http://www.cancer.gov/cancertopics/pdq/treatment/breast/Patient/page5#Keypoint24

122. National Cancer Institute. *Treatment option overview, targeted therapy.* Available at: http://www.cancer.gov/cancertopics/pdq/treatment/breast/Patient/page5#Keypoint25

123. U.S. National Library of Medicine, PubMed Health. *Cervical dysplasia.* Available at: http://www.ncbi.nlm.nih.gov/pubmedhealth/PMH0002461/

124. National Cancer Institute. *Stages of cervical cancer.* Available at: http://www.cancer.gov/cancertopics/pdq/treatment/cervical/Patient/page2

125. U.S. National Library of Medicine, accessed 2012, PubMed Health, Cervical Cancer. Available at: http://www.ncbi.nlm.nih.gov/pubmedhealth/PMH0001895/

126. National Cancer Institute. *Stages of cervical cancer.* Available at: http://www.cancer.gov/cancertopics/pdq/treatment/cervical/Patient/page2

127. US National Library of Medicine, PubMed Health. *Cervical Cancer.* Available at: http://www.ncbi.nlm.nih.gov/pubmedhealth/PMH0001895/

128. Centers for Disease Control and Prevention. *Cervical cancer screening guidelines.* Available at: http://www.cdc.gov/cancer/cervical/pdf/guidelines.pdf

129. Centers for Disease Control and Prevention. Human papillomavirus-associated cancer—United States, 2004–2008. *MMWR Report* 61(15): 258–261.

130. Medline Plus. *Cervical dysplasia.* Available at: http://www.nlm.nih.gov/medlineplus/ency/article/001491.htm

131. Mayo Clinic. *Uterine fibroids: Causes.* Available at: http://www.mayoclinic.com/health/uterine-fibroids/DS00078/DSECTION=causes

132. U.S. National Library of Medicine, PubMed Health. *Endometriosis.* Available at: http://www.ncbi.nlm.nih.gov/pubmedhealth/PMH0001913/

133. The American College of Obstetricians and Gynecologists. (2012). *Frequently asked questions: Endometrial hyperplasia.* www.acog.org/~/media/for%20patients/faq147.ashx

134. American Cancer Society. *Endometrial (uterine) cancer.* Available at: http://www.cancer.org/Cancer/EndometrialCancer/DetailedGuide/endometrial-uterine-cancer-risk-factors

135. National Cancer Institute. (2012). *Endometrial cancer treatment.* Available at: http://www.cancer.gov/cancertopics/pdq/treatment/endometrial/Patient/page4

136. American Cancer Society. *Treating endometrial cancer.* Available at: http://www.cancer.org/Cancer/EndometrialCancer/DetailedGuide/endometrial-uterine-cancer-treating-general-info

137. Medscape Reference, Drugs, Diseases & Procedures. *Benign lesions of the ovary.* Available at: http://emedicine.medscape.com/article/265548-overview#aw2aab6b3

138. Medline Plus. (2012). *Polycystic ovary syndrome.* Available at: http://www.nlm.nih.gov/medlineplus/ency/article/000369.htm

139. National Cancer Institute. (2012). *Ovarian cancer staging.* Available at: http://www.cancer.gov/cancertopics/wyntk/ovary/page7

140. National Cancer Institute. *Diagnosis and treatment.* Available at: http://www.cancer.gov/cancertopics/wyntk/ovary/page8

141. U.S. Cancer Statistics Working Group. *United States cancer statistics: 1999–2007 incidence and mortality web-based report.* Atlanta (GA): Department of Health and Human Services, Centers for Disease Control and Prevention, and National Cancer Institute; 2010. Available at: http://www.cdc.gov/uscs

142. Cancer.Net. (2009). *Women and lung cancer.* American Society of Clinical Oncology. Available at: http://www.cancer.net/patient/All+About+Cancer/Cancer.Net+Feature+Articles/Cancer+Screening+and+Prevention/Women+and+Lung+Cancer

143. National Cancer Institute. Cancer Progress Report 2003. U.S. Department of Health and Human Services, Public Health Service, National Institutes of Health, 2004.

144. Mesothelioma Cancer Alliance. (2012). *Mesothelioma and women.* Available at: http://www.mesothelioma.com/mesothelioma/information/women/

145. Roggli, V. A., Oury, T. D., & Moffat, E. J. (1997). Malignant mesothelioma in women. *Advances in Anatomic Pathology* 2: 147–163.

146. American Cancer Society. (2012). Cancer facts and figures, 2012: Lung cancer. Available at: www.cancer.org/research/cancerfactsfigures/acspc-031941

147. National Cancer Institute. *Lung cancer treatment.* Available at: http://www.cancer.gov/cancertopics/treatment/lung

148. American Cancer Society. *What is colorectal cancer?* Available at: http://www.cancer.org/Cancer/ColonandRectumCancer/OverviewGuide/colorectal-cancer-overview-what-is-colorectal-cancer

149. National Cancer Institute. *Colorectal cancer screening.* Available at: http://www.cancer.gov/cancertopics/factsheet/detection/colorectal-screening

150. National Cancer Institute (2012). *Stages of colon cancer.* Available at: http://www.cancer.gov/cancertopics/pdq/treatment/colon/Patient/page2

151. Colon Cancer Resource. *Cancer treatment diet.* Available at: http://www.coloncancerresource.com/cancer-treatment-diet.html

152. American Cancer Society. (2012). Colorectal cancer: Facts and figures 2011–2013. Available at: http://www.cancer.org/research/cancerfactsfigures/colorectalcancerfactsfigures/colorectal-cancer-facts-figures-2011-2013-page

153. National Cancer Institute. (2012). *Colorectal cancer, treatment options.* Available at: http://www.cancer.gov/cancertopics/pdq/treatment/colon/Patient/page4

154. National Cancer Institute. *General information about colon cancer.* Available at: http://www.cancer.gov/cancertopics/pdq/treatment/colon/Patient/page4

155. Centers for Disease Control and Prevention. *Colorectal cancer rates by race and ethnicity.* Available at: http://www.cdc.gov/cancer/colorectal/statistics/race.htm

156. Centers for Disease Control and Prevention. *Colorectal cancer rates by states.* Available at: http://www.cdc.gov/cancer/colorectal/statistics/state.htm

157. National Cancer Institute. (2012). *Skin cancer.* Available at: http://www.cancer.gov/cancertopics/types/skin

158. National Cancer Institute. (2012). *Types of skin cancer.* Available at: http://www.cancer.gov/cancertopics/wyntk/skin/page4

159. National Cancer Institute. (2012). *Common moles, dysplastic nevi, and risk of melanoma.* Available at: http://www.cancer.gov/cancertopics/factsheet/Risk/moles

160. Centers for Disease Control and Prevention. (2012). Sun-protective behavior rates. Available at: http://www.cdc.gov/cancer/skin/statistics/behavior.htm

161. National Library of Medicine, PubMed Health. (2011). Melanoma. Available at: http://www.ncbi.nlm.nih.gov/pubmedhealth/PMH0001853/

162. National Cancer Institute. *Treatment option overview.* Available at: www.cancer.gov/cancertopics/pdq/treatment/skin/Patient/page3

Chapter Eleven

Other Chronic Diseases and Conditions

Chapter Objectives

On completion of this chapter, the student should be able to discuss:

1. Major chronic diseases and their effects on women.

2. Differences between racial and ethnic groups in the incidence rates of chronic diseases.

3. The individual and societal costs of various chronic diseases.

4. Risk factors, screening tests, and preventive and treatment measures for osteoporosis.

5. The process of bone resorption, bone formation, and osteoporosis development.

6. The two major forms of arthritis that disproportionately afflict women.

7. Risk factors and symptoms of arthritis and methods for pain management.

8. How diabetes affects individuals and society as a whole.

9. Special risks that pregnancy presents to the diabetic mother.

10. Diabetes management and responding in emergency situations.

11. Symptoms, risk factors, and treatment of fibromyalgia.

12. Autoimmune diseases that most commonly affect women.

13. Types of lupus and the clinical manifestations of the disease.

14. The basics of Hashimoto's disease, Graves' disease, and other thyroid disorders.

15. The development of Alzheimer's disease and the resulting symptoms.

16. Methods for diagnosing Alzheimer's disease and ways to manage living with the disease.

17. Ways that a woman can recognize symptoms of a disease so as to seek treatment and prevent future disease-related complications.

womenshealth.jbpub.com

Women's Health Online is a great source for supplementary women's health information for both students and instructors. Visit

http://womenshealth.jbpub.com

to find a variety of useful tools for learning, thinking, and teaching.

Introduction

Chronic diseases persist or progress over a long time. They develop slowly, do not resolve spontaneously, and are rarely cured completely. While infections cause a few chronic diseases, genetics and lifestyle factors, such as diet, physical activity, and environmental exposures, play the biggest role in how chronic diseases appear and develop. Many of these diseases manifest themselves in young women, creating health issues that these individuals must learn to live with for the rest of their lives.

Living with a chronic disease can become an encompassing process, especially when the disease causes frequent illness and necessitates many visits to physicians. Some women begin to consider the management of their illness to be a full-time job. Others try to live as they did before diagnosis, not wanting their condition to become central to their lives. Women's responses to chronic disease are as individual as the women themselves. In all cases, however, active support networks via family, friends, healthcare providers, disease support groups, or therapy can help ease the burden of disease management. Support can help the woman cope with the physical, emotional, and financial ramifications of having a chronic disease.

Unhealthful diets, smoking, lack of exercise, continued stress, and other risks contribute to the appearance and progression of many chronic diseases. These lifestyle risk factors contribute to high blood pressure, high cholesterol levels, diabetes, obesity, arthritis, and other conditions, which in turn can lead to conditions such as stroke, heart attack, some forms of cancer, chronic bronchitis, and emphysema.

Chronic diseases are the leading cause of death in the United States and around the world. The World Health Organization (WHO) estimates that chronic diseases cause about 35 million, or 60%, of the 60 million deaths every year.[1] Cardiovascular disease and cancer (see Chapter 10) are by far the biggest killers in this category, but other chronic diseases, like the ones discussed in this chapter, still kill 10 million people every year—more than twice the number of annual deaths from AIDS and tuberculosis combined.[1]

This chapter reviews osteoporosis, arthritis, diabetes, fibromyalgia, major autoimmune diseases, and Alzheimer's disease—chronic diseases that have dramatic effects on the health of women in the world today. Discussions of some other chronic diseases, such as herpes and AIDS (Chapter 7), appear in other chapters.

Dimensions of Chronic Diseases

Epidemiological Overview

Understanding, preventing, and managing chronic conditions are important steps for maintaining satisfactory health. The prevalence of chronic conditions is difficult to ascertain because of differences and inconsistencies in diagnostic criteria and the lack of national reporting systems. Many chronic diseases affect women more often than they do men.

- Of the 10 million Americans estimated to have osteoporosis, 8 million are women and 2 million are men.[2]
- Osteoarthritis and rheumatoid arthritis, two of the most common health problems in the United States, are far more prevalent in women than in men.
- Diabetes affects 26 million people in the United States. Women make up almost half of this total; about 11% of adult U.S. women have diabetes.[3]
- About 75% of the people with autoimmune diseases are women. These diseases typically appear during women's childbearing years. **Table 11.1** shows the disproportionate female-to-male ratios in autoimmune diseases. Reproductive hormones appear to affect when (and how often) these diseases appear: Many autoimmune diseases improve during pregnancy and then reappear after delivery, appear after menopause, or get worse during pregnancy.[4]
- Women are more likely than men to develop Alzheimer's disease, primarily because women live longer than men and the likelihood of developing Alzheimer's disease increases as a person ages. Women are also most likely to be the primary caregivers for their parents, spouses, and other family members with the disease.

Table 11.1 Female–Male Ratios in Autoimmune Diseases

Sjögren's syndrome	18:1
Hashimoto's disease/hypothyroiditis	9:1
Lupus	10:1
Scleroderma	4:1
Rheumatoid arthritis	2:1
Multiple sclerosis	2:1
Type 1 diabetes	1:1.1

Source: Adapted from Fairweather, D., & Rose, N. (2004). Women and autoimmune diseases. *Emerging Infectious Diseases* 10(11): 2005-2011.

Racial/Ethnic and Socioeconomic Dimensions

Rates and severity of chronic diseases vary among racial and ethnic groups, often in complex ways. Black women, for example, typically have a higher bone mineral density than White and Asian American women. This puts Black women at a lower absolute risk of developing osteoporosis. However, due to other factors, such as general health status and reduced access to health care, Black women are more likely to die if they have a serious osteoporosis-related injury. Racial differences are also evident with arthritis. Although Black women are about as likely as White women to have arthritis, they are more likely (10.1% versus 7.9%) to have more serious symptoms that limit their daily activities. Overall, Black people with doctor-diagnosed arthritis have a higher prevalence of severe pain attributable to arthritis, compared with Whites (34.0% versus 22.6%).[5] Diabetes is also more prevalent among non-White populations. As **Figure 11.1** shows, non-Hispanic blacks, followed by Hispanics and Asian Americans, have the highest prevalence rates of diabetes in the United States.[6]

Economic Dimensions

In addition to harming individuals, chronic diseases have major effects on the economy. More than 90 million Americans live with chronic diseases, and chronic diseases (including cardiovascular disease and cancer) account for 70% of all deaths in the United States. More than 75% of America's $2 trillion in medical care costs (about $1.5 trillion) come from chronic diseases. Chronic diseases decrease life expectancy and account for one-third of the years of potential life lost before age 65.[7]

The costs associated with specific chronic diseases are huge. The total annual costs of diabetes are estimated to be $174 billion per year—about $116 billion in direct medical expenses, and about $58 billion in indirect costs like premature death, work loss, and disability.[8] Arthritis and related conditions create expenses of more than $128 billion a year.[9] Bone fractures caused by osteoporosis cost Americans $12 to $18 billion per year.[10] The costs of health care, home care, and hospice for people with Alzheimer's disease and other forms of dementia in 2011 were $183 billion; these costs are expected to increase to $1.1 trillion annually (in 2011 dollars) by 2050.[11]

People with chronic diseases often struggle to pay for appropriate medical care. Men and women with diabetes have, for example, more than twice the average medical expenses of people without diabetes.[8] Keeping a full-time job with a chronic disease may become increasingly difficult, so people who desperately need health insurance may not be able to receive it from their employers. This means that they may have to turn to public insurance programs such as Medicaid or Medicare for coverage or go without care. People with chronic diseases also experience costs in

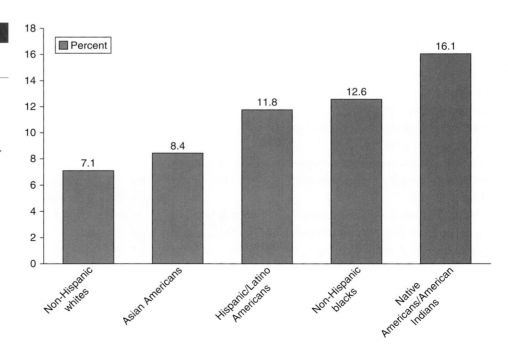

Figure 11.1

Age-adjusted total prevalence of diabetes in U.S. adults, 2010

Source: Data from Centers for Disease Control and Prevention. National diabetes fact sheet: national estimates and general information on diabetes and prediabetes in the United States, 2011. Atlanta, GA: U.S. Department of Health and Human Services, Centers for Disease Control and Prevention, 2011.

© Dee Breger/Science Source/Photo Researchers

© Pietro M. Motta/Science Source/Photo Researchers

Figure 11.2

Left to right, healthy bone vs. osteoporotic bone. "Osteoporosis" literally means "porous bone."

their personal relationships as the strain of dealing with chronic disease damages marriages, friendships, or other relationships.

Women are usually the primary caregivers for loved ones and family members with chronic diseases. Whether they or someone in their family is suffering, women carry the majority of the burden of care and support for patients.

Osteoporosis

Osteoporosis is an age-related disease characterized by a reduction in bone mass and structural deterioration of bone tissue. Bone is living, growing tissue that changes throughout life. **Bone remodeling** is the process that removes older bone (resorption) and replaces it with new bone (formation) to maintain a healthy skeleton. Until a woman's mid-20s, new bone forms faster than resorption occurs, until peak bone mass is reached—after age 30, bone resorption begins to exceed bone formation. The first few years after menopause are the most significant for bone loss. As bone is lost, the skeletal structure weakens, leading to an increased risk of fracture. Osteoporosis develops when bone resorption occurs too quickly or bone replacement occurs too slowly (**Figure 11.2**).

Osteoporosis is a major cause of bone fractures in post-menopausal women and a leading cause of frailty. It affects approximately 8 million women, with millions more at increased risk of developing osteoporosis due to low bone mass. This translates to one in two women older than age 50 having an osteoporosis-related fracture in her lifetime. Osteoporosis is responsible for more than 1.5 million fractures per year, including 300,000 hip fractures, 700,000 vertebral fractures, 250,000 wrist fractures, and more than

300,000 fractures at other sites.[2] **Table 11.2** outlines major risk factors for osteoporosis.

Hip fractures are especially serious. Only 25% of hip fracture patients will make a full recovery: 40% will require nursing home care, 50% will need a cane or walker, and 24% of those over age 50 will die within 12 months of the fracture.[12] Women have two to three times as many hip fractures as men, and White, postmenopausal women have a one in seven chance of hip fracture during their lifetime. The rate of hip fracture increases at age 50, doubling every 5 to 6 years. Nearly one-half of all women who reach age

Table 11.2   Risk Factors for Osteoporosis

Modifiable Risk Factors
- Diet low in calcium and vitamin D
- Sedentary lifestyle
- Cigarette smoking
- Estrogen deficiency
- Low weight and body mass index
- Certain medications, such as glucocorticoids, some anticonvulsants, and thyroid hormones
- Abnormal absence of menstrual periods (amenorrhea)
- Anorexia nervosa or bulimia

Nonmodifiable Risk Factors
- Being female
- Increased age/postmenopausal
- Small frame and thin-boned
- White or Asian race
- Family history of osteoporosis or fractures

Having one or more of these risk factors increases the risk of developing osteoporosis. The more risk factors a woman has, the greater her risk.

90 have suffered a hip fracture.[12] Hip fractures present long-term problems when they occur.

Risk Factors

Smoking is detrimental to bone health, as it can cause early menopause and increase the rate of bone loss. The effects of smoking on bone health have been difficult to analyze in more detail because possible confounding factors, such as lifestyle differences between smokers and nonsmokers, may also play a role. Smokers are often thinner, drink more alcohol, are more likely to lead sedentary lifestyles, and tend to have earlier menopause than nonsmokers do—all of which are risk factors for poor bone health. Additionally, inadequate calcium intake and a lack of regular weight-bearing exercise also increase the risk for developing osteoporosis.

Some medications used to treat other chronic conditions may also cause bone loss. For example, long-term use of glucocorticoids (medicines prescribed for diseases including arthritis, asthma, Crohn's disease, and lupus) can lead to a loss of bone density and increase in fractures. Anti-seizure drugs, gonadotropin-releasing hormone (GnRH) analogs, excessive use of aluminum-containing antacids, certain cancer treatments, and excessive thyroid hormone also may cause bone loss. The health benefits of these medications may be worth the risk of possible bone loss, however. Women using these medications should discuss their options for osteoporosis prevention and best treatment regimens with their healthcare providers.

Medical conditions, including diseases of the thyroid gland such as hyperthyroidism and hypothyroidism, may lead to bone loss. Amenorrhea (lack of menstrual periods) or diseases that lead to amenorrhea, such as anorexia nervosa, cause estrogen deficiencies, which in turn lead to accelerated bone loss (Table 11.2).

Signs and Symptoms

Osteoporosis is often called a "silent disease" because neither pain nor specific symptoms are associated with this condition. Only one out of four women who has osteoporosis is aware of the condition.[13] Some women notice a loss of height as the vertebrae weaken, collapse, and consequently fracture. When the bones in the spine fracture, a woman loses a small amount of height. The spine also begins to curve as multiple fractures occur.

Screening and Diagnosis

One red flag that signals a woman might have osteoporosis is a bone fracture that results from minimal trauma.

To test for osteoporosis, a bone mass measurement (also referred to as a bone mineral density test) must be taken.

Methods for measuring bone mineral density are painless, noninvasive, and safe. Traditional tests measure bone density in the areas most susceptible to fractures caused by osteoporosis: the spine, the hip, and the wrist. Newer machines measure density in the finger, the kneecap, the shin bone, and the heel.

My mother just found out that she has osteoporosis. I have watched my grandmother shrink with it. The doctor says that my mother can do some things to prevent further bone loss. The message for me is to prevent it from happening. I am now much more interested in diet and exercise.

26-year-old woman

Women who should be tested include:

- All postmenopausal women younger than age 65 who have one or more additional risk factors for osteoporosis besides menopause.
- All women age 65 or older.
- Postmenopausal women with fractures.
- Women who are considering therapy for osteoporosis or who want to monitor the effectiveness of certain osteoporosis treatments.

Prevention and Treatment

In the absence of a cure, prevention and management are the best strategies available for women with osteoporosis and for women at all stages of life. Lifestyle and personal behaviors are the key osteoporosis prevention strategies. A woman should not start smoking, and she should quit if she already smokes. An inadequate supply of calcium over a woman's lifetime is a major risk factor for developing osteoporosis. Calcium plays an important role in achieving peak bone mass, maintaining bone mass before menopause, and preventing bone loss in the postmenopausal years.

Vitamin D is necessary for intestinal absorption of calcium. Calcium and vitamin D reduce the risk of fracture of the spine, hip, and other sites. The typical diet of U.S. women contains less than 600 milligrams of calcium per day, about half the recommended amount for women. Dietary calcium is preferable; however, supplements can help a woman meet the recommended dose of 1,000–1,200 milligrams per day (see Chapter 9). The skin manufactures vitamin D after exposure to sunlight; vitamin D–fortified milk, cereal, egg yolks, saltwater fish, and liver can also provide vitamin D through the diet. Those people who

■ Osteoporosis in the vertebra can cause women to lose height and a curving of the spine.

cannot obtain enough vitamin D naturally should include 200–600 IU (International Units) in their diets per day.

Regular weight-bearing and muscle-strengthening exercise is important for osteoporosis prevention and overall health. These exercises improve agility, strength, and balance, thus reducing a woman's risk of falls and decreasing her risk of fractures. Weight-bearing exercises (exercises in which bones and muscles work against gravity) include

walking, hiking, jogging, stair-climbing, dancing, and tennis. Muscle-strengthening exercise, such as weight-lifting, improves muscle mass and bone strength.

Treatment involves managing osteoporosis-associated fractures, universal prevention measures, and medical treatment of the underlying disease. Current osteoporosis recommendations indicate that all persons who have had osteoporotic vertebral or hip fractures and those with a bone mineral density diagnostic of osteoporosis should receive treatment. In women with a bone mineral density above the osteoporosis range, treatment may be indicated depending on the number and severity of other risk factors.[14] The Food and Drug Administration (FDA) has approved several classes of medications that can help reduce or prevent the progress of osteoporosis; women with osteoporosis or at risk for developing osteoporosis should talk with their healthcare providers about these treatments.

Preventing fall-related fractures is a special concern for women with osteoporosis. Many factors can cause falls, including impaired vision or balance, certain chronic diseases, and certain medications. A woman with osteoporosis should be aware of any factors that may affect her balance or gait, and she should discuss these changes with her healthcare provider. Making some simple adjustments to one's living area and behaviors can also greatly lower risk of falls (**Table 11.3**).

■ Arthritis can be physically debilitating as well as painful.

Table 11.3 Tips for Fall Prevention

Outdoors
- Use a cane or walker for added stability.
- Wear rubber-soled shoes for traction.
- Walk on grass when sidewalks are slippery.
- In winter, carry salt to sprinkle on slippery sidewalks.

Indoors
- Keep rooms free of clutter, especially on the floors.
- Be careful on highly polished floors that become slick and dangerous when wet.
- Avoid walking in socks, stockings, or slippers without rubber soles.
- Be sure carpets and area rugs have skid-proof backing or are tacked to the floor.
- Keep stairwells well lit.
- Attach handrails on both sides of all stairwells.
- Install grab bars on bathroom walls near tub, shower, and toilet.
- Use a rubber bath mat in shower or tub.
- Keep a flashlight with fresh batteries beside the bed.

Arthritis

The term arthritis, which means "inflamed joints," includes more than 100 diseases and conditions that affect joints, the surrounding tissues, and other connective tissues. **Arthritis** affects about 50 million adults in the United States, making it the most common cause of disability in the country. Common forms of arthritis are osteoarthritis, rheumatoid arthritis, and gout. The underlying cause of arthritis can result from injury, wear and tear on the joints, an autoimmune response, or a bacterial or viral infection. No matter the cause, however, similar processes occur in the joints as the disease develops. Healthy joints are usually protected by cartilage, a flexible connective tissue, and synovial fluid, a viscous, protective fluid. Cartilage and synovial fluid cushion joints from impacts and allow them to move smoothly. If something damages or wears down the cartilage and synovial fluid, the bones may rub together, and stiffness, rigidity, and pain during movement may result. Eventually a scar between the bones may develop, resulting in joint deformity.

Arthritis and other rheumatic conditions (conditions affecting the joints and muscles) are among the most common chronic conditions and the leading causes of disability in the United States. Arthritis affects more than one out of five adults, most of whom are women, and limits the activity of more than 20 million Americans. The prevalence of arthritis will continue to increase as the population ages. Although aging is a risk factor, nearly three of every five people with arthritis are younger than 65 years of age. By 2030, 65 million Americans 18 years or older will have doctor-diagnosed arthritis.[15]

Osteoarthritis

Osteoarthritis, also called degenerative joint disease, is the most common form of arthritis, affecting more than 27 million people. A milder form of arthritis than rheumatoid arthritis, it is seen in all age groups but is most common among older adults. About one in seven adults, and about one in three adults over the age of 65, suffer from osteoarthritis. Osteoarthritis is more common in women than in men, especially after age 50.[16]

In osteoarthritis, the surface layer of cartilage erodes, causing bones under the cartilage to rub together. This friction causes joint pain, swelling, and loss of movement of the joints. This disease most often affects the knees, but it also affects the hips, hands, neck, lower back, and other joints. Hip and knee osteoarthritis are the leading causes of arthritis disability and the primary reasons for joint replacement surgery.

Rheumatoid Arthritis

Rheumatoid arthritis is a chronic inflammatory disease with increasing prevalence among older adults. It currently affects 1.5 million people in the United States, and is twice as common in women as in men.[17]

Rheumatoid arthritis is an autoimmune disease, meaning that the person's immune system attacks the body's own cells. The exact causes for this immune response are still unknown. In this condition, the immune system attacks the cells inside the synovial fluid and cartilage in the joint, causing inflammation, pain, and swelling. Eventually, the synovial fluid and cartilage may be mostly destroyed (**Figure 11.3**), which can lead to severe disability. In addition

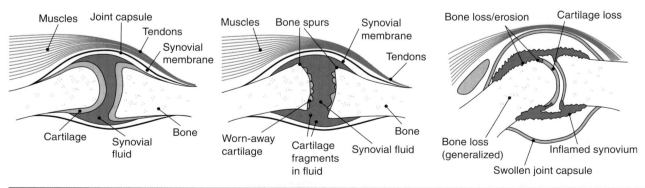

Figure 11.3

Left to right, healthy joint, joint affected by osteoarthritis, and joint affected by rheumatoid arthritis.

Courtesy of Jim Gathany/CDC

■ Infected deer ticks can transmit bacteria by biting humans, causing Lyme disease, which has many possible adverse outcomes, including arthritis.

to attacking the joint lining, the immune system may also attack other tissues. If a faulty immune response affects other organs, such as the lung and the heart, a person may be more likely to die from respiratory and infectious diseases. Rheumatoid arthritis generally occurs in a symmetrical pattern, meaning that it will involve both the left and right hands, not just one of them. The disease varies significantly between individuals: Some people have flareups followed by periods of remission, whereas others have severe disease that is continuously active. Rheumatoid arthritis can also go away and not return.

I am twenty-three, and I have arthritis. Sometimes I am frightened that I will end up with gnarled hands like my grandmother. I hope that new treatments will prevent my disease progression.
23-year-old student

Gout

Gout is a painful and potentially disabling form of arthritis that was first described more than 2,000 years ago by the Greek physician Hippocrates. Unlike other forms of arthritis, which are typically persistent, symptoms of gout can appear, typically for a few days or a few weeks, and then disappear for long periods. However, when symptoms are present they can be quite painful and debilitating.

Gout is caused by an excess of uric acid in the body. This excess can result from an increased production of uric acid due to a metabolic disorder or the inability of the kidneys to adequately clear uric acid. Consumption of certain foods (such as shellfish) and an excess of alcoholic beverages may increase uric acid levels and precipitate gout attacks, but studies are not conclusive on these associations. Some medications and transplant drugs can also increase uric acid levels. With time, elevated levels of uric acid in the blood

may be deposited around joints, especially in the feet and toes. Eventually, the uric acid may form needle-like crystals in joints, leading to acute painful gout attacks. Uric acid may also collect under the skin, where it is known as tophus, or in the urinary tract as kidney stones.

About 3 million people in the United States have gout.[18] While gout and its complications occur more commonly in men, gout is also common among women who have experienced menopause and people with kidney disease. Gout is strongly associated with obesity, hypertension, hyperlipidemia, and diabetes. Some families have a genetic predisposition to gout. African Americans and people with poor kidney function are more likely to have gout attacks.

Diagnosing gout can be difficult because infections or other kinds of arthritis can mimic a gout attack. Given that its treatment is specific to gout, proper diagnosis is essential. The definitive diagnosis of gout depends on finding uric acid crystals in the joint fluid during an acute attack. However, uric acid levels in the blood alone are often misleading and may provide "false positive" (indicating gout when it is not present) or "false negative" (missing gout when it exists) results.

Treatments can now control most cases of gout; however, because of their potential side effects, individual patients often work with their healthcare providers to find the treatment that is best for them. Colchicine has been a standard treatment for acute gout since the 1800s. However, while colchicine is effective, it can cause nausea, vomiting, diarrhea, and other side effects. Because of these side effects, nonsteroidal anti-inflammatory drugs (NSAIDs) have become the treatment of choice for most acute attacks of gout. NSAIDs may also have significant toxicity, but if used over a short term, they are generally well tolerated. However, some people are unable to take NSAIDs because of other medical factors such as ulcer disease, poor kidney function, or use of blood thinners. Elderly patients often cannot tolerate NSAIDs because of their multiple side effects. Corticosteroid-type medications are also used to treat gout attacks and can be given as pills or by injection. Decisions about appropriate treatments must be tailored to the individual and depend on his or her kidney function and other medical factors. With correct treatment, gout can be well controlled in almost all cases.

Risk Factors

Arthritis is the leading chronic condition among women and a major cause of activity limitation.[19] Women are two to three times more likely than men to have rheumatoid

Table 11.4   Risk Factors for Arthritis

Modifiable Risk Factors

- Overweight and Obesity: Obesity and overweight can contribute to both the appearance and development of knee osteoarthritis.
- Joint Injuries: Damage to a joint increases the likelihood that osteoarthritis will develop in that joint.
- Infection: Bacteria and viruses can infect joints and cause the development of some kinds of arthritis.
- Occupation: Jobs involving repetitive knee bending can lead to osteoarthritis of the knee.

Nonmodifiable risk factors

- Age: The risk of developing most types of arthritis increases with age.
- Gender: About 60% of arthritis cases develop in women.
- Genetics: Some genes are associated with rheumatoid arthritis (RA) and other types of arthritis.

Source: Modified from Centers for Disease Control and Prevention [CDC]. (2011). Available at http://www.cdc.gov/arthritis/basics/risk_factors.htm

arthritis.[20] Risk for arthritis increases with age, with nearly half of the elderly population being affected by some form of arthritis. Some people are genetically predisposed to arthritis, placing them at higher risk for developing the disease. Other risk factors are modifiable, although altering these factors does not guarantee prevention. Obesity, which increases the risk of many types of arthritis, is one such factor. Arthritis is nearly twice as common among people who are obese as it is among people of a healthy weight.[21] Joint injuries from sports, infectious diseases such as **Lyme disease**, and occupations that require repetitive joint use and knee bending are other factors that increase a person's risk of arthritis. **Table 11.4** summarizes the major risk factors associated with arthritis. Because women are more likely than men to have rheumatoid arthritis, researchers have been studying the role of hormones in the development of the disease, though investigations conducted to date have produced contradictory results.

Arthritis is not uniformly distributed across the United States. The reasons for the inequitable distribution are unclear, but are the subject of ongoing research. As **Figure 11.4** shows, arthritis is most common in the Midwest and the South, but arthritis affects at least one in five adults in every state.

Symptoms

Symptoms of arthritis depend on the specific disease affecting the joints. Osteoarthritis evolves slowly. Early in the disease, joints may ache after physical work or exercise. Small bony knobs may appear on the joints of the fingers, causing the fingers to become enlarged, gnarled, achy, stiff, and numb. Osteoarthritis in the knees or hips may make it difficult for a person to walk or bend.

Figure 11.4

Percentage of adults with arthritis, 2009.

Source: Reproduced from Centers for Disease Control and Prevention. Arthritis prevalence estimates by state, BRFSS, 2009. Available at http://www.cdc.gov/arthritis/data_statistics/state.htm

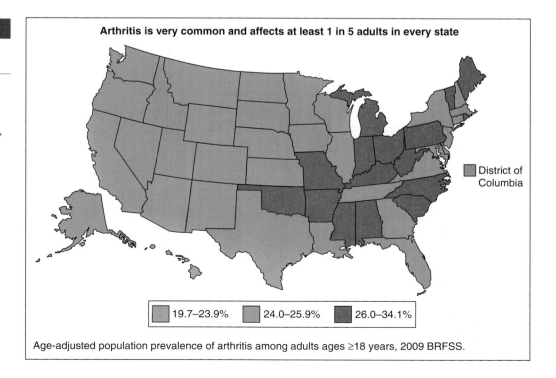

Arthritis is very common and affects at least 1 in 5 adults in every state

District of Columbia

19.7–23.9%   24.0–25.9%   26.0–34.1%

Age-adjusted population prevalence of arthritis among adults ages ≥18 years, 2009 BRFSS.

Rheumatoid arthritis is typically the most painful, disabling form of arthritis. Symptoms, which include pain, stiffness, and swelling of multiple joints, do not always respond to treatment. As a result of these symptoms, people with arthritis typically lead inactive or less active lives, placing them at greater risk for other diseases, including heart disease, hypertension, diabetes, colon cancer, obesity, depression, and anxiety.

Diagnosis

No single test can diagnose arthritis. Instead, healthcare providers use a variety of tools, such as a medical history, family history, and physical exams to check the joints, reflexes, and muscle strength. Radiographs can determine the amount of damage done to a joint by showing cartilage loss, bone damage, and bone spurs. In the early stages of arthritis, before damage is evident, radiographs are not useful; however, they are helpful in later stages for monitoring the progression of the disease. Blood tests to determine the cause of the symptoms, a test for rheumatoid factor (an antibody present in most rheumatoid arthritis patients), and a joint aspiration (drawing fluid from the joint for examination) may also be used for diagnosing arthritis.

Prevention and Treatment

Maintaining an appropriate weight is an important preventive measure. For people who are overweight or obese, losing weight through healthful eating and regular exercise also can help reduce the effects of osteoarthritis. Taking precautions during exercise can also reduce the chance of joint injury. Women should participate in warm-up and cool-down periods when performing any type of exercise or sports-related activities. They should also incorporate strength-training exercises into their routines. Other methods for preventing joint injury and damage to ligaments and cartilage, which in turn can prevent osteoarthritis, include avoiding contact sports and repetitive joint motion; wearing braces, pads, and proper shoes; and exercising on appropriate surfaces. Regular exercise decreases impairment by increasing muscle and joint function. Research has shown that weakness in a woman's quadricep muscles is a risk factor for osteoarthritis of the knee, and that exercise can significantly benefit knee osteoarthritis pathology.[22]

Another cause of arthritis is Lyme disease, a disease caused by the bacterium *Borrelia burgdorferi*. These bacteria are transmitted to humans by the bite of infected deer ticks and cause about 30,000 infections in the United States each year.[23] After several months of being infected, more than half of people who are not treated with antibiotics experience recurrent attacks of painful and swollen joints. About 10% to 20% of these people develop chronic arthritis.[24] Strategies to prevent Lyme disease include using insect repellants, wearing long-sleeved shirts and pants when walking in wooded areas, and checking one's body for ticks immediately upon return.

The goals of treating arthritis are to decrease pain, improve joint care by slowing down or stopping joint damage, and improve a person's sense of well-being and ability to function. Exercise is one of the best treatments for arthritis. Physical activity maintains healthy and strong muscles, preserves joint mobility, and maintains flexibility. It is important to exercise when pain is least severe and to recognize when rest is necessary. Resting the body reduces active joint inflammation and pain and prevents pain from overexercising. Canes, splints, or braces can temporarily take pressure off joints or provide extra support. Controlling body weight through a healthful diet also helps reduce stress on weight-bearing joints and limit further injury.

Many people with osteoarthritis or rheumatoid arthritis use medications to reduce pain and inflammation, as well as prevent joint damage. Medications include:

- NSAIDs, either in prescription or over-the-counter form, can reduce pain, swelling, and inflammation.

- Topical pain-relieving creams, rubs, and sprays, such as those containing capsaicin, can be applied directly to the skin to relieve pain.

- Corticosteroids (anti-inflammatory hormones) can provide short-term relief of pain, stiffness, and swelling and can reduce the risk of joint swelling.

- Hyaluronic acid, a medication for joint injection, can relieve pain associated with osteoarthritis of the knee.

- For rheumatoid arthritis, disease-modifying antirheumatic drugs (DMARDs) may produce significant improvement. DMARDs can alter the course of rheumatoid arthritis and prevent joint and cartilage destruction. These medications, however, can cause serious side effects, and are not appropriate for everyone.

- Biologic response modifiers (BRMs) inhibit proteins called cytokines that contribute to inflammation and joint damage in rheumatoid arthritis. BRMs must be injected under the skin or given as an infusion into a vein.

■ People with diabetes should check their blood sugar levels on a regular basis.

© Custom Medical Stock Photo/Alamy Images

■ Immunosuppressants appear to be very effective in restraining the active immune system, the causal factor behind rheumatoid arthritis. These medications can cause side effects, however, and their effectiveness appears to diminish over time.

Surgery can also be a treatment option for arthritis. Surgery can resurface and reposition bones, replace joints, remove loose pieces of bone or cartilage, reconstruct tendons, or remove inflamed synovial tissue. Alternative methods of treatment for arthritis, such as acupuncture and yoga, can also help relieve symptoms.

Diabetes

Diabetes is a disease characterized by abnormal glucose production or metabolism. A person with diabetes has either a deficiency of insulin (the hormone produced by the pancreas and needed to convert glucose to energy), or a decreased ability to use insulin. As a result, glucose builds up in the bloodstream, and, without treatment, will damage organs and contribute to heart disease. Cells without glucose also starve without their primary source of energy, leading to fatigue, irritability and other symptoms. Diabetes has become an extremely harmful and pervasive epidemic; it is now the seventh leading cause of death in the United States; additionally, every year, millions of people experience diabetes-related complications including blindness, nerve damage, amputations, heart disease, hypertension, or stroke.[3]

There are three major kinds of diabetes: type 1, type 2, and gestational diabetes. Type 1 diabetes is often classified as an autoimmune disease, though genetic and environmental factors can also influence its development. In this type of diabetes, the body's immune system attacks the cells that produce insulin, the hormone that regulates blood glucose. Type 1 diabetes often first appears in childhood or adolescence, and it accounts for about 5% of total cases of diabetes. About 90% to 95% of people with diabetes have type 2 diabetes. In this form of diabetes, cells develop insulin resistance, meaning that cells need increasing doses of insulin to absorb and use glucose. **Gestational diabetes** occurs when women become intolerant to glucose during pregnancy. After pregnancy, gestational diabetes usually goes away, but may return during later pregnancies or as type 2 diabetes. Women who have had gestational diabetes are at an increased risk of developing type 2 diabetes within the next 5 to 10 years.

Most people with type 1 diabetes develop the disease early in life, while type 2 diabetes generally occurs later in life; however, the rise in childhood obesity is leading to a dramatic surge in the incidence of type 2 diabetes among children and adolescents.

In 2011, 25.8 million people, or 8.3% of the U.S. population, had diabetes.[3] **Figure 11.5** shows the number of people diagnosed with diabetes over the past 30 years. Because many people with diabetes go undiagnosed, these numbers underestimate the true prevalence of the disease. According to the Centers for Disease Control and Prevention's (CDC's) most recent analysis:

■ Almost one-half of the people with diabetes are female. About 10.8% of women age 20 or older have diabetes.

■ Women of color are the hardest hit by type 2 and gestational diabetes; the prevalence is at least two to four times higher among Black, Hispanic, American Indian, and Asian/Pacific Islander women than among White women.

■ The risk of diabetic ketoacidosis (DKA), often called diabetic coma, is 50% higher among women than men.

■ Heart disease is the leading cause of diabetes-related deaths. Adults with diabetes have heart disease rates and risk for stroke rates about two to four times higher than adults without diabetes.

My grandmother had diabetes, but she was not always good about taking care of herself. She always loved taking us out for ice cream when I was a girl, and I worry that these habits may have contributed to her stroke. I also worry about myself and my father—a strong sweet tooth runs in our family, but I don't want either of us to suffer like my grandmother did.

24-year-old woman

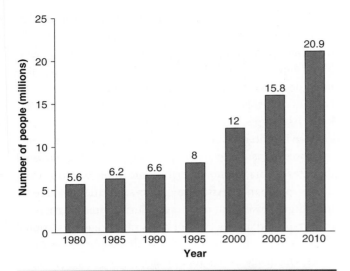

Figure 11.5

Number of Persons with Diagnosed Diabetes, United States. The number of people with diabetes in the U.S. has more than tripled over the past 30 years. Because this figure shows only diagnosed cases, the true number of cases in the U.S. is even higher than this estimate.

Source: Data from Centers for Disease Control and Prevention, National Center for Health Statistics, Division of Health Interview Statistics, data from the National Health Interview Survey. Statistical analysis by the Centers for Disease Control and Prevention, National Center for Chronic Disease Prevention and Health Promotion, Division of Diabetes Translation.

Researchers have also identified prediabetes, a condition in which a person has abnormally high blood-glucose levels, but does not have diabetes. An estimated 79 million adults in the United States—about one out of five adults—had prediabetes in 2010.[3] Prediabetes often progresses to type 2 diabetes, but weight loss and regular exercise can prevent or delay this progression.

I was diagnosed with diabetes at the age of five. I still remember being in the hospital and how scared I was. My father died young from diabetes complications. I am determined to learn as much as I can to take care of myself.

32-year-old woman

Risk Factors

Risk factors for diabetes include having a first-degree relative (mother, father, or sibling) with diabetes, and, for type 2 diabetes, being overweight, having hypertension, or abnormal high-density lipoprotein (HDL) or triglyceride levels. African Americans, Hispanics, and American Indians/Alaska Natives are at increased risk for developing

type 2 diabetes (see Figure 11.1). American Indians have the highest rate of diabetes in the United States—16% of American Indians and Alaska Natives age 20 years or older and receiving care from the Indian Health Services have diabetes.[3] **It's Your Health** provides a checklist of factors to ascertain personal risk for diabetes.

Symptoms and Complications

Symptoms of type 1 diabetes usually develop over a short period of time. Symptoms include increased thirst and urination, constant hunger, weight loss, blurred vision, and extreme fatigue. A person with type 1 diabetes needs insulin on a regular basis to survive. Without insulin, a person can lapse into a coma and eventually die. Symptoms of type 2 diabetes develop gradually. Although they are not as noticeable as symptoms of type 1 disease, type 2 symptoms are similar and include frequent urination, unusual thirst, weight loss, blurred vision, feelings of fatigue or illness, frequent infections, and slow healing of sores.

The most alarming part of diabetes is the severity of the complications associated with the disease (**Table 11.5**). Diabetes is the leading cause of new cases of blindness in adults 20 to 74 years of age: Each year, an estimated 12,000 to 24,000 people become blind because of diabetic eye disease. Early detection and treatment can prevent 90% of these cases of blindness.[3] Diabetes is also the leading cause of end-stage renal disease (ESRD) or kidney failure, accounting for about 44% of new cases. At least half of the new cases of diabetes-related kidney failure could be prevented each year. Severe complications of diabetes, however, should not be considered an unavoidable part of

Table 11.5   Complications of Diabetes

- Heart disease, including peripheral vascular disease, coronary heart disease, and cardiac failure
- Stroke
- High blood pressure
- Retinopathy (broken blood vessels in retina)/blindness
- End-stage renal disease (kidney failure)
- Damage of the nervous system
- Lower-extremity amputations
- Periodontal disease
- Congenital malformations/spontaneous abortions
- Neonatal mortality
- Macrosomia (large-birthweight babies)
- Diabetic ketoacidosis (coma)
- Susceptibility to infections and illness, such as pneumonia

Am I at Risk for Diabetes?

- I am 45 or older.
- I am overweight.
- I have a parent, brother, or sister with diabetes.
- My family background is Alaska Native, American Indian, African American, Hispanic/Latino American, Asian American, or Pacific Islander.
- I have had gestational diabetes, or I gave birth to at least one baby weighing more than 9 pounds.
- My blood pressure is 140/90 mmHg or higher, or I have been told that I have high blood pressure.
- My cholesterol levels are not normal. My HDL cholesterol ("good" cholesterol) is below 35 mg/dL or my triglyceride level is above 250 mg/dL.
- I am fairly inactive. I exercise fewer than three times per week.
- I have polycystic ovary syndrome (PCOS) (women only).
- On previous testing, I had impaired glucose tolerance (IGT) or impaired fasting glucose (IFG).
- I have other clinical conditions associated with insulin resistance (acanthosis nigricans).
- I have a history of cardiovascular disease.

The more items you checked, the higher your risk.

Anyone 45 years old or older should consider getting tested for diabetes. If you are 45 or older and overweight, getting tested is strongly recommended. If you are younger than 45, are overweight, and have one or more of the risk factors above, you should consider testing. Ask your doctor for a fasting blood glucose test or an oral glucose tolerance test. Your doctor will tell you if you have normal blood glucose, prediabetes, or diabetes.

Source: Centers for Disease Control and Prevention [CDC]. (2012). National diabetes fact sheet.

diabetes. With proper care and management, most diabetes complications can be prevented.

Because the high glucose levels of unregulated diabetes can literally thicken the blood, people with diabetes often develop complications relating to poor circulation. As a result, many people have trouble healing from injuries, especially in their extremities. About 60% to 70% of people with diabetes suffer damage to their nervous system, including impaired sensation or pain in the feet. If severe, the nerve damage can require lower-limb amputation. More than 60% of nontraumatic lower-limb amputations occur among people with diabetes.[25] Amputations are also caused by infection related to nonhealing diabetic foot ulcers. New treatments for nonhealing diabetic foot ulcers include genetically engineered replacement dermis, growth hormone products, and better wound management programs.

Adults with diabetes are two to four times as likely to develop heart disease or stroke as those without diabetes. The additional risk from diabetes is related to how well a person cares for his or her condition. A woman with diabetes who manages her blood glucose levels, gets regular exercise, and monitors her diet will have a much lower risk of heart disease than a women with poorly controlled glucose levels, eats an unhealthful diet and leads a sedentary lifestyle. Women with poorly controlled diabetes also are at risk of diabetic ketoacidosis (DKA), a serious condition in which acid levels increase in the blood. Diabetes is known to affect brain function and increase the risk for cognitive decline, dementia, depression, and stroke. These complications frequently occur together, leading to poor quality of life and compounding the need for medical care. Diabetes, often associated with high blood pressure, may contribute to cognitive decline in elderly diabetics as well as to increased frequency and severity of cerebral vascular events.[25,26]

Pregnancy presents special risks to diabetic women. Women are more likely to have healthy pregnancies if their diabetes is well controlled before they become pregnant and throughout the pregnancy. The risk of serious congenital malformations and macrosomia (large birthweight) in babies born to mothers with diabetes is greater than in the general population. Due to the increased incidence of babies with high birthweights, women with diabetes are three to four times more likely to have a cesarean delivery than are women without diabetes. In addition, 3% to 5% of pregnancies among women with diabetes result in death of the newborn, compared with 1.5% for women who do not have diabetes.[27]

Diagnosis

The routine test for diagnosing diabetes is a fasting plasma glucose test. A doctor may choose to perform an oral glucose tolerance test, which involves a fasting blood sample followed by numerous blood samples after glucose syrup is ingested. The "gold standard" for diagnosing diabetes is an elevated blood sugar level after an overnight fast (not eating anything after midnight). A value above 126 mg/dL on at least two occasions typically means a person has diabetes. People without diabetes have fasting sugar levels that generally run between 70 and 110 mg/dL. A fasting glucose level of 100 to 125 mg/dL indicates prediabetes, as well as a higher chance of developing type 2 diabetes in the future.[3]

Prevention and Treatment

Managing type 1 diabetes requires a regimen of multiple daily insulin injections, a carefully calculated diet, planned physical activity, and home blood glucose testing several times a day. Treatment of type 2 diabetes is also based on diet control, exercise, and blood glucose testing, and for some people may entail oral medications or insulin. Daily management is important to prevent blood sugar levels from going too high or too low. A person with diabetes should eat a healthful diet and monitor the amount of carbohydrates (starches and sugars) that he or she eats. Because simple carbohydrates, such as sugars and refined grains, can quickly raise blood glucose levels, their consumption should be limited. If blood sugar levels rise too high, as in **hyperglycemia**, a person may become very ill. Early signs of hyperglycemia include high blood sugar, high levels of sugar in the urine, frequent urination, and increased thirst. Hyperglycemia should be treated as an emergency situation and emergency services (such as 911) should be called immediately. The opposite problem, **hypoglycemia** (low blood sugar levels), may occur if a person with diabetes takes too much insulin. Hypoglycemia can cause a person to become nervous, shaky, confused, or even pass out. Consumption of food or drink with sugar in it can counteract low blood sugar.

Fibromyalgia

Fibromyalgia is a disease characterized by pain. People with fibromyalgia experience widespread pain throughout their bodies for most, if not all, of their waking lives. This pain lowers quality of life and reduces peoples' ability to function. Other symptoms associated with fibromyalgia include fatigue, depression, trouble sleeping, headaches, tingling or numbness in the limbs, and irritable bowel syndrome.[28] The causes of fibromyalgia are largely unknown. One theory is that people with fibromyalgia have a low pain threshold, meaning that the brain over-interprets stimuli as pain. Some evidence indicates that fibromyalgia may develop after some viral infections, as an autoimmune response, or through a combination of factors.

About 5 million people in the United States, or about 2% of the population, have fibromyalgia.[29] Accurate estimates are difficult, however, because the condition often goes undiagnosed. This may be because the symptoms are nonspecific or because providers believe that the condition is "all in the head" of the sufferer (it was not until 1990 that the medical community recognized fibromyalgia as a genuine, diagnosable condition). Diagnosis of fibromyalgia is made if a person feels pain in response to a firm touch in 11 out of 18 defined points on the head, legs, chest, and arms, and if other conditions are ruled out.

Fibromyalgia is about seven times more common in women than it is in men. It is most likely to appear during or after middle age, though it also appears among young adults. Other risk factors include obesity and having rheumatoid arthritis, lupus, or family history of fibromyalgia.[29]

Although fibromyalgia is rarely deadly, it can be an extremely debilitating condition. On average, working adults with fibromyalgia miss three times number the days from work due to illness as people without fibromyalgia. On average, people with fibromyalgia also incur about $3,500 a year in medical bills.[29]

Treatment for fibromyalgia focuses on managing and learning to live with symptoms. Medications, such as acetaminophen (Tylenol), antidepressants, and antiseizure drugs may help some people with fibromyalgia. However, the effects of these medications are modest, usually reducing pain by 30% to 50% in about one-half of patients.[30] Regular physical exercise appears to reduce pain, insomnia, and improve quality of life; exercise also provides the same benefits to people with fibromyalgia as it does to people without the condition. Cognitive-behavioral therapy (CBT), in which the patient works with a psychologist to develop and maintain healthful thoughts and behaviors, helps to reduce symptoms and helps people cope with them. A multimodal approach to treatment that includes medication, exercise, and CBT appears to provide the most overall benefits.

Autoimmune Diseases

Autoimmune diseases are those diseases in which the immune system attacks normal components of the body. More than 80 serious, chronic illnesses are collectively referred to as autoimmune diseases, and these diseases involve the nervous, gastrointestinal, and endocrine systems, as well as skin and other connective tissue, eyes, blood, and blood vessels. Autoimmune diseases are about three times more common in women than they are in men, and they most frequently first manifest during the childbearing years.[31] Autoimmune diseases include multiple sclerosis, type 1 diabetes, scleroderma, rheumatoid arthritis, thyroid disorders, Sjögren's syndrome, systemic lupus erythematosus (SLE), and Hashimoto's disease. Rheumatoid arthritis, type 1 diabetes, SLE, and thyroid disease are the most common autoimmune diseases. Together, autoimmune diseases represent the fourth-largest cause of disability among women in the United States.[31]

Lupus

Lupus is an autoimmune disease that is still not fully understood. In patients with lupus, the immune system forms antibodies that target healthy tissues and organs. Lupus can be a mild, moderate, or severe disease. Although lupus may affect men and women of any age, it is primarily a disease that affects women during their childbearing years. Lupus affects women 10 to 15 times more often than it does men, and it affects African American women 2 to 3 times more often than it does White women.[32]

Lupus presents in three forms. Discoid lupus, also known as cutaneous lupus, only affects the skin and causes a rash that usually appears on the face and upper body. Only about 10% of people with discoid lupus will progress to the systemic form of lupus, which can involve any organ or system of the body. Systemic lupus erythematosus (SLE) is the most common and more severe form of the disease; it is characterized by unpredictable periods of disease activity and periods of symptom-free remission. SLE can affect many parts of the body, including joints, skin, kidneys, lungs, heart, blood vessels, nervous system, blood, and brain. Drug-induced lupus is a reaction to some prescription medicines. The symptoms of this type of lupus are similar to SLE, but do not affect the kidneys or central nervous system. Drug-induced lupus usually disappears when the medication is discontinued.[32]

Risk Factors

The cause of lupus is unknown, although genetic, hormonal, and environmental factors appear to play a role. Lupus is known to occur within families, although no specific gene for it has been found. Environmental factors, including infections, exposure to sunlight, stress, and certain medications, play a role in triggering flare-ups of the disease. Because the cause of lupus is unknown, it has been difficult to determine its risk factors.

Symptoms

Lupus has been called "the great imitator" because of its varied symptoms, which often mimic other, less serious illnesses. Lupus is characterized by periods of remission when no symptoms are present. The two most common symptoms are painful, swollen joints and a skin rash. In addition to being nonspecific, symptoms of lupus vary from person to person because lupus can affect any organ or organ system. Although lupus can affect any part of the body, most people experience symptoms in only a few organs. **Table 11.6** summarizes the symptoms of lupus.

The origins of lupus remain a mystery and have been the subject of considerable speculation and research. Cigarette smoking is one of many environmental exposures, as are infectious agents, silica exposure, and hormonal and dietary factors such as vitamin D, which are hypothesized to be linked to the development of SLE.[33,34] However, the root causes of lupus likely involve more than these factors.

Table 11.6 Lupus Symptoms

Autoimmune Diseases Symptom	Percentage of Cases
Achy joints (arthralgia)	95%
Frequent fevers of more than 100°F	90%
Arthritis (swollen joints)	90%
Prolonged or extreme fatigue	81%
Skin rashes	74%
Anemia	71%
Kidney involvement	50%
Pain in the chest on deep breathing (pleurisy)	45%
Butterfly-shaped rash across the cheek and nose	42%
Sun or light sensitivity (photosensitivity)	30%
Hair loss	27%
Abnormal blood clotting problems	20%
Raynaud's phenomenon (fingers turning white and/or blue in the cold)	17%
Seizures	15%
Mouth or nose ulcers	12%

Source: Courtesy of Robert G. Lahita, MD, PhD, from the LFA brochure, "What Is Lupus?" Reprinted with permission from the Lupus Foundation of America, Inc. All rights reserved.

© NMSB/Custom Medical Stock Photo

■ A rash is a common symptom of lupus.

Diagnosis

The clinical diagnosis of systemic lupus involves noting potential symptoms, such as skin rash, joint pain, chest pain, seizures, and photosensitivity, and reviewing a person's history of medications. A complete blood count and urinalysis may provide evidence of the involvement of the kidneys and blood vessels. The antinuclear antibody (ANA) test may be used to rule out a diagnosis of lupus, as it is positive in virtually all people with lupus and is the best diagnostic tool available for lupus. Antinuclear antibody is not a definitive test, however, because other illnesses, certain medications, or other factors can produce a "false positive" ANA even in a person without lupus.

Treatment and Prevention

Lupus is characterized by periods of symptoms called "flare-ups." The symptoms are unpredictable and inconsistent when they present.

Women with lupus can take preventive measures to help prevent flare-ups. People who are photosensitive should avoid sun exposure and regularly use sunscreen to prevent rashes. Exercise is important to prevent muscle weakness and fatigue, while support groups, counseling, meditation, and other techniques can help to reduce stress. Treatment usually involves nonsteroidal anti-inflammatory drugs (NSAIDs) to ease muscle and joint pain. Corticosteroids are used on a short-term basis to treat skin rashes. Some people find antimalarial agents, such as Plaquenil or Aralen, helpful for skin and joint symptoms, as well as oral ulcers. Immunosuppressant drugs may be used in serious cases of lupus, when major organs are losing their ability to function. These drugs suppress, or turn down, the immune system to limit the damage done to the organ(s) and reduce inflammation. Serious side effects may occur with their use, including nausea, vomiting, hair loss, bladder problems, decreased fertility, and increased risk of cancer and infection.

Thyroid Disease

The thyroid is a small gland, shaped like a butterfly, located in the middle of the lower neck. Its primary function is to control the body's metabolism—the rate at which cells perform duties essential to living. To control body metabolism, the thyroid produces two hormones, T_4 and T_3, that regulate cell energy.

A properly functioning thyroid will maintain the right amount of hormones needed to keep the body's metabolism functioning at a steady state. The pituitary gland, located in the center of the skull below the brain, monitors and controls the quantity of thyroid hormones in the bloodstream. When the pituitary gland senses either a lack of thyroid hormones or a high level of thyroid hormones, it will adjust its own thyroid-stimulating hormone (TSH) and send messages to the thyroid to regulate hormone production.

Thyroiditis is an inflammation of the thyroid gland (**Figure 11.6**). When the thyroid produces too much hormone, the body uses energy faster than it should; this

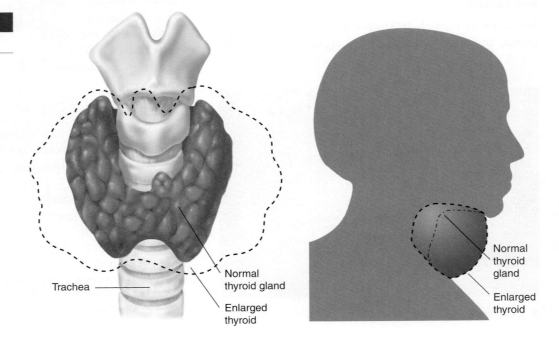

Figure 11.6

Thyroiditis.

Trachea

Normal thyroid gland

Enlarged thyroid

Normal thyroid gland

Enlarged thyroid

condition is called hyperthyroidism. When the thyroid doesn't produce enough hormone, the body uses energy slower than it should; this condition is called hypothyroidism. An estimated 27 million Americans have overactive or underactive thyroid glands, but more than half of them go undiagnosed.[33]

Hypothyroidism results from an underactive thyroid. Hypothyroidism can be caused by a lack of iodine in the diet. Another common cause is a condition known as Hashimoto's thyroiditis, or Hashimoto's disease. This autoimmune condition occurs when the immune system reacts against the thyroid gland. About 8 million Americans have this condition, and most of them are women.[34] Because people with hypothyroidism lack enough thyroid hormones to properly run their metabolisms, they often have symptoms associated with having low energy. (See **Table 11.7** for a full list of symptoms.)

Hyperthyroidism occurs when the body produces too much thyroid hormone. Because the excess of thyroid hormone increases the body's metabolism by as much as 60% to 100%, people with hyperthyroidism often feel symptoms associated with being overstimulated.[36] Graves' disease, an autoimmune disorder in which the immune system stimulates the thyroid, causes about 80% of hyperthyroid cases. Hyperthyroidism is 8 to 10 times more common in women than in men.[36] People with hyperthyroidism may develop moderate to severe eye problems, which may cause bulging of the eyes, blurring of vision, or damage to the eyes.

Risk Factors

Both Hashimoto's disease and Graves' disease are inherited conditions. Women over 20 years old are at an increased

Table 11.7	Symptoms of Hypothyroidism and Hyperthyroidism

Many people may have no symptoms.

Hypothyroidism

- Feeling tired and listless
- Fatigue
- Difficulty concentrating
- Sensitivity to cold
- Dry skin
- Dry, coarse hair and hair loss
- Constipation
- Heavy and irregular menses
- Slow-growing and brittle fingernails
- Feeling of fullness in throat
- Hoarse voice
- Slow heart rate
- Leg cramps
- Difficulty swallowing
- Sore muscles
- Depression
- For men, loss of interest in sex, erectile dysfunction
- Weight gain due to fluid retention, but usually no more than 3-4 pounds
- Goiter

Hyperthyroidism

Weight loss

Heat tolerance

Shakes and tremors of hands

Feeling nervous and irritable

Increased energy expenditure

Sweating more than normal

Fingernails growing faster

Muscle weakness, especially thighs and upper arms

Faster heart rate, sometimes irregular rhythms and an erratic pulse

Diarrhea

Vision problems, eye irritation

For women, lighter periods, as well as difficulties in becoming pregnant or in carrying the child to term

For men, loss of interest in sex, erectile dysfunction

Sleep disturbances

Eyes that appear larger than normal

© Chet Childs/Custom Medical Stock Photo

■ There are many symptoms of Graves' disease, including increased appetite, weight loss, nervousness, insomnia, and bulging appearance of the eyes.

risk for these conditions, though the disorder may occur at any age and does affect men. Other risk factors associated with thyroid disorders include a family history of thyroid disease, previous thyroid concerns (such as enlargement, goiter, or nodules), or a transient thyroid condition during pregnancy. Having one of these risk factors increases the risk of developing a thyroid disorder, but does not inevitably lead to one. Likewise, people without known risk factors can still develop thyroid disorders.

Symptoms

Table 11.7 summarizes clinical manifestations of Hashimoto's disease and Graves' disease. However, many people have no symptoms, and symptoms rarely occur all at once.

Screening and Diagnosis

Thyroid disease can be difficult to diagnose because its symptoms are easily confused with other conditions. A comprehensive history and physical examination are integral to a diagnosis of thyroiditis. An examination typically includes weight and blood pressure; pulse rate and cardiac rhythm; and examination of the thyroid, neuromuscular system, eyes, skin, and the cardiovascular and lymphatic systems.[36]

Laboratory testing is also important. The thyroid-stimulating hormone (TSH) test is generally used as a screening test because it can often identify thyroid disorders before the onset of symptoms. Blood tests measuring levels of thyroxine (T_4) can confirm the presence of thyroid disease.

If thyroid disease is caught early, treatment can control the disorder before symptoms become severe.

Treatment

Treatment for Hashimoto's disease is based on determining the correct amount of thyroid hormone (thyroxine) needed to stimulate the thyroid gland. Gradually increasing doses of thyroxine are given until a person's blood levels become normal. Annual checkups are necessary to confirm that the prescribed dose is still appropriate. During pregnancy, doses of thyroxine usually increase; as a person ages, doses usually decrease. Overtreatment of hypothyroidism with thyroid hormone can result in bone loss. Graves' disease is treated with antithyroid drugs to prevent the thyroid gland from manufacturing thyroid hormone.

Alzheimer's Disease

Alzheimer's disease is an irreversible, progressive brain disorder that affects thinking, memory, and behavior. The changes result from the death of brain cells and the breakdown of the connections between them. The progression of Alzheimer's disease and the resulting cognitive decline vary from person to person. People with this disease usually live anywhere from 3 to 20 years after first showing symptoms. Alzheimer's disease is the most common cause of **dementia**, with approximately 5.4 million people currently

■ Alzheimer's disease is a devastating disease that results in memory loss, behavior and personality changes, and a decline in cognitive abilities.

suffering from it.[11] This number will grow as the population ages. The risk of developing Alzheimer's disease increases with age; however, the disease and symptoms of dementia are not a part of normal aging.

Alzheimer's disease affects many areas of mental function, including memory, language, behavior, and thought processes. These changes are linked with distinct changes in the brain, most notably the development of amyloid plaques and neurofibrillary tangles. Plaques are dense deposits of protein and cellular material that form outside and around the brain's neurons. Researchers are not certain whether the plaques cause the disease or are simply a by-product of the disease process. Tangles are insoluble twisted fibers that build up inside neurons. A form of a protein called tau is the main component of the tangles. In healthy neurons, tau proteins help stabilize a cell's structure. In brains affected by Alzheimer's disease, the tau protein is chemically altered and cannot hold the structure together; the resulting collapse is responsible for malfunctions in communication.

There are two forms of Alzheimer's disease. Late-onset Alzheimer's disease is the most common form, usually occurring in people over the age of 60. This form of the disease progresses slower and has less of a genetic link than early-onset Alzheimer's disease. Early-onset Alzheimer's is less common, but more severe than the late onset form of the disease. Early-onset Alzheimer's disease can appear in a person's 40s or 50s and progress rapidly within a few years.

Risk Factors

The causes of Alzheimer's disease are not fully known. Multiple factors, including age, genetic background, and possibly lifestyle, influence its development and progression.

Some studies have implicated severe or repeated head injuries, lower education levels, and environmental agents as risk factors; however, more research is needed to determine the exact relationship among these risk factors and the development of Alzheimer's.

The risk of developing Alzheimer's increases with age. One out of every 10 persons 65 years or older is a victim of Alzheimer's disease, although early-onset victims may be in their 40s or 50s. Approximately 20% of Americans between the ages of 75 and 84, and almost one-half of those 85 years or older, suffer from Alzheimer's disease.[11]

Genetics plays a strong role in the development of early-onset Alzheimer's disease. As many as 50% of early-onset cases are caused by defects in three genes located on three different chromosomes. Even if only one of these mutations is inherited from a parent, a person will inevitably develop a form of early-onset Alzheimer's. Genetics play a role in late-onset disease as well; however, a person can inherit the gene associated with late-onset Alzheimer's and not get the disease. Similarly, people with late-onset Alzheimer's may not have any genetic factor.

Symptoms

Alzheimer's disease disrupts three key processes in the nerve cells of the brain: communication, metabolism, and repair. This disruption causes many nerve cells to stop functioning, lose connections with other nerve cells, and die. The disease advances by stages, from early, mild forgetfulness to severe loss of mental function (i.e., dementia). Symptoms usually first appear after age 65.

The disease first destroys neurons in parts of the brain that control memory; as a result, a person's ability to do easy and familiar tasks begins to decline. People in the initial stages of disease often think less clearly and forget the names of familiar people and common objects. Later in the disease, they may forget how to do simple tasks, such as brushing their teeth. The cerebral cortex, particularly the area responsible for language and reasoning, is affected next, disrupting a person's language skills and ability to make judgments. Personality changes also may occur. Emotional outbursts and disturbing behavior, such as wandering and agitation, become more frequent as the disease runs its course. Eventually, many other areas of the brain are involved. All of these brain regions atrophy, and the person becomes bedridden, incontinent, totally helpless, unresponsive to the outside world, and susceptible to a variety of illnesses and infections. People with Alzheimer's disease often die from pneumonia.

Diagnosis

In the absence of a conclusive diagnostic test, healthcare providers rely on symptoms, medical history, and physical and neurological examinations to diagnose Alzheimer's disease. These tests allow healthcare providers looking for Alzheimer's disease to diagnose it with up to 90% accuracy; however, many people with Alzheimer's disease are never diagnosed.[38] The only way to conclusively identify the disease is through autopsy, by examining the characteristic plaques and tangles in the brain.

It is important to rule out other illnesses or medications that can cause dementia. Severe depression in the elderly, which can often be treated successfully, is often accompanied by memory loss and therefore is often confused with Alzheimer's. However, depression and Alzheimer's disease do coexist in many patients.

Researchers are studying brain-imaging techniques to better detect biological changes or signs of dysfunction in the brain. The earlier an accurate diagnosis of disease can be made, the better the chance of managing symptoms and helping patients and their families plan for future care while the patient is still able to take part in the decision-making process.

My grandfather has Alzheimer's disease. My mother tries to take care of him but it is very difficult. Sometimes my sisters and I feel angry that she does not have time for us even when we understand that he needs her attention.

20-year-old woman

Treatment and Research

There is no cure for Alzheimer's disease. The FDA has approved several medications for its treatment; however, these medications usually provide little benefit, may cause harmful side effects, and do not stop the underlying degeneration of brain cells. In the absence of effective medication, treatment for Alzheimer's disease focuses on managing symptoms and making lifestyle changes to help the patients and their caregivers cope with the progression of the disease. Therapies include the management of problematic behaviors, home or "environmental" modifications, and the use of appropriate communication techniques. Support and education for caregivers and family members are also crucial to the best care of people with Alzheimer's.

The care of a person who has Alzheimer's disease is challenging on many fronts. More than 70% of people with Alzheimer's live at home, where family and friends provide their care.[38] Care can be emotionally devastating, physically demanding, and a financial burden. Caregivers are subject to high levels of chronic stress, and caregiver burnout is a major factor in the inability to continue caring for a person with Alzheimer's at home.

Physical activity, good nutrition, and social interaction are important for keeping Alzheimer's patients as functional as possible. Maintaining a calm, safe, structured environment also helps patients feel better and remain independent longer. Drugs can help soothe agitation, anxiety, depression, and sleeplessness, and may help boost participation in daily activities.

Genetic research is an important area of Alzheimer's disease study. Scientists have found genetic links to the two forms of Alzheimer's disease. In the 1980s, researchers found that mutations (or changes) in certain genes on three chromosomes cause early-onset disease. A person has a 50% chance of developing early-onset disease if one parent has any of these genetic mutations.[11] Certain forms of the apolipoprotein E (APOE) gene can also influence the development of late-onset disease. Scientists are now intensively searching for other genes that may be linked to Alzheimer's.

Informed Decision Making

Lifestyle changes are often the first step in preventing the development of chronic conditions or in slowing their progression. A healthy diet, regular exercise, and avoidance of harmful substances are standard methods for health promotion. Other important approaches toward disease prevention include being knowledgeable about chronic diseases and their symptoms and visiting one's healthcare provider regularly. A woman who knows her body may be able to recognize changes or problems readily and prevent or slow progression of disease before symptoms begin or complications arise.

For osteoporosis prevention purposes, a woman usually only needs to have a bone mineral density test two or three times during her lifetime. Preventive measures such as medication may be an appropriate option for women with decreasing bone density. A significant aspect of arthritis treatment involves learning ways to ease pain and perform daily activities. A diagnosis of arthritis should encourage women to become more active in their own health care and learn better ways to manage their diseases. Some diseases can cause significant damage if left undiagnosed and therefore untreated. Uncontrolled diabetes, for example, can lead to serious illness and possibly death. With appropriate treatment and by managing their condition, however, women with diabetes can live complete and satisfying lives.

A disease such as Alzheimer's presents different issues. Early diagnosis appears to have little effect on treatment or management of the disease. It does, however, afford both the patient and family members time to arrange for who will make future healthcare, financial, long-term care, and any other decisions necessary for the patient. Many issues need to be considered with Alzheimer's disease because as the disease progresses, a person will no longer be able to make rational decisions or care for himself or herself. A woman who is considering becoming a caregiver for a person with this disease needs to understand the time and commitment involved before making such a decision. Early diagnosis assists people in this preparation.

The Internet can help patients and their families learn more about chronic diseases, and cope with their effects. It provides individuals with information about symptoms, diagnosis, and treatment, and with support groups and individuals who understand first-hand what it is like to live with a chronic disease. As with all information sources, there are risks related to information received on the Internet, including claims for supposed "miracle cures" for certain disorders, and information that is misleading or inaccurate. As with all other topics, women should make every effort to go to trusted sources to get information about chronic diseases. (See the websites listed at the end of this chapter.)

■■■■

Summary

Chronic diseases are major causes of death and disability in the United States. While these diseases usually lack definitive cures, medical focus falls on preventing the diseases when possible, and managing them through medication and behaviors when they develop. In addition to cardiovascular disease and cancer, major chronic diseases include osteoporosis, arthritis, fibromyalgia, diabetes, lupus, thyroid disease, and Alzheimer's disease. Many chronic diseases are more common among women than among men. Women are also more likely than men to act as caregivers for other people living with chronic diseases.

Knowledge, healthful behaviors, and lifestyle modifications are the best measures by which a woman can reduce her chances of developing chronic conditions. In the cases of chronic diseases with genetic components, women can better understand their risks by learning about their family history. Health screenings can alert a woman to an

Mary Tyler Moore (1936–)

© s_bukley/ShutterStock, Inc.

Mary Tyler Moore began her career as a dancer and actress in TV commercials. After a series of unsuccessful TV series and specials, she landed a role on *The Dick Van Dyke Show* in the early 1960s. From that point, Moore's career took off. *The Mary Tyler Moore Show* ran from 1970 to 1977 and was followed by *Mary* (1978), *The Mary Tyler Moore Hour* (1979), and *Mary* (1985–1986). Moore won five Emmy awards for her roles on *The Dick Van Dyke Show* and *The Mary Tyler Moore Show*. Her career has continued with roles in movies and on Broadway.

Moore has overcome many obstacles in her personal life. Her son committed suicide at the age of 24; soon thereafter, she divorced her husband. She later checked herself into the Betty Ford Clinic with alcohol abuse problems.

Since early adulthood, Moore has also had diabetes. Over the course of her disease, she has experienced several flare-ups of diabetic retinopathy that have been kept under control with laser surgery. As the International Chairwoman of the Juvenile Diabetes Foundation (JDF), Moore has advocated for diabetes education, awareness, and increased funding for diabetes research. She has been featured in a series of public service announcements for the JDF. In June 1999, Moore led 100 child delegates in the first Juvenile Diabetes Foundation Children's Congress before the Senate Committee on Appropriations, Subcommittee in Labor, Health and Human Services, and Education. She and the children, as well as other advocates, called on lawmakers to increase funding for diabetes research to help speed up the discovery of a cure. Moore has continued to lead the Children's Congress to Capitol Hill every other year, making the event one of the largest media and grassroots efforts held in support of finding a cure for juvenile diabetes, raising national awareness, and representing personal advocacy. Moore continues her fight against the disease that affects her life and the lives of the more than 26 million people with diabetes.

increased risk of disease, allowing her to make decisions on lifestyle changes and treatment options. Although prevention is the first step, chronic diseases can affect a woman who has followed a healthy lifestyle and has adhered to screening guidelines for various conditions. The next step is understanding how to control or treat a condition, through lifestyle modifications and appropriate treatment.

Topics for Discussion

1. What type of ethical issues may arise with testing for genetic predisposition to various chronic diseases?

2. Have you, close friends, or family members ever been diagnosed with a chronic disease? How has that diagnosis changed your or his or her life?

3. How can lifestyle changes affect chronic disease management?

4. What differences exist between chronic diseases that occur early in life versus those that manifest later in life?

5. In what ways does early diagnosis help a woman and her family to cope with her disease?

Key Terms

Arthritis: Inflammation of the joints. Arthritis encompasses more than 100 diseases and conditions that affect joints, the surrounding tissues, and other connective tissues.

Bone remodeling: The process that removes older bone (resorption) and replaces it with new bone (formation) so as to maintain a healthy skeleton.

Dementia: Cognitive decline, often occurring in old age. This mental deterioration and decline in intellectual functioning is severe enough to interfere with routine daily activities.

Diabetes: A disease characterized by abnormal glucose production or metabolism. A person with diabetes has either a deficiency of insulin (the hormone produced by the pancreas needed to convert glucose to energy) or a decreased ability to use insulin. As a result, glucose builds up in the bloodstream and, without treatment, may damage organs, contribute to heart disease, or cause coma, and, eventually, death.

Fibromyalgia: A chronic illness characterized by constant, unexplained pain throughout the body.

Gestational diabetes: A form of diabetes that develops in 2% to 5% of all pregnancies, but usually disappears when the pregnancy is over.

Hyperglycemia: High blood sugar levels, whereby a person may become very ill. Early signs of hyperglycemia include high blood sugar, high levels of sugar in the urine, frequent urination, and increased thirst.

Hyperthyroidism: Thyroid disease resulting from an overactive thyroid, most commonly caused by Graves' disease.

Hypoglycemia: Low blood sugar levels that can cause a person to become nervous, shaky, and confused and can result in the person passing out.

Hypothyroidism: Thyroid disease resulting from an underactive thyroid, most commonly caused by Hashimoto's disease.

Lupus: A complex chronic inflammatory disorder in which the immune system forms antibodies that target healthy tissues and organs. Lupus can be a mild, moderate, or severe disease.

Lyme disease: A type of inflammatory arthritis that is caused by a tiny, tick-borne bacterium. If Lyme disease is not treated, it can lead to cardiac problems, neurological disorders, or infectious arthritis (usually of the knees).

Osteoarthritis: A disease in which the surface layer of cartilage erodes, causing bones under the cartilage to rub together. This friction results in joint pain, swelling, and loss of movement of the joints. Also called degenerative joint disease.

Rheumatoid arthritis: Chronic inflammatory disease of the joints that results from an autoimmune response.

Thyroiditis: An inflammation of the thyroid glad. Chronic thyroiditis frequently results in lowered thyroid function (hypothyroidism).

■■■■
Websites

Alzheimer's Association: http://www.alz.org

Alzheimer's Disease Education and Referral Center (ADEAR): http://www.alzheimers.org

American Diabetes Association: http://www.diabetes .org

Arthritis Foundation: http://www.arthritis.org

Lupus Foundation of America: http://www.lupus.org

National Institute of Arthritis and Musculoskeletal and Skin Diseases: http://www.niams.nih.gov

National Institute of Diabetes and Digestive and Kidney Diseases: http://www.niddk.nih.gov

National Institutes of Health, Osteoporosis and Related Bone Diseases National Resource Center: http://www.niams.nih.gov/bone

National Multiple Sclerosis Society: http://www.nmss .org

National Osteoporosis Foundation: http://www.nof.org

■■■■
References

1. World Health Organization. (2005). *Preventing chronic diseases: A vital investment.* Department of Chronic Diseases and Health Promotion. WHO Library. Geneva, Switzerland: WHO Press.

2. National Osteoporosis Foundation. (2011). *Osteoporosis fast facts.* Available at: http://www.nof.org/osteoporosis/node/40

3. Centers for Disease Control and Prevention [CDC]. (2011). National diabetes fact sheet: National estimates and general information on diabetes and pre-diabetes in the United States, 2011. Atlanta, GA: U.S. Department of Health and Human Services, Centers for Disease Control and Prevention.

4. National Institutes of Health. (2005). Progress in auto-immune disease research: Report to Congress. Available at: http://www.niaid.nih.gov/dait/pdf/ADCC_Final.pdf

5. Centers for Disease Control and Prevention [CDC]. (2005). Racial/ethnic differences in the prevalence and impact of doctor-diagnosed arthritis—United States, 2002. *Morbidity and Mortality Weekly Report* 54(5): 119–123.

6. Centers for Disease Control and Prevention [CDC]. (2005). *National diabetes fact sheet.* National Center for Chronic Disease Prevention and Health. Available at: http://www.cdc.gov/diabetes/pubs/estimates .htm#prev4

7. Centers for Disease Control and Prevention [CDC]. (2005). Chronic disease overview. Available at: http://www.cdc.gov/nccdphp/overview.htm

8. Centers for Disease Control and Prevention [CDC]. (2012). National diabetes statistics. Available at: http://diabetes.niddk.nih.gov/dm/pubs/statistics/#Diagnosed20

9. Centers for Disease Control and Prevention [CDC]. (2007). National and state medical expenditures and lost earnings attributable to arthritis and other rheumatic conditions. *Morbidity and Mortality Weekly Report* 56(1): 4–7.

10. Centers for Disease Control and Prevention [CDC]. (2004). Improving the clinical use of biochemical bone marker in metabolic bone diseases. Available at: http://www.cdc.gov/nceh/dls/osteoporosis.htm

11. Alzheimer's Association. (2011). Alzheimer's facts and figures. Available at: http://www.alz.org/AboutAD/statistics.asp

12. American Academy of Orthopaedic Surgeons. (2001). Falls and hip fractures. Available at: http://orthoinfo.aaos.org/fact/thr_report.cfm?Thread_ID=77&topcategory=Hip

13. Delaney, M. F. (2006). Strategies for the prevention and treatment of osteoporosis during early menopause. *American Journal of Obstetrics and Gynecology* 194(2 suppl): S12–S23.

14. Cosman, F. (2005). The prevention and treatment of osteoporosis: A review. *Medscape General Medicine* 7(2): 73.

15. Centers for Disease Control and Prevention [CDC]. (2012). *Arthritis: Meeting the challenge of living well at a glance 2012*. Available at: http://www.cdc.gov/chronicdisease/resources/publications/aag/arthritis.htm

16. Centers for Disease Control and Prevention [CDC]. (2011). Arthritis-related statistics. Available at: http://www.cdc.gov/arthritis/data_statistics/arthritis_related_statistics.htm#1

17. Arthritis Foundation. (2012). Osteoarthritis fact sheet. Available at: http://www.arthritis.org/conditions/fact_sheets/OA_Fact_Sheet.asp

18. Helmick C. G., Felson, D. T., Lawrence, R. C., et al. (2008). Estimates of the prevalence of arthritis and other rheumatic conditions in the United States: part I. *Arthritis and Rheumatism* 58(1): 15–25.

19. Lawrence R. C., Felson, D. T., Helmick, C. G., et al. (2008). Estimates of the prevalence of arthritis and other rheumatic conditions in the United States: part II. *Arthritis and Rheumatism* 58(1): 26–35.

20. Leveille, S. G., Wee, C. C., & Iezzoni, L. I. (2005). Trends in obesity and arthritis among baby boomers and their predecessors, 1971–2002. *American Journal of Public Health* 95(9): 1607–1613.

21. Messier, S. P., Loeser, R. F., Miller, G. D., et al. (2004). Exercise and dietary weight loss in overweight and obese older adults with knee osteoarthritis: the Arthritis, Diet, and Activity Promotion Trial. *Arthritis and Rheumatology* 50(5): 1501–1510.

22. Miyaguchi, M., Kobayashi, A., Kadoya, Y., et al. (2003). Biochemical change in joint fluid after isometric quadriceps exercise for patients with osteoarthritis of the knee. *Osteoarthritis and Cartilage* 11: 252–259.

23. Centers for Disease Control and Prevention [CDC]. (2004). Lyme disease—United States, 2001–2002. *Morbidity and Mortality Weekly Report* 53(5): 365–369.

24. National Institutes of Health. (2005). *Lyme disease: The facts, the challenge*. National Institute of Allergies and Infectious Diseases and National Institute of Arthritis and Musculoskeletal and Skin Diseases. NIH Publication #05-7045.

25. Bauduceau, B., Bourdel-Marchasson, I., Brocker, P., et al. (2005). The brain of the elderly diabetic patient. *Diabetes Metabolism* 2: 92–97.

26. Kumari, M., & Marmot, M. (2005). Diabetes and cognitive function in a middle-aged cohort: Findings from the Whitehall II study. *Neurology* 65(10): 1597–1603.

27. National Institutes of Health. (2008). *Diagnosis of diabetes*. National Diabetes Information Clearinghouse. Available at: http://diabetes.niddk.nih.gov/dm/pubs/diagnosis/

28. Navarro, R. P. (2009). Contemporary management strategies for fibromyalgia. *American Journal of Managed Care* 15(7 suppl): S197–218.

29. Centers for Disease Control and Prevention [CDC]. (2011). Fibromyalgia. Available at: http://www.cdc.gov/arthritis/basics/fibromyalgia.htm

30. Arnold, L. (2009). Strategies for managing fibromyalgia. *The American Journal of Medicine* 122(12 Suppl): S31–S43.

31. American Autoimmune Related Diseases Association. (2012). Autoimmune disease in women—the facts. Available at: http://www.aarda.org/women_and_autoimmunity.php

32. Lupus Foundation of America. (2012). Lupus fact sheet. Available at: http://www.lupus.org/

webmodules/webarticlesnet/templates/new_news-roomnews.aspx?articleid=351&zoneid=59

33. Kamen, D. L., Cooper, G. S., Bouali, H., et al. (2006). Vitamin D deficiency in systemic lupus erythematosus. *Auto-Immune Review* 5(2): 114–117.

34. Costenbader, K. H., & Karlson, E. W. (2005). Cigarette smoking and systemic lupus erythematosus: A smoking gun? *Autoimmunity* 38(7): 541–547.

35. Blackwell, J. (2004). Evaluation and treatment of hyperthyroidism and hypothyroidism. *Journal of American Academy of Nurse Practitioners* 16(10): 422–425.

36. MayoClinic. (2012). *Hyperthyroidism*. Available at: http://www.mayoclinic.com/health/hyperthyroidism/DS00344

37. American Association of Clinical Endocrinologist Thyroid Task Force. (2002). American Association of Clinical Endocrinologists medical guidelines for clinical practice for the evaluation and treatment of hyperthyroidism and hypothyroidism. *Endocrinology Practice* 6: 457–469.

38. American Health Assistance Foundation. (2012). *Alzheimer's: Risk factors and prevention*. Available at: http://www.ahaf.org/alzdis/about/adrisk.htm.

Chapter Twelve

Mental Health

Chapter Objectives

On completion of this chapter, the student should be able to discuss:

1. The importance of maintaining good mental health, as well as reasons why objectively defining "mental health" is difficult.

2. How biological, social, and environmental factors contribute to and affect mental health.

3. Epidemiological, economic, legal, and political dimensions of mental health.

4. Basic categories of mental disorders, including mood, anxiety, and eating disorders, as well as their symptoms, treatment, and effects on women.

5. Risk factors for suicide among adults, adolescents, and children.

6. Major factors that influence a woman's overall mental health.

7. Strategies for coping with life's daily stresses and improving mental health in general.

8. When to consider seeking treatment for mental illness.

9. Different methods of treating mental disorders, including pharmaceutical treatments and counseling.

womenshealth.jbpub.com

Women's Health Online is a great source for supplementary women's health information for both students and instructors. Visit

http://womenshealth.jbpub.com

to find a variety of useful tools for learning, thinking, and teaching.

Introduction

Mental health is at least as important as physical health for a happy, meaningful life. Poor mental health can interfere with maintaining relationships, having a sense of satisfaction in one's self and one's work, and functioning in day-to-day life. Mental illnesses can dull or block even our basic interests in food, sleep, and sexual contact.

So how should a topic as important, yet as nebulous, as "mental health" be defined? One definition of mental health is "how we think, feel, and act as we cope with life."[1] By this definition, good mental health could be considered a state of well-being that allows a person to be productive, have fulfilling relationships, adapt to changes, and cope with difficult circumstances. Mental disorders can be defined as health conditions marked by changes or abnormalities in mood, thinking, or behavior (or a combination of the three) that produce distress or impair functioning.[2]

Making more specific definitions without going into extensive detail is difficult. *The Diagnostic and Statistical Manual of Mental Disorders, fourth edition* (DSM-IV-TR), the manual the American Psychological Association uses to classify mental disorders, uses more than 140 words to define "mental disorder," and 943 pages (17 major diagnostic classes along 5 axes) to define every recognized mental disorder.

Defining terms like "mental health," "mental disorders," and "mental illness" is also difficult because the distinction between mental and physical health is largely artificial. The brain governs our ability to think, feel, and respond—everything we think of as "mental health." But the brain, like any other organ, requires nutrients and oxygen. It can be damaged or otherwise affected by nutritional deficiencies, thyroid problems, tumors, or physical trauma. Mental health also influences physical health. Depression, for example, makes people less likely to exercise, more likely to engage in substance abuse, and less able to take good care of themselves, greatly increasing their risk for heart disease and other conditions. The environment also affects a person's mental health. Just as if you restrict a person's vitamin C intake, that person will be very likely to develop scurvy even if that person is otherwise "healthy," if you prevent a person from getting enough oxygen, he or she will have a panic attack, even if that person is otherwise a brave, disciplined person in good mental health.

Social context also influences how cultures conceptualize mental health. The DSM once, but no longer, classified homosexuality as a mental illness. Today, suicide is considered the ultimate symptom of mental illness, but in feudal Japan, this act was expected of an honorable person under some circumstances. Freud said the mark of a mentally healthy individual was the ability to love and to work, but even this definition carries certain social judgments about what is important for a good life.

Finally, mental health is difficult to define because it is a matter of degree. People normally considered "mentally healthy" may engage in behaviors that, if taken further, are associated with mental illness. A woman may be considered mentally healthy, and even sensible, for washing her hands several times a day during cold or flu season, but if that same woman washes her hands 30 or 40 times a day and her hand washing interferes with her ability to work, she could be diagnosed with obsessive-compulsive disorder (OCD). Drawing a line between the mentally healthy and people with mental disorders requires a judgment call that may vary from person to person. (Similarly, people have different definitions about at what point water turns from "hot" to "cold," even if everyone agrees that boiling water is hot and ice is cold.)

Mental illness is extremely common. Just as a person's physical health varies throughout his or her lifetime, so, too does his or her mental health. Most people with mental disorders are otherwise normal people who love and are loved, and who contribute to society. People with mental illnesses can be politicians, artists, bus drivers, accountants, doctors, or any other profession. They may seek treatment and recover fully, or they may cope with their disorder as best they can by themselves. In some cases, the perspectives people gain from dealing with mental illness may be of great value to society; some historians have argued that Abraham Lincoln and Winston Churchill were better leaders because of their depressive tendencies.

Half of all Americans experience mental illness in their lifetimes, but most of these people will not seek professional treatment.[2] Many factors contribute to this lack of care. Sometimes good mental health care is not available or affordable, or people do not know where they can find it. The stigma associated with mental illness—many people are afraid to seek help because they are afraid of being thought of as "crazy"—prevents people from seeking needed care. Even as science continues to make enormous strides in mapping the brain and understanding cognitive function, the basic problem of improving access to mental health care remains one of the major health challenges of the 21st century.

Factors Affecting Mental Health

Biological, psychosocial, and environmental factors, and even the food a person eats, all influence mental health. Genetics, for example, clearly predispose some people to mental illness. Studies following separated identical twins find that if one twin has bipolar disorder, the other twin has about a 59% chance of also developing the disease—clearly greater than the proportion of bipolar disorder in the general population.[2] Yet genes are clearly not the only factor: Since identical twins share the same genetic code, some other factor in their environment is responsible for the other 41%. Psychosocial and cultural factors influence how a woman views herself, responds to stress, interacts, and is treated by other people. Factors such as low self-esteem and experiences such as abuse or trauma, all of which women are more likely than men to experience, can make a person more vulnerable to mental illness.

Biological Factors

Biological factors vary among mental illnesses, but they often include genetic predisposition to a disease, abnormal brain structure or function, irregular levels or activity of neurotransmitters or hormones, head or brain injuries, or prenatal exposure to illegal drugs or alcohol.

Many studies have examined patterns in twins and families to determine genetic factors that create vulnerability to certain types of mental illness. Most people with mental disorders have a history of mental illness in their family, providing evidence of a genetic link. Other studies have found that if one identical twin has a mental illness, the other one often has the same illness.

The influence of hormones during reproductive-related events is another important biological factor in women's mental health. Although studies have produced conflicting findings, it appears that changes in hormone levels affect mental well-being and may be a factor in depression during premenstrual syndrome, postpartum depression, and postpartum psychosis. Brain structure and function, as well as neurotransmitter levels, also have been studied to identify gender-related differences and differences between people with and without mental illness.

Social and Psychosocial Factors

Social and psychosocial factors change throughout a woman's lifetime and influence the way a woman views herself and interacts with others. Women with low incomes; who work in difficult, stressful, and low-status jobs have higher rates of mental illness than do women who have a higher socioeconomic status, higher education level, and higher-status job. These higher rates likely result from a combination of the undervalued or nonvalued roles that these women fill and the financial difficulties that accompany such roles. Women in roles that society does not highly value, such as full-time homemakers, often suffer from low self-esteem. Women who are trying to fill multiple roles as career women, mothers, and caretakers often feel overwhelmed, which may lead to low self-esteem, increased stress, and, in some cases, depression.

Societal expectations and the way parents treat their children also influence mental health. Modern American society, for example, expects men to be aggressive, independent, stoic, and strong, and women to be passive, dependent, emotional, and weak. Consequently, many parents interact with girls and boys differently; parents may encourage girls to be delicate, nurturing, nonaggressive, and sensitive to the feelings of others, and teach boys to be assertive, aggressive, and dominant. For many women, aggression can turn inward, resulting in aggression directed at themselves rather than at others, and manifested as depression or another mental illness.

As children reach puberty, gender differences, both physically and culturally, become more apparent. A girl's success often comes from popularity and attractiveness, while a boy's success is often based on athleticism and academic achievement. Factors such as these lead many girls to base their self-esteem on their physical appearance and body weight. These pressures, along with the physical and

© Amy Sancetta/AP Photos

■ In most parts of the U.S., rates of depression are much greater in women than in men. In Amish society, rates of depression are equal by gender. Social and cultural factors are the likely cause for the difference.

Gender Dimensions: Health Differences Between Men and Women

Gender Differences in Mental Illness

Strong gender differences exist both in the prevalence of specific mental disorders and in the way the diseases manifest themselves. Some of these differences are:

- Women have twice the rate of clinical depression as men.
- Women have four times the incidence of seasonal affective disorder as men.
- Women experience more of the depressed phase of bipolar disorder and have more rapid cycling between mania and depression.
- Women are nine times more likely to suffer from anorexia nervosa and bulimia nervosa.

- Twice as many women suffer from panic disorder.
- Women are more likely to have phobias and experience more intense symptoms.
- Borderline personality disorder and histrionic personality disorder are diagnosed in more women.
- Men are more than three times as likely to be diagnosed with anti-social personality disorders than women.
- More women attempt suicide, although more men die from their attempts.

---

hormonal changes of puberty and other stressors, make adolescence an especially difficult period.

Research shows that at all grade levels, girls continue to receive less attention than boys in academic settings. Girls generally make better grades than boys do, but despite this academic success, girls experience more internal costs— worry, anxiety, and depression. As the authors of one study note, "Although girls may have the edge over boys in terms of their performance in school, this edge is lost when it comes to the experience of internal distress."[3] Another study showed that women tend to attribute their successes to luck and their failures to lack of ability, whereas men

© AbleStock

■ Young girls often lag behind boys in self-esteem and they are more likely to experience depression.

tend to attribute their successes to ability and their failures to bad luck.[4]

During and after adolescence, girls must create an identity for themselves, deal with their sexuality, make education and career choices, and become independent. For adolescents, risk factors for mental disorders include lack of parental support, sexual abuse, low self-esteem, and weak relationships with friends or family. Some teens may not exhibit obvious signs of emotional distress and may express their lack of mental wellness through substance abuse, disordered eating, behavior problems, and sexual promiscuity.

Teenage girls are more likely than teenage boys to experience depression. Studies show that female high school students have significantly higher rates of anxiety disorders, eating disorders, and adjustment disorder than their male counterparts, who have higher rates of disruptive behavior disorders, attention deficit disorder, autism, and learning disabilities.

Early adulthood brings many decisions, including those concerning career choices, relationships such as marriage or intimate partnerships, and childbearing. Reproductive events at this time in a woman's life, such as pregnancy, child care, infertility, or the decision not to have children, may create personal stress and relationship tension. Many women also experience increased independence at this time in their lives, as well as increased financial obligations and responsibilities at work and at home. All of these factors can affect a woman's mental health.

Many women begin to experiment with recreational drug use during adolescence and early adulthood. Among women with mental health disorders, substance abuse is a common occurrence. Substance abuse may occur when these women attempt to self-medicate and cope, or from the fact that their mental disorders inhibit their reasoning skills. The prolonged use of illicit drugs can put people at higher risk for developing mental disorders and can make existing disorders worse, causing people to self-medicate with drugs more intensely or more frequently. This pattern creates a vicious cycle in the relationship between drug use and mental disorders.

Studies have shown that between 30% and 60% of drug abusers have mental health disorders; depression and attempted suicide are especially common among female substance abusers. For many of these abusers, their depressive symptoms predated their use of alcohol and other drugs. Rates of drug abuse or dependence among anorexics range from 5% to 19%; among bulimics, these rates are significantly higher, ranging from 8% to 36%.[5] These women may abuse cocaine, heroin, or methamphetamines to lose weight because these substances act as appetite suppressants. Between 30% and 60% of patients with bipolar disorder also have a substance abuse problem. In fact, substance abuse is more likely to be present with bipolar illness than with any other disorder. Individuals with bipolar disorder who abuse drugs or alcohol may have an earlier onset and worse course of illness than those who do not.

As women reach midlife, many continue to deal with career issues and financial burdens while struggling to balance their many roles of mother, wife, daughter, friend, sibling, employer, employee, and self. Women also may be dealing with stress from growing children and aging parents. The support and joy that good relationships offer a woman are often important counterbalances to the stress of managing her everyday life. As she nears late adulthood, a woman may be fortunate enough to feel satisfied with her accomplishments and be financially secure. Women who struggle with retirement issues, physical health, unaccomplished areas of their lives, ill parents, or adult children with difficulties, however, may feel overwhelmed by stressors not fully within their control.

Depression and **dementia** resulting from Alzheimer's disease (Chapter 11) are serious mental health issues affecting the elderly. A majority of people with Alzheimer's disease are women, in part because women constitute a larger percentage of the elderly population than men. Depression is widely underdiagnosed and undertreated in the elderly population. One in every 14 Americans age 65 or older currently has a diagnosable depressive illness. Older adults in the United States are also about 40% more likely to commit suicide than the general population.[6]

Poor physical health, limited independence, loss of privacy and freedom, and loss of one's partner or friends all contribute to stress and poor mental health in older women. Cognitive impairments in the elderly often result from some form of dementia, but may also result from severe depression. In many cases, depression occurs concurrently with chronic medical conditions such as heart disease, diabetes, cancer, and dementia. Because of the common occurrence of depression in the elderly, many healthcare providers, as well as patients and caregivers, believe that symptoms of depression are a normal part of aging or a normal consequence of chronic disease. Depression in older women can lead to disorientation, loss of short-term memory, verbal difficulty, and inappropriate reasoning skills. Personality changes also may result from dementia or depression or from a decrease in overall physical health.[7]

Discrimination—being singled out by others based on sexual, ethnic, or physical characteristics, including the presence of a mental disorder—is another risk factor for mental illness that women of all age groups experience. Discrimination can affect any aspect of a woman's life, including her work, marriage, and social status. Both mental and physical abuse put women at high risk for developing depression, posttraumatic stress disorder, or obsessive-compulsive disorder. Many people with mental disorders suffered from childhood abuse or traumas, and their disorders represent a response to their repressed emotions. This factor may partly account for women's increased incidence of certain mental disorders, because women are at

© Marmaduke St. John/Alamy Images

■ Six out of 10 female inmates in federal prisons are mentally ill; more than 7 in 10 female inmates in state prisons and jails are mentally ill.

a higher risk of being victimized through rape, abuse, and sexual harassment.

Other reasons that women suffer from mental disorders may relate to their individual personality traits. Women who are prone to pessimistic thinking, have low self-esteem, feel they have little control over life events, and worry excessively are at higher risk for depressive and anxiety disorders. Many women also have a heightened sense of sympathy and empathy, which leaves them more vulnerable to suffering from depression after tragic events, even if they were not directly affected by the events themselves.

Stress

Stress is the physical, mental, or emotional response that a person experiences when subjected to any type of stressor, a situation that produces tension or requires a difficult decision. Stressors can range from daily hassles to life-altering events, and people experience and react to them in different ways. Today's women face special stressors. A national recession, along with continuing high rates of unemployment, have increased financial insecurity and made it harder for women to earn a living wage. More women, especially those with young children, are becoming members of the paid workforce. However, women continue to do more housework and spend more time caring for dependent family members than men, often creating a "second shift" after a woman returns from her day job. Domestic chores, child care, and running errands can sap women of their energy and cause stress that affects both their home life and their work life.

It's Your Health

Methods of Coping

Maintain a good support system.

Make time for pleasurable activities.

Avoid using food, drugs, or alcohol for mood enhancers.

Try to get 30 minutes or more of physical activity per day.

Develop positive thinking techniques.

Learn to control anger, but do not suppress it.

Practice body acceptance.

Get a good night's sleep.

Say NO to excessive responsibilities.

Use relaxation techniques to control stress.

Acute stress can be helpful for energizing and motivating a person, but chronic stress can overload a person and cause emotional symptoms such as edginess and distorted thinking. Chronic stress also can lead to physical symptoms

such as increased heart rate and blood pressure, and lowered immune defense to common colds and other illnesses.[8] Women and men often perceive, evaluate, and respond to stress in different ways. Men may respond positively with physical activity, but negatively through aggression and substance abuse. In contrast, women often internalize their stress, which can cause feelings of failure and self-blame.

People adopt different strategies to cope with the stress in their lives. Because stress levels change over time, individuals may adjust their coping mechanisms accordingly. Positive ways of coping with stress include relaxation techniques; supportive, positive interactions with friends and family; and exercise (see the **It's Your Health** boxes in this chapter). People with better coping skills are less distressed overall and suffer from less pain, anxiety, depression, illnesses, and "burnout."

Nutrition

The food that people eat can also affect their mental health. Certain foods tend to increase stress levels, whereas others help to calm the physiological effects of stress. "Food stressors" include chocolate, caffeine, sugar, and alcohol. Foods that can provide a calming effect include water, vegetables, fruit, and oil-rich fish. Eating regular, healthful meals also appears to have a positive effect on mental health. The effects of nutrition on mental health are considered secondary, however, to other physiological and environmental factors.[9]

Perspectives on Mental Health

Epidemiological Data

More than one out of four American adults—about 58 million people—experience a diagnosable mental disorder in a given year.[10] About 13 million, or 1 out of 17 American adults, will suffer from a severe mental illness that seriously disrupts their day-to-day activities, and about half the people who have one mental disorder also have at least one other. Taken together, mental illnesses are responsible for 4 of the top 10 causes of disability. Among adults ages 15–44, mental illnesses cause more death and injury than cancer.[10]

Men and women are equally likely to suffer from mental disorders, but the frequencies of specific mental disorders vary by gender. Men and women may also experience the same disorder in different ways, including the average age that disorders appear, frequency of psychotic symptoms, course of disease progression, social adjustment, and long-term outcome.[11] Variations in mental illnesses may be partially a result of distinct brain structures and the presence of different brain hormones in males and females, which cause neurons to act differently. Evidence shows that the development of brain hemispheres differs by gender, possibly resulting in males and females using their brains in different ways when decoding words, deciphering emotion, and performing other basic tasks. Other differences in how men and women experience mental illness may be due to how men and women cope with problems, view themselves, and express emotions. The **Gender Dimensions** box lists gender differences in common mental health disorders.

■ Mentally ill homeless people present a host of legal and ethical dilemmas for society.

Economic Dimensions

In addition to their harmful effects on individual health, mental illnesses carry a great economic cost. One major study found that lost earnings from serious mental illnesses cost Americans $193 billion a year.[12] This estimate does not include the billions of dollars spent on medical care such as medications, clinic visits, and hospital visits; nor does it include the time and resources spent by families and caregivers of people with mental illnesses or the cost of social problems such as increased crime and threats to public safety.

Treating mental illness is often a costly undertaking. Prescription drugs can be very expensive, especially for people who don't have health insurance or who are **underinsured**. Because individual responses to medications vary and medications sometimes have serious side effects, time and medical care must often be spent on determining, often by trial and error, the correct medication and dosage for a person's individual needs. Inpatient and outpatient mental healthcare services are also expensive and require commitments of time and resources for patients and facilities providing care. Because people with serious mental illnesses sometimes have difficulty holding down jobs for long periods of time, they are at increased risk for being both uninsured and economically vulnerable.

Legal Dimensions

Most people with mental disorders are law-abiding citizens. With access to proper treatment, people with mental disorders are not more likely to commit crimes than the general population. However, if mental illnesses are left untreated or are not treated properly, a correlation between mental illness and crime does exist, especially among individuals with psychotic and mood disorders. Many people are not identified as suffering from a mental disorder during the legal and criminal process. The Bureau of Justice Statistics estimates that more than half of prison and jail inmates suffer from at least one mental disorder, most often mania, depression, and psychotic disorders. Female inmates are more likely to have some form of mental illness than male inmates: 73% of women in state prisons, 61% of women in federal prisons, and 75% of women in jails had a significant mental disorder. Less than one-third of prisoners who had a mental health problem had received treatment since they were incarcerated.[13] These numbers likely reflect both a link between untreated mental disorders and crime as well as increased rates of mental illness that result from the trauma related to committing a crime, going to trial, and adjusting to a life in prison.

Mentally ill homeless people also create legal and ethical dilemmas for society. During the 1980s, thousands of mentally ill people became homeless after cuts in federal and state funding to inpatient mental facilities and outpatient mental health clinics. These funding cuts forced facilities to release thousands of patients who were not capable of caring for themselves, and also removed a source of mental health care for thousands of others who were caring for themselves but were economically vulnerable. Without appropriate care and access to consistent medications and treatment, and with continued exposure to the stress of living on the street, over time many mentally ill homeless people have become less healthy, both mentally and physically. For this and other reasons, homeless people with mental disorders have a high incidence of arrests and encounters with the law for threatening behavior, substance abuse, or other disorderly conduct. They also face numerous health problems that develop from their unhealthy living conditions. The connection between the inability of many mentally ill people to access appropriate care and the incidence of criminal behavior underscores the continued need for social programs that improve the quality of life for the mentally ill in the United States.

Political Dimensions

The National Institute of Mental Health (NIMH) is the largest research organization in the world dedicated to improving mental health. Part of the National Institutes of Health, which itself is part of the federal government, the NIMH researches new ways to understand the mind, brain, and behavior; examine, treat, and prevent mental disorders; and promote and maintain good mental health. The Substance Abuse and Mental Health Services Administration (SAMHSA), another agency of the federal government, is responsible for preventing death and preventing, treating, and rehabilitating disability caused by mental illness and substance abuse. Whereas the NIMH tends to focus more on research and furthering scientific understanding, SAMHSA focuses on aid and research that more directly helps people who suffer from poor mental health or substance abuse.

Federal, state, and local policies and laws have enormous, far-reaching effects on mental health. The connections between the two are not always obvious, however. If more effective drug-enforcement laws are enacted, they could reduce rates of underage drinking and illegal drug use among pregnant women, which in turn could prevent cases of mental illness resulting from fetal exposure to drugs and alcohol. An overseas conflict that sends U.S. armed forces into combat will inevitably increase rates of post-traumatic stress disorder (PTSD) as those troops react to injuries and their experiences on the battlefield. A program offering low-interest loans to small businesses could reduce rates of depression if it lifted large numbers of people out of poverty and reduced the stresses and risk factors associated with living under the poverty line.

Laws and policies affect the affordability of mental health care. For years, people who had health insurance often found that the plans charged more for mental health services than for other services, or that the plans did not cover mental health services at all. This discrepancy often resulted in people being unable to afford mental health care and contributed to the false idea that mental health services are either unimportant or a luxury. In 2008, Congress passed legislation requiring health insurance plans that offered mental health services to give those services the same coverage they offer for other physical health services; however, this law only affected insurance plans that offered mental health coverage to begin with.[14]

Preventing mental illnesses can minimize suffering and loss of productivity associated with the disorders, and eliminate the costs of diagnosing and treating the disorders after they develop. Simple, cost-effective ways to prevent mental illness include enacting policies to reduce head injuries by mandating the use of motorcycle helmets; reducing childhood exposure to lead by replacing old plumbing in public schools; and preventing fetal exposure to alcohol, tobacco, and other drugs by offering rehabilitation programs for pregnant women. Programs that support good parenting, such as ample maternity and paternity leave programs, or providing classes and support to new parents, have especially powerful mental-health-promoting effects for both children and parents.

Clinical Dimensions of Mental Illness

Mood Disorders

Mood disorders (also known as **affective disorders**) are mental disorders characterized by extreme disturbances of mood, the dominant emotion (or emotional tendency) a person feels at any given moment. Many factors including genetics, out-of-balance neurotransmitters, a person's life experiences, and other environmental factors can contribute to a mood disorder or influence how a given disorder progresses. Depression and dysthymia are associated with persistent sadness, whereas bipolar disorder is associated with rapid mood changes or sustained elevations in mood.[2]

Depression

Depression is a medical illness affecting the mind as well as the body. Usually triggered by stressful life events, depression is characterized by persistent, inescapable feelings of sadness. These emotions are often accompanied by feelings of inadequacy and hopelessness, physical exhaustion, and other symptoms (**Table 12.1**). Symptoms of depression are so intense that they usually disrupt a person's basic

Table 12.1 Symptoms of Depression

Persistent sad mood
Constant feelings of sadness
Excessive crying
Low energy
Feelings of worthlessness or hopelessness
Difficulty concentrating or making decisions
Loss of interest in pleasurable activities
Sleep disturbances
Appetite and weight changes
Thoughts of death or suicide
Physical symptoms that do not respond to treatment

Table 12.2 Symptoms of Postpartum Depression

Anxiety
Feelings of hopelessness and guilt
Panic attacks
Insomnia
Lack of interest in the baby
Thoughts of suicide
Thoughts of hurting self or baby

activities, including eating, sleeping, maintaining relationships, and taking pleasure in life.[15] People with depression often feel undesirable and inadequate. They anticipate rejection and dissatisfaction from their interactions and experiences, and they blame themselves when their negative expectations are fulfilled. People with depression often know their feelings are unhealthy and unproductive, and want desperately to feel better, but are unable to do so. This inability to "snap out of it" makes them feel even more weak and inadequate.[16] Feelings of hopelessness and worthlessness also make people with depression unlikely to seek professional help. Less than one-third of people with depression seek help from a mental health professional.[17]

Depression often coexists with other physical and mental illnesses. Among the elderly, for example, depression is often mistaken for, or present with, Alzheimer's disease. Medical conditions, such as thyroid disease, multiple sclerosis, and cancer, also increase a person's risk of getting depression. Depression also may arise as a response to a serious illness, a consequence of substance abuse, or a side effect of certain medications. In addition, depression frequently accompanies chronic diseases, including coronary heart disease, diabetes, stroke, cancer, and HIV/AIDS.

Hormonal shifts during reproductive-related events and their link to mental illness have been the subject of much controversy. For example, it was previously believed that hormones were solely responsible for depression during premenstrual syndrome (PMS); however, research now shows that hormones may trigger, but are not solely responsible for, PMS-related depression. Severe depression during PMS, called premenstrual dysphoric disorder (PMDD), affects 3% to 7% of menstruating women.[18]

Postpartum depression is a type of depression that affects 10% to 15% of all new mothers.[15] This condition is different from the "baby blues," or postpartum blues, which occurs

in the first 10 days after delivery and are quite common and typically mild. Postpartum depression typically begins 3 to six 6 after delivery and is much more severe (**Table 12.2**), although less severe than **postpartum psychosis**. Postpartum depression is more common in women with a history of depression, marital issues, lack of social support, or a history of negative life experiences. Although it often goes unnoticed and untreated, postpartum depression can greatly affect the mother and child as well as damage the relationship between the parents. For women who are already at risk, menopause can be another hormone-related event that can trigger depression.

My grandmother suffered from severe depression. My mother also had it, and now I've got it too. I've been in counseling for six years and on antidepressants for three years. I feel I've finally gained control of my life, but I'm scared for my children. I don't want my daughter to have to suffer like all of the other generations in my family have suffered.

33-year-old woman

Levels of the neurotransmitter **serotonin** are lower in people with major depression. Medications that boost levels of serotonin, called selective serotonin reuptake inhibitors (SSRIs), can often relieve symptoms of depression. One study found that men's brains make 52% more serotonin than do women's brains, possibly explaining why depression can manifest differently in men and women.[19]

Genetics also play a major role in depression. Someone with a family history of depression is significantly more likely to develop depression than someone with no family history of the disease. Studies have shown that children with one depressed parent are two to three times more likely to experience depression by age 18 than are children without depressed parents. The risk doubles if both parents suffer from depression.[20]

Seasonal shifts in daylight hours, which affect a person's circadian rhythm or sleep–wake cycle, can cause a

© luxorphoto/ShutterStock, Inc.

■ Depression is characterized by persistent, intense feelings of sadness, inadequacy, and hopelessness.

particular form of depression called **seasonal affective disorder (SAD)**. Seasonal affective disorder often affects women in their reproductive years, producing symptoms such as increased appetite, lethargy, and carbohydrate cravings. Researchers believe the cause of SAD may be related to melatonin disturbances. Therapeutic doses of bright light in the morning can help to relieve this condition.

Depression is the most common mood disorder among women and is about twice as common in women as it is in men. Depression affects 1 in 10 women at any given moment, but more than 1 in 5 women will experience at least one depressive episode during their lives.[17,21] Adolescent females have especially high rates of depression. Before puberty, boys are more likely than girls of the same age to be diagnosed with depression or depressive symptoms. After puberty, however, girls are far more likely to

be diagnosed with depression.[17] Between the ages of 30 and 44—typically the years of childbearing and childrearing—rates of depression are three times greater for women than they are for men. Elderly women, especially women who are widowed, are in poor physical health, or have lost some or all of their independence, are also at risk for developing depression. Medical illness and the effects of multiple medications in the elderly make diagnosing depression especially difficult.

Rates of depression vary significantly by race/ethnicity and socioeconomic characteristics (see **Figures 12.1 and 12.2**). People of color are significantly more likely to be depressed than White people. Education, employment status, and poverty are also predictors for depression. People without a high school diploma are 2.5 times more likely to be depressed than people who have gone to college; people who are unemployed or unable to work are 3 to 5 times more likely to be depressed than people who work, and people living in poverty are about twice as likely to be depressed as people who are not poor.[17,21] The reasons for these correlations are complex and not fully understood. However, these higher rates of depression can be traced in part both to reduced access to health care and other resources, and to increased vulnerability to negative life events and the stress resulting from this vulnerability.

Researchers are examining whether the higher rates of depression in women truly represent a greater incidence of depression or whether the rates reflect gender-based differences in the acknowledgment of mental illness or ability to recognize symptoms. Rates of depression in men may be underestimated because women are more likely than men to discuss feelings associated with being depressed, to

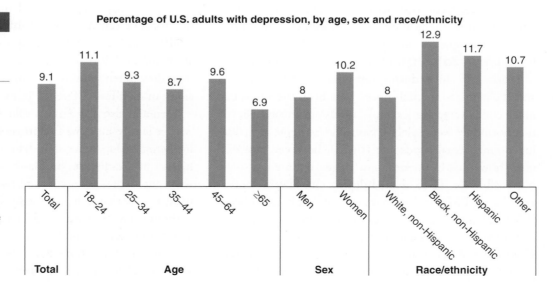

Figure 12.1

Percentage of U.S. adults with depression, by Age, Sex and Race/Ethnicity

Source: Data from Centers for Disease Contol and Prevention. (2010). Current Depression Among Adults—United States, 2006 and 2008. Available at http://www.cdc.gov/features/dsdepression/revised_table_estimates_for_depression_mmwr_erratum_feb-2011.pdf

Percentage of U.S. adults with depression, by age, sex and race/ethnicity

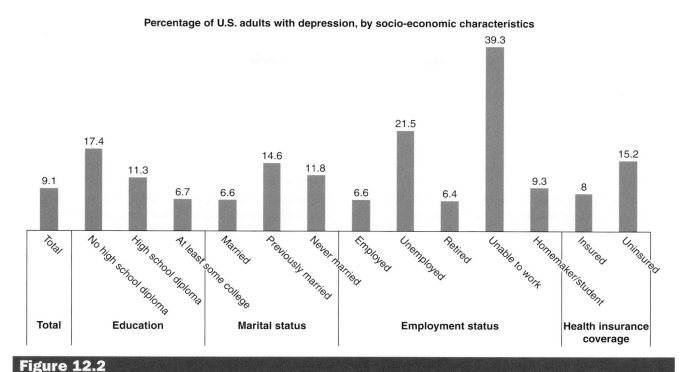

Figure 12.2

Percentage of U.S. adults with depression, by Socio-Ecnomic Characteristics

Source: Data from Centers for Disease Contol and Prevention. (2010). Current Depression Among Adults–United States, 2006 and 2008. Available at http://www.cdc.gov/features/dsdepression/revised_table_estimates_for_depression_mmwr_erratum_feb-2011.pdf

admit to feeling depressed, and to seek help. Men are also more likely to direct negative feelings outward rather than inward, toward the self. (These same tendencies make men more likely to engage in self-destructive behaviors such as substance abuse and violent behavior directed at others.) In Amish culture, where women's roles as mothers and homemakers are more highly valued than in U.S. society as a whole and society frowns on self-destructive "macho" behaviors and alcohol consumption, rates of depression are equal for men and women.[16] Women also have higher rates of victimization from physical abuse, sexual harassment, and rape. Acts of violence such as these not only cause trauma, but foster low self-esteem, a sense of helplessness, social isolation, and, ultimately, depression. Being a caregiver for young children, aging parents, or ill family members—roles often filled by women—also has been noted as a risk factor for depression.

Dysthymia

Dysthymia is a milder but persistent form of depression. Even though dysthymia's symptoms are less severe than other forms of depression, dysthymia is still a serious, debilitating disease. It is diagnosed when symptoms last at least 2 years in adults or 1 year in adolescents and children. People with dysthymia exhibit a depressed mood and at least two other symptoms of depression, such as poor appetite, overeating, sleep difficulties, or low self-esteem. Dysthymia often begins in childhood or adolescence, but can occur at any age. Because it often develops at a young age, the depressed state becomes integrated within the woman's personality, often not only affecting her self-esteem and motivation, but also her ability to live a satisfying life and function normally. Dysthymia affects about 1.5% of the adult population (about 3.3 million adults) in any given year.[10]

Bipolar Disorder

Bipolar disorder, sometimes also referred to as **manic-depressive disorder**, is somewhat like depression in that it affects a person's emotions and ability to function, but bipolar disorder is characterized by shifts in emotion, not by a single mood.[22] A person with bipolar disorder experiences episodes of both mania ("highs") and depression ("lows"). During manic episodes a person with bipolar disorder typically has an excess of energy, activity, and restlessness. At this point, a person could feel wonderful and euphoric, or overly stimulated and easily irritated. Other symptoms of a manic phase include racing thoughts, extreme distractibility, overconfidence, and an increased sex drive. People experiencing depressive episodes typically have deep, persistent feelings of sadness, anxiety, hopelessness, or guilt; they might also have low energy, a reduced sense of pleasure, a lowered sex drive, and thoughts of suicide.[21] In between manic and depressive episodes, a person with bipolar disorder could have extended periods of being within the normal range of moods. People with bipolar disorder are at great risk for abusing alcohol and other drugs and engaging in other self-destructive behaviors.

About 2.6% of the adult population (5.7 million people) will be affected by bipolar disorder in any given year. Bipolar disorder typically first appears during a person's 20s.[10] Gender differences influence the manifestation of the disease, however, with women typically having more depressed episodes and more rapid cycling between depression and mania than do men.

Treatment

The good news is that treating mood disorders can provide great benefits, allowing people to live satisfying, functional, and healthy lives. The bad news, however, is that mood disorders have no "quick fix." Between 70% and 80% of people who experience one episode of depression will experience depression again at some point in their lives[22]; bipolar disorder typically requires ongoing treatment for a person to stay within a stable mood range. Short-term treatments for either of these illnesses are unlikely to be effective.[2] For both depression and bipolar disorder, the earlier a person seeks treatment, the better chance that person will have of making a recovery and of preventing further episodes.

Mood disorders can be treated with medications, psychosocial treatment (some form of "talk therapy"), or both of these forms used together. A combined approach usually works better than either form used alone.[15,21] Medications are a powerful, yet imperfect tool to treat people with mood disorders. Medications can gradually bring a person with depression or bipolar disorder back into a normal range of moods, but they may take days or even weeks to have any noticeable effects. Individuals respond differently to treatments and treatments may have side effects, so a person with a mood disorder taking medications should work with his or her psychiatrist to find the specific pharmaceutical drug and dosage that provides the most benefit while reducing side effects to a low, or at least acceptable, level. Because some medications for depression or bipolar disorder may affect fetal development, a woman with a mood disorder should talk with her psychiatrist about her medication routine if she is pregnant or wishes to conceive.

Antidepressant medications attempt to restore a depressed person's levels of **neurotransmitters**, particularly serotonin, norepinephrine, and dopamine, to a normal level. There are several types of antidepressant medications. The two newest, most commonly used types are called selective serotonin reuptake inhibitors (SSRIs) and serotonin and norepinephrine reuptake inhibitors (SNRIs). Older forms of antidepressants, including tricyclics or monoamine oxidase inhibitors (MAOIs), are more likely to have side effects, though these medications may be best for some individuals. Possible side effects of antidepressant medications include headaches, nausea, insomnia, constipation, and reduced sexual desire and function.

Bipolar disorder is usually treated with one or more of several kinds of medications known as "mood stabilizers." Mood-stabilizing drugs include lithium and several classes of anticonvulsant drugs. These drugs help to keep a person's mood within a consistent, central range. To be effective, these drugs should be taken on a regular basis. Sometimes a person with bipolar disorder can "feel" a mood shift approaching; if a person notices this and talks with his or her psychiatrist, a temporary change in his or her treatment plan can often prevent an episode from occurring.[22]

Psychosocial treatment for depression can provide benefits on either a short-term (around 10–20 weeks) or a continuous basis, depending on the individual's needs and desires. The two most popular forms of psychotherapy used to treat depression are cognitive behavioral therapy (CBT) and interpersonal therapy (IPT). Cognitive behavioral therapy teaches a depressed person to recognize patterns of thinking and behaving that contribute to depression, and helps that person find new thoughts and behaviors that support recovery, while IPT helps people to understand and improve their own personal relationships and interactions with other people. Psychotherapy is often the best treatment option for people with mild to moderate depression; for people with major depression, psychotherapy can be combined with antidepressant medications.[15]

For people with bipolar disorder, psychosocial treatment includes:

- Cognitive behavioral therapy, which helps patients to recognize and change harmful thought patterns and behaviors associated with the disorder
- Psychoeducation, which teaches patients (and sometimes relatives or loved ones) about the effects, treatment, and management of bipolar disorder

- Family therapy, which works on improving family interactions to improve harmful relationships or patterns of interaction that contribute to or result from the patient's symptoms

- Interpersonal and social rhythm therapy, which helps patients improve their personal interactions and establish regular daily routines[22]

Anxiety Disorders

Anxiety is an adaptive mental function that helps us live safe, productive lives. At healthy levels, anxiety can motivate a person to study for a test, look both ways before crossing the street, double-check that the front door is locked, or refrain from stealing or committing some other crime. **Anxiety disorders** occur when anxiety grows to unhealthy levels, or when anxiety appears in situations in which no risks exist. People with anxiety disorders often know that the worries, fears, or behaviors caused by the disorders are unhelpful and unrealistic, but this knowledge does not eliminate the symptoms (see **Table 12.3**). Anxiety disorders include generalized anxiety disorder (GAD), social phobias (also known as social anxiety disorder), specific phobias, panic disorder, obsessive-compulsive disorder (OCD), and posttraumatic stress disorder.[24]

Anxiety disorders affect about 40 million American adults (about 1 out of 5 adults) during a given year. Women are two to three times more likely than men to suffer from anxiety disorders. People with an anxiety disorder are disproportionately likely to experience some form of depression, another anxiety disorder, or engage in substance abuse in efforts to self-medicate. Anxiety disorders usually appear early as compared to other mental illnesses: Three-fourths of people with an anxiety disorder experience their first symptoms before they turn 21.[10]

Table 12.3 Symptoms of Anxiety Disorder

Feelings of terror and dread
Feelings of apprehension and uncertainty
Nervousness
Irritability
Rapid heartbeat
Chest pain
Fainting
Difficulty breathing
Sweating
Belief that feelings are signs of a heart attack

Generalized Anxiety Disorder

Generalized anxiety disorder (GAD) is characterized by chronic and exaggerated worry and tension that lasts for at least 6 months. People with GAD may worry about disasters befalling themselves or their loved ones, or about routine events of everyday life. This constant worrying eventually affects the body in many ways, producing symptoms such as an inability to relax, nausea, muscle tension or pain, trembling, or having to go to the bathroom frequently. The worrying can also interfere with concentration and memory. The severity of GAD varies from person to person: It can be relatively mild, or the anxiety can be intense and disabling enough to prevent a person from carrying out daily activities, holding a job, or interacting with others. Generalized anxiety disorder currently affects 6.8 million adults in the United States, two-thirds of whom are women.[24]

Social Phobia

Phobias are intense fears of something that poses little or no threat. A person with social phobia, or social anxiety disorder, experiences a powerful, lasting fear of interacting with other people. People with this mental disorder become very self-conscious in social settings, often imagining that they are being watched or judged, or that they are doing something embarrassing. A social phobia may create anxiety surrounding all human interactions, or it may be limited to specific situations, such as eating or drinking in public, or speaking in front of a group. Anxiety can last for days or weeks before a social event and can continue after. Fifteen million U.S. adults experience social phobia; about half of them are women.[10]

Other Phobias

People can develop phobias about specific animals, objects, places, or events other than social interactions. Phobias may involve heights, closed spaces, flying, spiders, elevators, the sight of blood, or other things or situations. A phobia involves more than a moderate level of fear—a person can be afraid of any of the previously mentioned things without having a phobia. Phobias involve powerful, overwhelming fear that occurs not only when the object of the phobia appears, but also often when it is merely even thought about. Phobias can be especially disabling if the object of the phobia is common or difficult to avoid in a person's daily life. About 20 million U.S. adults, including 14 million women, have a phobia of some kind.[24]

■ Therapeutic doses of bright light in the morning can help relieve depression caused by seasonal affective disorder (SAD).

Panic Disorder

Panic disorder affects about 6 million U.S. adults and is twice as common in women as in men. This disorder is characterized by panic attacks—periods of intense fear accompanied by physical and emotional distress that may last anywhere from 5 to 20 minutes.[24] The panic attack often strikes without warning. Its symptoms have often been mistaken for a heart attack, and include a pounding heart, sweating, faintness, dizziness, chest pain, nausea, and emotional symptoms such as a feeling of impending doom or of losing control. In many cases the intensity of the symptoms, as well as their unexplainable nature, makes the panic attacks themselves a major source of anxiety.

An initial panic attack usually occurs in a person's 20s. A panic attack may occur during transition periods, times of considerable stress, or crises and often sends the individual to the emergency room. Some women have an isolated attack without ever developing the disorder; nevertheless, repeated panic attacks are a definitive sign of panic disorder. Panic attacks can be extremely disabling if they occur on a regular basis.

Obsessive-Compulsive Disorder

Obsessive-compulsive disorder (OCD) is an anxiety disorder in which a person develops intense, persistent fears, worries, or superstitions (obsessions), and uses specific rituals (compulsions), often repeated over and over again on a daily basis, for relief. One of the classic obsessions in OCD is an overwhelming fear of germs; a woman with this obsession might wash her hands dozens of times a day, or be afraid to touch a doorknob or any item that someone else has touched. Other obsessions include fear of social embarrassment, thoughts about having harmed a loved one, worries about having forgotten something or left something out of place, and intrusive sexual thoughts. The ritual adopted to find relief varies from person to person, but some common themes emerge. Rituals often involve repeatedly checking, counting, or touching things in a specific pattern or order. The rituals are distracting and time-consuming and do not actually bring pleasure, just, at most, short-lived relief from symptoms.[24]

Slightly more than 2 million adults in the United States have OCD, which affects men and women in equal numbers. Obsessive-compulsive disorder usually appears in the first 20 to 30 years of a person's life, often appearing in childhood. It also runs in families, suggesting that genetics can predispose a person to the disorder.[24]

Posttraumatic Stress Disorder

Posttraumatic stress disorder (PTSD), also referred to as posttraumatic stress injury, is an extremely debilitating disorder that occurs after an exposure to a terrifying event involving violent harm or the threat of violent harm. PTSD can result from situations such as armed combat, a car accident, sexual assault, mugging, or natural disaster. A person can develop PTSD if he or she was threatened directly, or if he or she witnessed a threat to a friend or family member. People with PTSD may be easily startled or may be constantly anxious and hyper-vigilant. Situations that remind them of the traumatic event can trigger "flashbacks" in which they relive part or all of their experience. Flashbacks can also occur in dreams or for no apparent reason while the person is awake. People with PTSD can also become emotionally numb, unable to maintain personal relationships or take pleasure from daily life. People with PTSD may become violent or aggressive; they may also become depressed, or turn to substance abuse for relief.

PTSD was originally identified in male Vietnam veterans, but PTSD is a major public health concern for women as well. Women are more than twice as likely as men to develop PTSD after exposure to a traumatic event, in part because they are more likely to blame themselves. Women are also more likely than men to be victims of sexual assault, a major trigger event for PTSD. Women are more likely to experience PTSD if they have more than one traumatic experience, had or have a mental disorder before the trauma, or do not have good social support.[25] One bit of good news for women, however, is that they tend to recover from PTSD more easily than men, because they are more likely to be comfortable talking about their feelings and difficult personal issues. At least 7.7 million U.S. adults have PTSD,[24] but this number may be an underestimate.

Over the past decade, millions of women have been subject to traumatic events that have made them more vulnerable to PTSD. Hundreds of thousands of women and have lost their jobs, homes, or financial security as a result of the 2007–2008 global economic crisis. Women living in and around New Orleans have had their lives, homes, and families ravaged by the flooding of (and slow government response to) Hurricane Katrina; one study found that almost one in four residents of Mississippi directly affected by Hurricane Katrina exhibited some signs of PTSD.[26] Women veterans have had to adjust to coping with daily life after returning from the wars in Iraq and Afghanistan—about one out of seven military personnel who have experienced combat in Iraq are women.[25] Women soldiers are much more likely than men to be victims of sexual assault or violence from their fellow soldiers and from superior officers. Although a male soldier may have to deal with significant stress from fighting enemy combatants, he might be able to have a deep sense of trust around his fellow troops; a woman who has been sexually assaulted not only has to deal with the direct trauma of the experience, but can never fully relax.

Treatment

Like many other mental illnesses, anxiety disorders can be treated with medications, psychotherapy, or a combination of the two, depending on individual needs and preferences. Without treatment, people with anxiety disorders may find themselves making serious life decisions based on their likelihood of encountering a phobic or anxiety-producing object or situation. Treatment can provide great benefits for people living with anxiety disorders, but time and effort are necessary to see improvements; people sometimes believe that they can't be treated, or that the treatment doesn't work for them, when more time or an adjustment to the treatment is all that is needed.[24] Commonly prescribed medications for anxiety disorders include antidepressants, antianxiety medications, and beta blockers, a type of drug originally developed to treat heart conditions. Cognitive behavioral therapy can help people with anxiety disorders learn to recognize and change thoughts and behaviors associated with the disorder. Another form of therapy used for anxiety disorders is called exposure/response therapy. Exposure/response therapy aims to desensitize sufferers to their fears by supporting them in staying calm while gradually confronting more and more anxiety-producing situations. Certain forms of group therapy can also help people

■ Rates of post-traumatic stress disorder among women have increased as more women have joined the U.S. military.

with anxiety disorders, especially people with PTSD or social phobia. If a person with an anxiety disorder is experiencing another form of mental illness or has a substance-abuse problem, these issues will also need to be treated.

Eating Disorders

Eating disorders are serious mental illnesses characterized by dysfunctional eating patterns. But an eating disorder is much more than an unhealthy eating habit or a desire "not to eat." Like other mental illnesses, eating disorders have biological and environmental causes, distinct symptoms, and harmful consequences for the body.[27] People with eating disorders are also likely to have other mental illnesses, including depression, anxiety disorders, and substance-abuse problems. At some point in their lives, between 0.5% and 3.7% of women will have anorexia, and between 1.1% and 4.2% of women will have bulimia.[28] Eating disorders are treatable, but success requires the person to acknowledge the seriousness of the issue and seek professional medical help.

There is no single explanation for why an eating disorder evolves. Eating disorders often begin with dieting; however, before dieting, other factors have already affected a person's mindset. Some women may have a biological vulnerability to eating disorders. Levels of neurotransmitters and hormones that affect one's mood, appetite, and eating behavior may be altered in women with eating disorders. For example, the hormone serotonin, which creates feelings of satiety after eating, may be present at lower levels in women with bulimia. Therefore, these individuals tend to not feel as satisfied after eating and may binge as a result. Poor self-image, depression, anxiety, loneliness,

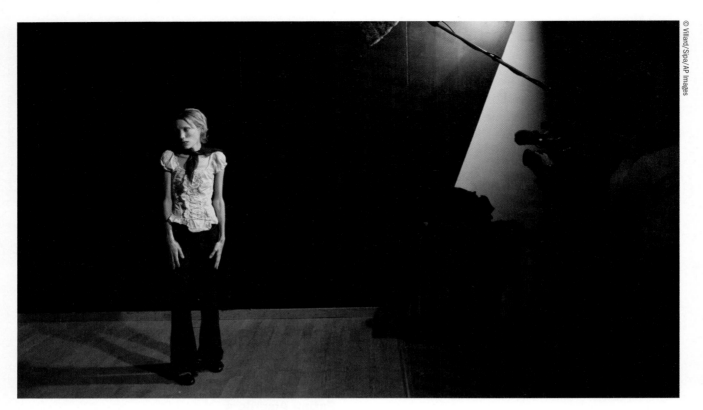

© Villard/Sipa/AP Images

■ Anorexia creates numerous problems for physical and mental health.

and certain family and personal relationships may contribute to the development of an eating disorder, too. The stresses associated with adolescent and adult life also can precipitate anorexia or bulimia.[29]

Our culture, with its unrelenting idealization of thinness, "the perfect body," and its presentation of weight loss as an accomplishment, is also partly to blame. Consider the rise in pro-eating-disorder websites that share information among those with eating disorders on how to better meet their disordered goals of weight loss and behavior control. Women (and men) use personal blogs and webpages such as Pinterest to share photographs, stories, and techniques in an effort to create a sense of support and community among people of like thinking. Many health professionals, however, believe these websites encourage harmful eating habits and have mounted campaigns with Internet service providers to have the sites removed.

Eating disorders have harmful consequences for the mind and the body. People with eating disorders are more likely to suffer from other mental illnesses; they can also develop health complications including dental problems, kidney failure, and heart conditions.[27]

The female athlete triad is a particularly harmful interrelationship between disordered eating, **amenorrhea** (the absence of a regular menstrual cycle in a woman of reproductive age), and **osteoporosis**. The triad usually begins with disordered eating. Poor nutrition and intense athletic training cause weight loss and a decrease in or shutdown of estrogen production. These stresses on the body lead to a cessation of the menstrual cycle. The final condition in the triad, osteoporosis, may follow if estrogen levels remain low and the woman's diet is lacking in calcium and vitamin D. Although the triad can occur in any athlete, those at greatest risk are endurance athletes such as distance swimmers and runners, and athletes in sports where slim appearance is highly valued, such as gymnasts and figure skaters.

Anorexia Nervosa

Anorexia nervosa is characterized by deprivation of food and a body weight of at least 15% below the normal weight for a person's height and age. The *DSM-IV* classifies anorexia as an eating disorder associated with the following factors:

- Refusal to maintain an adequate weight
- Intense fear of gaining weight
- Distorted body image

- In women, three consecutive missed periods without pregnancy

Physical symptoms of anorexia nervosa include a significant loss of weight, a refusal to eat, amenorrhea, and a denial of unusual eating behaviors or weight change. As an anorexic person's metabolism slows to adjust to the lack of nourishment, other symptoms, such as muscle weakness, constipation, brittle hair and nails, lethargy, and a lowering of the body temperature, which causes a constant feeling of coldness and slowness, occur. Psychological symptoms of this eating disorder include a distorted body image, confusion of selfimage, a sense of being incompetent, depression, and withdrawal from others.[27] Individuals also tend to become socially withdrawn as the disorder progresses. Researchers note that the most notable belief shared by women with anorexia is that weight, shape, or being thin is the predominant reference for establishing personal value or self-worth.[30] Other identified psychological features of the illness include:

- A frustration over becoming overweight
- A fear of losing control over eating
- A loss of judgment relative to the requirement of food as a basic need for the body
- An unrealistic sense of body image

I look in the mirror and see myself as grotesquely fat—a real blimp. My legs and arms are really fat and I can't stand what I see. I know that others say I am too thin, but I can see myself and I have to deal with this my way.

100-pound anorexic girl

Women with anorexia often display obsessive-compulsive behaviors, such as obsessing about becoming fat and, consequently, compulsively exercising or practicing odd eating rituals to avoid becoming fat. Other compulsive activities may include constant weighing, looking in the mirror, and taking body measurements. Women with anorexia also are obsessed with food and eating, and will often cook, prepare, and purchase food for others. They will eat in secret and reject food in public.

Anorexia nervosa usually strikes in early to late adolescence. A general characteristic of the anorectic personality is a feeling of overall ineffectiveness as a person. The typical anorexic woman is highly critical of herself, has poor self-esteem, and believes that she is quite inadequate in most areas of personal and social functioning. She often feels powerless and unable to control many areas of her life, so she establishes power over her food intake and weight.

Because of her perfectionist tendencies, the woman with anorexia believes that the ultimate sign of control is a "perfect" body. Symptoms of depression, with large mood swings, are commonly seen in individuals with the disorder. The increased risk for heart and kidney failure, suicide, and other serious consequences makes people with anorexia about 10 times more likely to die early than people without this condition.[27]

Bulimia Nervosa

Bulimia nervosa is an eating disorder characterized by cyclic binge eating (**bingeing**) followed by purging. Prevalence rates for bulimia range from 1% to 16%, with the highest rates occurring in adolescents and young adults.[25]

The *DSM-IV* associates four distinguishing characteristics of bulimia:

- Recurrent episodes of binge eating (at least 2 episodes per week for at least 3 months)
- A feeling of lack of control over eating behavior during the binge
- Regular engagement in purges
- Persistent overconcern with body shape and weight

Bulimia is a progressive disorder that usually begins with extreme hunger as a result of long periods of food deprivation from fasting or dieting. This hunger is followed by attempts at eating while still trying to control weight. Women with this eating disorder often maintain normal body weight but are extremely dissatisfied with their bodies. Some bulimics have reported that in their preadolescent years, they gained feelings of control and power through this self-denial. The situation progresses to out-ofcontrol binges/purges because the artificial elimination methods have relieved the feeling of being "stuffed," and the bulimic believes it is a good way to lose weight.

Binges often occur when bulimics feel that they have passed a self-imposed limit on acceptable food intake. Consequently, they feel defeated and generally gorge until they are interrupted or the food runs out. During such binges, the caloric intake may range from 2,000 to 3,000 calories. Binges generally lasts for less than 2 hours but have been reported to last as long as 8 hours. The binge foods of choice are usually highcalorie, easily ingested "junk" food that requires little preparation and can be obtained while keeping the binge secret from others. Bulimics may use several modes of purging, including induced vomiting, diuretics, laxatives, fasts, enemas, diet pills, chewing for hours and then spitting out the food, and excessive exercise.

The number of different methods of purging is a stronger index of the severity of the woman's condition than is the frequency of use of any one type.

The binge–purge cycle may occur anywhere from once or twice weekly to several times daily. The cycle often begins in response to a strong emotion, either positive or negative. These emotions can come from a food craving, stress, sleeplessness, anxiety, joy, excitement, physical or emotional pain, helplessness, hopelessness, loneliness, or sadness. After the binge, some women say they initially feel relaxed and soothed, but these feelings turn to shame, guilt, and self-hatred. The women then feel the need to purge to relieve the fear of weight gain and to regain a sense of control and purity. After the purge, bulimics may feel relieved that they have controlled their weight but guilty and negative about succumbing to the cycle again. These feelings of guilt invariably lead the bulimic to perpetuate the behavior.

People with bulimia are often independent high achievers and of normal weight. Bulimia has traditionally afflicted adolescent and young adult females from middle-class backgrounds, but it affects other groups of women and men as well. Bulimics are often perfectionist, obsessive-compulsive, depressed, intense, insecure, sensitive to rejection, anxious to please, and dependent on others. They may be socially isolated as a result of their all-consuming preoccupation with food and weight and their struggle to hide their eating behavior. The majority of women who suffer from bulimia are aware that their eating habits are abnormal, but may believe that they have the ultimate weight control secret of being able to "have their cake and eat it, too." Other factors thought to contribute to the development of bulimia include family problems, maladaptive behavior, self-identity conflicts, history of sexual abuse, and cultural overemphasis on physical appearance. In addition to the psychological problems, bulimia nervosa can cause a variety of physical problems, including hypoglycemia, a slowed metabolism, spontaneous regurgitation, erosion of tooth enamel or tooth loss, bleeding and sores in the mouth and esophagus, and mineral deficiencies. **Table 12.4** compares the symptoms of anorexia nervosa with those of bulimia nervosa.

Binge Eating Disorder

Binge eating disorder (BED) is characterized by compulsive overeating without attempting to purge. Defining factors of BED include recurrent episodes of binge eating at least 2 days per week for a minimum of 6 months, as well as an overall sense of loss of control over the binges.

Table 12.4 Symptoms of Anorexia Nervosa/Bulimia Nervosa

Symptoms of Anorexia Nervosa

Loss of at least 15% of body weight

Intense fear of weight gain

Distorted body image (feeling fat even when too thin)

Absence of three consecutive menstrual periods (amenorrhea)

Insistence on keeping weight below a healthy minimum

Symptoms of Bulimia Nervosa

Repeated (usually secretive) episodes of bingeing and vomiting

Feeling out of control during a binge

Purging after a binge (vomiting, use of laxatives or diuretics, excessive exercise)

Frequent dieting

Extreme concern with body weight and shape

Women with BED also have a preoccupation with food and weight, as well as a distorted body image.

Binge eating disorder is different from nonpurging bulimia nervosa, because people with nonpurging bulimia binge after periods of fasting and use excessive exercise as a way to compensate for their binges. Most people who suffer from BED are obese and have a long history of weight fluctuations. Women who suffer from BED are at high risk for medical problems associated with obesity, as well as depression and anxiety due to guilt and feelings of self-disgust. Many people with BED have histories of major family dysfunction and childhood abuse.

My friends confronted me about my anorexia in my senior year of high school. By that point it had gotten so bad that even I had to admit it—I got lost on the way to school because I couldn't think straight. It was really tough for the first year, and was still difficult after that, but now I'm really okay with it. In fact, I'm eating a healthier diet than I ever was before, even though I don't think about food nearly as much.

22-year-old woman

Treatment

People with eating disorders are usually intensely secretive about them. However, observant friends and family members often have an idea when an eating disorder is occurring. Many people try to ignore their suspicions so as to protect the privacy of their friend or family member or out of a wish not to interfere. Women with bulimia and BED are often able to identify the disorder themselves. In contrast, women with anorexia are often in denial about their condition and usually are brought to treatment by concerned family members. Many women enter therapy to treat an eating disorder only after being persuaded to do so by people in their lives. It thus becomes extremely important for people to confront the women in their lives when they suspect disordered eating, and to provide them with support in finding the appropriate help. As with all health interventions, sensitivity and care need to be taken when discussing eating disorders with individuals, and one needs to have an understanding of the very central and painful role the disorder may play in an individual's life.

Several approaches are used to treat eating disorders, including motivating the patient, enlisting family support, and providing nutrition counseling and psychotherapy. Behavior modification therapy and drug therapy, such as antidepressants, may also be used. Hospitalization may be required for those patients with life-threatening complications or extreme psychological problems. If the patient's life is not in danger, treatment may be provided on an outpatient basis and may last for a year or longer.

Treatment is often a lengthy and difficult process, with many women suffering from relapses. Stopping the pattern of dysfunctional eating is essential for successfully treating an eating disorder, but this is not the only requirement. Healthful eating habits must be learned and established to replace the harmful behaviors. Additionally, people with eating disorders also need professional help to develop a realistic body image, develop positive self-esteem, and resolve the underlying control issues that may have contributed to the eating disorder.

Other Disorders

Personality Disorders

Personality disorders are characterized by distorted and inflexible thoughts and behaviors that make it impossible for a person to live a productive life or establish fulfilling relationships. These types of disorders have created controversy in the field of psychiatry because it is often difficult to decide when the personality style of a person becomes clinically deviant. For a woman to be diagnosed with a personality disorder, she must experience long-term patterns of the distorted thoughts and behaviors and these behaviors must cause interpersonal trouble. Several personality disorders exist (**Table 12.5**), with histrionic and borderline personality disorders being the most commonly diagnosed in women.

Table 12.5 Types and Symptoms of Personality Disorders
Antisocial: disrespectful of others; often in trouble with authorities
Avoidant: extremely inhibited socially; low self-esteem; intense fear of rejection
Borderline: poor self-image; unstable relationships; mood swings; impulsive behavior; extreme fear of being abandoned; self-destructive behaviors such as drug abuse, casual sex, and binge eating
Dependent: submissive; feelings of worthlessness; allows others to make important decisions; common in women who have suffered domestic abuse
Histrionic: seeks attention; acts overly emotional to attract desired attention; constantly seeks approval; is demanding and needy in relationships
Narcissistic: needs constant admiration and attention; has low self-esteem and an exaggerated sense of her own importance; constantly worried what others think of her
Obsessive-compulsive: obsessive about certain areas of life, including work; perfectionist tendencies; controlling personality
Paranoid: extremely distrustful; suspicious of others; extremely jealous, unforgiving, and quick to anger
Passive-aggressive: passively resists taking on responsibilities; consistently fails to live up to demands placed on her; often is irritable and complaining, resulting in problems in relationships
Schizoid: cannot form close relationships; has a very limited range of emotions; may lead to schizophrenia
Schizotypal: cannot form close relationships; eccentric in behavior; experiences distorted thinking and strange speech and behavior patterns; suffers from extreme social anxiety; often suspicious of others

People with histrionic personality disorder are deeply emotional, have low self-control, and feel a strong need for attention. People with this mental disorder feel uncomfortable and unappreciated unless they are constantly the center of attention. Because people with this disorder are very sensitive, they can be easily hurt by real or imagined slights. People with histrionic disorder often have a difficult time maintaining stable jobs, living arrangements, and relationships. Additionally, their suggestibility, and need for attention and approval, can lead people with histrionic disorder to engage in risky sexual behaviors.[31] Borderline personality disorder (BPD) is also characterized by instability in moods, relationships, identity, and behavior. People with BPD may develop intense feelings of anxiety, anger, or depression that appear and disappear within several hours. The intensity of these feelings makes people with BPD more likely to hurt themselves, engage in substance abuse, and commit suicide. The same intense, changing emotional pattern also makes it very difficult for people with BPD to build and maintain stable relationships.[32] A combination of environmental and genetic factors likely play a part in whether a person develops histrionic personality disorder or BPD.

Many people with personality disorders never enter treatment. Those who do usually seek help for depression or anxiety. Treatment often involves long-term psychotherapy, cognitive behavioral therapy, and/or family or group therapy. Medications may be given with psychotherapy to relieve symptoms of depression or anxiety.

Schizophrenia

Psychosis is a severe mental disorder characterized by loss of contact with reality and severe personality changes. Although mood disorders primarily affect how a person feels, psychosis disorders primarily affect how a person thinks and perceives the world. **Schizophrenia**, a type of psychosis, represents an extraordinarily complex group of disorders and is the most chronic and disabling of the severe mental disorders. Many subtypes of schizophrenia exist, each of which is characterized by specific symptoms and a certain degree of disease severity. Although the word "schizophrenia" comes from the Greek word for "split," it does not mean that a schizophrenic person has a "split" or multiple personality. Instead, this meaning describes the splitting of coherent thoughts in those who suffer from the illness.

My brother had schizophrenia. He just started hearing voices when he was in his twenties. He was married, in graduate school, and he just fell apart. I took care of him, but my family was too embarrassed to deal with him. He hated the way the medication made him feel and he hated how he was when he was off the drugs, so he took his own life. I was so angry with him for doing that, at myself for not being able to prevent it, and at my family for not helping him. But now I feel that I need to do something—to educate people about mental illness, to advocate for research to get better treatment, and to help erase the stigma that goes along with mental disorders.
26-year-old woman

Schizophrenia afflicts about 2.4 million U.S. adults (about 1% of the adult population), with men and women being affected equally. Gender differences are apparent in the development of the disease, however. Men are more likely to be affected between the ages of 16 and 25, whereas women are more likely to have a disease onset between the ages of 25 and 30. Women typically start with a milder form of the disease, experiencing more mood symptoms than psychoses. A significant proportion of women with schizophrenia experience an increase in symptoms during pregnancy and the postpartum period.

Living with schizophrenia can be terrifying. People with schizophrenia experience hallucinations (usually voices and other sounds, but also smells and sights that are not there) and delusions (beliefs that are not true, such as that people are reading the person's mind, planning to harm or trap the person, or controlling the person's thoughts). To the person experiencing them, these hallucinations and delusions appear utterly real.[2] These and other symptoms can appear suddenly or gradually over a period of years. Other symptoms of schizophrenia include disordered thinking, difficulty interacting with others, and difficulty thinking clearly. Some women with schizophrenia may experience symptoms for years or decades at a time, whereas others may experience random episodes of symptoms throughout life.

Treatments for schizophrenia are improving and can provide some relief, but most people with schizophrenia experience symptoms throughout their lives.[33] Fewer than half of people with schizophrenia get adequate treatment. New medications that cause fewer side effects have been developed over the last decade. A newly developed class of drugs, the atypical antipsychotics, are more effective than older types of drugs, but have much more severe side effects. Psychotherapy and support groups also may help some patients. Schizophrenia is a difficult disease; only 1 in 5 people recovers completely and 1 in 10 eventually takes his or her own life.[33]

Dissociative Disorders

Dissociative disorders develop as an unconscious way to protect oneself from emotional traumas by detaching from a part of one's personality. These disorders occur as a response to a severe childhood trauma. While the created defense appears helpful to the individual, it is actually detrimental to the process of recovery.

Several types of dissociative disorders exist, with the most common being dissociative identity disorder, also known as multiple personality disorder. Dissociative identity disorder is associated with early childhood abuse and usually begins in late adolescence or early adulthood. The disorder is progressive and often coexists with personality disorders. Women with this disorder are unable to process their thoughts, feelings, memories, and actions into a complete and single state of consciousness. Signs of dissociative identity disorder include amnesia, detachment from reality, and detachment from oneself through depersonalization. People with dissociative identity disorder often hurt themselves intentionally in acts of self-mutilation. Treatment includes psychotherapy to integrate the various personalities and to resolve feelings surrounding the traumatic event.

Dissociative amnesia, another form of a dissociative disorder, is loss of memory resulting from trauma. Depending on the form of dissociative amnesia, either some or all of the experiences from various time periods are blocked out. Therapy is used to help the person adjust to the current situation rather than to resolve the past.

Suicide

The taking of one's own life can be considered the most harmful symptom of mental illness. There are almost always warning signs that a person is at risk of suicide. More than 90% of people who kill themselves have depression, another diagnosable mental illness, or a substance abuse disorder. Adverse life events like a death in the family, a relationship breakup, or financial ruin, along with other risk factors, also may make a person more likely to take his or her own life. However, suicide is not a normal or acceptable response to stress. Many people have considered suicide at some point in their lives when they were depressed or experienced something very bad; however, most would never act on these thoughts, and are thus not considered suicidal.

Risk factors for someone committing suicide include the following:

- Adverse life events along with other factors such as depression
- Prior suicide attempt
- Family history of mental disorder or substance abuse
- Family history of suicide
- Family violence, including physical or sexual abuse
- Firearms in the home
- Incarceration
- Exposure to suicidal behavior of others, including family members, peers, and even the media

Although more women than men report attempts at suicide, more men complete the act. Suicide is the 11th leading cause of death in the United States—the 9th leading cause of death for males, and the 16th leading cause of death for females.[34] For many people, an attempt at suicide is a "cry for help." In adults, the strongest risk factors for attempting suicide are depression, substance abuse, and separation or divorce. Risk factors for children and adolescents include depression, substance use, and aggressive behavior. Friends and family members of people with known depression or with one of the risk factors mentioned earlier should pay close attention to their loved ones. If they demonstrate suicidal behaviors or discuss suicidal wishes, seek professional psychiatric, social work, or medical help immediately.

Suicide has become a major problem in many developing countries and Eastern European countries. Among rural communities in China and many former Soviet bloc countries, it is one of the leading causes of death for young women.

Preventive interventions for suicide are often intensive. They typically require learning new coping skills, recognizing the underlying factors causing distress, and receiving appropriate treatment for existing mental and substance abuse disorders.

Informed Decision Making

People have different vulnerabilities to mental disorders based on their genetic inheritance, physical condition, social situation, and life experiences, but mental health is a concern for everyone. No one is immune to mental disorders. Even if you are fortunate enough to never experience one, it is almost certain that you will know and care for someone who has experienced one, has one now, or will have one.

Good mental health is more than the absence of mental illness, just as good physical health is more than the absence of disease. There may be no perfect definition of good mental health, but being able to engage in rational thought and decision making; feeling a variety of emotions

■ Women can improve their mental health by integrating physical activity into their day.

without being controlled by those emotions; being able to maintain stable, fulfilling relationships; and being able to cope with difficult circumstances are all signs of a healthy mind.

To maintain emotional well-being, it is essential to take care of oneself. Some women tend to put other people's needs before their own. If a woman does this on a consistent basis, it can put her under great stress and make her more likely to experience and suffer from mental illness. Finding appropriate coping mechanisms can help women deal with stressful situations and difficult circumstances. Some good coping mechanisms include taking time to relax, and having a trusted friend, family member, or mentor to talk to. Other basic healthy behaviors, like getting a good night's sleep, eating a nutritious diet, and integrating physical activity into one's daily routine, benefit the mind as well as the body. In particular, regular exercise yields enormous benefits for people suffering from depression and anxiety disorders. The **It's Your Health** box lists healthful activities that can relieve stress and promote good mental health.

If a woman does notice a pattern of disturbing thoughts, finds herself unable to cope with life's daily challenges, or finds herself anxious or unhappy most of the time, she should seek professional help. Seeking help is not always easy. Many people who could benefit from mental health services decide not to seek care out of fear that they will be labeled "crazy" or "unstable." Other people believe either that "things will get better on their own" or that treatment would be useless. Millions of Americans already benefit from (or would benefit from) some form of mental health treatment. Although some mental disorders may go away on their own, others do not, and treatment can often dramatically shorten the course of a disorder. **Self-Assessment 12.1** can help a woman determine whether she, or someone she cares about, needs to seek help.

Psychiatrists, clinical psychologists, and social workers are all trained, certified practitioners who have been

It's Your Health

Helpful Ways to Promote Good Mental Health and Relieve Stress

Here is a list of common activities that can provide relief from stress, anxiety, and depression, as well as promote good mental health.

- Watching a funny movie or show, telling and listening to jokes, or other activities that bring laughter
- Exercise (30 minutes or more a day is best, but any amount of exercise brings benefits—for more information, see Chapter 9)
- Meditation or prayer
- Gardening
- Spending time with a pet or pets
- Getting a massage
- Visualization (imagining yourself on a calm beach, in a quiet meadow, or in some other peaceful, relaxing situation)
- Listening to music
- Napping or simply lying down, closing one's eyes, and relaxing
- Creative endeavors (writing, drawing or painting, dancing, singing, etc.)

educated in helping people with mental health problems. Many colleges and universities have professional mental health services available, or at least can give referrals to nearby services. A good match between a patient and provider that includes mutual trust is key. Asking a mental health provider questions about his or her training, number of years in practice, experience treating someone with a similar problem, fees, types of insurance accepted, and methods of therapy can all help a woman decide whether that provider is best for her.

There are four basic forms of psychotherapy:

- Traditional psychotherapy, which deals with psychosocial aspects of depression and is often referred to as "talk therapy"

Self-Assessment 12.1

Determining One's Need to Seek Professional Help

Experiencing any of the following symptoms for several weeks may be an indication that a person needs to seek professional help.

- Feelings of sadness, hopelessness, or worthlessness
- Loss of energy and drive
- Behavioral changes, such as restlessness, irritability, or self-destructive behavior
- Physical symptoms, such as headache, nausea, backache, or unexplained pain without another medical explanation

- Prolonged worry or anxiety without any identifiable cause or reason
- Sudden episodes of intense and overwhelming fear for no apparent reason
- Irrational and uncontrollable fear or panic when exposed to a particular object or situation
- Frequent thoughts or talk about death or suicide

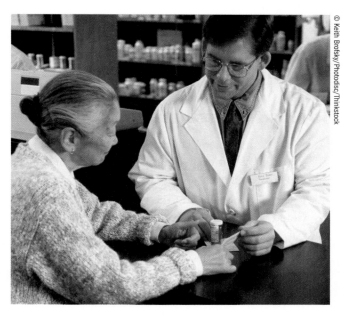

New medications have made it easier to bring relief to people with mental disorders.

- Psychodynamic psychotherapy, which deals with experiences from childhood to resolve rooted problems
- Cognitive behavioral therapy, which works to identify and correct patterns of thinking and behaviors

- Interpersonal psychotherapy, which focuses on present problems and helps with improving relationships, communication skills, and coping skills

New medications have made it easier to bring relief to people with mental disorders. However, although medications can be of great benefit, they should not be thought of as a "magic bullet" that can instantly fix or eliminate mental illness. Medications usually take days or weeks to have any effects, may require professional help and personal observation to determine the correct choice of medication and dosage, and may cause unpleasant or dangerous side effects. Medications for mental illness include antidepressants, lithium (used for bipolar disorder), antianxiety medications, and antipsychotic medications. For dealing with a persistent issue, a combination of therapy with medication often works better at treating mental illness than either medication or therapy alone.

Summary

Mental health is a difficult concept to define, yet it is nevertheless essential for both individuals and societies to function. Mental health includes a person's ability to find

Profiles of Remarkable Women

Dorothea Lynde Dix (1804–1887)

Dorothea Lynde Dix was a nurse and humanitarian who was instrumental in the reform of treatment of the mentally ill in the 19th century. Dix became interested in this issue when she visited a prison in Massachusetts that housed mentally ill people. She saw naked prisoners in chains being kept in filthy quarters, with visible signs of harsh treatment and abuse. Dix spent the next 2 years researching the situation and then reported her findings to the Massachusetts legislature. Responding to her plea for humane care for the mentally ill, Massachusetts took action and moved the mentally ill people to an asylum. Dix sought change all over the United States through legislative reform, and her work prompted the establishment of 32 mental health hospitals across the United States. Dix also made an international impact, recommending reforms for prisons in Italy, France, Russia, Scotland, and Turkey.

peace in life, feel emotions without being controlled by them, build and maintain stable relationships, and cope with difficult circumstances. Biological, social, psychological, and environmental factors all influence mental health.

Mood disorders, anxiety disorders, and eating disorders are three kinds of mental disorders affecting women. These and other mental illnesses affect the way people feel, think, perceive reality, and interact with the world. Mood disorders, such as depression, dysthymia, and bipolar disorder, interfere with a person's ability to feel and control their emotions. Anxiety disorders, including GAD, phobias, panic disorder, OCD, and PTSD, occur when anxiety grows to unhealthy levels, or appears in situations where no danger exists. Eating disorders, such as anorexia, bulimia, and BED, are characterized by dysfunctional eating patterns. Left alone, mental illnesses cause a variety of harmful effects, perhaps the worst of which is suicide. Treatment for mental disorders may involve psychotherapy, medications, or a combination of both. Mental health should involve not just avoiding and treating mental disorders, but also practicing behaviors that reduce stress and promote good mental health.

■■■■
Topics for Discussion

1. Freud defined mental health as "the ability to love and to work." What do you think of this definition? Can you create a better one?

2. If you were president of the United States, what laws would you change to promote better mental health?

3. Why does stigma around mental illness exist? What can be done to reduce this stigma?

4. What are some of the advantages and disadvantages of prescribing medication for a mental disorder?

5. A young woman suspects that her friend has an eating disorder. What can she do? What if her friend denies the disorder in spite of overwhelming evidence?

Profiles of Remarkable Women

Joanne Rowling (1965–)

© Everett Collection Inc/Alamy Images

Joanne "J.K." Rowling is the author of the *Harry Potter* series of novels, the best-selling book series in history. More than 400 million copies of the seven-part *Harry Potter* books have been sold, and the movies based on the series have grossed almost $6 billion worldwide. Rowling's journey from a poor, single working mother to a billionaire and world-famous author has become a well-known rags-to-riches story. What is less well-known, however, is that Rowling suffered from severe depression for a 3-year period during her mid-20s.

Rowling first became depressed shortly after the breakdown of her first marriage in 1993. This time was an especially traumatic one for her: Rowling was left without a job after her marriage ended, and she struggled to support herself and her 1-year-old daughter. Rowling's own mother had also died the year before.

Rowling described her time with depression as the worst part of her life. "We're talking suicidal thoughts here, we're not talking 'I'm a little bit miserable,'" Rowling said in a 2008 interview. Rowling's concern for her daughter eventually convinced her to seek counseling. With time and help, Rowling eventually overcame her depression. During this period, Rowling also completed the manuscript for *Harry Potter and the Sorcerer's Stone*.

Rowling's time with depression had at least one silver lining: Rowling was able to incorporate her experiences with depression into the *Harry Potter* series. Dementors, evil wraith-like creatures in the books, induce a state much like permanent depression after consuming the souls of their victims. One character describes Dementors as "drain[ing] peace, hope, and happiness out of the air around them ... Get too near a Dementor and every good feeling, every happy memory will be sucked out of you ... . You will be left with nothing but the worst experiences of your life."

Rowling continues to speak about her time with depression and recommends that anyone experiencing the disease not blame themselves and seek help instead. "The funny thing is, I have never been remotely ashamed of having been depressed," Rowling said in a 2010 interview.

6. A young woman suspects that her grandfather is depressed. What can she do? What if her grandfather tells her he doesn't know what "being depressed" means?

7. What are steps that you can take (as a class or as individuals) to promote good mental health?

■■■■
Key Terms

Amenorrhea: Absence of the menstrual period in a woman by age 16 (primary amenorrhea) or absence of the menstrual period for 3 to 6 consecutive months in a woman who has had regular periods since the onset of menstruation (secondary amenorrhea). It often is caused by stress, acute weight loss, or excessive strenuous exercise.

Anxiety disorders: Group of conditions that share extreme or pathological anxiety as the principal disturbance of mood. Anxiety disorders include panic disorder, agoraphobia, generalized anxiety disorder, specific phobia, social phobia, obsessive-compulsive disorder, acute stress disorder, and posttraumatic stress disorder. Anxiety disorders are the most common mental disorder in the United States and affect a significant number of people worldwide.

Binge eating disorder (BED): An eating disorder characterized by a lack of control in overeating and overeating in secret. Victims do not force themselves to vomit, however, as with bulimia nervosa.

Bingeing: The consumption of large amounts of food that is characteristic of bulimia nervosa.

Bipolar disorder (manic-depressive disorder): A mental disorder that is characterized by wide mood swings that can occur within hours or days and that features abnormally euphoric or irritable moods.

Dementia: Cognitive decline, often occuring in old age. This mental deterioration and decline in intellectual functioning is severe enough to interfere with routine daily activities.

Depression: A mental condition in which a person feels extremely sad, worthless, and hopeless. In more severe cases, the person may experience thoughts of suicide. Types of depression include clinical depression, bipolar depression, seasonal affective disorder (SAD), dysthymia, and postpartum depression.

Dissassociative disorders: Disorders that develop as an unconscious way to protect oneself from emotional traumas by detaching from a part of one's personality. These disorders occur as a response to severe childhood trauma.

Dysthymia: A form of depression that is milder and less disabling than major depression, but more chronic in nature.

Generalized anxiety disorder (GAD): An anxiety disorder that causes an ongoing general feeling of intense worry and fear, often for no apparent reason.

Mood disorders (affective disorders): Conditions characterized by extreme disturbances of mood.

Neurotransmitters: A group of chemicals found in the brain and nervous system that transmit and modulate communication between neurons.

Obsessive-compulsive disorder (OCD): An anxiety disorder that causes a person to have disturbing repetitive thoughts (obsessions) and to perform rituals or routines (compulsions) to get rid of the obsessions. The disorder is diagnosed only when the repetitive behaviors consume many hours each day and interfere with daily life.

Osteoporosis: An age-related debilitating disorder characterized by a general decrease in bone mass and structural deterioration of bone tissue.

Panic disorder: An anxiety disorder characterized by periods of intense fear, known as panic attacks, that are accompanied by physical symptoms (pounding heart, sweating, dizziness, chest pain, and so on) and emotional distress.

Personality disorders: Mental disorders that are characterized by distorted and inflexible thoughts and behaviors that make it impossible for a person to live a productive life or establish fulfilling relationships.

Phobia: An anxiety disorder characterized by a powerful and irrational fear of a particular object or situation.

Postpartum psychosis: The most severe of the psychiatric disorders that can develop in women after delivery. Symptoms of postpartum psychosis include depression, anxiety, irritation, tiredness, and sleep disturbances, as well as behavior that tends to change throughout the day from clear consciousness to total loss of reality.

Posttraumatic stress disorder (PTSD): An anxiety disorder that usually begins with 3 months after a traumatic event. Its symptoms include flashback episodes, nightmares, and emotional numbness.

Psychosis: A severe mental disorder characterized by a loss of contact with reality and severe personality changes.

Seasonal affective disorder (SAD): A form of depression caused by seasonal shifts in daylight hours that affect a person's sleep–wake cycle.

Schizophrenia: A type of psychosis representing a complex group of diseases with symptoms that may appear gradually or suddenly and include hallucinations or delusions, disordered thinking, and an impaired ability to manage emotions and interact with others. Schizophrenia is the most chronic and disabling of the severe mental disorders.

Serotonin: A neurotransmitter (brain chemical) known to affect appetite.

Underinsured: For the purposes of this book, a person who technically has health insurance but whose coverage is not enough to cover his or her regular medical expenses or whose coverage would not allow a person to afford adequate care in the event of a serious disease or illness.

■■■■
Websites

American Psychological Association: http://www.apa.org

Anxiety Disorders Association of America: http://www.adaa.org

Depression and Bipolar Support Alliance: http://www.dbsalliance.org

Medline Plus: Mental Health: http://www.nlm.nih.gov/medlineplus/mentalhealth.html

National Association of Anorexia Nervosa and Associated Disorders: http://www.anad.org

National Eating Disorders Association: http://www.nationaleatingdisorders.org

National Institute of Mental Health: http://www.nimh.nih.gov

National Mental Health Information Center: http://www.mentalhealth.org

Substance Abuse and Mental Health Services Administration: http://mentalhealth.samhsa.gov

Swamp Nurse: What's the best hope for the first child of a poor mother? (article): http://www.newamerica.net/publications/articles/2006/swamp_nurse

■■■■
References

1. Kellogg, R. (2008). Quoted in *What is mental health?* [Press Release]. Available at: http://www1.dshs.wa.gov/mediareleases/2008/pr08057.shtml

2. U.S. Department of Health and Human Services. (1999). Mental health: A report of the Surgeon General. Rockville, MD: U.S. Department of Health and Human Services. Available at: http://www.surgeongeneral.gov/library/mentalhealth/home.html

3. Pomerantz, E., Rydell Altermatt, E., & Saxon, J. (2002). Making the grade but feeling distressed: Gender differences in academic performance and internal distress. *Journal of Educational Psychology* 94(2): 396–404.

4. Stewart, W. F., Ricci, J. A., Chee, E., et al. (2003). Cost of lost productive work time among U.S. workers with depression. *Journal of the American Medical Association* 289(23): 3135–3144.

5. Vitiello, B., & Lederhendler, I. (2000). Research on eating disorders: Current status and future prospects. *Biological Psychiatry* 47(9): 777–786.

6. Centers for Disease Control and Prevention [CDC], National Center for Injury Prevention and Control. (2011). Web-based injury statistics query and reporting system (WISQARS). Available at: http://www.cdc.gov/ncipc/wisqars

7. Nadien, M. (1996). Aging women: issues of mental health and maltreatment. *Annals of the New York Academy of Sciences: Women and Mental Health* 789: 129–145.

8. Brydon, L., Walker, C., Wawrzyniak, A., et al. (2009). Synergistic effects of psychological and immune stressors on inflammatory cytokine and sickness responses in humans. *Brain, Behavior, and Immunity* 23(2): 217–224. doi:10.1016/j.bbi.2008.09.007.

9. Lawson, W. (2003). Eat right to fight stress. *Psychology Today*. Available at: http://www.psychologytoday.com/articles/pto-2633.html

10. National Institute of Mental Health [NIMH]. (2008). The numbers count: Mental disorders in America. Washington, DC: NIMH. Available at: http://www.nimh.nih.gov/health/statistics/index.shtml

11. Lapine, J. P. (2001). Epidemiology, burden and disability in depression and anxiety disorders. *Journal of Clinical Psychology* 62(suppl 13): 148–160.

12. Kessler, R.C., Heeringa, S., Lakoma, M. D., et al. (2008). Individual-level and societal-level effects of mental disorders on earnings in the United States: Results from the National Comorbidity Survey Replication. *American Journal of Psychiatry* 165(6): 703–711.

13. James, D., & Glaze, L. (2006). *Mental health problems of prison and jail inmates*. Bureau of Justice Statistics. Available at: http://www.ojp.usdoj.gov/bjs/abstract/mhppji.htm

14. 110th Congress of the United States. (2008). Mental Health Parity and Addiction Equity Act of 2008. Available at: http://www.govtrack.us/congress/bill.xpd?bill=h110-1424

15. National Institute of Mental Health [NIMH]. (2008). *Depression*. Washington, DC: NIMH. Available at: http://www.nimh.nih.gov/health/publications/depression/complete-index.shtml

16. O'Connor, R. (1997). *Undoing depression*. New York, NY: Brown, Little and Company.

17. Pratt, L., & Brody, D. (2008). *Depression in the United States household population, 2005–2006*. NCH Data Brief 7. Rockville, MD: U.S. Department of Health and Human Services.

18. Halbreich, U., Borenstein, J., Pearlstein, T., et al. (2003). The prevalence, impairment, impact, and burden of premenstrual dysphoric disorder (PMS/PMDD). *Psychoneuroendocrinology* 28(3): 1–23.

19. Nishizawa, S., Benkelfat, C., Young, S. N., et al. (1997). Differences between males and females in rates of serotonin synthesis in the human brain. *Proceedings of the National Academy of Science* 94(10): 5308–5313.

20. Silberg, J., Pickles, A., Rutter, M., et al. (1999). The influence of genetic factors and life stress on depression among adolescent girls. *Archives of General Psychiatry* 56: 225–232.

21. Centers for Disease Control and Prevention [CDC]. (2010). Current depression among adults—United States, 2006 and 2008. *Morbidity & Mortality Weekly Report* 59(38): 1229–1235.

22. National Institute of Mental Health [NIMH]. (2008). *Bipolar disorder*. Washington, DC: NIMH. Available at: http://www.nimh.nih.gov/health/publications/bipolar-disorder/complete-index.shtml

23. Scott, J. (2006). Depression should be managed like a chronic disease. *British Medical Journal* 332: 985–986.

24. National Institute of Mental Health [NIMH]. (2009). *Anxiety disorders*. Rockville, MD: U.S. Department of Health and Human Services. Available at: http://www.nimh.nih.gov/health/publications/anxiety-disorders/summary.shtml

25. Vogt, D. (2006). *Women, trauma and PTSD*. National Center for Posttraumatic Stress Disorder, U.S. Department for Veteran's Affairs. Available at: http://www.ncptsd.va.gov/ncmain/ncdocs/fact_shts/fs_women_lay.html

26. Galea, S., Tracy, M., Norris, F., et al. (2008). Financial and social circumstances and the incidence and course of PTSD in Mississippi during the first two years after Hurricane Katrina. *Journal of Traumatic Stress* 21(4): 357–368.

27. National Institute of Mental Health [NIMH]. (2007). Eating disorders. Washington, DC: NIMH. Available at: http://www.nimh.nih.gov/health/publications/eating-disorders/nimheatingdisorders.pdf

28. American Psychiatric Association Work Group on Eating Disorders. (2000). Practice guideline for the treatment of patients with eating disorders. *American Journal of Psychiatry* 157(1 Suppl): 1–39.

29. Vitiello, B., & Lederhendler, I. (2000). Research on eating disorders: current status and future prospects. *Biological Psychiatry* 47(9): 777–786.

30. Blank, S., Zadik, Z., Katz, I., et al. (2002). The emergence and treatment of anorexia and bulimia nervosa. A comprehensive and practical model. *International Journal of Adolescent Medicine and Health* 14(4): 257–260.

31. American Psychiatric Association. (2000). *Diagnostic and statistical manual of mental disorders* (4th ed.). Washington, DC: American Psychiatric Association.

32. National Institute of Mental Health [NIMH]. (2010). Borderline personality disorder. Washington, DC: NIMH. Available at: http://www.nimh.nih.gov/health/publications/borderline-personality-disorder/complete-index.shtml

33. National Institute of Mental Health [NIMH]. (2009). Schizophrenia. Washington, DC: NIMH. Available at: http://www.nimh.nih.gov/health/publications/schizophrenia/complete-index.shtml

34. Heron, M. (2007). Deaths: Leading causes for 2004. *National Vital Statistics Reports* 56: 5.

Part Four

Interpersonal and Social Dimensions of Women's Health

4

Chapter Thirteen

Substance Abuse

Chapter Objectives

On completion of this chapter, students should be able to discuss:

1. The difference between proper and improper drug use, and the effects drug use and abuse have on individuals and society.

2. Biological, cultural, and legal factors that influence how and why women use drugs.

3. Health consequences of smoking, including cardiovascular disease, cancer, other chronic diseases, and risks during pregnancy.

4. The significance of secondhand and third-hand smoke.

5. Nicotine's role as an addictive drug and the reasons why women continue to smoke.

6. Basic strategies for quitting smoking and smoking cessation methods.

7. Epidemiological trends and various perspectives on alcohol use and abuse.

8. The physiological effects of alcohol on the body.

9. Alcoholism, the symptoms of alcoholism, and approaches to understanding and treating alcoholism.

10. The most common illicit drugs and their effects on the body.

11. Links between drug use and mental illness.

12. The development of drug dependency, tolerance, and basic approaches to drug abuse treatment.

womenshealth.jbpub.com

Women's Health Online is a great source for supplementary women's health information for both students and instructors. Visit

http://womenshealth.jbpub.com

to find a variety of useful tools for learning, thinking, and teaching.

Introduction

A **drug** is any substance other than food taken to affect body processes. The development of medical drugs has been one of modern society's greatest advances. Drugs prevent or cure diseases, alleviate pain, treat a variety of conditions, and perform many other functions. **Recreational drugs**—or drugs taken for pleasure—such as alcohol and caffeine, can provide relief or enjoyment when used in moderation, and their use has become an important part of many cultures.

Drug Use and Abuse

However, drugs can also cause serious harm or death. **Drug abuse** is the overuse or misuse use of any drug. Any drug has the potential for abuse, including tobacco, alcohol, medications purchased over-the-counter (OTC) or with a prescription, and illegal drugs. Substance abuse, and problems related to substance abuse, are among society's most pervasive health and social concerns. Tobacco use is the greatest preventable cause of death, disability, and disease in the United States; every year, it kills more than 440,000 people through cardiovascular disease, cancer, and other conditions. Chronic alcohol use harms every system in the body. In addition, drunk driving is a factor in one-third of all automobile accidents.[1] Illegal drugs directly cause about 38,000 deaths a year and contribute to deaths from accidents, homicides, and other causes.

Other drugs also cause great harm. Every year, millions of people abuse or misuse drugs purchased over the counter

■ Opium (extracted from the poppy flower as seen here) was used both therapeutically to induce calm and relieve pain and recreationally to induce euphoric dream states.

or via prescription, sometimes on purpose and sometimes accidentally. Individuals who abuse illegal drugs may experience addiction, cardiac illness and death, neurological damage, numerous mental illnesses, fetal and infant morbidity and mortality, infection with HIV and hepatitis, and other consequences. On a societal level, illegal drug use contributes to accidents and violent crime, and causes billions of dollars in medical expenses and lost productivity.

Although many people consider legal and illegal drugs as separate categories, the line between the two from a health perspective is not always distinct. Many drugs that are illegal today were originally developed for legitimate medical purposes. In addition, the legal status of some drugs has changed with time, and even varies by country or state. In the 1920s and 1930s, for example, alcohol was illegal and marijuana was legal. Today, the reverse is true. In the early 1900s, opium, morphine, and cocaine were openly advertised and sold as "remedies" in the form of tonics, syrups, and elixirs. Coca-Cola contained cocaine until 1906, when the cocaine was replaced by caffeine. Today, marijuana use is tolerated in the Netherlands and in small amounts in most of Europe. In the United States, federal law prohibits the sale or possession of marijuana under any circumstances. However, state laws are more complicated. Eighteen states allow some form of marijuana use with a doctor's approval, and, in 2012 two states, Colorado and Washington legalized the sale and possession of marijuana. Under federal law, however, marijuana technically remains illegal in all of states: In 2005, the Supreme Court ruled that the federal government can override state laws on patient use. The age at which a person can legally purchase and use alcohol varies throughout Europe and much of the Americas. Many predominately Muslim countries have laws that either outlaw alcohol or severely restrict how it can be bought and sold.

Legal drugs in the United States include alcohol, nicotine, caffeine, OTC drugs, and drugs obtained with a medical prescription. Prescribed medications are legal drugs that can be obtained only through the authorization of a licensed physician or dentist. Besides marijuana, drugs that are illegal include cocaine, methamphetamines, and heroin. Despite a declared "war on drugs," drug availability continues to grow. Nearly one-half of Americans over the age of 12 have tried at least one illegal drug.[3]

The use of a drug for a purpose for which it was not originally intended is called **drug misuse**. Drug misuse can be accidental or deliberate, and includes taking more or less of a prescribed or OTC drug or using an outdated or a friend's prescribed medication. Sleep aids, antihistamines, and cough suppressants containing dextromethorphan (DXM) are frequently misused OTC drugs. Deliberate drug use inconsistent with or in excess of accepted medical practice constitutes drug abuse. The most frequently abused prescribed medications include pain relievers, tranquilizers, stimulants, and sedatives.

The dangers of misusing or abusing a particular drug are often associated with the drug's ability to cause addiction. Addiction can cause physical dependence, where the body adjusts to having a drug in its system and goes through observable negative changes when the drug is removed. Many legal drugs—including barbiturates, tranquilizers, analgesics, opiates, alcohol, and tobacco—can cause physical dependence. Besides physical dependence, drugs can create a **psychological dependence**, called habituation. A combination of physical and psychological dependence can greatly increase a person's risk for addiction. Some people can become so consumed by their addictions that they direct all their energies to compulsive drug-seeking behavior, even as those drugs provide increasingly less pleasure or relief.

Drugs typically enter the body through one of three ways:

- *Oral administration.* Swallowing a drug in capsule, tablet, or liquid form is the most common way of consuming a drug. Drugs taken orally do not reach the bloodstream as quickly as those taken by other means.

- *Through the lungs.* The user sniffs a powder, such as cocaine; inhales gases, aerosol sprays, or fumes from solvents or other compounds that evaporate quickly; or smokes a substance.

- *Use of a syringe.* Drugs may be injected subcutaneously (under the skin), intramuscularly (into the muscle tissue), or intravenously (directly into a vein). An intravenous injection immediately introduces the drugs into the bloodstream. Intramuscular and subcutaneous injections are slower in action.

In addition to the dosage and the route of ingestion, several factors influence the intensity and the duration of a drug's effects:

- Physical conditions such as a cold, pregnancy, or menstruation may make the body more vulnerable to the effects of a drug.

- Genetic differences among individuals may account for varying drug responses. Some people appear to be more sensitive than others to specific classes of drugs, or to drugs in general.

■ There are several ways that drugs can enter the body.

Courtesy of Orange County Police Department, Florida

- Mindset can also influence a drug's effects. Someone who snorts cocaine to enhance sexual pleasure may feel more stimulated simply because that is what she expects to happen.

- Social setting may influence drug effects. Drug effects at a noisy, crowded party are different from the effects produced at an intimate, subdued event.

Tolerance is the body's ability to withstand the effects of a drug. Continued use of certain drugs increases tolerance even as they lower the effects of a drug. As a person becomes tolerant, increasingly large doses may become necessary to produce the same effects. Larger doses also increase the risk of toxicity—the level at which a drug becomes poisonous to the body. Toxicity-related damage may be temporary, permanent, or deadly, depending on the drug, dose, and individual.

Many people with substance abuse problems may be abusing more than one drug at once; the average user who enters treatment is on five different drugs. The more drugs used, the greater the chance of side effects, complications, and possible life-threatening situations.

Sociocultural Dimensions

The path toward drug abuse is often complex for women, yet certain patterns emerge. A person may become more likely to abuse drugs when there is a breakdown of protective factors, such as family, friends, or a supportive environment. Harmful events such as trauma, a disrupted financial situation, abrupt changes in living conditions, or failed relationships can also increase the likelihood of drug abuse. Several factors increase the likelihood of drug abuse in women[3,4]:

- Significant life stresses, such as divorce, loneliness, and dissatisfaction with a career

- Sexual abuse and physical abuse, beginning before the age of 11 and occurring repeatedly

- Mental illnesses such as anxiety, depression, or personality disorder

Society's double standard for women prevails in drug use. Women face greater stigma for drug abuse than men, sometimes because of their potential position as mothers, sometimes because perceived irresponsibility is forgiven more easily in men than in women, and sometimes for other reasons. These social sanctions against addiction can make it harder for women to seek help, or make their friends and families less willing to recognize the addiction and intervene. Females also have a higher rate of substance abuse co-occurring with other psychiatric disorders, such as depression, anxiety, posttraumatic stress disorder, eating disorders, and borderline personality disorder. The connection between mental illness and drug abuse is not always clear. Some women with mental illness may use drugs in an attempt to self-medicate their symptoms, while in other cases, women may develop mental illnesses as a result of the consequences of drug abuse. In some cases, both mental illness and drug abuse may result from the same trauma or event.

Pregnant drug users are at increased risk for miscarriage, ectopic pregnancy, stillbirth, low weight gain, anemia, hypertension, low-birthweight babies, and other medical problems. HIV infection, a possible consequence of intravenous drug use, is another risk among pregnant drug users. Approximately 4.4% of pregnant women between the ages of 15 and 44 use illicit drugs, less than half of the rate of women who were not pregnant in the same age group (10.9%). However, rates of drug use vary considerably among pregnant women of different age groups: 16.2% of pregnant women between the ages of 15 and 26 reported currently using illegal drugs, nearly 10 times the rate (1.9%) of pregnant women between the ages of 26 and 44.[3]

Legal Dimensions

In addition to the legal (or illegal) status of specific drugs, several laws and legal realities affect drugs and women's health. Chief among these is how criminalizing drug use disproportionately affects people of color. While White, Black, and Hispanic Americans use drugs at roughly equal rates, Black and Hispanic Americans are much more likely to be arrested for using or selling drugs. For example, whereas African Americans constitute 14% of marijuana

users in general, they account for nearly one-third of all marijuana arrests. Hispanic and African American drug offenders both have a greater chance of being sentenced to prison than White drug offenders (40% and 20% greater, respectively). African Americans also receive longer prison terms for drug offenses than Whites, serving nearly as much time in prison for a drug offense as Whites do for a violent offense.[5] These disparities may not always be the result of deliberate racism; instead they may be due in large part to a focus on making arrests in urban, low-income areas where Black and Hispanic people live. Harsher sentences for Blacks and Hispanics arrested for drug possession may be due either to unconscious or conscious bias on the part of judges, or due to White arrestees being more likely to live in areas where there are more lenient judges. Whatever their origins, however, racial drug-related disparities have had numerous consequences for the people who are arrested, their families, and their communities.

While men are still more likely than women to be sentenced to prison, the number of women in prison has increased at nearly double the rate for men over the past 35 years. There are now nearly seven times as many women in state and federal prisons as in 1980; in particular, the number of women incarcerated for drug offenses has risen by more than 900% since that year. African American and Hispanic women represent a disproportionate share of this increase. Minority women are also least likely to receive effective drug treatment. Once arrested, many addicts are incarcerated, where their addiction is either left untreated or worsens due to the widespread underground availability of drugs in many prisons.

Other legal considerations affecting women are associated with drug use during pregnancy. Several states are now dealing with prenatal substance abuse through their legal systems. This approach shifts the focus to punishment and away from the urgent need to provide appropriate drug treatment programs. These states may require healthcare professionals to report prenatal drug exposure; others have amended their child welfare laws to include prenatal substance abuse, using this as evidence of child abuse to end or diminish parental rights. Only a few states have viewed drug use by pregnant women as a sign of the need for treatment, forcing pregnant users into inpatient treatment programs. Punitive reproductive health policies have an especially negative effect on low-income women and women of color. Most pregnant women charged with crimes for drug abuse are women of color, and drug testing of newborns is implemented almost exclusively by public hospitals that predominantly serve low-income women.

Such policies often discourage women from seeking needed prenatal care or drug treatment. The threat of criminal punishment fosters a climate of fear and mistrust between doctors and patients, potentially causing harm to the health of both women and their future children.

Economic Dimensions

The use and abuse of illicit drugs has a tremendous impact on American society, causing about $200 billion dollars a year in economic damages.[6] Alcohol and tobacco also cause hundreds of billions of dollars every year in medical expenses, accidents, lost productivity at the workplace, and other factors. Drug use has economic consequences at both the individual and the societal level.

Individual effects include:

- Physiological changes
- Mental dependence
- Conflicts in relationships

Societal costs include:

- Burden of drug-related crime
- Creation of treatment facilities
- Loss of individual productivity
- Care for children of drug-dependent parents
- The policing of illicit drug availability
- Treatment of medical complications resulting from inappropriate drug use

The federal government budgeted $25.6 billion for drug control in 2013.[7] The government will use this money to reduce and prevent illicit drug use, and deal with the consequences of illegal drug use. Under President Obama, the Office of National Drug Control Policy shifted its approach to acknowledge drug control as both a public health concern and matter for law enforcement. Under this policy, the nearly $26 billion will focus on six major areas[7]:

- Preventing illicit drug use and addiction
- Allowing offenders for drug abuse to end their abuse and rebuild their lives while maintaining public safety
- Stopping drug trafficking within the United States
- Allowing Americans who use drugs to get needed treatment
- Securing U.S. borders against illicit drugs
- Working with other countries to improve their drug enforcement laws, reduce corruption, and improve human rights and democratic institutions.

Across the board, drug use is more prevalent among people of lower socioeconomic status. Use of certain drugs, such as crack cocaine, is more common among poorer people than among affluent people. These drugs tend to be relatively affordable on a per-dose basis. Most often drugs are exchanged for money, but they may also be exchanged for sex. This practice is most common among poor female drug users, with crack addiction being a prevalent precursor to such behavior. Exchanging drugs for sex puts women at heightened risk for acquiring HIV and other sexually transmitted infections, and for becoming a target for sexual violence.

Regular tobacco use also imposes serious economic costs. Today, the price of a pack of cigarettes averages around $5 to $7, with state and city taxes bringing the cost up to more than $10 per pack. State, federal, and local taxes often make up half or more of the price of cigarettes sold in stores. State taxes on a package of cigarettes range from $4.35 in New York to $0.17 in Missouri.[8] As a result, a pack-a-day smoker may spend anywhere from $2,000 to $4,000 annually to fund her habit. In response to the price increase, an underground trade of cigarettes is thriving. Some street vendors sell black-market cigarettes for below-market prices, pocketing the money that would otherwise go to taxes. Untaxed cigarettes are available on Indian reservations, in countries outside of the United States, and on the Internet for as little as $2.50 a pack. Organized crime and large-scale smugglers are now participating in the underground cigarette market. In addition to the cost of purchasing cigarettes, smokers may have to pay higher premiums for their health insurance coverage. Some companies have even implemented policies against hiring smokers in states where it is legal to do so.

Tobacco

The health consequences of smoking are devastating to women's health. Tobacco causes 10 times as many deaths as illicit drug use, and more than the total deaths from accidents, illicit drug use, HIV, murders, and suicides combined. Half of all Americans who smoke will die from a smoking-related disease. Lung cancer is the leading cause of cancer death among U.S. women and men; roughly 90% of all lung cancer deaths and 30% of all cancer deaths are attributable to smoking.[9] Environmental exposure to smoke exhaled from a cigarette (secondhand smoke) as well as leftover chemicals that accumulate in a room where someone has smoked (third-hand smoke) also increase the risk for lung cancer, asthma, and other conditions.

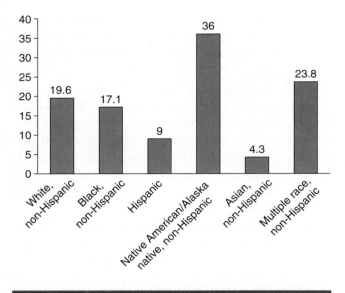

Percentage of U.S. women who smoke cigarettes in the last month by race and ethnicity, 2010

Source: Data from Centers for Disease Control and Prevention. (2011). Current Cigarette Smoking Among Adults Aged ≥ 18 Years—United States; 2005–2010. Available at http://www.cdc.gov/mmwr/preview/mmwrhtml/mm6035a5.htm

Epidemiological Trends and Issues

Native Americans first cultivated and smoked tobacco in North America thousands of years ago. Tobacco became popular in Europe about 450 years ago, when Spanish explorers brought it to their colonies and Europe from the New World. Tobacco became an accepted component of early colonial life, though its use was largely limited to men. Through the next century, tobacco was also snuffed (inhaled), dipped, and chewed.

Cigarette smoking gradually increased in popularity throughout the 19th century. During this time, a few doctors noted that tobacco seemed to cause a number of diseases, but this information was not widely spread or believed. Most people believed that tobacco use either posed no harm or actually improved health. Over the course of the 1800s, a series of technological additions to cigarettes enhanced the ease of inhalation and modified their flavor and aroma.

The 1920s were a critical period of change for women, characterized by new social and cultural patterns, a Constitutional ability to vote, and a push for greater rights and emancipation. In an extremely effective series of advertising campaigns, the tobacco industry took advantage of this women's rights movement. Cigarette companies marketed smoking as a symbol of rebellion, romance, and emancipation for women—women could now smoke cigarettes alongside men as well as vote. Women began to smoke openly in public settings, and female cigarette smoking prevalence rates rose from 2% in 1930 to 34% in 1965.[10]

Just over one in six women (17.3%) currently smoke in the United States. While this number represents tremendous progress—current smoking rates are half of what they were 50 years ago—this decline has not affected all groups of women equally.[11] Large disparities exist based on race, ethnicity, and other factors (see **Table 13.1** and **Figure 13.2**).

Table 13.1 **Percentage of U.S. Women Who Smoke,* 2010**

Characteristic	Percentage of Women
Age (Years)	
18–24	17.4
25–44	19.8
45–64	19.1
≥ 65	9.3
Education‡	
Some high school or less	21.8
GED§ diploma	44.1
High school graduate	20.6
Associate degree	16.4
Some college	21.6
Undergraduate degree	9.5
Graduate degree	5.4
Region	
Northeast	16.3
Midwest	20.8
South	18.3
West	13.0
Poverty Status	
At or above poverty level	16.4
Below poverty level	25.7
Total	**17.3**

Source: CDC (2010) *Current cigarette smoking among adults aged ≥ 18 Years—United States 2005–2010.*

*Persons who reported smoking ≥100 cigarettes during their lifetime and at the time of interview reported smoking every day or some days.

†Does not include Native Hawaiians or other Pacific Islanders.

‡Persons aged ≥ 25 years.

§General Educational Development.

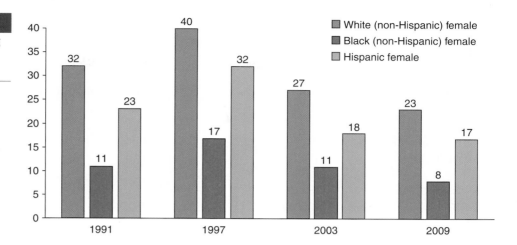

Figure 13.2

Current* cigarette smoking among female high school students by race and ethnicity, 1991–2009

Source: Data from Centers for Disease Control and Prevention. MMWR. (2010). Youth Risk Behavior Surveillance, United States, 2009. Available at http://www.cdc.gov/mmwr/pdf/ss/ss5905.pdf

Among adult women in the United States, smoking rates are by far the highest among people of Native American descent (36%). This is twice the national average, and nine times the smoking rate of Asian Americans, the racial group least likely to smoke. After Native Americans, the ethnic and racial groups most likely to smoke are people of mixed race, Whites, African Americans, and Hispanics. Smoking also varies by education and poverty level, with higher rates of smoking corresponding to lower levels of education and incomes below the poverty level.[11]

Even though tobacco use is illegal for people under the age of 18, many teenagers and adolescents have tried tobacco. This tobacco use often becomes a lifelong habit. Almost one-half (46%) of all high school students have tried smoking, establishing a pattern for becoming smokers as adults. About one in five (19%) of female high school students reported smoking in the past month, slightly less than the smoking rate among male high school students

(20%).[12] White high school students are most likely to smoke, followed by Hispanic and Black high school students (Figure 13.2).

Waterpipes, also known as hookahs, have become popular among some adolescents, college students, and young professionals. An old custom among some cultures in the Middle East, hookahs can now be found in fashionable clubs, restaurants, and cafes in many cities. Hookah smoking appears to be just as harmful as cigarette smoking.[13] In fact, it may be even more dangerous because the waterpipe is used over a longer period of time than smoking a cigarette (about 40 to 45 minutes compared to 5 to 10 minutes). This longer period of inhalation and exposure may lead a smoker to inhale as much smoke as consuming 10 or more cigarettes during a single hookah session.[14]

Societal Costs of Smoking

The human costs are the greatest toll associated with smoking. Annual tobacco-related deaths exceed the number of deaths from alcohol, illegal drugs, homicide, suicide, car accidents, fire, and AIDS combined. Each year, approximately 443,000 deaths in the United States are attributed to cigarette smoking.[11] Women make up 174,000 (about 40%) of these deaths (**Table 13.2**). These deaths translate into more than two million years of women's lives lost every year. The economic costs of smoking in the United States are estimated at $167 billion per year, including costs from lost productivity and medical expenditures.[15]

Legal Dimensions of Tobacco Use

Federal and state governments share responsibility for controlling how tobacco products are bought and sold.

© Simone van den Berg/ShutterStock, Inc.

■ Females are beginning to smoke at younger ages, increasing their risk for suffering from smoke-related deaths.

Table 13.2 Annual Deaths, Years of Potential Life Lost, and Productivity Losses Attributable to Smoking Among U.S. Women

Causes of Death	Deaths from Smoking	Potential Years of Life Lost	Productivity Losses (in millions of dollars)
Cancer	56,400	922,000	16,300
Cardiovascular Disease	49,400	612,000	1,000
Respiratory Diseases	49,500	527,000	6,350
Perinatal Diseases	331	26,419	*
Residential Fires	320		*
Secondhand Smoke	18,012		*
Total	174,000	2,100,000	32,611

*= not available

Source: CDC. (2008). Smoking-attributable mortality, years of potential life lost, and productivity losses—United States, 2000-2004.

In 2009, the U.S. Food and Drug Administration (FDA) gained the authority to regulate tobacco products. With this authority, the FDA issued new rules about how tobacco products could be sold, distributed, and marketed. Most of these changes were made to prevent people younger than 18 from purchasing or receiving tobacco products. These FDA requirements included:

- Banning the sale of tobacco products to people younger than 18
- Prohibiting the distribution of free cigarettes or the sale of packages containing fewer than 20 cigarettes
- Limiting the sale of cigarettes in vending machines to select locations where only adults are present
- Prohibiting tobacco company names from appearing as a sponsor of athletic, musical, or cultural events
- Requiring that audio advertisements use words alone rather than music or sound effects
- Banning the sale or distribution of promotional items with tobacco company brands or logos

State governments may tax cigarettes or place additional restrictions on when or where smoking is allowed. All 50 states and the District of Columbia impose a cigarette excise tax; the national average for state cigarette excise taxes is $1.63 per pack. City taxes can occasionally add to these taxes: New York City taxes each package $1.50, for a combined state-local tax rate of $5.85 per package.[8] These taxes have become a valuable revenue source for many state budgets. Many of these taxes were enacted to pay for state medical bills associated with smoking. However, as other sources of income have declined, some states are using cigarette tax revenues to pay for their general expenses.

Smoking and Women Worldwide

Around the world, an estimated one billion people, or one-seventh of the total population, are smokers.[16] The World Health Organization (WHO) estimates that tobacco use kills almost 6 million people each year, with about 5 million dying as a direct result of tobacco use and about 600,000 dying as from exposure to secondhand smoke. Even as smoking rates have fallen in the developed world, smoking

■ Tobacco companies are savvy in the ways they lure new smokers, particularly women.

has increased in developing countries, where there is typically less government regulation, and people are generally less educated and have fewer medical resources. Four in five of the world's smokers now live in low and middle-income countries. Because tobacco smoking has primarily been a custom and addiction of men, women and children represent the majority of the world's passive or **involuntary smokers**.

Tobacco companies are savvy in the ways they lure new smokers, particularly women. Many tobacco companies have cleverly linked the emancipation of women in the developing world with smoking, similar to methods that were used in Western countries in the early 20th century. According to the Institute for Global Tobacco Control, governments in developing countries may be less aware of the harmful effects of tobacco use on women and children and are often preoccupied with other health issues; they mostly see tobacco as a problem confined to men. If no dramatic changes in prevention and cessation occur, tobacco-related deaths could rise to 8 million a year by 2030.[16] To reduce these deaths, WHO has an initiative to counteract campaigns from tobacco companies, obtain more accurate data through surveillance, encourage governments to implement tighter tobacco-control laws, and help people who want to stop smoking quit successfully.

Health Consequences for Women Who Smoke

Tobacco use kills roughly 50% the people who use it. Cigarette smoke causes numerous health problems, primarily for the lungs, but also for almost every system in the body. Health risks to smokers vary depending on the amount smoked, the depth of cigarette inhalation, the tar and nicotine content of cigarettes, and the duration of smoking. Inhalation patterns and puffing behavior affect the degree of exposure to carbon monoxide and other toxic compounds.

The health consequences of smoking also depend largely on when a person starts smoking, and when, if ever, he or she quits. On average,

women who smoke will lose 14.5 years of life from smoking. Symptoms of smoking-related illness usually take years to develop, although irritation symptoms such as watery eyes, nasal irritation, squinting, and coughing develop fairly soon after a woman starts (**Figure 13.3**). In addition, smoking causes premature signs of aging including wrinkles, blotchy skin, and discolored teeth.

Cigarette smoking increases the risk of coronary heart disease, the number-one cause of death among both men and women in the United States. Smoking doubles a woman's risk of myocardial infarction (heart attack) and doubles to quadruples her risk of sudden cardiac death. Young and middle-age women who smoke have substantially higher rates of both fatal and nonfatal stroke than nonsmokers. Each year, more than 8,800 deaths from stroke and 40,000 deaths from coronary heart disease are attributed to smoking in women (see **Figure 13.4**).[15] Smoking is also a major risk factor for arteriosclerosis and peripheral vascular disease.

Cigarette smoking is a major risk factor for cancers throughout the body. Cancer accounts for about one-third

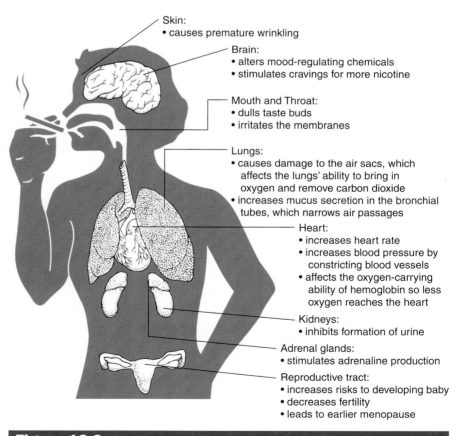

Skin:
• causes premature wrinkling

Brain:
• alters mood-regulating chemicals
• stimulates cravings for more nicotine

Mouth and Throat:
• dulls taste buds
• irritates the membranes

Lungs:
• causes damage to the air sacs, which affects the lungs' ability to bring in oxygen and remove carbon dioxide
• increases mucus secretion in the bronchial tubes, which narrows air passages

Heart:
• increases heart rate
• increases blood pressure by constricting blood vessels
• affects the oxygen-carrying ability of hemoglobin so less oxygen reaches the heart

Kidneys:
• inhibits formation of urine

Adrenal glands:
• stimulates adrenaline production

Reproductive tract:
• increases risks to developing baby
• decreases fertility
• leads to earlier menopause

Figure 13.3
Physiological effects of cigarette smoking

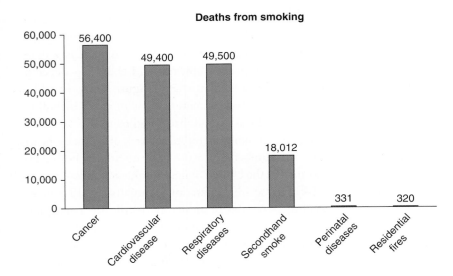

Deaths from smoking

Figure 13.4

Annual U.S. Deaths of Women Attributable to Cigarette Smoking

Source: Data from Centers for Disease Control and Prevention. (2008). Smoking-Attributable Mortality, Years of Potential Life Lost, and Productivity Losses—United States, 2000–2004. Available at http://www.cdc.gov/mmwr/preview/mmwrhtml/mm5745a3.htm#tab

of all smoking-related deaths (Figure 13.4).[15] Smoking is associated with an increased risk of at least 15 types of cancer, including cancers of the lung, larynx, pharynx, mouth, esophagus, kidney, pancreas, cervix, and bladder in women (see **Figure 13.5**). Smoking accounts for more than 80% of lung cancer deaths—lung cancer is an especially deadly form of cancer, and it now is the leading cause of cancer-related deaths among women.[9] Both cigar and cigarette smoking are associated with cancers of the lung, oral cavity, and esophagus.

In addition to increasing the risk for heart disease and cancer, cigarette smoking severely damages the respiratory system. **Chronic obstructive pulmonary disease (COPD)** is characterized by permanent airflow obstruction and extended periods of disability and restricted activity. Cigarette smoking is the major risk factor for developing COPD, with 80% to 90% of COPD deaths being attributed to smoking. Over the past few years, more women than men have died from COPD (66,000 females compared to 61,000 males).[17] Females who smoke also are nearly 13 times more likely to die from COPD than are female nonsmokers.

COPD encompasses many conditions, including emphysema and chronic bronchitis, which usually occur together. With **emphysema**, the limitation of airflow results from gradual, irreversible disease changes in the lung tissue after years of assault. The air sacs in the lungs are destroyed, which compromises the lungs' ability to bring in oxygen and remove carbon dioxide from the body. As a result, breathing becomes labored, and the heart must work harder to transport oxygen. **Chronic bronchitis** is characterized by constant inflammation of the bronchial tubes. The inflammation thickens the walls of the bronchi, and the production of mucus increases, resulting in a constricting or narrowing of the air passages.

Women who smoke face an increased risk of osteoporosis and early menopause, with smokers reaching spontaneous menopause one to two years earlier than nonsmoking women. The age differences in menopause appear to be smoking-dose dependent. Smoking reduces fertility and may increase back pain. In addition, cigarette smoking can worsen the symptoms or complications of allergies, asthma, and existing disorders of the pulmonary and circulatory system.

Smoking as an Addiction

Although tobacco smoke contains thousands of compounds, the most significant from a health perspective are nicotine, tar, and carbon monoxide.

- **Nicotine** is the addictive element in cigarettes. It has several effects on the body, including increasing blood pressure, increasing heart rate, and negating hunger. Nicotine stimulates the pleasure centers of the brain, causing physical addiction. While nicotine can harm the body over the long term, it also appears to have short-term benefits: many smokers state that nicotine helps them relax, concentrate, or complete some tasks more easily. These benefits, along with nicotine's addictive potential, help explain why many people continue to smoke despite knowing tobacco's harmful nature. Two studies published in 2007 found that the nicotine available in cigarettes steadily increased from 1997 to 2005, suggesting that cigarette manufacturers have deliberately increased the amount of nicotine available in cigarettes.[18]

- Tar is a thick, sticky, dark fluid produced when tobacco is burned. Tar consists of hundreds of compounds, many of which are **carcinogenic** (capable of promoting growth of cancerous cells) in their own right. Through

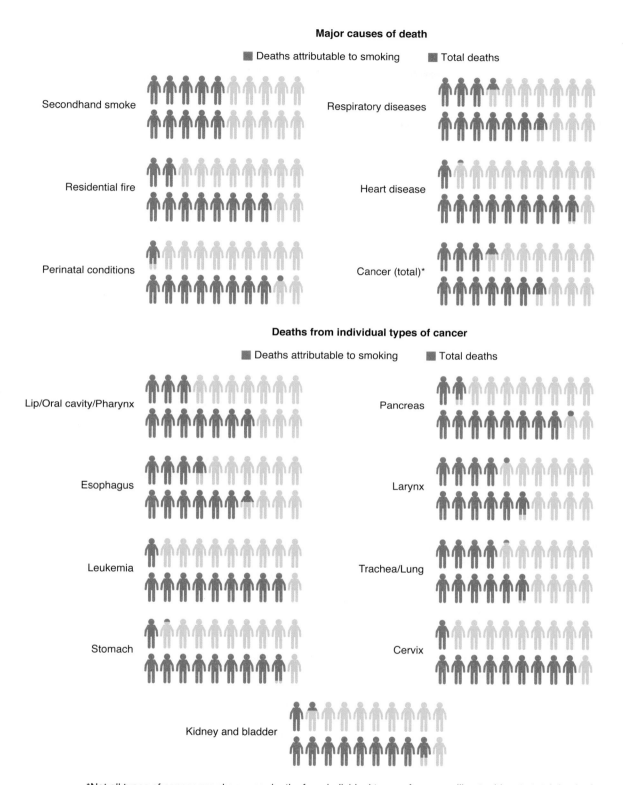

Major causes of death

■ Deaths attributable to smoking   ■ Total deaths

Secondhand smoke

Residential fire

Perinatal conditions

Respiratory diseases

Heart disease

Cancer (total)*

Deaths from individual types of cancer

■ Deaths attributable to smoking   ■ Total deaths

Lip/Oral cavity/Pharynx

Esophagus

Leukemia

Stomach

Pancreas

Larynx

Trachea/Lung

Cervix

Kidney and bladder

*Not all types of cancer are shown, so deaths from individual types of cancer will not add up to total deaths from cancer.

Figure 13.5

Proportion of major causes of death attributable to smoking among U.S. women

Source: Data from Centers for Disease Control and Prevention. (2008). Smoking-Attributable Mortality, Years of Potential Life Lost, and Productivity Losses—United States, 2000–2004. Available at http://www.cdc.gov/mmwr/preview/mmwrhtml/mm5745a3.htm#tab

Are You Addicted to Cigarettes?

Self-Assessment 13.1

Carefully read and answer each of the following questions honestly.

1. Have you ever failed in an attempt to give up cigarettes?   yes   no

2. Have you ever failed in an attempt to cut back on cigarettes?   yes   no

3. Have you ever failed in an attempt to switch to a lower-tar and lower-nicotine cigarette?   yes   no

4. When you have not smoked a cigarette for a while, do you feel any withdrawal symptoms, such as an urge for a cigarette, irritability, anxiety, difficulty concentrating, or drowsiness?   yes   no

5. Have you developed any smoking-related side effects, such as a morning cough or a hoarse voice, yet continue to smoke?   yes   no

If you answered "yes" to any of these questions, you are probably hooked on cigarettes and have an addiction to tobacco. Consider quitting cigarettes, seeking help from your healthcare provider if necessary.

---

inhalation, tar settles and accumulates throughout the oral cavity and pulmonary system. The combination of tar and smoke further compromises the cardiopulmonary system.

■ Carbon monoxide is another deadly by-product of cigarettes. This gas interferes with the blood's ability to carry oxygen, impairs normal functioning of the nervous system, and contributes to degradation of the cardiopulmonary system.

Smoking is an addictive behavior, with nicotine being the primary addictive pharmacological component. **Self-Assessment 13.1** provides an opportunity to assess whether an individual is addicted to cigarette smoking. Smoking cessation results in withdrawal, an adverse reaction characterized by unpleasant symptoms and an intense psychological and physiological demand for nicotine. Symptoms of withdrawal usually include the following:

■ Cigarette craving

■ Irritability

■ Restlessness

■ Anxiety

■ Difficulty in concentrating

■ Headache

■ Drowsiness

■ Depression (deep, overwhelming feelings of apathy, sadness, or anger)

■ Varied gastrointestinal disturbances such as diarrhea and constipation

The physical and psychological withdrawal symptoms that occur with cigarette smoking cessation vary in their duration and intensity. For heavy smokers, withdrawal symptoms may occur within 2 hours of the last cigarette. The peak period of physiological symptoms from smoking cessation is usually 24 to 48 hours into abstinence, but many smokers report "craving" cigarettes for years.

Why Women Smoke

Women often initiate cigarette smoking in adolescence in the context of social interactions with peers. Adolescents are more likely to be smokers if their parents, older siblings, or peers smoke. Many smokers report that their

It's Your Health

Strategies to Quit Cigarettes Gradually

Wait 15 minutes after the initial urge for a cigarette. This delay gives a feeling of control, and sometimes the urge will simply go away.

Distract yourself when you want to smoke by drinking water, making a phone call, chewing gum, taking a short walk, or brushing your teeth.

Avoid the places where the smoking habit has thrived—a favorite chair, lingering after a meal, a coffee break.

Establish nonsmoking hours and gradually extend them.

Buy cigarettes only by the pack. Never buy the same brand twice in a row.

Try to buy cigarette brands with successively lower levels of tar and nicotine.

Ask that other smokers do not light up around you. Have friends and family help you fight the urge to smoke again.

Make it harder to get your cigarettes. Keep them in a locked drawer or with a friend.

Declare former smoking areas to be nonsmoking areas, such as the car, house, and office.

Don't empty ashtrays.

Keep a daily record to document and reinforce progress with quitting. Write down reasons why you want to quit.

Be willing to try again. Many people are able to quit after several attempts.

Consider nicotine replacement therapy (NRT) or other medications to help reduce the physical addiction of cigarettes.

primary reason for smoking is to give them something to do in social situations and/or to "fill time." The social situations in which smoking occurs, as well as the physical effects of nicotine, strongly affect smoking dependence in women. (See **It's Your Health 13.2**.)

Many women hesitate to quit smoking over a fear of unwanted weight gain. Even many pregnant women who smoke indicate that their reason for doing so is to avoid weight gain. Smokers do tend to weigh less than nonsmokers. There is no scientific consensus yet regarding the physiological or biochemical mechanism that is responsible for this relationship between weight regulation and smoking behavior. Some evidence indicates that nicotine elevates the body's basal metabolic rate (BMR). The average person gains between 4 and 10 pounds upon quitting smoking, but exercise combined with a smoking cessation program can decrease this weight gain and increase rates of abstinence from smoking.

Women's concerns about weight gain and the maintenance of their smoking behavior sadly reflect their willingness to risk long-term detrimental—and potentially catastrophic—consequences in exchange for dealing with body image and weight-control issues. Teenage girls, in particular, often believe that smoking helps them control their weight, and this belief dissuades many from quitting this behavior. Health professionals, educators, mothers, and other female role models must strike a balance between recognizing that girls have concerns about their weight, while trying to refocus them on healthy behaviors, self-esteem, and safer coping strategies.

Smoking and Pregnancy

Quitting smoking may be one of the most significant things a pregnant woman can do to optimize the well-being of her baby. It is estimated that smoking during pregnancy is responsible for 11% of stillbirths and a 5% of newborn deaths.[19] Smoking is believed be a factor in 17% to 30% of low-birthweight babies, 14% of preterm deliveries, and 10% of all infant deaths. The prevalence of smoking during pregnancy has declined steadily over the past 20 years, with about one in seven pregnant women smoking during the last 3 months of pregnancy. About 45% of smoking women who become pregnant quit during pregnancy; half the women who quit during this time relapse within 6 months of delivery.[20]

Cigarette smoking during pregnancy retards fetal growth and is associated with miscarriage, stillbirth, sudden infant death syndrome (SIDS), and infant mortality.

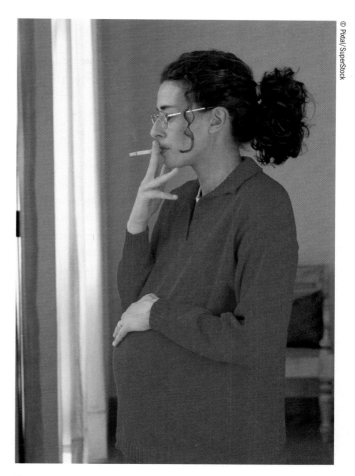

■ Smoking presents many risks to a woman and her unborn child.

Pregnant women who smoke more are at additional risk. Nicotine and carbon monoxide are considered the two most important components in cigarettes that constitute major hazards to the fetus:

- Nicotine reduces fetal breathing movements and uterine blood flow, and increases fetal heart rate.
- Carbon monoxide reduces the amount of oxygen available to the fetus by as much as 25%.

Secondhand and Third-Hand Smoking

Smokers are not the only ones affected by cigarette smoke. Secondhand smoke, or environmental tobacco smoke (ETS), is air contaminated with chemicals from cigarette smoke. Nonsmokers who breathe secondhand smoke are at increased risk of developing asthma, lung cancer, heart disease and other conditions; secondhand smoke also increases smokers' exposure to carcinogens and dangerous chemicals. Secondhand smoke nearly 50,000 adults each year in the United States—about 46,000 from heart disease and about 3,000 from lung cancer.[11]

Secondhand smoke is also a concern for babies and young children, whose lungs are more sensitive than the lungs of adults. Secondhand smoke increases a child's risk of low birthweight; sudden infant death syndrome (SIDS); acute lower respiratory tract infections, such as bronchitis and pneumonia; induction and exacerbation of asthma; chronic respiratory symptoms; and middle-ear infections.

The greatest source of exposure to secondhand smoke for children, infants, and most adults is the home. For adults living in households where no one smokes, the workplace is the greatest source of exposure to ETS. The separation of smokers and nonsmokers within the same airspace reduces, but does not eliminate, exposure to ETS. As of 2012, 27 states and the District of Columbia prohibit smoking in restaurants, bars, and government buildings, and seven states prohibit smoking in restaurants; the remaining states have weaker laws that allow smoking in at least some pub-lic locations. Many states have also legally mandated that most workplaces follow a nonsmoking policy.

"Third-hand smoke," or the leftover nicotine and other chemicals that accumulate on walls, furniture, clothing, and other surfaces in areas where smoking has occurred, also creates health risks. These chemicals may last on sur-faces for weeks or months. While third-hand smoke does not appear to be as dangerous as secondhand smoke, it still may increase the risk for asthma, lung cancer, and other conditions. More research is needed to fully understand the risks of third-hand smoke.

Quitting Smoking

Quitting smoking is often the most significant personal behavior that a person can undertake to improve one's health. Some health benefits of quitting begin shortly after the last cigarette. After a few weeks, a person's lungs and circulatory system improve; coughing and shortness of breath usually decline within a few months. The risk for car-diovascular disease and cancer also drops over time. A year after quitting, a person's risk of coronary heart disease falls by 50%. A person's risk of mouth, throat, and lung cancers also usually fall by 50% within 5 to 10 years. A person will experience greater benefits the earlier she or he quits, but quitting at any age improves health in many ways.

Quitting smoking is not an easy process. Some people are able to quit on their first attempt, others are able to quit after several efforts, and some people are never able to quit.

It's Your Health

Common Rationalizations of Women Smokers

It can't be as bad as they say.

The government wouldn't let them sell cigarettes if they were that harmful.

My aunt lived to be 80 and she smoked.

We all have to die sometime.

I have so much stress in my life.

I really need cigarettes to make things better.

I DON'T want to gain weight.

It is okay if I smoke because I eat well and exercise every day.

I only smoke at work, not at home.

I only smoke low-tar cigarettes.

I am too busy to eat, and smoking helps me to control my hunger.

Typically, only about 8% to 10% of smokers who attempt to quit on their own are successful on any given attempt. The most difficult period is usually the first 3 months, when a person's physical and psychological addiction to tobacco is the strongest. After that period, some people have an easy time staying away from smoking, while others continue to feel cigarette cravings for years.

Some people decide to quit by going "cold turkey," or making a sudden, decisive break from cigarettes. Some people find that they are able to go cold turkey if they do it one day at a time. They promise themselves to be smoke free for 24 hours; at the end of that day, they reaffirm their commitment to another smoke-free day. Another approach involves gradually reducing the amount of nicotine the body receives. A person can do this either by reducing the num-ber of cigarettes he or she smokes, or by switching from smoking to an alternate form of nicotine, such as nicotine replacement therapy (NRT) or electronic cigarettes, and then gradually reducing their use.

Some smokers are able to quit by enlisting the help of other people. Counseling can help smokers identify their motivations for smoking and "triggers" that make them more likely to smoke. Support groups, conducted either online or in person, can help a person meet with and get sympathy, advice, and help from other people trying to quit. A person's own friends and family can be a valuable source of assistance by providing sympathy and gently but persis-tently encouraging them to continue their efforts to quit.

Various forms of treatment are also available to help people quit tobacco use. Nicotine replacement therapy allows a person to gradually reduce feelings of withdrawal by providing an alternate source of nicotine. It is available as a patch, gum, lozenge, spray, or inhaler. Although these forms all provide the same drug, they differ in the speed in which it is delivered. The nicotine patch provides a slow, steady dose of nicotine that lasts all day. Kept in the mouth, nicotine gum and lozenges may take about 30 minutes to take effect. Nicotine sprays (sprayed into the nose like some allergy medicines) and inhalers provide a strong, short-lasting dose of nicotine within a few minutes. Studies have found that NRT improves a person's chances of quitting by 50% to 70% for the first 3 to 6 months.[21] However, the long-term effectiveness of NRT—whether they help people quit tobacco for good—is still unknown.

The FDA has also approved two medications to help people quit smoking: bupropion (Zyban) and varenicline (Chantix). Both of these medications appear to reduce cravings for tobacco and to block the pleasurable effects nicotine has within the brain. After taking these medications for a few weeks, a person who does smoke a cigarette may feel little or no enjoyment from the experience. Both of these medications are about as effective as NRT in helping people to quit; like NRT, there are still questions as to their long-term efficacy.[21] A small percentage of people who take varenicline may experience disturbing psychological symptoms, ranging from changes in mood, to altered dreams and thoughts of violence or suicide; women who experience any of these symptoms should contact their healthcare providers immediately.

Electronic cigarettes occupy a gray area between a method of quitting and a new habit. These electronic devices, shaped like cigarettes, deliver a breathable vapor containing nicotine. Some people use electronic cigarettes to taper down their nicotine intake. However, electronic cigarettes do not have FDA approval as quitting devices and are instead sold as "alternatives to cigarettes." In addition, fewer studies have examined electronic cigarettes' effectiveness as a quitting tool.

I had smoked for years before I became pregnant with my first child. I quit smoking while I was pregnant, but as life became more stressful, I started again—just having a cigarette after a bad day or if my friends were over. Gradually, I began to smoke more and more. Four years later, my daughter told me that my mouth smelled bad, like I "lit a fire in it." I knew then that I had to quit this disgusting habit. Although I don't smoke anymore, I still want one after lunch, when I have a drink, just at certain times of the day. I will always be addicted.

—32-year-old woman

Alcohol

Pure **alcohol** is a colorless liquid obtained by fermentation of a sugar-containing material. Ethyl alcohol (ethanol) is the type of alcohol found in alcoholic beverages. The amount of alcohol varies from beverage to beverage. Roughly the same amount of alcohol is present in a 12-ounce bottle or can of beer (4% alcohol), 5-ounce of table wine (10% alcohol), and 1.25 ounces of distilled spirits (40% alcohol). For most people, drinking moderate amounts of alcohol (no more than one drink a day for women or two drinks a day for men) is unlikely to cause any health problems and may even slightly lower the risk of heart disease. However, when a person drinks larger amounts of alcohol on a regular basis, or engages in irresponsible drinking behaviors, numerous health consequences can result.

Blood Alcohol Concentration

Blood alcohol concentration (BAC) is a physiological indicator that clinicians and law enforcement officials use to determine whether a person is legally "drunk." Blood alcohol concentration represents the percentage of alcohol in the blood. A BAC of 0.10 indicates the presence of approximately one part of alcohol per 1,000 parts of other blood components. As **Table 13.3** shows, a BAC of 0.10

Table 13.3 Blood Alcohol Concentrations

BAC	Effects
0.02–0.04	No overt effects; feelings of muscle relaxation and slight mood elevation
0.05–0.06	Relaxation and warmth; slight decrease in reaction time and slight decrease in fine muscle coordination
0.08–0.10	Balance, speech, vision, and hearing slightly impaired; euphoric feelings; increased loss of motor coordination
0.11–0.12	Difficulty with coordination and balance; distinct impairment of mental facilities and judgment
0.14–0.15	Major impairment of mental and physical control; slurred speech, blurred vision, and lack of motor skill
0.20	Loss of motor control; substantial mental disorientation
0.30	Severe intoxication with minimum conscious control of mind and body

Greater levels lead to unconsciousness, coma, and death from respiratory failure.

Source: Substance Abuse and Mental Health Services Administration.

results in significant compromise of mental and psycho-motor capabilities. In all 50 states, driving with a BAC of 0.08 or higher is illegal. The punishment for violating this limit, as well as the number and kinds of other laws related to driving while intoxicated, vary from state to state.

Many factors affect BAC and an individual's response to alcohol. For example, BAC increases more quickly when alcohol is consumed at a faster rate and without food. Stronger drinks, smaller body size, older age, or being of Asian or Native American descent can also lead to increased BAC levels when drinking. In addition to higher BACs, some people of Native American or Asian descent experience effects such as nausea, headaches, and flushing of the skin when they drink.

With regular alcohol consumption, additional alcohol is required to achieve the same desired psychological effect, although motor coordination and judgment are impaired at the same level. After years of heavy drinking, damage to the liver can sometimes cause "reverse tolerance." Reverse tolerance occurs when a person lacks enough liver enzymes to break down alcohol at normal rate; if this happens a person can quickly become intoxicated after drinking only a small amount of alcohol.

Epidemiological Trends and Issues

Although alcohol consumption is generally considered a personal and private issue, its effects permeate all sectors and dimensions of society. Alcohol has been a constant component of American life since the colonial period. Attempts to control, restrict, or abolish alcohol in the United States have all met with failure. In 1919, the 18th Amendment to the Constitution was ratified in an attempt to stop the rapid growth of alcohol addiction. This amendment prohibited the manufacture, sale, and transportation of alcohol, ushering in the Prohibition era. During this time, illegal sales of bootlegged beverages and alcoholic prescription "medications" prevailed as people sought ways around the ban. Prohibition was officially repealed in 1933 by the 21st Amendment.

During the 19th and early 20th centuries, most people believed that alcoholics were morally weak. Today, there is a greater awareness of the complex nature of alcoholism. Public admissions of alcoholism by well-known women such as Betty Ford, Drew Barrymore, Lindsay Lohan, and Nicole Richie have reinforced the fact that alcoholism is a personal and pervasive health problem that affects women from all walks of life.

According to the National Survey on Drug Use and Health, 47% of females age 12 and older had at least one drink within the past month; this rate increased to 57% among women between the ages of 18 and 25. American Indian/Alaska Native women are most likely to have alcohol dependence or abuse issues (14%), compared to White women (6%), Black women (4%), Latina women (4%), or Asian women (2%).[3] In general, women are less likely to drink, drink less, and are less likely to become alcohol dependent than men.

Although underage drinking is also more common among males than females, it occurs for both genders. In 2010, an estimated one in four (24%) female teenagers drank within the past month, one in seven (14%) had engaged in binge drinking, and one in 25 (4%) had drank five or more drinks on at least five separate occasions in the past month.[3]

Cultural factors influence the prevalence of alcoholism. In cultures where drinking is a part of family rituals or ceremonies or where there is great disapproval of public drunkenness, there appears to be lower prevalence of heavy drinking. Gender-based social norms often contribute to alcohol consumption patterns. For example, in some cultures, men are drinkers while women generally abstain.

Adult alcohol use is most common in the Northeast (58%), followed by the Midwest (55%), West (51%), and South (48%); the rate of alcohol use is also higher in large metropolitan areas (54%) as compared with small metropolitan and nonmetropolitan areas (51% and 46.0%, respectively).[3]

Social Dimensions

Many cultural factors affect women's drinking patterns or behavior. Society's double standard for women often prevails where alcoholism is concerned. Folklore and popular media may portray male drinkers as comical, lovable, or noble but a drunken woman as loose, weak, and immoral. Additionally, greater social sanctions applied to alcoholism make some women less willing to seek help and others less willing to recognize that they need help. Because alcoholic women violate the stereotype of feminine behavior, they often distress their families and friends and even the health professionals who might support them. For both women and men, depression is associated with excess alcohol consumption. In some cases alcohol may be a symptom of depression; in others alcohol use may be a consequence of it.

Victimization is also associated with alcohol-related problems. Women who are sexually abused in childhood or physically abused as adults are more likely to experience alcohol-related problems as adults. The relationship between victimization and alcohol may be confounded by the fact that victimization often leads to depression, which in turn is associated with alcohol use.

Although the literature includes few studies on alcohol and drug use among lesbians, it has been suggested that lesbians consume more alcohol for longer periods and are more likely than heterosexual women to use alcohol with other drugs.[22] Lesbian women may be at greater risk of alcohol problems because of the social disapproval directed at their sexual orientation.

■ Alcohol is an accepted and often traditional part of many social events.

Societal Costs of Alcohol Use and Alcoholism

With more than 126 million Americans reporting current use of alcohol and 17 million calling themselves heavy drinkers, the economic, social, and personal costs of alcohol-related crimes, accidents, illnesses, and deaths are profound.[3] One estimate of cost of alcohol abuse and alcoholism in the United States is $224 billion per year, or about $750 per person.[23] Most of these costs come from binge or heavy drinking. This estimate includes healthcare costs of people who use or are affected by alcohol, lost productivity, law enforcement and criminal justice expenses, and motor vehicle accidents caused by drunk driving.

The costs to society from alcohol cannot be measured just in terms of dollars. More than 75,000 deaths in the United States are attributed to alcohol every year; just under one-third (21,000) of these deaths are women. About half of alcohol-related deaths are a result of chronic conditions, while the other half are a result of falls, homicides, motor vehicle accidents, suicides, and other acute conditions.[24] Chronic alcohol use contributes to several often-fatal illnesses, most notably liver disease, cancer, and cardiovascular disease, and can damage most organs in the body (**Table 13.4**). Drunk driving, or driving under the influence of alcohol, affects not only the people who drink, but their passengers and other drivers. Alcohol is a factor in one in three automobile-related fatalities, causing an estimated 11,000 deaths a year.[25] While men make up the majority (80%) of drunk drivers, both sexes drink and drive, and both sexes are injured or killed as a result of drunk driving.

Table 13.4 Complications from Chronic Alcohol Consumption	
Cancer:	Cancer of the liver, larynx, esophagus, stomach, colon, breast, and skin (malignant melanoma)
Cardiovascular effects:	Hypertension, stroke, and cardiovascular disease
Organ damage:	Brain, stomach, colon, pancreas, and kidneys
Diabetes	
Fetal alcohol syndrome	
Impotency and infertility	
Diminished immunity	
Sleep disturbances	

Legal Issues of Alcohol Use and Alcoholism

There are many legal issues related to drinking. During Prohibition (1920–1933), alcohol was illegal in the United States. Although the 21st amendment made alcohol legal again, both states and the federal government have since enacted laws that limit its use. Nationally, alcohol is legally restricted to people 21 and older; most other countries have legal drinking ages of 18 or 19.

In addition to setting age limits on alcohol use, states have enacted laws governing drinking and driving, drunk and disorderly behavior, purchase of alcohol for a minor, and driving with an open container of alcohol. Most of the penalties associated with alcohol abuse or misuse involve misdemeanor charges or fines, but some—for example, drunk driving violations—entail mandatory jail time in many states.

Effects of Alcohol

Alcohol is a central nervous system depressant that effectively impairs all major body systems. When consumed in small quantities, it has a mild, relaxing effect. Consumption of larger quantities results in compromised sensory motor coordination, judgment, emotional control, and reasoning capabilities. Once ingested, alcohol circulates throughout the body, affecting nearly every bodily function (**Figure 13.6**). Alcohol usually takes about 15 minutes to reach the bloodstream, and the peak effect occurs in 1 hour. Once in the bloodstream, alcohol quickly reaches the liver, heart, and brain.

The liver is the organ that metabolizes alcohol and removes it from the body. This exposure makes the liver the organ most vulnerable to alcohol. Heavy drinking may lead to alcoholic hepatitis, which is characterized by inflammation and destruction of liver cells, and **cirrhosis**, which produces progressive scarring of liver tissue. More than

90% of heavy drinkers develop fatty liver, a type of liver disease; 20% will develop liver cirrhosis.[26] Compared with men, women develop alcohol-induced liver disease over a shorter period of time and after consuming less alcohol.[27]

Chronic heavy alcohol consumption is also associated with cardiovascular damage. Consuming one or two alcoholic drinks per day may slightly lower the chances of developing coronary heart disease; however, heavier drinking greatly increases the risk. Chronic heavy alcohol use also increases the risk for cancers of the liver, mouth, throat, colon, and breast.

To an observer, the most noticeable effects of alcohol are on the brain and behavior. Alcohol alters the activity of brain neurons, impairing sensory, motor, and cognitive function. Moderate amounts of alcohol also lower perception, judgment, and psychomotor skills. Alcohol's anesthetic effect may cause diminished perception of pain and temperature, possibly leading to serious injury or exposure to extreme temperatures. Although drinking may decrease judgment, increase interest, and reduce inhibitions in sex, it also impairs a man's ability to achieve or maintain an erection and a woman's ability to achieve orgasm. Additional drinking progressively reduces behavioral activity, which may lead to sleep, general anesthesia, coma, and even death.

Figure 13.6

Physiological effects of alcohol

Blood:
• decreases white blood cells for fighting infection
• causes anemia
• interferes with blood clotting

Pancreas:
• leads to inflammation of the pancreas

Immune System:
• increases susceptibility to infections such as pneumonia and tuberculosis

Brain:
• damages brain cells
• impairs perception and judgment
• impairs motor skills

Bones:
• increases risk of osteoporosis

Heart:
• weakens the heart muscle
• increases blood pressure and risk of stroke
• causes heart rhythm irregularities

Stomach:
• triggers bleeding and peptic ulcers

Liver:
• damages liver cells

Reproductive Tract:
• causes birth defects
• leads to gynecological and obstetrical problems

Alcohol is particularly dangerous when combined with other drugs, such as depressants and antianxiety medications. Of the 100 most frequently prescribed drugs, more than half contain at least one ingredient that interacts adversely with alcohol. Combining alcohol with drugs may heighten the effect of either drug or produce additional harmful effects (**Table 13.5**). Acetaminophen (brand name Tylenol) can be especially toxic to the liver when taken with many drinks, and in rare cases can lead to acute hepatic failure.

Heavy alcohol consumption typically leads to several nutritional problems for the chronic user. Because alcohol dulls the senses of taste and smell, heavy drinkers often skip meals and develop nutritional deficiencies. Alcohol consumption also has been associated with osteoporosis due to alcohol's ability to block the absorption of calcium. Chronic consumption disrupts normal digestive processes, resulting in gastritis (inflammation of the stomach lining), stomach ulcers, and intestinal lesions, which interfere with the metabolism of vitamins and minerals. In addition, alcoholism has been associated with thiamine (vitamin B_1) deficiency, which can increase the risk for diseases of the nervous, digestive, muscular, and cardiovascular systems.

Physiologically, women appear to have less body water than men of similar body weight and produce less alcohol dehydrogenase, the enzyme responsible for ethanol metabolism. As a result, women absorb about 30% more alcohol than men do into the bloodstream before it can be metabolized in the liver.[27] Alcohol reaches women's brains and other organs more quickly than it does in men, resulting in more rapid intoxication as well as more organ-specific ethanol toxicity. For a woman of average size, one drink has roughly the same effect as two drinks have on the average-sized man. Women alcoholics also are more likely to suffer liver damage than men.

Hormone levels affect alcohol metabolism. Studies have found that both the menstrual cycle and the use of oral contraceptives influence blood alcohol levels. The rate of alcohol metabolism and peak BAC attained with a standard dose of alcohol may vary depending on estrogen levels. Moderate alcohol consumption may increase the risk of breast cancer in postmenopausal women taking hormone replacement therapy.[28] These variances may help explain why some women have difficulty predicting their response to alcohol and their feelings of loss of control over their responses.

Alcohol can also cross the placental barrier to affect reproductive health and pregnancy. Alcohol's effects on the developing fetus vary depending on the degree and timing of exposure, genetic differences in maternal metabolism of alcohol, maternal nutritional status, and possible interaction with other drug compounds. Women who are alcoholics or who drink heavily during pregnancy are more likely to miscarry. A direct effect of alcohol in pregnant

Table 13.5 Alcohol and Drug Interactions

Type of Drug	Examples	Possible Effects
Analgesics (narcotic)	codeine, Demerol, Percodan	Increased CNS* depression possibly leading to respiratory arrest and death
Analgesics (nonnarcotic)	aspirin, acetaminophen, ibuprofen	Gastric irritation and bleeding Increased susceptibility to liver damage
Antidepressants	Tofranil, tricyclics (Elavil)	Increased CNS depression, decreased alertness
Antianxiety drugs	Valium, Librium, Xanax, Ativan	Increased CNS depression, decreased alertness
Antihistamines	Actifed, Dimetapp, cold medications (prescribed and over-the-counter)	Increased drowsiness
Antibiotics	penicillin, erythromycin	Nausea, vomiting, headache Some antibiotics are rendered less effective
CNS* stimulants	caffeine, Dexedrine, Ritalin, Adderall	Somewhat counter depressant effect of alcohol but do not influence level of intoxication
Diuretics	Lasix, Diuril, Hydromox	Reduction in blood pressure with possible lightheadedness
Psychotropics	Tindal, Mellaril, Thorazine	Increased CNS depression possibly leading to respiratory arrest
Sedatives	Dalmane, Nembutal, Quaalude	Increased CNS depression possibly leading to respiratory arrest and death
Tranquilizers	Valium, Miltown, Librium	Increased CNS depression, decreased alertness and judgment

*CNS: Central nervous system.

women is fetal alcohol syndrome (FAS). This syndrome causes physical and mental abnormalities in infants born to mothers who drank alcohol during pregnancy (see Chapter 6). Fetal alcohol syndrome has the following symptoms:

- Small body size and weight
- Slower than normal development and failure to catch up
- Skeletal deformities
- Facial abnormalities
- Organ deformities
- Central nervous system handicaps[30]

Alcohol consumption may inhibit the release of oxytocin and prolactin, two hormones important for initiation and maintenance of lactation. It also may alter the composition of a woman's breast milk and inhibit milk production.[31]

Alcohol plays an indirect role in many unwanted pregnancies and sexually transmitted infections (STIs). Because of impaired judgment and reasoning from intoxication, a woman may forget or ignore contraception, make judgments she later regrets, or miss signs of danger. In addition to unwanted pregnancies and STIs, alcohol is often a factor in acquaintance rape cases and incidents of pressured sex.

Alcoholism

An alcoholic is a person who is addicted to alcohol and whose consumption of alcohol interferes with a major aspect of her or his life. Until the early to mid 20th century, dependence on alcohol was largely seen as a sign of weakness or moral failure. Since then, however, **alcoholism** has been recognized as a chronic disease with genetic, psychological, and environmental components. Alcoholism has a generational cyclic effect. Children of alcoholics are more likely to suffer abuse, to have psychological or emotional problems, to become alcoholics, and to marry alcoholics. Approximately one in five U.S. adults have lived with an alcoholic relative while growing up.[32]

Chronic alcohol abuse usually manifests itself as one of the following patterns:

- Daily intake of large amounts of alcohol
- Regular heavy drinking on weekends
- Periods of sobriety between binges of daily heavy drinking that may last for weeks or months

Alcoholism most often appears between ages 20 and 40, but can present in childhood or early adolescence. Alcohol becomes a problem when an individual is no longer able to control when and how much drinking takes place.

I used to think that I couldn't be an alcoholic. I had a good job and I drank only wine. I certainly don't look like an alcoholic, whatever that look is. It took a long time for me to admit that I really was dependent on that wine. I needed it every day just to dull the world.
—30-year-old woman

Clinical diagnosis of alcoholism is based on the presence of at least three of the following symptoms, persisting for a month or more or occurring repeatedly over a longer period of time:

- Large amounts of alcohol (5 or more drinks per day)
- Persistent desire to quit drinking or one or more unsuccessful attempts to cut down or quit alcohol
- Considerable time spent obtaining, using, or recovering from alcohol
- Continued drinking despite social, psychological, or physical harm
- Withdrawal symptoms, such as physical trembling, sweating, high blood pressure, delusions, and hallucinations, when alcohol intake is curbed
- The avoidance or relief of withdrawal symptoms by drinking
- Desire or need for a drink to start the day
- Denial of an alcohol problem
- Sleep problems
- Trying, but being unable to stay away from alcohol
- Depression and paranoia
- Failure to recall what happened during a drinking episode
- Dramatic mood swings
- Behaviors or activities while drinking that are regretted later
- The experience of the following symptoms after drinking: headaches, nausea, stomach pain, heartburn, gas, fatigue, weakness, muscle cramps, irregular or rapid heart rate

Risk Factors for Alcoholism

A family history of alcohol problems, early initiation of drinking, and victimization may increase a woman's risk for alcohol abuse or alcoholism. Identical twins, for example, have closer rates of alcohol dependence, abuse, and heavy consumption than fraternal twins, suggesting a genetic component to alcoholism. There is also a significant association between alcoholism in people who were adopted and their biological parents, further reinforcing this hypothesis.[33] Women who were sexually, verbally, or physically abused also reported more alcohol-related problems.

Alcoholism is associated with personality disorders, depression, and other mental illnesses. This association appears to be a two-way street: It may result if a person resorts to alcohol abuse to cope with the symptoms of a mental illness or if a person becomes depressed as a result of alcohol abuse. Alcoholism is also associated with antisocial behavior and low self-esteem.

Treating Alcoholism

The most difficult and significant step for an alcoholic is admitting to an alcohol problem. Often well-intended friends or family members, out of fear, embarrassment, loyalty, or hope, help shield the alcoholic from the truth. Confrontation—either personal or via an accident or drunk-driving conviction—that makes the individual acknowledge the alcohol problem is often a turning point in seeking assistance (**Self-Assessment** 13.2). Recovery from alcoholism is more likely when the person has a strong

---

Self-Assessment 13.2

National Council on Alcoholism Self-Test: Do You Have a Drinking Problem?

1. Do you occasionally drink heavily after a disappointment or a quarrel, or when your parents give you a hard time? yes no
2. When you have trouble or feel pressured at school, do you always drink more heavily than usual? yes no
3. Have you noticed that you are able to handle more liquor than you did when you were first drinking? yes no
4. Did you ever wake up on "the morning after" and discover that you could not remember the evening before, even though your friends tell you that you did not pass out? yes no
5. When drinking with other people, do you try to have a few extra drinks that others don't notice? yes no
6. Are there certain occasions when you feel uncomfortable if alcohol is not available? yes no
7. Have you recently noticed that when you begin drinking you are in more of a hurry to get the first drink than you used to be? yes no
8. Do you sometimes feel guilty about your drinking? yes no
9. Are you secretly irritated when your family or friends discuss your drinking? yes no
10. Have you recently noticed an increase in the frequency of your memory blackouts? yes no
11. Do you often find that you wish to continue drinking after your friends say that they have had enough? yes no
12. Do you usually have a reason for the occasions that you drink heavily? yes no
13. When you are sober, do you often regret things you did or said while drinking? yes no
14. Have you tried switching brands or following different plans for controlling your drinking? yes no
15. Have you often failed to keep the promises you've made to yourself about controlling or cutting down on your drinking? yes no
16. Have you ever tried to control your drinking by changing jobs or moving to a new location? yes no
17. Do you try to avoid family or close friends while you are drinking? yes no
18. Are you having an increasing number of financial and academic problems? yes no
19. Do more people seem to be treating you unfairly without good reason? yes no
20. Do you eat very little or irregularly when you are drinking? yes no
21. Do you sometimes have the shakes in the morning and find that it helps to have a little drink? yes no
22. Have you recently noticed that you cannot drink as much as you once did? yes no
23. Do you sometimes stay drunk for several days at a time? yes no
24. Do you sometimes feel very depressed and wonder whether life is worth living? yes no
25. Sometimes after periods of drinking, do you see or hear things that aren't there? yes no
26. Do you get terribly frightened after you have been drinking heavily? yes no

Those who answer "yes" to two or three of these questions may wish to evaluate their drinking in these areas. "Yes" answers to several of these questions indicate the following stages of alcoholism:

Questions 1–8: Early Stage: Drinking is a regular part of your life.

Questions 9–21: Middle Stage: You are having trouble controlling when, where, and how much you drink.

Questions 22–26: Beginning of the Final Stage: You no longer can control your desire to drink.

Source: National Council on Alcoholism and Drug Dependence, Inc. http://www.ncadd.org.

emotional support system, including concerned family, friends, and employers.

Alcoholism is a complex problem. Each case must be treated with sensitivity and recognition of its unique situation and contributing factors. Standard treatment programs focus on the relief of physiological dependence but do not eliminate the underlying disease. Individual personality, psychological factors, and sociocultural factors must be addressed to help the alcoholic regain control of her life. Alcohol treatment programs often follow three steps in the treatment of alcoholism:

1. Managing acute intoxication episodes
2. Correcting chronic health problems associated with alcoholism
3. Changing long-term behavior

The most successful treatments combine different approaches and provide ongoing support as a person learns to live without alcohol. Many alcohol treatment facilities assist clients in overcoming their physical addiction to alcohol and helping them deal with their withdrawal symptoms (**Table 13.6**) through detoxification programs. Detoxification programs are generally available in medical or psychiatric hospitals.

Psychological addiction is usually addressed shortly after the detoxification process is completed. Programs such as Alcoholics Anonymous (AA), which is entirely run by volunteers who are also recovering alcoholics, provide help and support for people trying to maintain their abstinence from alcohol. Studies conducted by Alcoholics Anonymous show that the average length of sobriety for its members is more than 8 years; 50% of members have been sober for more than 5 years, 24% for between 1 and 5 years, and 26% for less than 1 year. Since the organization began in 1935, AA has supported more than 100,000 groups and

had over 2 million members in 150 countries.[33] Alcoholics Anonymous meetings can now be found in towns and cities across the country almost every day of the week.

Women alcoholics who enter treatment programs have special needs. Their treatment programs must be culturally sensitive and incorporate issues such as age, socioeconomic status, drug use, and sexual orientation into their format. Strategies that can help women address their alcohol problems include using culturally appropriate, nonstigmatized language; supportive case management; mentoring or buddy systems; childcare services; and multimedia campaigns that educate and welcome women.

Illicit Drugs

Illicit drugs include drugs that are either banned outright, such as heroin, cocaine, and marijuana, as well as legal drugs used for nonlegal means, such as prescription drugs used such as by someone for whom they were not intended or for nonmedical purposes. Every year, about 2 million Americans end up in the emergency room as a result of

Table 13.6	Alcohol Withdrawal Symptoms
Irritability	Dry mouth
Agitation	Elevated blood pressure
Depression	Headache
Lack of concentration	Anxiety
Body tremors	Puffy, blotchy skin
Nausea and vomiting	Fitful sleep with nightmares
Generalized weakness, achiness	Brief hallucinations
Sweating	Delirium tremens (DTs)
Fever	

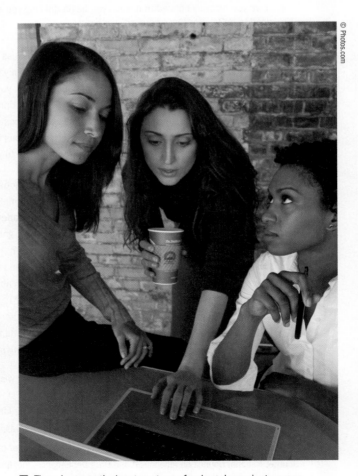

© Photos.com

■ There is no particular stereotype of a drug-dependent woman.

Figure 13.7

Emergency Department Visits Due to Drug Abuse or Misuse, 2009

Source: Data from Substance Abuse and Mental Health Services Administration, Drug Abuse Warning Network, 2009: National Estimates of Drug-Related Emergency Department Visits. HHS Publication No. (SMA) 11-4659, DAWN Series D-35. Rockville, MD: Substance Abuse and Mental Health Services Administration, 2011.

U.S. emergency department visits due to drug abuse or misuse, 2009*

- Pharmaceuticals alone
- Illicit drugs alone
- Illicit drugs and alcohol
- Pharmaceuticals and alcohol
- Pharmaceuticals and illicit drugs
- Alcohol alone (underage)
- Pharmaceuticals, alcohol, and illicit drugs

*Thousands of visits

overdosing, accident, or injury related to drug use (**Figure 13.7**). In addition to the directly causing physiological harm, drugs may have additional consequences based on how they are taken. For example, sharing needles to inject drugs can transmit hepatitis B and C, and HIV. **Table 13.7** summarizes the effects and risks of illicit drugs.

Epidemiological Trends and Issues

In 2010, 22.6 million Americans aged 12 or older, or 8.9% of the population, had used at least one illicit drug within the past month. Women are less likely to use illicit drugs, including marijuana, cocaine, crack, hallucinogens, and inhalants, than men.[3] Users of illicit drugs are more likely to be young, with rates for both 12-to-17 year olds (10.1%) and 18-to-25 year olds (21.5%) significantly above the national average.

With 17.4 million users over the age of 12, marijuana is by far the most commonly used illicit drug, followed by prescription drugs used for nonmedical purposes (7.0 million users), and cocaine (1.5 million users).[3]

Among older women, drug overuse and misuse are particular problems. Although they are generally not users of illicit drugs, older women may be likely to be consumers of

Table 13.7 Summary of Effects and Risks of Drugs

Cocaine and Crack	
Names	"Coke," "snow," "Aunt Nora," "lady," "rock," "blow"
Physiological effects	Speed up physical and mental processes; create sense of heightened energy and confidence
Health effects	Headaches, exhaustion, shaking, blurred vision, nausea, seizures, loss of appetite, loss of sexual desire, impotence, impaired judgment, hyperactivity, babbling, paranoia, violence
Long-term risks	Nasal damage (if snorted); lung damage (if smoked); hepatitis and HIV (if injected); damage to heart and blood vessels; chest pain; heart attack; disruptions in cardiac rhythm; stroke; damage to liver
Special risks to women	Increased danger of miscarriage and physical and mental impairment of the fetus; increased risk of congenital malformations, fetal deaths, and SIDS
Amphetamines	
Names	Benzedrine ("bennies"), dextroamphetamine (Dexedrine, "dex," Adderall), methamphetamine (Methedrine, "meth," "crank"), Desoxyn ("copilots"), methylphenidate (Ritalin), pemoline (Cylert), phenmetrazine (Preludin), "black beauties"
Physiological effects	Speed up physical and mental processes; lessen fatigue; boost energy; sense of excitement
Health effects	Loss of appetite; blurred vision; headache and dizziness; sweating; sleeplessness; trembling; anxiety and paranoia; delusions and hallucinations
Long-term risks	Cardiovascular damage—hypertension, stroke, heart failure; malnutrition, vitamin deficiencies; skin disorders; ulcers; sleeplessness; fever; brain damage; depression; violent behavior; fatal overdose
Special risks to women	Increases risk for low birthweight babies, premature birth, and other health issues

(continues)

Table 13.7   Summary of Effects and Risks of Drugs *(Continued)*

Barbiturates

Names	Pentobarbital (Nembutal, "yellow jackets"), secobarbital (Seconal, "reds"), thiopental (Pentothal), amobarbital (Amytal, "blues," "downers"), phenobarbital (Luminal, "phennies"), methaqualone ("love drug," Quaalude, "ludes," "Q"), sopor ("Sopors")
Physiological effects	Mild intoxication, drowsiness, lethargy, decreased alertness
Health effects	Drowsiness, poor coordination, slurred speech, impaired judgment, hangover, confusion, irritability; cold skin; depressed respirations; rapid heart rate
Long-term risks	Disrupted sleep; impaired vision; increased risk of fatal overdose with increased use
Special risks to women	Risk of birth defects and subsequent behavioral problems if used during pregnancy

Antianxiety Drugs

Names	Benzodiazepines: chlordiazepoxide (Librium), diazepam (Valium), oxazepam (Serax), flurazepam (Dalmane); dicarbamates: meprobamate (Equanil, Miltown), alprazolam (Xanax), lorazepam (Ativan)
Physiological effect	Slows down central nervous system
Health effects	Slurred speech, drowsiness, stupor
Long-term risks	Physical and psychological dependence; possible fatal overdose; withdrawal can lead to coma, psychosis, and death
Special risks to women	Menstrual irregularities and failure to ovulate have been reported

Marijuana and Hashish

Names	Marijuana ("pot," "grass," "weed," "Mary Jane"), hashish ("hash")
Physiological effects	Relaxes the mind and body; heightens perceptions
Health effects	Increased heart rate; dry mouth and throat; impaired perceptions and reactions; lethargy; nausea; disorientation, possible hallucinations, heightened anxiety
Long-term risks	Psychological dependence; impaired thinking, perception, memory, and coordination; increased heart rate and hypertension; compromised immunity
Special risks to women	Prenatal use may lead to fetal effects, including small head, poor growth, lower birthweight

Psychedelics

Names	LSD ("acid"), mescaline, PCP ("angel dust," "peace pill")
Physiological effects	Alters perceptions and produces hallucinations
Health effects	Increased heart rate, hypertension, fever, headache, nausea, sweating, and trembling; delusions and unpredictable violence
Long-term risks	Possible flashbacks, psychological dependence; stupor, coma, convulsions, heart and lung failure; brain damage
Special risks to women	Effects on fetus unknown

Inhalants

Names	Depends on specific product
Physiological effects	Temporary feelings of well-being; giddiness; hallucinations
Health effects	Nausea, sneezing, coughing, nosebleeds, loss of appetite, decreased heart and breathing rates; impaired judgment; loss of consciousness
Long-term risks	Hepatitis, liver and kidney failure; respiratory impairment; blood abnormalities; possible suffocation
Special risks to women	Not yet determined

Opiates/Synthetic Narcotics

Names	Opium, morphine, codeine; heroin ("horse," "junk," "smack," "downtown"); methadone (Dolophine, "meth," "dollies"); hydromorphone (Dilaudid, "little D"); oxycodone (Percodan, "perkies"); meperidine (Demerol, "demies"); propoxyphene (Darvon)
Physiological effects	Relaxation of the central nervous system; pain relief; temporary sense of well-being
Health effects	Nausea and vomiting; restlessness; reduced respirations; lethargy; weight loss; slurred speech; mood swings; sweating
Long-term risks	Physical dependence; malnutrition; compromised immunity; hepatitis; HIV; skin lesions; fatal overdose
Special risks to women	Higher risk for preterm labor, intrauterine growth retardation, and preeclampsia

high levels of medications. Women age 65 or older represent 12% of the general population, but they receive more than 25% of all written prescriptions.[3] Sedatives, hypnotics, antianxiety drugs, antihypertensive drugs, vitamins, analgesics, diuretics, laxatives, and tranquilizers are prescribed for elderly women at a rate that is 2.5 times the prescription rate for elderly men. Women are diagnosed with anxiety and depression disorders more often than men, and so are prescribed drugs more often to treat these disorders. Gender differences in weight, body composition, gastric emptying time, cerebral blood flow, and use of hormones in contraception and hormone therapy can influence the effects of these drugs.

Although many use prescribed medication appropriately, some older women develop a dependency on sleeping pills, muscle relaxants such as Valium, or diet pills. In the 1950s and 1960s, many middle-class women were prescribed these medicines, which were widely viewed as acceptable coping tools. Rather than using these drugs therapeutically, many of these women used them to dull emotions, anxiety, or stress caused by the demands of everyday life and became dependent on them.

Stimulants

Stimulants affect the central nervous system and increase heart rate, blood pressure, strength of heart contractions, blood glucose level, and overall muscle tension. Collectively, these effects place additional stress on the body.

Caffeine, one of the most widely used stimulants in the world, is found in many different sources. It has a variety of effects:

- Relief of drowsiness
- Help in the performance of repetitive tasks
- Improved mental capacity for work
- Increased basal metabolic rate

Caffeine can also cause anxiety, insomnia, irregular heartbeat, faster breathing, upset stomach and bowels, dizziness, and headaches in some women. Women who drink a lot of caffeine and then suddenly stop may experience headaches, irritability, and fatigue. Caffeine may temporarily increase the blood pressure, so some women with high blood pressure or heart disease may be advised to limit their consumption. For most women, however, moderate amounts of caffeine are not likely to cause health problems.

Cocaine is a popular stimulant made from the leaves of the coca plant (unrelated to the cocoa plant used to make chocolate). About 1.5 million people, or 0.6% of the population, use cocaine on a regular basis.[3] Cocaine can be snorted (inhaled as a powder through the nose), injected, or smoked. Cocaine increases levels of dopamine, a neurotransmitter that creates feelings of pleasure in the body, creating intense feelings of euphoria. With repeated use, the brain becomes tolerant to cocaine, and users need more of it to get high.

Crack is a smokable mixture of cocaine and baking soda. Because it causes a person to feel intense highs and lows, this drug produces a powerful chemical and psychological dependence. Crack users often need another "hit" within minutes of the previous one. Smoking cocaine in its "freebase" form also delivers a concentrated high that can disappear within seconds.

As a powerful stimulant, cocaine has many negative effects on the body. Cocaine constricts blood vessels and increases the heart rate and blood pressure, increasing the risk for heart attacks or strokes. Cocaine use can cause feelings of paranoia, a loss of judgment, and an intense need to get high again. Cocaine causes additional health problems for pregnant women and their unborn babies; its use can cause miscarriages, premature labor, low birthweight babies, and babies with small head circumferences. Women who use cocaine while pregnant are more likely to miscarry in the first 3 months of pregnancy than women those who do not use drugs as well as those who use heroin or narcotics. Infants born to cocaine and crack users suffer major complications, including drug withdrawal and permanent disabilities. Cocaine can deprive the fetal brain of oxygen or cause brain vessels to burst, so that the fetus experiences the prenatal equivalent of a stroke, resulting in permanent physical and mental damage. In addition, cocaine babies are more likely to have respiratory and kidney problems. Visual problems, low birthweight, seizures, depression, lack of coordination, and developmental retardation are common among cocaine babies as well.

Amphetamines are manufactured stimulants sold under a variety of names. Generally found in pill form, they may also be ground and sniffed or made into a solution for injection. Amphetamines were once widely prescribed for weight control because they suppress the appetite and stimulate the central nervous system. These drugs place serious stress on the cardiovascular system, which can lead to severe cardiovascular damage.

Methamphetamine, also known as "meth," "crystal meth," "crank," or "ice," is a stimulant with a chemical structure similar to amphetamine. Use of methamphetamine greatly increases dopamine levels in the brain, producing strong feelings of pleasure. Unfortunately, methamphetamine appears to also change the brain in other ways. Prolonged use may reduce a person's motor skills, learning capacity, and ability to feel pleasure from any activities other than using methamphetamine. An estimated 353,000 people (0.1% of the population) regularly use this drug.[3]

Anabolic steroids are synthetic derivatives of the male hormone testosterone. These powerful compounds are legitimately prescribed for treatment of burns and injuries, but some athletes and bodybuilders who want to appear muscular and quickly gain muscle mass also use them. Women who take anabolic steroids risk development of a deepened voice, breast reduction, enlargement of the clitoris, changes in or cessation of the menstrual cycle, and growth of facial hair. Other potential effects include an increased risk of heart disease or stroke, liver tumors and jaundice, acne, bad breath, aching joints, and increased aggression. Anabolic steroids can also be addictive, creating some of the same problems with dependence and withdrawal as other drugs.

Depressants and Antianxiety Drugs

Drugs that relax the central nervous system are called depressants, sedatives, or hypnotics. The most widely used depressant is alcohol. Depressants have synergistic effects when they are mixed together, causing a combined effect greater on the body than both drugs would have taken individually. As the user builds tolerance, the likelihood of a potentially fatal overdose increases.

Barbiturates are depressants used medically for inducing relaxation and sleep, relieving tension, and treating seizures. They may also be administered intravenously as a general anesthetic. Low doses of barbiturates produce mild intoxication and euphoria, and decrease alertness and muscle coordination. With a higher dose, the person may suffer slurred speech, decreased respiration, cold skin, weak and rapid heartbeat, and unconsciousness. Side effects of these drugs include drowsiness, impaired judgment and performance, and a hangover that may last for hours or days. Regular barbiturate use leads to physical dependence. Barbiturate addicts tend to be sleepy, confused, or irritable.

Barbiturates also present problems in pregnancy. These drugs easily cross the placenta and can cause birth defects and behavioral problems. Babies born to mothers who abused sedatives during pregnancy may be physically dependent on the drugs and are more prone to respiratory problems, feeding difficulties, disturbed sleep, sweating, irritability, and fever.

Barbiturate withdrawal is a time-consuming process and medically difficult to manage. Withdrawal symptoms include anxiety, insomnia, delirium, and convulsions. Systemic dependence is so critical that occasionally an abrupt ending of barbiturate use leads to death.

Antianxiety drugs, such as benzodiazepines, are primarily prescribed to treat tension and muscular strain. The most commonly used benzodiazepines are alprazolam (Xanax) and diazepam (Valium). These drugs act quickly, creating effects in less than an hour. Drowsiness and loss of coordination are the most common side effects. When used with other substances, such as alcohol, benzodiazepines can cause serious, possibly life-threatening complications. When taken with benzodiazepines, medications such as anesthetics, antihistamines, sedatives, muscle relaxants, and some prescription painkillers may increase central nervous system depression. Similar to the barbiturates, high doses of these drugs result in slurred speech, drowsiness, and stupor. Physiological and physical dependence on antianxiety

It's Your Health

Indications of Drug Use

Abrupt change in attitude, including a lack of interest in previously enjoyed activities

Frequent vague and withdrawn moods

Sudden decline in work or school performance

Sudden resistance to discipline or criticism

Secret telephone calls and meetings with a demand for greater personal privacy

Increased frustration levels

Decreased tolerance for others

Change in eating and sleeping habits

Sudden weight loss

Frequent borrowing of money

Stealing

Disregard for personal appearance

Impaired relationships with family and friends

Disregard for deadlines, curfews, or other regulations

Unusual temper flare-ups

New friends, especially known drug dealers, and strong allegiance to these friends

Source: National Institute on Drug Abuse (NIDA), National Institutes of Health.

drugs may occur within 2 to 4 weeks. Withdrawal symptoms from antianxiety drugs may include coma, psychosis, and death.

Cannabis (Marijuana)

Cannabis, known as marijuana, "pot," or "weed," is by far the most used illicit drug. More Americans use marijuana than the number using nonmedical prescription drugs, cocaine, heroin, inhalants, and hallucinogens combined. Marijuana consists of a mixture of crushed leaves and flower buds of the *Cannabis sativa* plant; this drug is usually smoked, but it is also occasionally cooked and eaten. **Hashish** is an extract of cannabis that is 2 to 10 times as concentrated as marijuana. Tetrahydrocannabinol (THC) is the primary psychoactive ingredient in both drugs.

When taken in low to moderate doses, the effects of marijuana are similar to the effects of alcohol and some tranquilizers. In contrast to alcohol, however, marijuana at low doses does not dull sensation, but rather may cause slight alterations in perception. Its immediate physical effects include an increased heart rate, bloodshot eyes, and dry mouth and throat. High doses diminish the ability to perceive and react and cause sensory distortion. Hashish users may experience vivid hallucinations and LSD-like psychedelic reactions, and some people experience acute panic attacks.

> *I don't really know how I got into heroin. It started with friends and was fun. I was curious and thought it was something I could easily handle. It ran away with me. I didn't realize how desperate I had become until I was arrested for stealing. I couldn't believe that I was in jail.*
>
> **—22-year-old woman**

Marijuana use has grown over the past decade, in part because of the belief that it is not a dangerous drug.[6] Marijuana does not typically cause the same rapid deterioration of mind and body seen in users of drugs like heroin, methamphetamine, or cocaine. Studies show conflicting results regarding smoking marijuana and its relationship to cancer. However, medical evidence does indicate that marijuana, especially when used chronically, is a harmful drug. In the short term, marijuana impairs problem-solving and lowers coordination; over the long term, marijuana may increase the risk for heart disease and cause respiratory problems. On a personal level, chronic marijuana use is associated with reduced physical and mental health, a lower career status, and absenteeism in school and at work.[6]

In women, chronic use of marijuana appears to suppress ovulation and alter hormone levels. Frequent use of this drug during pregnancy may result in lower-birthweight infants and may be associated with impaired verbal, perceptual, and memory skills, as well as difficulties with decision making and sustained attention in children.[2]

Marijuana for medical use has been a subject of controversy for many years. The drug has been studied for its possible analgesic effect; its potential for reducing spasms and spasticity produced by multiple sclerosis and partial spinal cord injury; its use for chemotherapy-related nausea and vomiting; its ability to lower intraocular pressure to treat glaucoma; and its work as an appetite stimulant for wasting syndrome due to HIV infection, anorexia, and cancer. Some believe that evidence for the prescription of marijuana remains inadequate and that other medications produce similar results without the side effects. Others believe that marijuana provides relief for a variety of medical purposes.

Psychedelics and Hallucinogens

Hallucinogenic drugs create changes in perceptions and thoughts. Some of their more common effects are changes in mood, sensation, perception, and relations. These drugs produce tolerance to the **psychedelic** effects, but do not create physical dependence or produce symptoms of withdrawal, even after long-term use. As with most psychoactive drugs, however, there is a danger of psychological dependence.

Peyote, lysergic acid diethylamide (LSD), and phencyclidine (PCP) are the three most common hallucinogens in the United States. Mescaline is the active ingredient in peyote, a spineless cactus with a small crown, or button, that is dried and then swallowed. LSD ("acid") also is ingested orally and produces hallucinations, including bright colors and altered perceptions of reality. The hallucinogenic experience, or "trip," increases the body temperature, heart rate, and blood rate; it also causes sweating, chills, and sometimes headaches and nausea. A "bad trip" may result in an acute anxiety reaction that may trigger panic, depression, confusion, fear of insanity, and distorted thoughts and perceptions. The most common delayed reaction of LSD is a "flashback," in which individuals re-experience the perceptual and emotional changes originally produced by the drug. PCP, or "angel dust," is a synthetic drug that can be smoked, snorted, or eaten. PCP not only causes a person to see and hear things that do not exist, but also alters a person's own perception of herself, often producing symptoms similar to those of schizophrenia. About 500,000 Americans over the age of 12 (0.2% of the population) use hallucinogens.[3]

Narcotics

Narcotics include the opiates—opium and its derivatives, morphine, codeine, and heroin—and some other nonopiate synthetic drugs. All narcotics have sleep-inducing and pain-relieving properties. Some opiates may be used medically for pain relief, but they have a high potential for abuse. Narcotics relax the user and, when injected, may produce an immediate rush. They also may result in restlessness, nausea, and vomiting. With large doses, the skin becomes moist, cold, and bluish, and the pupils become smaller. Respiration slows, and the user may become unresponsive. Death is possible. Over time, opiate users may develop heart infections, skin abscesses, and congested lungs. Infections from unsterile equipment increase the risk of hepatitis, tetanus, and HIV infection. Roughly 200,000 Americans, or 0.06% of the population, use heroin.[3]

Although narcotics such as heroin affect a woman's ability to conceive, many addicts still can become pregnant. Use of heroin during pregnancy may affect the developing brain of the fetus or cause behavioral abnormalities in childhood. A baby of a heroin addict is born an addict as well and often suffers severe withdrawal symptoms after birth.

Inhalants

Inhalants are chemicals that produce vapors with psychoactive effects. Inhalants are most common among young adolescents and teenagers, in part because the chemicals that produce inhalants may be easily obtainable (or already present in the homes) of people in these age groups. Common products used as inhalants include solvents, aerosols, cleaning fluids, and petroleum products. Most inhalants produce the same effects as anesthetics—namely, they slow down bodily functions. Roughly 700,000 Americans over the age of 12, or 0.25% of the population, use inhalants on a regular basis.[3]

At low doses, users may feel slightly stimulated; at higher doses, they may feel less inhibited. Inhalants may cause serious medical complications, such as brain damage and memory loss, hepatitis with liver failure, kidney failure, respiratory impairment, destruction of bone marrow and skeletal muscles, blood abnormalities, and irregular heartbeat.

■ Many products that are used as inhalants are not meant for inhalation and are extremely dangerous.

Designer Drugs

Designer drugs—sometimes referred to as "club drugs" because they are often sold at nightclubs or raves—are produced in chemical laboratories and then sold illegally. Such synthetic narcotics are particularly dangerous because they are more powerful than those derived from natural substances. The risk of brain damage or fatal overdose from ingestion is correspondingly higher.

MDMA (3,4-methylenedioxymethamphetamine), commonly known as "Ecstasy," is the most common designer drug, with about 700,000 users (0.3% of the population).[3] Ecstasy has features of both hallucinogens and stimulants. Other "club drugs" include GHB, Rohypnol, Ketamine, and methamphetamine. In the United States, the drug has been associated with a predominantly White, middle-class population. Immediate effects of the drug include a feeling of warmth and openness. Delayed responses, usually within a day, include insomnia, muscle aches, fatigue, and difficulty concentrating. Chronic use of MDMA can cause brain damage with the extent of damage directly correlated to the extent of MDMA use. Heavy users also have significant impairments in visual and verbal memory.[6]

I had a knee injury from playing tennis and was given a prescription for Percocet. A few weeks later, after I had stopped taking the medicine, a friend and I decided to take some Percocet just for fun. The next night, we took more. Before I knew it, I was taking pills every night. I needed more each night to make me feel good. When I ran out of pills, I panicked and called the doctor for a refill. I didn't even realize how quickly I had become addicted.

—28-year-old woman

Prescription Drugs

The three classes of prescription drugs most commonly abused are opioids prescribed for pain, which include morphine, codeine, and oxycodone (e.g., OxyContin, Percodan, Percocet); central nervous system depressants for anxiety and sleep disorders such as barbiturates and benzodiazepines (e.g., Valium, Librium, and Xanax); and stimulants for sleep disorders and attention-deficit hyperactivity disorder (e.g., Dexedrine and Ritalin). Any of these medications, when used improperly, can lead to serious health consequences and even death. Prescription drug use and abuse are on the rise in the United States, especially among older adults, adolescents, and women. In 2010, more than 7 million Americans over the age of 12 (about 3% of the population) reported currently using prescription drugs for nonmedical purposes, more than any illicit drug besides marijuana.[3]

Drug Dependency

Drug dependency refers to the attachment—physical, psychological, or both—that a person may develop to a drug. Physical dependence occurs when physiological changes in the body's cells cause an overpowering, constant need for a drug. If the drug is not taken, the user develops withdrawal symptoms, such as intense anxiety, extreme nausea, and deep craving for the drug. Tranquilizers, painkillers, barbiturates, and narcotics may produce physical dependence. Psychological dependence, also referred to as habituation, results in a strong craving for a drug because it produces pleasurable feelings or relieves stress or anxiety. Physical and psychological dependence do not always coexist. For example, marijuana and LSD may not create physical dependence, but their continued use has been demonstrated to cause psychological dependence.

Cross-tolerance, or cross-addiction, often presents with drug dependency. In this condition, a state of physical dependence exists in which psychological need for one psychoactive substance leads to dependence on similar substances.

Treatment Dimensions of Drug Dependency

There are three basic approaches to drug-abuse treatment: detoxification, therapeutic communities, and outpatient drug-free programs. The best type of treatment program for any woman may depend on her circumstances, preferences, drug use, and history.

- *Detoxification* is the supervised withdrawal from drug dependence, either with or without medication, in a hospital or outpatient setting.

- *Therapeutic communities* are highly structured, drug-free environments in which abusers live under strict rules while participating in group and individual therapy.

- *Outpatient drug-free programs* are available through community and treatment facilities. Self-help programs include Narcotics Anonymous and Pills Anonymous, which follow the philosophy of Alcoholics Anonymous. In these programs, users admit to their helplessness and put their faith in a "higher power." Many people do not recognize their own drug problems, and require intervention by friends and family before they will seek treatment (see **Self-Assessment 13.3**).

Self-Assessment 13.3

Do I Have a Drug Problem?

Carefully read and honestly respond to the following statements:

1. Sometimes I am preoccupied with getting and taking a drug. — yes   no

2. Sometimes I don't go to an important event at school or work, or a social or recreational event, so that I can get or take a drug instead. — yes   no

3. I continue to use a drug despite the fact that it makes things with my family or friends worse, or it interferes with school or work activities. — yes   no

4. I have developed a specific physical or mental condition from my drug use (example, irritated nose from cocaine). — yes   no

5. I have repeatedly tried to cut down or eliminate my use of a drug. — yes   no

6. I am sometimes unable to fulfill my obligations (to family, friends, work, or school) because of my drug use. — yes   no

7. I feel specific symptoms when I cut back or eliminate the drug. — yes   no

8. I sometimes take another drug to relieve withdrawal symptoms. — yes   no

9. I sometimes use the drug in larger doses or over a longer period than recommended. — yes   no

10. I need to take more of the drug now than I did before to get the same effect. — yes   no

If you answered "yes" to any of these statements, it is important to seek help now with your drug problem.

Informed Decision Making

Many outside and environmental factors affect whether a person eventually uses or becomes addicted to alcohol, tobacco, or other drugs. While these factors cannot always be controlled, all individuals have responsibility for their own decisions. Personal responsibilities regarding drugs include:

- Understanding the effects that a particular substance can have on a person's physical and psychological well-being
- Being aware of how substance abuse affects personal behaviors and the assessment of reality
- Being able to ascertain and acknowledge that a problem when substance abuse may be present

Recognizing the warning signs of addiction and seeking early treatment intervention are important first steps when someone has a problem. Maintaining abstinence after treating the problem is an ongoing process. This process may get easier after the first few weeks or months, but for some people, the desire to use a drug never goes away. If a person does have a relapse, he or she should start on the recovery process from the beginning.

Tobacco

Quitting smoking is the single most significant step most women who smoke can to improve their chances of wellbeing. Regardless of the difficulty—and breaking any addictive behavior is undeniably difficult—smoking causes serious damage to the body and shortens the life span. Quitting smoking at any point brings serious health benefits. Many options to help women quit smoking are available, including counseling, enlisting the help of friends and family, nicotine replacement therapy, electronic cigarettes, and bupropion or varenicline.

Avoiding secondhand smoke is not always simple. Although legislation now restricts smoking in many areas, smoking still occurs in some restaurants, bars, and smoking lounges; women who work or otherwise spend lots of time in these areas may be at risk for asthma or other lung conditions. Some children of smoking parents may be exposed to tobacco smoke in their own homes, cars, and even in the womb before birth. Nonsmokers' desire for a "smoke-free" environment presents a potential threat to smokers, who feel that their rights to smoke are violated. The challenge for nonsmokers is to assert their right to a smoke-free environment in a nonviolent but assertive manner. Much of the resistance by smokers is defensive, as they are reminded of their own need to quit and their fear of failure and frustration with the process.

Women often do not consider tobacco to be a drug. In reality, tobacco can decrease the effects of certain medications such as acetaminophen, antidepressants, and insulin taken for diabetes. Smoking also increases the risk of heart and blood vessel disease when taking oral contraceptives. When relevant, women should mention tobacco when healthcare providers inquire about medications or drug use.

Alcohol

For women who choose to drink, drinking in a responsible manner can improve their health. Drinking to excess has numerous direct effects on health. Excessive drinking also indirectly increases the risk of death, injury, or trauma through drunk driving and potential sexual assault.

Gender Dimensions: Health Differences Between Men and Women

Treatment Programs

Drug dependency treatment programs must address the spectrum of physical and psychosocial issues that confront the addict. These challenges are especially difficult for female addicts, who experience concerns such as contraception, pregnancy, motherhood, childrearing, and health problems in addition to the underlying drug dependency. Women are generally less likely to seek treatment for drug abuse, and they respond differently than men to drug treatment. Female addicts often are caregivers and are reluctant to seek care for themselves because of the needs of others. In addition, they more often need specialty treatment than males. These types of services include prenatal treatment, mental health services, domestic violence counseling, and childcare assistance. Substance abuse treatment facilities providing special programs or services for women are becoming more common, but these programs are still unavailable or unaffordable for many women. Some programs also provide activities for children, housing and transportation assistance, and services for pregnant women.

Psychosocial and behavioral treatment programs that emphasize increased self-esteem and choosing positive life options help many women more than programs originally developed for men. Unfortunately, few programs focus on the special needs of women or acknowledge the barriers that women must overcome to obtain treatment. These barriers include lack of day care for children, lack of safe drug-free housing, fear of losing their children, financial and legal difficulties, lack of transportation, and health problems requiring services beyond drug treatment. In addition, treatment needs of women should be evaluated with the realization that women do not constitute a homogenous group, but rather run the gamut of pregnant women, adolescent users, older women, single professionals, housewives, and others.

For those with a propensity toward excessive drinking, it is important to set a limit and stick to it. For most women, drinking no more than one drink a day may provide some health benefits; drinking beyond this level on a regular basis may cause serious harm. It is also critical to have healthy coping strategies to avoid turning to alcohol when upset or depressed. Alcohol neither fixes a problem nor provides an escape. When drinking becomes the primary focus of an activity, a significant risk for serious long-term alcohol problems arises.

Communication skills are an important component of responsible drinking. Learning to say, "No thanks, I've had enough," is an important step in exercising personal power and control over drinking behavior. Pacing alcohol consumption is important as well. Drinking a week's worth of alcohol on a Friday night is not the same as moderately paced drinking throughout the week. Alcoholic beverages are not good or wise thirst quenchers, as alcohol increases dehydration. Food should be consumed before drinking, so it is a good idea to eat something before going to a party or meeting someone for a drink.

I feel responsible for [my husband] Joe's drinking. He really has no one else who understands and helps him. I try to be patient each time he is drunk and clean up the mess. I keep thinking that if I just try harder in understanding maybe he won't have this problem.
35-year-old woman

Helping others to drink in moderation is also a personal responsibility issue. It is not wise to push drinks or refill empty glasses quickly. Food helps to slow the absorption of alcohol and should be encouraged first, particularly if guests have not eaten for a while. Nonalcoholic beverages should always be available alongside alcoholic ones. Perhaps the most important responsibilities are never to serve alcohol to a guest who seems intoxicated and never to permit an intoxicated person to operate a vehicle. Assuming responsibility includes making contingency plans for intoxication. The early identification of designated drivers helps ensure safe transportation home for guests. If intoxication occurs despite efforts to prevent it, assume responsibility for the health and safety of guests by providing transportation home or overnight accommodations. Women should stay with their female friends who appear overly intoxicated and be aware of men who may try to take advantage of an intoxicated woman. Stay with the person if he or she is vomiting. If the person is lying down, turn his or her head to the side and protect the person from swallowing the vomit. Monitor the person's breathing status. If there

Table 13.8	How to Handle a Friend Who Is Intoxicated

- Try to find out what the person was drinking and if she took any other drugs or medicines.
- Help your friend get home safely; don't let her drive, get in a car with another friend who has been drinking, or walk home alone in an unsafe area.
- Encourage your friend to go to sleep; the only way to sober up is to give it time.
- Position your friend on her side to prevent her from choking if she vomits. Check on her regularly to be sure she is responsive and breathing.
- Avoid giving your friend any medication, including aspirin, ibuprofen, or acetaminophen.
- Call for help if she is unresponsive or vomiting while unconscious; call for help if you fear being alone with the intoxicated friend.

Source: Reprinted by permission of Julie Barnes, coordinator, Substance Abuse Services, University of Northern Iowa.

are any signs of unconsciousness or respiratory problems, seek immediate medical attention. Remember that the only thing that sobers a drunk person is time. (See **Table 13.8**.)

Other Drugs

Understanding the short- and long-term negative effects that drugs can have, while also developing personal strengths and self-confidence, is the foundation that enables a woman to resist drugs effectively. Knowing how to cope with stress in a healthy way can minimize the likelihood that a woman will turn to drugs as a coping mechanism.

Early identification and treatment offer hope to the person who is using drugs. Unfortunately, many people either miss or refuse to see the signs that a person is using drugs. Many treatment and counseling centers offer free online or telephone services that provide advice on assessing the situation and helpful resources for action. Confronting the substance abuser is sometimes best handled by a group of loved ones and in the presence of a trained counselor. Outlining how the abuse has affected each person in the abuser's life and how much each person cares about the abuser helps to balance the information. It is unrealistic to expect the abuser to quit without assistance. Although offering support is beneficial, the abuser needs to know that treatment and therapy are necessary.

Informed decision making is also an essential responsibility with prescribed and OTC medication use. Many women have little or no idea why they take certain prescribed

It's Your Health

Codependency

A person (friend, spouse, partner, parent) may, without meaning to, allow or help the addict to remain dependent on drugs through enabling behaviors. These enabling behaviors may include the following activities:

- Rescuing: displaying overprotective behavior that permits the addict to use drugs at home to avoid being discovered or at risk elsewhere.
- Rationalizing: accepting and explaining the addict's behavior; making excuses for the behavior.
- Shielding: covering up for addicts; running interference for them at work, school, and for obligations.
- Controlling: personally attempting to control the addict's use of drugs with bribes or rewards (money, favors, sex).
- Covering: taking over chores, assuming job responsibilities, paying bills, or giving/loaning money to the addict so that he or she can buy drugs.
- Cooperating: becoming involved in buying, selling, testing, preparing, or using the drug.

medications, or they have multiple and vague reasons for using complex OTC medications. Drugs, whether prescribed or self-medicated, can have powerful adverse reactions with other drugs, certain foods, alcohol, tobacco, and caffeine. Older women are often subject to dangerous and possibly fatal drug interactions due to the numerous medications and supplements they are taking. Because many of the most serious effects of drugs are often wrongly attributed to "being depressed" or "growing old," women should know about possible adverse drug reactions and side effects so such events can be recognized and reported. They should also know which foods and other drugs interact with the medications being taken and whether specific dietary recommendations have been identified for the medications.

Codependency

The concept of codependency is important for many women who become embroiled within the chaos of another person's life.

The term "co-dependent" describes a person obsessed, tormented, or dominated by the behavior of others. The term grew out of the older notion of "co-alcoholic," a term once applied to the wives of heavy drinkers. The premise of codependency is that everyone in a user's or abuser's family is diseased. Consciously or unconsciously, and to their lifelong detriment, codependents interact with the user and "enable" this person to partake in her addiction. Codependents often feel helpless, miserable, hopeless, and angry as they accept the victim role. A woman may be codependent in a relationship with a lover, spouse, parent, child,

Profiles of Remarkable Women

Drew Barrymore (1975–)

© Helga Esteb/ShutterStock, Inc.

Drew Barrymore was born into an acting family; her kin include the actors Lionel, John, and Ethel Barrymore. Drew Barrymore began her career appearing in a Puppy Choice dog food commercial when she was 11 months old. She got her first movie role at the age of two, playing a boy in *Suddenly Love*. At age five, she appeared in *Altered States*, and she was turned into a household name when she starred in the blockbuster *E.T.: The Extraterrestrial*. She continued her appearances in films, including Stephen King adaptations *Firestarter* (1984) and *Cat's Eye* (1985).

Barrymore tried alcohol for the first time at age 9 and marijuana at age 10. She then turned to cocaine, stirred controversy with her near-nude appearances in *Far from Home*, and was forced into ASAP Family Treatment Center, a drug rehabilitation clinic. Following rehab, Barrymore published a memoir entitled *Little Girl Lost* and made a comeback in Hollywood in the early 1990s.

Barrymore's persistence and energy have helped her recover from the difficulties of growing up in front of the camera and in the public eye, and have shaped her into a strong and determined woman. She has not only appeared in numerous successful movies, but has also become active as a producer for movies such as *He's Just Not That Into You*, *Never Been Kissed*, *Charlie's Angels*, and *Donnie Darko*. A dedicated philanthropist, Barrymore is actively involved in volunteering for and supporting animal rights issues and anti-fur campaigns, urging young people to vote, and advocating for children's rights.

or friend. A codependent typically feels responsible for the behavior and mood of the other.

The codependent must learn how to separate her own life from that of the addicted person's. The recovery from codependence is similar to recovery from alcohol or drug dependence in that only the codependent can take the necessary steps toward her own recovery. A codependent must learn not to try to control someone else's life and to stop playing the victim role. Many codependents have received useful support and encouragement from programs such as the twelve-step program of Al-Anon, a support group for family and friends of alcoholics.

Summary

Tobacco, alcohol, and other drugs directly and indirectly harm women, their children, and others in their environment in many ways. Staying away from tobacco, or quitting smoking, will greatly improve a woman's health and reduce her risk of dying early. Women also must exercise caution and wisdom with alcohol and legal drug use. Knowing the consequences of drinking alcohol and assuming personal responsibility for one's drinking are the first steps in controlling alcohol use. Reducing and having control over the kinds and amounts of drugs taken, including recreational drugs, prescribed medications, OTC medications, and substances such as caffeine, should also be an important health goal.

Topics for Discussion

1. Should pregnant women be permitted to drink alcohol, use drugs, or smoke? How, if at all, should states intervene in cases of maternal substance use?

2. Is it a sign of personal weakness or strength for a woman to admit that she has a problem with alcohol or drugs?

3. What should a woman do or say when she knows her friend has a problem with drugs or alcohol, but the friend does not think so?

4. Can smokers' rights and nonsmokers' rights both be protected at the same time? What are those rights?

5. How can young girls be educated to resist peer and advertising pressure to smoke?

6. Discuss how the presence of drugs in a neighborhood affects a community. What type of social action is needed to help keep this community safe and become drug free?

7. List all chemicals and substances that you use to change your state of consciousness, such as caffeine, tobacco, alcohol, prescription drugs, over-the-counter drugs, and illegal drugs. Try to give up one or more of these substances for a period of time, and replace it with a healthy behavior such as exercise. Keep a record of how you feel and any changes that you notice in your health or behavior.

8. Should natural substances and over-the-counter medicines be regulated in the same way as prescription drugs?

9. Is it better to put drug addicts in prison or to send them to mandatory drug treatment programs?

10. Is there any validity to the arguments to legalize marijuana? What about other illicit drugs? Discuss the pros and cons of a change in policy in this area.

Key Terms

Alcohol: A colorless liquid obtained by fermentation of a sugar-containing liquid. Ethyl alcohol (ethanol) is the type of alcohol found in alcoholic beverages.

Alcoholism: Traditionally, the disease of an alcoholic, who is a person whose consumption of alcohol interferes with a major aspect of his or her life. Alcoholism has since been redefined as a primary, chronic disease with genetic, psychological, and environmental factors influencing its development and manifestations.

Amphetamines: Synthetic stimulants that increase energy and alertness, produce euphoria, and suppress appetite. Excessive use can cause headaches, irritability, dizziness, insomnia, panic, confusion, and delirium.

Barbiturates: A class a sedatives that have a depressant effect on the central nervous system.

Blood alcohol concentration (BAC): A physiological indicator used by clinicians and law enforcement officials to determine whether a person is legally "drunk." BAC is expressed in terms of the percentage of alcohol in blood.

Carcinogenic: The ability to cause cancer.

Chronic bronchitis: Constant inflammation of the bronchial tubes. The inflammation thickens the walls of the bronchi, and the production of mucus increases, resulting in a constricting or narrowing of the air passages.

Chronic obstructive pulmonary disease (COPD): A disease characterized by permanent airflow obstruction and extended periods of disability and restricted activity.

Cirrhosis: Alcohol-induced liver disease.

Drug: Any chemical other than food that is purposely taken to affect body processes.

Drug abuse: The excessive use of a drug that has dangerous side effects.

Drug dependency: The attachment—physiological or psychological (or both)—that a person may develop to a drug. Physical dependence occurs when physiological changes in the body's cells cause an overpowering constant need for the drug.

Drug misuse: The use of a drug for a purpose other than its original intent.

Emphysema: The limitation of airflow as the result of irreversible disease changes in the lung tissue after years of assault on that tissue. The air sacs in the lungs are destroyed, and the lungs are compromised in bringing oxygen and removing carbon dioxide from the body. As a result, breathing becomes compromised, and increased demand is placed on the heart.

Hallucinogenic drugs: Drugs that create changes in perceptions and thoughts. A common feature of a hallucinogenic experience is that the drug suspends normal psychic mechanisms that integrate the self with the environment.

Hashish: An extract of cannabis that is 2 to 10 times as concentrated as marijuana.

Inhalants: Chemicals that produce vapors with psychoactive effects and are predominantly abused by pre-adolescents and young adults.

Involuntary smokers: Nonsmokers who have to breathe air contaminated by smokers. Also known as passive smokers.

Narcotics: A class of drugs that includes the opiates—opium and its derivatives, morphine, codeine, and heroin—and some nonopiate synthetic drugs. All narcotics have sleep-inducing and pain-relieving properties.

Nicotine: The addictive element in cigarettes. Nicotine has several effects on te body, including increasing blood pressure, increasing heart rate, and negating hunger.

Psychedelic: A heightened sense of reality with visual hallucinations and, sometimes, psychotic-like behaviors.

Psychological dependence: An emotional or mental attachment to the use of a drug. Also called habituation.

Recreational drugs: Drugs taken purely for fun.

Stimulants: Drugs that affect the central nervous system and increase the heart rate, blood pressure, strength of heart contractions, blood glucose level, and overall muscle tension.

Tolerance: The body's ability to withstand the effects of a drug. Continued use of a drug may result in increased tolerance and decreased responsiveness.

■■■■
Websites

Alcoholics Anonymous: http://www.aa.org

College Drinking: Changing the Culture: http://www.collegedrinkingprevention.gov

National Institute on Alcohol Abuse and Alcoholism: http://www.niaaa.nih.gov

National Institute on Drug Abuse: http://www.nida.nih.gov

Recovery Services: http://www.soberrecovery.com

Substance Abuse and Mental Health Services Administration's National Clearinghouse for Drug and Alcohol Information: http://www.health.org

Substance Abuse and Mental Health Services Administration: http://www.samhsa.gov

Surgeon General's Guide to Quitting Smoking: http://www.surgeongeneral.gov

■■■■
References

1. U.S. Department of Transportation. (2010). *National Highway Traffic Safety Administration (NHTSA). Traffic safety facts 2009: Alcohol-Impaired Driving.* Washington, DC: NHTSA.

2. Office of National Drug Control Policy. (2011). *Fact sheet 2010.* Available at: http://www.whitehouse.gov/sites/default/files/ondcp

3. Substance Abuse and Mental Health Services Administration. (2011). *Results from the 2010 National Survey*

on Drug Use and Health: Summary of national findings. NSDUH Series H-41, HHS Publication No. (SMA) 11-4658. Rockville, MD.

4. National Center on Addiction and Substance Abuse, Columbia University. (2003). *The formative years: Pathways to substance abuse among girls and young women ages 8–22.* New York, NY: Columbia University.

5. The Sentencing Project. (2005). *Briefing: The federal prison population: A statistical analysis.* Washington, DC: The Sentencing Project.

6. Office of National Drug Control Policy (2012). *National drug control strategy.* Washington, DC: Office of National Drug Control Policy.

7. Office of National Drug Control Policy. (2012). *National drug control strategy FY2013 budget summary.* Washington DC: Office of National Drug Control Policy.

8. Campaign for Tobacco-Free Kids. (2012). *State cigarette excise tax rates and rankings.* Available at: http://www.tobaccofreekids.org/research/factsheets/pdf/0097.pdf

9. American Cancer Society. (2012). *Cancer facts & figures 2012.* Atlanta, GA: American Cancer Society.

10. National Cancer Institute. (1999). *Smoking and tobacco control monograph.* Available at: http://cancercontrol.cancer.gov/tcrb/monographs/1/m1_3.pdf

11. Centers for Disease Control and Prevention [CDC]. (2011). Cigarette smoking among adults aged ≥18 years—United States, 2005–2010. *Morbidity and Mortality Weekly Report 53*(20): 427–431.

12. Eaton, D., Kann, L., Kinchen, S., et al. (2011). *Youth Risk Behavior Surveillance—United States, 2009.* Atlanta, GA: CDC.

13. Centers for Disease Control and Prevention [CDC]. (2011). *Smoking and tobacco use: Hookahs.* Available at: http://www.cdc.gov/tobacco/data_statistics/fact_sheets/tobacco_industry/hookahs/

14. World Health Organization [WHO]. (2005). Waterpipe tobacco smoking: Health effects, research needs and recommended actions by regulators. Geneva, Switzerland: WHO.

15. Centers for Disease Control and Prevention [CDC]. (2005). Annual smoking-attributable mortality, years of potential life lost, and economic costs—United States, 1997–2001. *Morbidity and Mortality Weekly Report 54*: 625–628.

16. World Health Organization [WHO]. (2012). *Tobacco fact sheet.* Available at: http://www.who.int/mediacentre/factsheets/fs339/en/index.html

17. Murphy, S., Xu, J., & Kochanek, K. (2012). Deaths: Prelinary data for 2010. *National Vital Statistics Reports 60*(4). Hyattsville, MD: National Center for Health Statistics.

18. Connolly, G., Alpert, H., Wayne G., et al. (2007). *Trends in smoke nicotine yield and relationship to design characteristics among popular U.S. cigarette brands, 1997–2005.* Harvard School of Public Health. Available at: http://www.hsph.harvard.edu/nicotine/trends.pdf

19. U.S. Department of Health and Human Services. (2004). *The health consequences of smoking: A report of the Surgeon General, 2004.* Atlanta, GA: Centers for Disease Control and Prevention, Office on Smoking and Health.

20. Centers for Disease Control and Prevention [CDC]. (2011). *Tobacco use and pregnancy.* Available at: http://www.cdc.gov/reproductivehealth/tobaccousepregnancy/index.htm

21. Stead, L., Perera, R., Bullen, C., et al. (2008.) Nicotine replacement therapy for smoking cessation. *The Cochrane Library.* Available at: www.thecochranelibrary.com

22. Gruskin, E. P., Hart, S., Gordon, N., et al. (2001). Patterns of cigarette smoking and alcohol use among lesbians and bisexual women enrolled in a large health maintenance organization. *American Journal of Public Health 91*(6): 976–979.

23. Brouchery, E., Harwood, H., Sacks, J., et al. (2011). Economic costs of excessive alcohol consumption in the U.S., 2006. *American Journal of Preventive Medicine 41*(5): 516–524.

24. Centers for Disease Control and Prevention [CDC]. (2004). Alcohol-attributable deaths and years of potential life lost—United States, 2001. *Morbidity and Mortality Weekly Report 53*(37): 866–870.

25. Centers for Disease Control and Prevention [CDC]. (2011). Vital signs: Alcohol-impaired driving among adults—United States, 2010. *Morbidity and Mortality Weekly Report 53*(37): 866–870.

26. National Institute on Alcohol Abuse and Alcoholism [NIAAA]. (2007). *Alcohol Alert No. 72: Cirrhosis.* Rockville, MD: NIAAA.

27. Caithers, R. L., & McClain, C. (2006). Alcoholic liver disease. In: Feldman, M., Friedman L. S., & Brandt,

L. J. Feldman: *Sleisinger & Fordtran's gastrointestinal and liver disease* (8th ed.). Philadelphia, PA: Saunders Elsevier, Chapter 81.

28. Nelson, H. D., Humphrey, L. L., Nygren, P., et al. (2002). Postmenopausal hormone replacement therapy: scientific review. *Journal of the American Medical Association 288*: 872–881.

29. Levy, D. T., Stewart, K., & Wilbur, P. M. (1999). *Costs of underage drinking.* U.S. Department of Justice, Office of Juvenile Justice and Delinquency Prevention.

30. Bertrand, J., Floyd, R. L., Weber, M. K., et al. (2004). Fetal Alcohol Syndrome: Guidelines for Referral and Diagnosis. Atlanta, GA: U.S. Department of Health and Human Services, CDC. Available at: http://www.cdc.gov/ncbddd/fas/documents/FAS_guidelines_accessible.pdf.

31. American Academy of Pediatrics. (2005). Breastfeeding and the use of human milk. *Pediatrics 115*(2) 496–506.

32. American Academy of Child and Adolescent Psychiatry. (2011). *Facts for families: Children of alcoholics. No. 17.* Available at: http://www.aacap.org/cs/root/facts_for_families/children_of_alcoholics.

33. Alcoholics Anonymous [AA]. (2011). *Alcoholics Anonymous 2011 membership survey.* Washington, DC: AA.

Chapter Fourteen

Violence, Abuse, and Harassment

Chapter Objectives

On completion of this chapter, the student should be able to discuss:

1. Self-directed, interpersonal, and collective violence, and how these forms of violence affect women.

2. How sociocultural, economic, and historical factors influence violence and its consequences.

3. How poverty, alcohol, drugs, and the media influence violence.

4. How violence affects women throughout the world.

5. Types of family and intimate violence.

6. Common forms of stalking and actions a woman can take to protect herself.

7. Forms of domestic violence, including physical, sexual, property, psychological, and social violence.

8. How domestic violence during pregnancy affects women and prenatal development.

9. How domestic violence affects lesbians, women with disabilities, and other groups.

10. Forms, common causes, and effects of child abuse and elder abuse.

11. Basic facts about rape and sexual assault.

12. How rape affects physical health, mental health, sexual intimacy, and relationships.

13. Common forms of violence toward women by strangers and how women can protect themselves.

14. How sexual harassment acts as a form of social control and its effects on women in the workplace.

15. Strategies to prevent and cope with with intimate violence and sexual harassment.

womenshealth.jbpub.com

Women's Health Online is a great source for supplementary women's health information for both students and instructors. Visit

http://womenshealth.jbpub.com

to find a variety of useful tools for learning, thinking, and teaching.

© Maria Teijeiro/Photodisc/Thinkstock

Introduction

Violence has always been part of human society. Today, violence continues to affect millions of women around the world. The World Health Organization [WHO] classifies violence into three categories, based on who commits the violent act: self-directed violence, interpersonal violence, and collective violence.[1] Self-directed violence includes suicidal behavior and **self-mutilation** (see **It's Your Health**). Chapter 12 discusses suicide in further detail.

Interpersonal violence includes violence toward a child, partner, relative, or elder, as well as community violence toward an acquaintance or a stranger. Family and intimate violence—including stalking, domestic battering, child abuse, elder abuse, and rape in many cases—are major facets of the violence epidemic. Although most intimate violence qualifies as a crime, historical and cultural traditions have often condoned violence within the family setting. Violence by strangers—such as robbery, carjackings, aggravated assault, rape, and homicide—affects women when they are the victims of crime and when a partner or family member is a victim. Sexual harassment is considered a form of violence as well, because it also usually involves threats or an unjust use of power.

Collective violence is violence committed against a group of people to achieve social, political, or economic objectives. It can take a variety of forms, including armed conflicts, genocide, repression, terrorism, and organized violent crime. Many acts of violence toward women evolve as a result of women's subordinate status in society. Around the world, women face collective violence through female genital mutilation, female infanticide, trafficking of women and girls for sexual exploitation, rape during war, and other acts. These forms of abuse have traditionally been associated with the developing world; however, collective violence also occurs in the United States, Canada, and Europe.

From a legal perspective, most violent crime can be categorized into one of four categories: rape or sexual assault, robbery (taking something from someone through threats or force), simple assault (attacking someone and causing physical harm, or threatening to attack someone), and aggravated assault (a more extreme form of assault, often using a weapon). **Figure 14.1** shows the number of violent crimes committed against women in the United States in 2010, as well as the relationship between the victim and aggressor.

Violence has mental and physical consequences for its victims, the most serious of which are long-term disability or death. Each year, more than 1.6 million people worldwide lose their lives to violence. Indeed, violence is among the leading global causes of death for people ages 15 to 44 years old.[1] More than 2.5 million females experience some form of violence each year. On average, one in three females is abused by an intimate partner during her lifetime, and several global studies suggest that half of all women who die from homicide are killed by current or former husbands or partners.[2] This chapter provides an overview of violence, focusing on interpersonal violence and the issues that contribute to violence and victimization. This chapter also reviews informed decision-making

It's Your Health

Self-Mutilation

Self-harm, self-injury, self-inflicted violence, or self-mutilation is any self-directed, repetitive behavior that causes physical injury. These acts are not usually suicide attempts but rather behaviors that express or release emotional turmoil. They are often referred to as parasuicidal behaviors. Examples include the following acts:

- Skin cutting with razors or knives (the most common pattern)
- Burning, branding, or biting oneself
- Picking one's skin or hair
- Hitting with hammer or other object; bone breaking
- Extreme injuries such as auto-enucleation (self-removal of the eye), castration, or amputation

There are several known risk factors for self-injury:

- Female gender
- Adolescence and college age
- Substance abuse or personality disorders
- History of parasuicidal behavior

People who self-harm are unable to identify or express difficult feelings in a healthy way. They use self-harm as a coping mechanism. They often feel increasing tension or physical arousal before the act and release of pleasure or gratification after the act. Little is known about the cause of self-mutilation, but studies are looking at biological, psychological, and social contributions to the disease. Medications, psychotherapeutic approaches, and crisis interventions are all forms of treatment. See the websites at the end of this chapter for more information.

Source: Adapted from Fong, T. (2003). Self-mutilation: Impulsive traits suggest new drug therapies. *Current Psychiatry* 2(2).

Figure 14.1

Violent crimes committed against women and girls, by crime and victim-offender relationship, 2010.

Source: Data from U.S. Department of Justice. Bureau of Justice Statistics. (2011). National Criminal Victimization Survey, 2010.

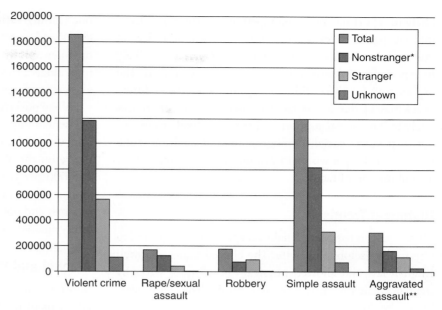

*Nonstrangers include intimate partners, relatives, friends, and acquaintances.

**Aggravated assault is a stronger form of attack than simple assault and often involves the use or threat of a deadly weapon.

criteria and ways that women can prevent or cope with violence and its consequences.

Perspectives on Violence, Abuse, and Harassment

Sociocultural Issues

I feel like it was my fault that I was raped. I had a little too much to drink and I went back to my apartment with him. I wanted to kiss him, but I didn't want to have sex. When he started forcing me to do more than kiss, I asked him to stop. But he wouldn't listen. I probably shouldn't have invited him back with me and I feel guilty for leading him on.

19-year-old college sophomore

Cultural attitudes about violence toward women may be based on how society accepts the idea of male dominance. In some cultures, both men and women believe that a man has the right to control his wife's and daughters' behaviors and that a disobedient woman should be punished. By legitimizing these behaviors, cultures perpetuate violence against women. Women are particularly vulnerable to abuse by their partners in societies where there are marked inequalities between men and women, rigid gender roles, weak sanctions against violent behavior, and cultural norms that support a man's right to sex regardless of a woman's

feelings. Violence in intimate relationships can be triggered by a woman not obeying her husband, not having food ready for him, refusing him sex, or simply being a woman.[3]

Society's tolerance of rape between intimate partners, especially married partners, is an important dimension of violence. For years, many people believed that marriage gave men the right to have sex with their wives at any time. In these settings, if the wife refuses, the husband can force her to have sex or punish her through violent means. Tendencies to "blame the victim" influence how women and communities cope with relationship violence. Women who feel they are at fault or that they "deserved" punishment may not report a rape or other crimes. Certain factors, including a woman's style of dress, her relationship with the assailant, evidence of resistance, presence of alcohol or drugs, and location of the incident, may affect a third party's attitude toward the rape and contribute to his or her belief that the rape may actually be "excusable" or "understandable."

Reported rates of rape and sexual assault vary by race and ethnicity. Native American women are significantly more likely to report rape and physical assault than were women of other backgrounds, while women of Asian and Pacific Islander descent are less likely to report rape victimization. Hispanic women are less likely than non-Hispanic women to report having been raped by strangers, but were more likely to report having being raped by a current or former intimate partner.[4] Native Americans, who are victimized at rates twice as high as the national average, are more likely to experience violence from a non-Native American. The explanation for these differences is unclear. These differences may be due to the fact that women of color are less likely to have social support and are more likely to be living in poverty; social, demographic, and environmental factors that keep a woman from reporting an incident; or a combination of factors.

Historical Trends

Historically, it has been socially acceptable for a husband to physically discipline his wife. The United States followed English law and allowed physical discipline of wives by their husbands until U.S. courts criminalized wife beating in the 20th century.[5]

Rape has been documented in American history since the arrival of the Europeans. Spanish explorers used female Native American captives for sexual services and raped Native American women whose tribes they conquered. Native American cultures, however, prohibited rape, and it had rarely occurred until the arrival of the explorers. Fears of brutal rapes by Native American men were found to be unsubstantiated during colonial-era "Indian" wars. Indeed, English women who had been held captive reported no such treatment.[5]

In 17th-century New England in particular, female servants were at high risk of rape and sexual harassment. During that era, an estimated one-third of rape victims were female servants, even though that group represented only 10% of the total population.[6] Later, in the South, where slave labor was increasingly used instead of indentured servants, African female servants and slaves found themselves victimized by white owners and overseers who viewed them as property—available for service of their sexual needs. Some historians assert that rape was used to dominate female slaves in a system that otherwise treated them as equals to male slaves.[6]

Poverty Influences

Poverty and joblessness are strongly connected with violence, including violence that occurs within the family. The relationship between violence, poverty, and joblessness may result from feelings of inadequacy and low self-esteem brought on by unemployment, stress associated with financial instability, and/or an inability to provide for one's family. Often, these emotions turn to frustration and anger, and eventually lead to fighting within the household or violence toward one's partner or children. Unemployed individuals also spend significantly more time in the home, allowing greater opportunities for tensions to rise.

When poverty inspires violence, women and children are overwhelmingly the victims. Women often remain trapped in abusive relationships because of their financial dependence on the abuser. In households with incomes under $15,000 per year, one in three (35.5%) of women suffer violence from an intimate partner.[7] Living in circumstances of stress and poverty can also lead some women to act violently against their children, spouses, or family members.

Alcohol and Drug Influences

Substance use and abuse are consistently associated with all forms of relationship violence. It is unclear whether a direct cause-and-effect relationship exists between the use of drugs or alcohol and violence, or whether this situation involves two overlapping social epidemics. Violence in a home may cause depression and lower self-esteem, possibly leading to an increased use of alcohol abuse. Conversely, conflicts in interpersonal relationships may arise as a consequence of substance use and abuse and lead to violent behavior.

Data from the National Crime Victim Survey, an ongoing nationally representative survey on crime, highlight the strong association between interpersonal violence and substance use. Among victims able to tell whether there was substance use by the perpetrator, 30% reported alcohol use by the offender at the time of the crime. Two-thirds of victims who suffered violence by a current or former partner reported alcohol use by the offender.[8] Alcohol can play a significant role in violence. For example, 62% of Native American victims report an offender who was under the influence of alcohol, compared to 42% for the national average.[9]

Media Influences

Media access through television, movies, video and computer games, and the Internet is a major influence in the lives of Americans, especially for children and adolescents. Media can be a powerful tool for positive learning and entertainment, but can also pose a threat to emotional and physical safety.

Violence and sex on television and in other media are important, often unrecognized, influences on children and adolescent health and behavior. Research is conflicting as to whether exposure to violent media actually causes violent behavior. However, exposure to violent television, movies, and video games does appear to desensitize children and adolescents, or make them more accepting, towards violent behavior. Exposure to violent media also creates a "mean world effect," causing people to believe the world is a more violent, cruel place than it actually is.[10]

Costs of Victimization

Violent crime directly causes financial losses, such as healthcare costs for treating any physical and mental injuries, as well as lost wages for missed workdays. The annual health-related costs of rape, physical assault, stalking, and homicide by intimate partners are more than $5.8 billion. Victims of intimate partner violence lose nearly 8 million days of work as a result of violence.[11] Other costs may include stolen property in burglaries and expenses for repairing or replacing damaged property. Police services, fire services, and state victims' services that deal with violent crime impose a financial burden on society as well. Each year, federal, state, and local governments in the United States spend about $228 billion and employ 2.5 million people for police protections, corrections, and judicial and legal activities.[12]

I cannot describe how I felt when it was over. I was wondering if it would have been better if I had died. I was humiliated, angry, hurt, and so violated. He had been someone I had trusted—I thought that he was a friend. Looking back, though, there were clues to his violent nature. I had ignored them. It was a mistake for which I paid dearly.
18-year-old student

But violence causes much more than just financial losses. Intangible losses, such as long-term pain and suffering and reduced quality of life, are more difficult to quantify but no less real. Studies show a significant relationship between intimate partner violence and chronic pain, headaches, vaginal infections and bleeding, digestive problems, depression, low self-esteem, and substance abuse.[13] All of these findings lead to higher direct medical costs and consequently more losses for the victim. Many studies have found that the intangible loss of quality of life exceeds the tangible losses for victims of all crimes.

Legal Dimensions

The number of violent crimes by intimate partners against females has significantly decreased over the past 20 years.

This decrease has been attributed to the Violence Against Women Act (VAWA) of 1994, which includes these provisions:

- Making it a crime to cross state lines to continue to abuse a spouse or partner
- Creating tough new penalties for sex offenders
- Prohibiting anyone facing a restraining order for domestic abuse from possessing a firearm
- Providing a substantial commitment of federal resources for police, prosecutors, and prevention service initiatives in cases involving sexual violence or domestic abuse
- Requiring sexual offenders to pay restitution to their victims
- Requiring states to pay for rape examinations
- Providing funds for federal victim-witness counselors
- Extending rape shield laws to protect crime victims from abusive inquiries into their private conduct
- Requiring that released offenders report to local enforcement authorities

Global Issues

In 2005, the World Health Organization conducted a study of more than 24,000 women in 10 countries from different geographical areas, cultures, and rural and urban settings. This landmark study allowed researchers, for the first time, to estimate the frequency and predominant forms of violence against women around the world. The study found that violence against women exists in every culture and every setting, but the frequency of that violence varies sharply. Violence against women was typically, but not always, more common in rural settings and the developing world.[14]

Among other findings, the study found that:

- The proportion of women who had ever suffered physical violence from an intimate partner ranged from 13% in urban Japan to 61% in rural Peru.
- The proportion of women who had ever experienced sexual violence from an intimate partner ranged from 6% in urban Japan and Montenegro to 59% in rural Ethiopia.
- More than 75% of women in urban parts of Serbia, Namibia, Japan, and Brazil said that violence against women was never justified, while fewer than 25% of women in rural Peru, Ethiopia, and Bangladesh thought the same.

- In two-thirds of interview settings, at least 5% of women reported that their first sexual encounter was forced. Rates of forced first sexual encounters were highest in Bangladesh, rural Peru, rural Ethiopia, and Tanzania.[14]

Partner violence can and does lead to death. In many countries, about half of female murder victims were killed by a husband or a boyfriend, often during an ongoing abusive relationship. These deaths may sometimes be concealed as accidents. For example, some deaths of women in India that were recorded as "accidental burns" may actually be murders where women were doused with kerosene and set on fire.[1]

Even in healthcare settings, tens of thousands of women each year are subjected to sexual violence, including sexual harassment by providers, genital mutilation, forced gynecological exams, and obligatory inspections of virginity. Rape is also used as a documented weapon of war. Before the country split into North and South Sudan in 2011, civil war raged in Sudan from 1983 to 2005. During this time, Janjaweed militias from the North systematically used rape as tools of intimidation (by scaring individuals and villages into submission), destruction (by harming and killing thousands of women), and genocide (by reducing the proportion of the ethnic tribes that existed in southern Sudan).[15] During the Bosnia–Herzegovina conflict from 1992 to 1995, soldiers raped between 10,000 and 60,000 women.[1]

Worldwide data on child abuse are scarce; nevertheless, about 57,000 children younger than 15 years of age die from homicides every year. Nonfatal child abuse also occurs in virtually every country. In a study conducted in South Korea, for example, 67% of parents admitted whipping children to discipline them and 45% reported hitting, kicking, or beating their children. In Ethiopia, 21% of urban schoolchildren and 64% of rural schoolchildren reported bruises or swelling from parental punishment.[1]

In Southeast Asia, hundreds of thousands of children are involved in the sex trade, and poverty in those countries continually drives more boys and girls into this arena. Although the demand is driven mostly by local clients, sex tourism (travel for the purposes of finding a sex partner) continues to grow and fuel the market in countries such as Thailand, Cambodia, and Vietnam. In Cambodia, almost all of the girls in prostitution are the main providers for their families. Children as young as age 12 from poor families are sold by parents or agents into the sex trade.

Elder abuse also occurs around the world. In some countries, rapid socioeconomic change weakens family networks that once supported older generations. Twenty years after the collapse of the Soviet Union, thousands of elderly men and women from Russia and other former Soviet republics have been left to fend for themselves with only minimal stipends from the government, resulting in numerous cases of elder neglect.

Family and Intimate Violence

Family and intimate violence refers to violence directed toward former or current spouses or partners, dates, elders, and children. Most violence against women is intimate violence. In the United States, one out of every four women will experience violence by an intimate partner at some point during her life. Family and intimate violence includes many forms of mental and physical harm, as well as threats of injury (see **Self-Assessment 14.1**).

Stalking

Stalking is a violent behavior directed at a specific person, involving:

- repeated sightings or encounters
- nonconsensual communication;
- written, verbal, or implied threats; or

Self-Assessment 14.1

Recognizing a Potentially Abusive Partner

1. Did the person grow up in a violent family? Was he or she abused as a child?
2. Is the person jealous of your friendships? Does he or she try to control the time you spend with other people?
3. Does the person lose his or her temper frequently and overreact to minor problems and frustrations?
4. Does the person abuse alcohol or drugs?
5. Does the person control the finances and make all the decisions within the household?
6. If male, does he have a distorted concept of manhood? Does he have traditional ideas about women's roles versus men's roles?
7. Do you fear the person when he or she is angry?
8. Has the person used physical or psychological coercion to pressure you for sex? Has he or she ever physically assaulted you?

If you answered "yes" to one or more of these questions, you may be at risk of abuse. Talk to your healthcare professional about ways to prevent abuse before it happens.

- a combination of the previous factors that would cause a reasonable person to feel afraid.[16]

Stalkers are frequently a current or former spouse, cohabiting partner, or love interest from some point in the stalked women's lives.[3] Stalking is associated with other forms of violence in intimate relationships. One survey found 81% of women stalked by a current husband, former husband, or cohabiting partner were physically assaulted by that partner; 31% also were sexually abused by that partner.[4]

Although every stalking case is different, a stalker's behavior typically becomes increasingly threatening, serious, and violent. The behavior may begin with the stalker making harassing calls, watching or following the victim, sending unwanted letters or messages, or making verbal threats. The activity generally escalates from what initially may be bothersome and annoying to the level of obsessive, dangerous, violent, and potentially fatal acts. Some stalkers may not begin with violent intentions, but still may cause harm if jealousy or anger is involved.

All 50 states have passed laws to prevent stalking and punish people who engage stalking. California passed the first anti-stalking laws in 1990 in response to several high-profile cases in which the perpetrators stalked and eventually killed their victims. In each case, the victim had notified the police of the stalker's threatening behavior, yet the police were unable to do anything legally unless the stalker acted on the threats. The California law gave law enforcement officers the right to intervene in stalking cases before the stalker acted. Since then, all states have passed similar laws.

Restraining or protection orders can be issued against stalkers to protect citizens against stalking situations. A woman who believes she is being stalked should take action by recording stalking behavior, letting others know about the stalker, and taking proper safety precautions (see **Table 14.1**).

Stalking can also be conducted from a distance. Threatening behavior or unwanted advances directed at another using the Internet and other forms of online communications is called cyberstalking. **Cyberstalking** can be conducted through email, social media sites such as Facebook, cellular phones, global positioning systems (GPS), and other technologies. The stalker may use emails, text messages, wall posts, or online comments to send obscene, threatening or unwanted messages. Online stalking often turns into offline stalking, bringing a real threat of physical

Table 14.1 Guidelines for Women Who Are Being Stalked

These guidelines provide practical information for a woman who believes she is being stalked, but is not in imminent danger. The guidelines do not guarantee her safety, but may reduce her risk of harm.

- Record each incident of stalking with great detail. Save any messages a stalker leaves, and write details of any conversations or encounters. These records can be used as evidence against the perpetrator if necessary.
- Let family and friends know about the stalker. This protects not only the victim, but also those close to the victim.
- Be extremely alert when away from home; carry a whistle to alert others nearby, or a cellular phone to report suspicious behavior or to contact someone for help if necessary.
- Seek protection, restraining, or stay-away orders.
- Inquire about the state's stalking laws because each state's laws differ, and see how they apply to this specific case.
- Note any illegal acts by the stalker, such as entering the residence without permission, destroying property, and so on. By reporting these acts to the police, the acts are not only documented for future evidence, but also may require that the stalker be incarcerated or ordered to stay away from the woman.
- Create a safety plan. Keep a list of important numbers, such as law enforcement, legal representation, and safe places. Victims may want to keep important items and extra money in one place to grab in a rush if necessary.
- Other preventive measures include changing the locks on doors; adding extra outside light around the residence; maintaining an unlisted phone number; varying regular routes; staying in public places when out of the house; and informing neighbors so they can alert someone if they see something suspicious

harm to the victim. Law enforcement agencies estimate that cyberstalking is a factor in 20% to 40% of all stalking cases. Although current state laws encompass any type of unwanted communication with the victim, in many cases, the gap between new technologies and existing laws have created "gray areas" where stalking or stalking-like behaviors can legally occur.[17]

Women can lower their chances of being stalked online by sharing their personal information carefully and responsibly. By adjusting their personal and account settings on sites like Facebook, women can control who has access to their posts and contact information. Safety experts generally advise women either to limit this information to the "friends" they know and trust, or to only add trusted friends and acquaintances as Facebook friends.

Women who write or contribute to websites or personal blogs have a difficult choice about whether to reveal their real names. Revealing a personal name can help a woman build a reputation and readership, but it may also allow cyberstalkers to begin looking up a person's personal information, city of residence, and other information. Whether or not they use their real names, women who contribute to websites may receive angry or romantic emails, messages, or posts. Many of these messages can be safely ignored. However, women should report any message that contains a threat (whether direct or indirect) or that feels potentially dangerous to the police or other authorities.

Domestic Violence

Domestic violence, also referred to as **battering**, occurs when a person subjects a current or former romantic partner to forceful physical, social, and psychological behavior. Battering includes five types of interpersonal violence: physical, sexual, property, psychological, and social. Physical violence includes slapping, choking, punching, kicking, pushing, and using objects as weapons. Forced sexual activity constitutes sexual violence. Property violence denotes threatened or actual destruction of property. Psychological and social forms of violence include threats of harm; physical isolation of the woman; extreme jealousy; mental degradation; and threats of harm to children, pets, or other loved ones.

Battering occurs in families of all racial, economic, educational, and religious backgrounds. Violence in a home

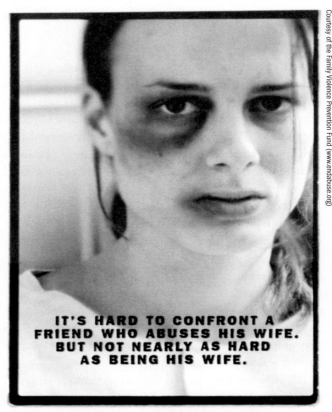

IT'S HARD TO CONFRONT A FRIEND WHO ABUSES HIS WIFE. BUT NOT NEARLY AS HARD AS BEING HIS WIFE.

So you know your friend is an abuser. Do you ignore it or bring it up? Ignoring it is easy. Bringing it up is awkward. You could lose a friend. But maybe bringing it up is the only way to really be a friend. Telling him you know, telling him it's wrong, telling him it's a punishable crime, could be doing him a big favor. Maybe he needs someone to talk to. Maybe he needs someone to say, "No, it's not OK." But more important than his feelings, his wife's well-being, her very life may be in your hands. We can give you some information that may help. Call us at 1-800-END ABUSE.

THERE'S **NO** EXCUSE for Domestic Violence.

Family Violence Prevention Fund

■ At least one out of every three murdered women is killed by her husband or boyfriend. Reprinted with permission from the Family Violence Prevention Fund.

■ Sudanese women and girls march to improve awareness of violence against women.

often involves more than the adult couple. More than 15 million children in the United States live in families in which partner violence occurred at least once in the past year; nearly half of these families experienced severe partner violence.[18] Research suggests that almost all of these children are aware of the violence in their homes; even if they do not see it, they hear the screams and see the bruises, broken bones, and abrasions sustained by their mothers.[19]

Domestic violence is more common among immigrant women than among U.S. citizens. Immigrants from some cultures condone the use of violence from a man toward his wife or other women in the family. A more important factor, however, is that immigrant women are typically more vulnerable than other women and have less access to legal and social services, as well as extended family or other support networks. Immigrant women also may not feel that they are protected by the U.S. legal system or may feel that they are unable to seek help from authorities if their immigrant status is unstable.[20] Studies involving Latina, South Asian, and Korean immigrants found that 30% to 50% of these women have been sexually or physically victimized by a male intimate partner.[21]

My boyfriend always put me down when we were alone and when we were out without friends. He told me that I needed to lose weight, I should shave more often, and I should change my hair. I always tried to make him happy, but he would still find something that he didn't like about me. Even when he cheated on me, he blamed me for pushing him away. I didn't even realize how abusive he was until he finally left me for another woman.

24-year-old woman

Although domestic violence occurs at all levels of society, intimate violence against women generally becomes more common as household income levels decrease (**Figure 14.2**).[22] Spousal abuse perhaps appears more frequently in poorer households because educated, middle-class, and affluent women tend to have more resources with which to avoid or leave violent relationships. For example, affluent women may seek confidential professional help and are more likely to be able to afford and get to a safe location, such as a hotel or friend or relative's house in another city or state.

Relationship violence can and often does lead to death. An intimate (or formerly intimate) partner kills about 33% of female murder victims. In the United States, more than three women are murdered every day by an intimate partner.[23] Battering is often underdiagnosed during medical visits because both the patient and her healthcare provider may be reluctant to initiate or discuss the topic. One study showed that 92% to 98% of women did not discuss their experiences of abuse with their healthcare providers.[24] Although most states have mandatory reporting requirements for child abuse or elder abuse, only a few have a corresponding requirement for healthcare providers to report battering of women.

Domestic Violence in Same-Sex Relationships

Gay men and lesbians also have to contend with domestic abuse, and often face difficulties that other people dealing with domestic abuse do not. Many lesbians perceive battering as a heterosexual phenomenon and therefore may not recognize the patterns of abuse within their own relationships. Additionally, fewer protective measures from the legal system are available to lesbians. In 2010, one out of every four gay, lesbian, or transgendered people reporting domestic violence were either arrested themselves or were arrested along with their battering partners.[25] In the same year, more than half of gay, lesbian, and transgender survivors of violence were turned away from shelters. Most battering-related services are designed for heterosexual female victims and heterosexual male offenders, making it difficult for lesbians to find support. This lack of services

Figure 14.2

Victimization rates for persons age 12 and older, by annual family income.

Source: Greenfield L. (2005). National Crime Victimization Survey, 2003

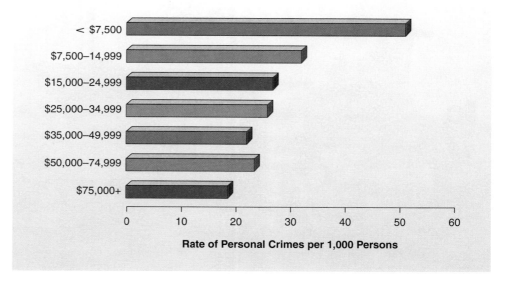

further contributes to the lack of recognition of lesbian, bisexual, and gay domestic violence.

Domestic Violence During Pregnancy

Women are not immune to battering during pregnancy. Each year, as many as 335,000 pregnant women experience intimate partner violence.[26,27] Battering during pregnancy is linked to an increased risk of miscarriage, premature labor, fetal distress, and low birthweight. Blunt abdominal trauma can lead to fetal death or low birthweight by provoking preterm delivery. Battering during pregnancy has numerous consequences. Women who are battered may be less likely to seek prenatal care and gain sufficient weight. They also may be more likely to engage in harmful behaviors such as smoking or alcohol use. Excessive stress and anxiety caused by being in an abusive relationship may also have physical consequences for the mother and her developing fetus.[28]

Domestic Violence Women with Disabilities

Women with disabilities are about as likely as other women to experience physical, sexual, or emotional abuse at some point in their lives. Women with disabilities, however, were more likely to report multiple perpetrators, longer duration of abuse, and more intense experiences of abuse.[29]

Disabled women are most likely to be abused by an intimate partner, followed by a family member, a personal care attendant, a stranger, or a healthcare provider. The abuse often begins subtly, as the abuser tries to determine how much violence will remain unnoticed. Abuse may take the form of psychological, physical, or financial abuse, or it may involve neglect by withholding care, medication, or mobility devices.

Many people with disabilities are especially vulnerable to victimization because of their real or perceived inability to fight, flee, or to tell anyone about the abuse. Many battered women's shelters may be inaccessible or lack attendant care or personnel trained in working with women with disabilities; a woman, therefore, may find herself trapped in an abusive situation. Consequently, healthcare practitioners should find ways to conduct at least part of their visit with a woman with disabilities in private. This opportunity allows a woman to answer questions and confide in her practitioner without a caretaker or family member being present.

Child Abuse and Neglect

Legally, **child abuse or neglect**, often referred to as maltreatment, consists of any act, or failure to act, that causes serious harm, or that creates an imminent risk of harm, to a child. Child maltreatment includes physical, emotional, and sexual abuse, as well as neglect (failure to provide for a child's basic physical, educational, medical, or emotional needs).

© Photodisc

■ Women with disabilities who are in abusive relationships often have a difficult time finding help.

In 2010, 695,000 children were reported as victims of abuse and neglect. This number is likely an underestimate, since many cases go unreported. Of these children, 51% were girls and 49% were boys. More than 80% of these children were maltreated by one or both parents, most commonly the female parent; women represented nearly 60% of all perpetrators of such violence. Women are more likely than men to commit neglect, but men are more likely to commit sexual abuse.[30]

Neglect is the most common type of child maltreatment, followed by physical abuse, sexual abuse, emotional abuse, and medical neglect (**Figure 14.3**). Many abused children suffer more than one type of maltreatment. Younger children are most likely to be abused or neglected (**Figure 14.4**). Common reasons for child abuse and neglect include substance abuse by one or both of the parents, poverty or other economic strain, parental capacity and skill, and other incidents involving domestic abuse.

Children who experience abuse or neglect often develop behavioral and psychological problems, relationship problems, low self-esteem, depression, suicidal behavior, alcohol and substance abuse, sexual dysfunction, and sexual risk-taking later in life.[3] About 1,500 children die from abuse and neglect in the United States each year; about 80% of children who die as a result of abuse are younger than 4 years old.[30]

Substance abuse is a often major problem in families with suspected child maltreatment.[31] Although children from all socioeconomic levels suffer from abuse and neglect, children from families with annual incomes of less than $15,000 are more than 25 times more likely than children from families with annual incomes of $30,000 or more to suffer abuse or neglect.[32] Many problems associated with poverty contribute to child maltreatment, including more transient residence, poorer education, and higher rates of substance abuse and emotional disorders. Moreover, families at the lower socioeconomic levels have less adequate social support systems to assist parents in their childcare responsibilities.

Abuse and battering tend to perpetuate themselves in cycles. Almost all abusive parents were themselves abused or neglected as children, and battered children often grow up to become battering adults. Child abuse is frequently a symptom of family violence. One large study revealed that women who had both witnessed violence between their parents and been victims of parental abuse themselves were twice as likely to abuse their partner or children than were women who had been exposed to only one or the other type of violence. Women appeared to be most strongly influenced by their mother's behavior. With every witnessed incident in which the woman's mother had attacked her father, there was an increased likelihood that the woman would:

- abuse her child;
- abuse her partner; or
- become the victim of her current partner.[33]

Several psychological traits are associated with child abusers:

- Immaturity and dependency
- A sense of personal incompetence
- Difficulty in seeking pleasure and finding satisfaction as an adult
- Social isolation
- A reluctance to admit the problem and seek help
- Fear of spoiling children
- A strong belief in the value of punishment

Figure 14.3

Frequency of Reported Child Abuse and Neglect Cases, 2010.

Source: Data from U.S. Department of Health and Human Services, Administration for Children and Families, Administration on Children, Youth and Families, Children's Bureau. (2011). Child Maltreatment 2010. Available from http://www.acf.hhs.gov/programs/cb/stats_research/index.htm#can

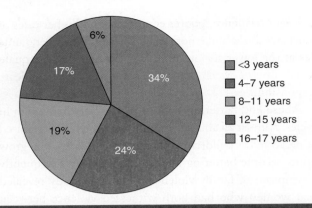

Figure 14.4

Victims of child abuse and neglect by age, 2010

Source: Data from U.S. Department of Health and Human Services, Administration for Children and Families, Administration on Children, Youth and Families, Children's Bureau. (2011). Child Maltreatment 2010. Available from http://www.acf.hhs.gov/programs/cb/stats_research/index.htm#can

- Unreasonable and age-inappropriate expectations of children
- Low personal self-esteem

Any combination of these traits results in an inability to cope and problem-solve effectively when a problem or crisis evolves. In such cases, the outcome may ultimately be abuse.

Elder Abuse

As the U.S. population has aged over the past 20 years, so has the number of abuse cases involving elderly victims. In most cases, elders become increasingly dependent on others for their care as they get older. It is estimated that 1 to 2 million Americans age 65 or older have been victimized by someone who provided care for them. **Elder abuse** is in part a serious problem for women because they tend to live longer than men. However, even after accounting for their larger share of the aging population, women still account for two-thirds of all elder abuse reports.[34] There are three major situations for abuse of the elderly:

- Domestic abuse (maltreatment by someone who has a relationship with the victim)
- Institutional abuse (maltreatment by staff in a residential facility)
- Self-neglect (failure to care for oneself)

Within these situations, the National Center on Elder Abuse defines seven types of elder abuse:

- Physical elder abuse is the use of physical force that results in bodily injury, physical pain, or impairment.
- Sexual elder abuse is nonconsensual sexual contact of any kind with an elderly person.
- Emotional or psychological elder abuse is the infliction of anguish, pain, or distress through verbal or nonverbal acts.
- Financial or material exploitation occurs when an abuser misuses or misappropriates an elder's funds, property, or assets.
- Neglect refers to a caretaker's refusal or failure to perform his or her obligations or duties to an elderly person. Neglect can be active, when the failure or refusal to acknowledge an obligation is deliberate, or passive, when the failure is unintentional.
- Self-neglect is the failure to provide oneself with adequate food, water, clothing, shelter, safety, personal hygiene, and medication, thereby threatening the elderly person's own health or safety.
- Abandonment, also known as "granny dumping," occurs when a caretaker or guardian of an elderly person deserts the elder.

Elder abuse occurs among people of all racial, ethnic, and economic backgrounds. In general, elders who are unable to care for themselves are more likely to suffer abuse. Researchers have found that in 90% of substantiated cases, perpetrators of elder abuse were family members, with two-thirds being adult children or spouses. Men were more likely to commit abandonment, physical abuse, emotional abuse, and financial and material exploitation, while women were slightly more likely to neglect elders. In self-neglect cases, approximately two-thirds of elders were female, 75 or older, and white.[35]

My granddaughter and her boyfriend always take money from me. The other day, when I asked them to leave my house, they pushed me. They're always yelling at me and telling me how much they hate caring for me. My daughter who lives with me pretends she doesn't see it. But who can I tell? If I report them, I'll end up in a nursing home all alone.

82-year-old woman

In one survey, 36% of nursing-home staff reported having witnessed at least one incident of physical abuse of an elderly patient in the previous year, 10% admitted having committed at least one act of physical abuse themselves, and 40% said that they had psychologically abused patients.[34] Institutional abuse includes physically restraining patients, depriving them of dignity and choice over daily affairs, and providing insufficient care (allowing them to develop pressure sores, for example).

Factors that increase stress in a caretaker's life may increase the likelihood of that caretaker committing abuse. These factors include stressful life events, impairment of the dependent elder, and resentment of dependency, especially as the level of dependency increases. Abusive caregivers are often unprepared, unable, or unwilling to provide the care that an elderly person needs. Elder abuse is also related to emotional problems, such as alcohol or drug use by the abuser, social isolation of the abuser and the abused, and lack of community support. In some cases, an abuser may be repeating a cycle of violence, similar to the cycle identified in cases of child abuse and neglect; the abuser of an elderly parent may have been abused by the parent in childhood, or the abuser may have witnessed the same type of elder abuse by the parent against the abuser's grandparent.

Rape and Sexual Assault

Rape and sexual assault are violent crimes of aggression. Rape is a nonconsensual event, involving the use of force or the threat of force to sexually penetrate the victim's vagina, mouth, or rectum.[4] Sexual assault often refers to forced sexual contact, but this term frequently acts as an all-encompassing descriptor for any type of unwanted sexual advances, including rape. The National Institute of Justice and the Centers for Disease Control and Prevention estimate that one in six women and one in 33 men in the United States have been the victim of attempted or completed rape as a child or an adult.[4] More than 9 out of every 10 rape victims are female.

Determining an accurate estimate of how often rape occurs is difficult given the significant underreporting of the crime. Fortunately, rates of rape and sexual assault have fallen over the past decade. In 2010, there were 184,400 reported victims of rape, attempted rape, or sexual assault in the United States, a drop of about 24% compared to 2001.[36]

Rape may occur among strangers or intimates. Acquaintance rape, or **date rape**, occurs when the victim and the rapist either previously knew each other or have interacted in some socially appropriate manner. About three-fourths of rape victims in the United States know their assailant: Approximately 48% were raped by a friend or acquaintance,

17% by a current intimate partner, and 8% by another relative (see **Figure 14.5**).[36] Rape by a coworker, teacher, professor, a husband's friend, or boss—anyone the individual knows—is considered acquaintance rape.

Many victims of rape are children and adolescents; about 44% of rape victims are younger than age 18 and about 15% are younger than age 12.[36] Although physical abuse and neglect account for the greatest portion of child abuse incidents, child sexual abuse is another tragic dimension of child abuse in general. Sexual abuse accounts for about 1 in 10 cases of child abuse.[37] It is difficult to determine the incidence rate of sexual abuse among children. One report found that 13% of girls and 3.4% of boys had been sexually abused.[38] In reported cases, three-fourths of adolescent sexual assault victims knew their attackers—21% were family members and 33% were acquaintances or friends.[38] Males are reported to be the abusers in most sexual abuse cases involving children.

My stepfather started fondling me when I was 6. It evolved into sex by the time I was 12. I think my mother knew, but she had so many other problems to deal with. I had three younger sisters and I was so afraid for them. He said that he wouldn't touch them if I wouldn't tell "the secret." I was trapped. Eventually I found out that he was telling them the same thing. I have been in therapy for a year. I am still so hurt and so angry. The feelings and memories just won't go away.
21-year-old woman

In many cases of date or acquaintance rape, aggressors use drugs to render the victim unconscious or incapacitated. Flunitrazepam, commonly known as Rohypnol, is one type of "date rape drug." This drug is 10 times as strong as Valium and is tasteless and odorless. It dissolves in liquid, takes effect quickly, and produces memory loss for as long as 8 hours. Rohypnol is especially popular on high school and college campuses, as well as in nightclubs. Many women have been raped after consuming a drink with the drug dissolved in it. The use of the drug is extremely dangerous and can cause death. Gamma hydroxybutyrate (GHB) and gamma butyrolactone (GBL) are found in liquid form and have also been associated with sexual assault. Abuse of GHB and GBL can lead to coma and seizures. Ketamine, used as a tranquilizer in veterinary medicine, is another common date rape drug that is snorted or injected. It is referred to as "special K" and can cause death.

Rape also happens in marriages, during legal separation, or after divorce. Rape in marriage is often called spousal rape or marital rape. Historically, husbands had unlimited sexual access to their wives and, therefore, rape within marriage was not recognized as a crime: Marital rape has only been a crime in all 50 states since 1993. Many states provide exemptions for certain situations, such as mental or physical impairment of a woman rendering her unable to consent, that protect husbands from being prosecuted for rape. In addition, rape can occur between people of the same sex. The National Violence Against Women Survey found that 10.8% of women rape or sexual assault victims were assaulted by a female.[4]

Rape is often characterized as not being a "clear-cut" crime such as murder. Societal pressures and norms have reinforced beliefs that rape is sometimes justifiable, depending on the circumstances. For various reasons, about 6 in 10 rapes are never reported to the police.[36] Unreported rapes can harm more than the victim, because if the rapists are not stopped, their violent behavior may continue. The underreporting of rape is due to a number of factors, including the pattern of "blaming the victim." Many women fear unwanted publicity from making a formal complaint, and others distrust hospital and law enforcement agencies. Feelings of shame or guilt, fear of not being believed, and fear of reprisal or punishment if the rapist is an acquaintance or employer are other reasons why women do not report rape.

Around the world, countless women in prisons and jails are at risk of rape and other forms of sexual violence. Reporting procedures in prisons are often ineffectual, and complaints are routinely ignored. To make matters worse, punishment for the crime is rare and some inmates face retaliation from the offender if a report is made.

Reducing Risk of Rape/Sexual Assault

Society as a whole, as well as individuals of both genders, need to act together to prevent rapes and sexual assault. Women are never "at fault" when a rape occurs; women

■ Most rapes go unreported.

© George Doyle/Stockbyte/Thinkstock

It's Your Health

Information About "Date Rape Drugs"

Rohypnol (roofies, ruffies, roach, R2, rophies, la roche, rib, mind eraser, the forget pill, the date rape drug)

- Characteristics: small white pill (often has "ROCHE" on one side for Hoffmann-La Roche, its manufacturer, and a circled "1" or "2" on one side); can be swallowed as a pill, dissolved in a drink, or snorted; tasteless and odorless
- Effects: may feel dizzy, disoriented, nauseated, sleepy, extremely relaxed, or drunk; can cause difficulty speaking or moving, unconsciousness, and loss of memory; effects may last from 2 to 8 hours

Gamma Hydroxybutyrate (GHB, liquid ecstasy, easy lay, liquid X, energy drink, somatomax, scoop, Georgia Home Boy, grievous bodily harm, goop)

- Characteristics: white powdered material or liquid form
- Effects: may feel drowsy, dizzy, or nauseated; may cause unconsciousness, seizures, severe respiratory depression, and coma

Ketamine (special K, vitamin K, cat tranquilizer, k)

- Characteristics: white powdered material, similar to cocaine; can be snorted, smoked with marijuana, or dissolved in beverages
- Effects: short-acting hallucinatory effects; can affect the senses, judgment, and coordination for 18 to 24 hours

Ways to Protect Yourself

- Don't leave a beverage unattended or accept a drink from an open container.
- Don't drink from someone else's drink.
- Don't drink any beverage with a funny taste, odor, residue, color, or consistency.
- Go to parties with trusted friends; watch out for each other and leave together.

---

can, however, lower their risk by being careful and clearly communicating what they are, and what they are not, comfortable with.

Response to Rape/Sexual Assault

If a rape or sexual assault occurs, a woman's first concern should be finding safety and calling the police. The police will assist the victim in seeking medical attention, which is important for treating any physical injuries, testing for sexually transmitted infections (STIs) and HIV/AIDS, and collecting medical evidence for prosecution. It is important to report the assault to the police immediately; the decision about whether to prosecute the offender can be made later. A woman also should contact her local rape crisis center to inquire about counseling and support.

It's Your Health

Reducing the Risk of Date Rape

Be wary of a relationship that is operating along classic stereotypes of dominant male and submissive, passive female. The dominance in ordinary activities may extend to the sexual arena.

Be wary when a date tries to control behavior or pressures others in any way.

Be explicit with communication. Don't say "no" in a way that could be interpreted in any way as a "maybe" or "yes."

Avoid ambiguous messages with both verbal and nonverbal behavior. Saying "no" and permitting heavy petting implies confusion or ambiguity.

First dates with an unknown companion may be safer in a group.

Avoid remote or isolated spots where help is not available.

Limit alcohol and illegal drug use.

The recovery process from rape depends on the individual and the circumstances in which the rape occurred. Victims of rape often suffer from mental health problems, gynecological issues, negative health behaviors, chronic health conditions, and higher risk for suicide. Rape also may lead to unwanted pregnancies and STIs, including HIV/AIDS. Being tested immediately after the incident for STIs may help a woman prevent long-term consequences from disease. Postexposure prophylactics, including antibiotics, emergency contraceptive pills, hepatitis B vaccination, and antiretroviral drugs, can reduced the likelihood for some sexually transmitted infections or unwanted pregnancy.

Posttraumatic stress disorder (PTSD; see Chapter 12) is another common reaction to rape. At some point during their lifetimes, 32% of all rape victims develop PTSD, compared with 9% of victims of non-crime-related trauma, such as car accidents.[39]

Rape trauma syndrome is another condition associated with rape victims. It is usually described as having two phases. The first phase, or acute phase, includes the immediate emotions following the event, which include shock, anger, numbness, guilt, disbelief, embarrassment, shame, feelings of being unclean, anxiety, denial, fear, self-blame, and restlessness. This phase is often characterized by significant disruption in a woman's life. The second phase of rape trauma syndrome includes attempts at reorganizing one's life and lifestyle, and learning to cope again. Victims may decide to change schools, jobs, or routes to school or work

It's Your Health

Myths and Facts About Rape

Myth: Rape only occurs in the dark alleys, not in homes or good neighborhoods.

Fact: Six out of 10 sexual assaults take place at the victim's own home or at the home of a friend, neighbor, or relative.

Myth: Rape occurs only late at night, in the dark.

Fact: Forty-three percent of rapes occur between 6 P.M. and midnight; 24% of rapes occur between midnight and 6 A.M.; and the other 33% take place between 6 A.M. and 6 P.M.

Myth: If a person pays for a date, he or she has the right to expect something back, such as sex.

Fact: No one ever owes anyone sex or sexual favors.

Myth: If a person returns to his or her date's apartment or house, the date has the right to expect sex.

Fact: Consent for sexual contact is not defined by one's willingness to enter someone else's home or inviting someone into his or her home, including a date.

Myth: People who commit rapes are unable to control their sexual urges.

Fact: Rapists are not driven by uncontrollable sexual urges, but rather by the need to feel powerful and in control. Forcing someone to engage in sexual intercourse against her or his will is an act of violence and aggression. Sex is the weapon used to humiliate and control the victim.

Myth: Rapists are always strangers to the victim.

Fact: Almost three-fourths of rape victims know their assailants.

Myth: Rapists are usually African American men who rape white women.

Fact: In most rapes, the victim and the offender are members of the same race.

Myth: All rapists are men.

Fact: Although men commit 99% of forcible rapes, women do commit rape and other sexual assault offenses.

Myth: Only promiscuous women or women wearing provocative clothing are victims of rape.

Fact: Neither provocative dress nor promiscuous behavior is an invitation for unwanted sexual activity. Forcing someone to engage in nonconsensual sexual activity is sexual assault, regardless of the way the person dresses or acts.

Myth: All rape victims are women.

Fact: About one in every 10 rape victims is male.

Myth: Women who are raped were asking for it.

Fact: No one deserves to be raped. A victim should never be blamed for the actions of the perpetrator.

Source: Data from National Crime Victimization Survey, 1999; National Crime Victimization Survey, 2000; Sex Offenses and Offenders. Bureau of Justice Statistics, U.S. Department of Justice, February 1997.

in an attempt to remove reminders of the event from their daily lives. Overwhelming feelings often develop that the victim may not directly link to the rape. Even if a woman successfully represses her emotions about a rape, the feelings can persist, sometimes for years. Depression, guilt, and loss of self-esteem are common reactions. Other psychological problems include suicide attempts, eating disorders, substance abuse, social phobia, and other anxiety disorders. Being a victim of rape can also affect a woman's sexual health and intimacy.

Violence by Strangers

Victimization rates of women are lower than those of men in all types of violent crimes committed by strangers, except rape and sexual assault. However, the proportion of crimes committed by strangers against women has grown over the past 20 years. These crimes include carjacking, robbery, murder, gang violence, sexual assault, and rape. In general, women are more likely to be victimized by an intimate than by a stranger, except in cases of robberies. Strangers also commit about 53% of the aggravated assaults against females.[2011]

Hate crimes are a form of collective violence often committed against strangers. Hate crimes consist of arson, vandalism, assault, murder, and other offenses that are motivated by hatred or prejudice towards a person's race, religion, sexual orientation, or ethnicity. Hate crimes account for less than 1% of total reported crimes, but the damage they can cause is immense. In addition to harming their victims directly, hate crimes also affect the victims'

families and communities. At heart, hate crimes are acts of terrorism—a systematic use of fear to change the way other persons behave. The number of hate crimes has fallen over the past decade. In 2009, 148,400 hate crime incidents were reported to U.S. law enforcement, a 38% decline since 2003. About 40% of victims of hate crimes are female. Most hate crimes are committed based on a person's race or ethnicity, followed by a person's perceived association with a community or group, sexual orientation, perceived characteristics, religion, and disability (see **Figure 14.5**).[40]

Although violence cannot always be avoided, people can take measures to protect themselves. Women (and men) can walk with at least one other person or stick to populated, well-lit areas, especially at night, to avoid being caught alone. When alone, women should avoid isolated areas and carry a whistle or cellular phone in case of emergency. When visiting potentially dangerous areas, women can avoid carrying flashy jewelry or large sums of money.

Self-defense classes can also give women the knowledge and confidence to survive or escape a violent attack. The goal of any practical self-defense class should not be to destroy an opponent, but rather to allow a person to get home safely if he or she is attacked. A good self-defense class can teach women the ways they are most likely to be attacked, as well as different responses to those attacks. Regular practice striking and grappling can give a person "muscle memory" that he or she can call upon and use quickly if needed. In addition, learning and practicing self-defense can give a person the confidence and will to use her body effectively, rather than to panic, in a dangerous situation.

Figure 14.5

Suspected motivations of hate crimes, 2003–2009.

Source: Modified from Bureau of Justice Statistics. (2011). Hate crime, 2003–2009.

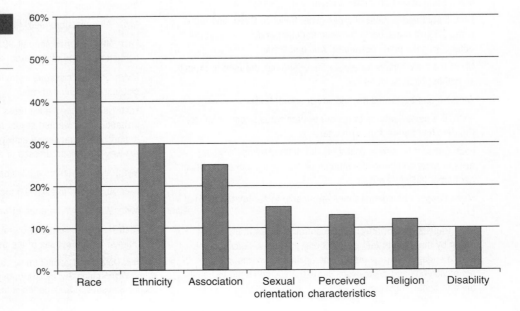

Women who are aware of their surroundings and use common sense can greatly reduce their risk of victimization; this does not mean, however, that women who are victimized are at fault. The circumstances and characteristics of each violent crime and each victim are unique, and it is not practical or realistic to imagine that these strategies alone could prevent all types of violence. Prevention is just one useful but limited tool available to women.

Sexual Harassment

Sexual harassment is an illegal, violent act involving unwanted sexual attention, requests of sexual favors, or the use of sexual language or behaviors to create a hostile environment. Although sexual harassment can occur in any setting, it most commonly occurs in the workplace. Sexual harassment often involves a male harasser and a female victim. However, sexual harassment recognizes no gender boundaries—a female may harass a male, and the victim and the harasser may be the same sex.

There are three types of harassment:

- Gender harassment constitutes behavior that conveys a degrading or hostile attitude toward women.

- Unwanted sexual attention or advances include behaviors such as staring, commenting, touching, or repeated requests for dates or sexual favors.

- Sexual coercion, also referred to as quid pro quo (defined as an "equal" exchange or substitution), is the use of threats or bribery to obtain sexual favors.

Any type of harassment may interfere with a woman's ability to perform her regular duties at work and often creates an intimidating or hostile working environment. Women who are at the greatest risk for sexual harassment are those in careers traditionally considered to be male occupations. Any person may initiate sexual harassment, but a harasser is most likely to be someone with more power or authority than the recipient. In addition to suffering physical and emotional victimization, the threat of economic vulnerability often leaves the victim with the feeling that she has few real options in the situation.

For years, workplaces and individuals trivialized sexual harassment and refused to recognize it as a violation of rights or personal dignity. This practice sometimes persists in the present day. Harassers may rationalize their behavior or offer excuses, but these rationalizations perpetuate power disparities and further dehumanize women. As with other forms of sexual victimization, harassment operates as an instrument of social control.

It's Your Health

Common Excuses for Sexual Harassment

"Sexual harassment is a trivial distraction from the real work."

Sexual harassment has serious, long-term emotional consequences for the victim. The emotional and economic impact of sexual harassment is not trivial in nature or form.

"I didn't mean any harm. I was just having fun."

Sexual harassment is similar to poking someone with a stick. The fun is one-sided and unfair.

"She should take it as a compliment that we like her when we say things like that."

Unwanted and unsolicited sexual advances and innuendoes, particularly from others in positions of power, can be frightening. The victim can hardly feel "complimented" when she feels threatened and put down.

"She just wanted to make trouble here with a complaint."

Women are caught between the proverbial rock and a hard place. If they accept the harassment, they perpetuate the behavior and risk further, and perhaps worse, harassment. If they file a complaint, they may be labeled as troublemakers, with no guarantees that the situation will be corrected. Filing a complaint may also place a woman's job security or career in jeopardy.

Whatever form it appears in, sexual harassment is a harmful, legally punishable offense. A common situation involves a boss or supervisor who requires sexual services from an employee as a condition for keeping a job or getting a promotion. Less blatant forms of workplace sexual harassment include being subjected to obscenities or being made the target of sexual jokes and innuendoes. However deep a harassed person's feelings of humiliation, anger, and shame, the financial consequences of not complying with sexual coercion on the job may be devastating. Many victims, especially if they are supporting families, cannot afford to be unemployed. Also, many find it difficult to seek other work while they are employed. Thus, a person who quits or is fired as a result of sexual harassment faces the prospect of severe financial difficulties.

Employers have become more sensitive to the issue of sexual harassment, in part because of court decisions that have awarded large payments to victims. Employers paid more $52 million in damages to victims of sexual harassment in 2011.[41] It is an employer's responsibility to maintain a workplace that is free of sexual harassment by educating employees about which behaviors constitute harassment and taking appropriate measures if these behaviors occur. The U.S. Department of Labor Employment and Training Administration provides training guidelines for the workplace.

Reported cases of sexual harassment have fallen over the past 20 years, dropping by nearly 30% from 1997 to 2011 (see **Figure 14.6**). While women continue to make up the vast majority of victims of harassment, the percentage of males filing claims of sexual harassment grew from 11.6% to 16.3% over the same period.[41]

> *A guy I worked with would always come up behind me and start rubbing my shoulders. When I asked him to stop, he told me that I needed to relax, that he was just trying to help by giving me a massage. I didn't know who to tell, but it made me really uncomfortable, especially because he continued to do it even after I asked him to stop. Eventually, I went to our Human Resources department and it turned out that another coworker had just reported him for making lewd comments to her. Within a week, he was fired. Although I felt bad at first for turning him in, it just made me too uncomfortable and nervous to work with him. I think I did the right thing.*
>
> **26-year-old computer programmer**

Sexual harassment is not limited to the workplace. A report from the American Association of University Women found that nearly two-thirds of college students have encountered some type of sexual harassment while at college. More than half of female students have been subjected to sexual comments and jokes, and about 35% have experienced physical harassment by being touched or grabbed in a sexual manner. Students who are lesbian, gay, bisexual, or transgender are more than twice as likely to be harassed as heterosexual students. Only 7% of students reported the harassment. Many students actually admit to sexually harassing other students; the reason more than half gave for the harassment was "I thought it was funny."[42]

Common reactions to sexual harassment include anger, humiliation, shame, embarrassment, nervousness, irritability, and lack of motivation. Guilt is another common feeling, with a victim often questioning whether she (or he) has done something wrong to encourage the harassment. The sense of alienation and helplessness many victims of sexual harassment feel is similar to that experienced by many rape victims. Sexual harassment victims may also experience headaches, stomach pain and nausea, back and neck pain, and a variety of other stress-related ailments.

Dealing Effectively with Harassment

Individuals who have been sexually harassed have several options. First, the victim should recognize that criminal charges can be filed against the perpetrator. If the coercion falls short of attempted rape or assault, it is often wise to confront the person responsible for the harassment. The confrontation should be stated in clear terms, and the specific behaviors should be identified as sexual harassment. The victim should make it clear that the behavior is unwelcome, will not be tolerated, and that, if it continues, charges will be filed through appropriate channels. Some victims carefully document what has occurred and provide a written confrontation rather than undertake a verbal discussion. Others may choose to seek out the assistance of their human resources department if the sexual harassment occurs within a work setting.

If the behavior does not stop, the next step is to discuss it with the supervisor of the person responsible for the harassment. It is often helpful to talk to other employees—many times there is more than one victim. Discussing the matter with other employees provides peer support and pressure for the behavior to stop. Official complaints can be filed with local or state Human Rights Commissions or Fair Employment Practice Agencies.

If legal action is necessary, victims can file lawsuits in federal courts under the Civil Rights Act. Lawsuits can also be filed under city or state laws prohibiting employment

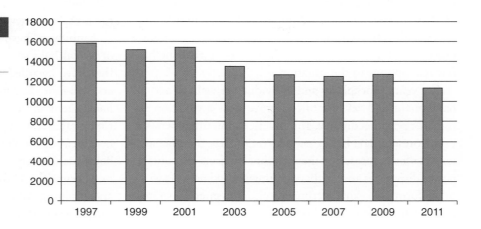

Figure 14.6
Number of Sexual Harassment Charges Filed, 1997–2011
Source: Data from U.S. Equal Employment Opportunity Commission. (2012) Sexual harassment charges EEOC & FEPAs combined: FY1997–FY2011.

discrimination. A person who has been the victim of sexual harassment is more likely to receive a favorable court ruling if attempts were made to resolve the problem within the organization before taking the issue to court

Informed Decision Making

Knowing the facts about violence can lead to a certain level of paranoia and anger, both unhealthy conditions. Identifying the factors that contribute to violence and working to eliminate them are much more constructive reactions to potential or perceived threats of violence.

The stereotype that men should be aggressive and that women should be passive, compliant, and pleasing to others continues to exist and influences people's behavior. When people—whether male or female—buy into these stereotypes, it sets the stage for problems. For example, women who have been socialized to be passive may not think that they have a right to express their opinions openly and freely. Men who have been socialized to live up to a macho image may think that they need to "score" with women or control women to be "real" men. They may expect women to go along with their need to prove themselves or believe that a woman means "yes" when she says "no."

To address these stereotypes, a woman must take several steps:

- Recognize the inherent limitations in any stereotype
- Be open in discussing values with respect to relationships and sexuality
- Decide for herself and be explicit about when she will or will not have sex
- Understand that coercion and violence are never acceptable or deserved within a relationship
- Avoid situations where inebriation by one or both parties makes open and clear communication difficult

Some women find talking openly about relationships and sexuality difficult. Instead of using clear communication, they rely on assumptions, hints, innuendoes, and considerable hope that their partner understands. Unfortunately, such indirect communication is highly unreliable. Expectations and values about relationships and sexuality should be explicitly expressed. Communication is bidirectional: In a relationship, each person must carefully listen to the other person and confirm what has or has not been said.

Finally, "no" means "no."

Sources of Help

Women in abusive relationships first need to identify and acknowledge the presence of the problem. Denial, avoidance, and protection of the abusive partner often prevent or delay such acknowledgment, particularly for women who may have grown up in a dysfunctional family situation.

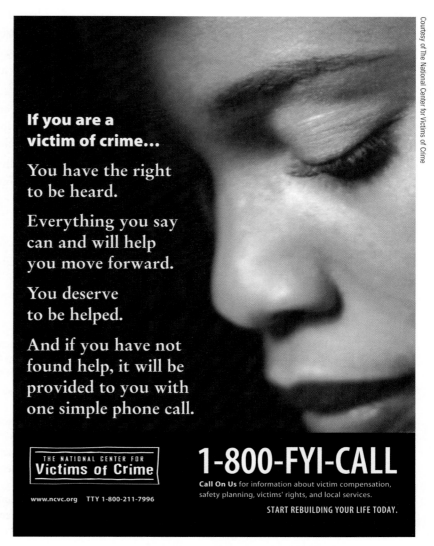

■ Reaching out for help can be the most important step. Reprinted with permission from the National Center for Victims of Crime.

Professional counseling and support can help a woman cope with and recover from a violent relationship. Most communities have services and facilities to support female victims of violence, including local crisis hotlines. Hotline counselors can help callers find counseling, supportive services, and emergency shelter. Shelters provide physical safety, psychological counseling, and referral services. Many local organizations have been started by women who have been battered themselves and recognize the need for sensitive and protected outreach services. Support groups allow women to share common concerns, fears, and information. For many women, the most important step in taking control of a violent situation is admitting there is a problem and reaching out for help.

causes psychological harm, such as a loss of self-esteem, depression, anxiety disorders, and suicide. Children in battered households may experience illness, emotional problems, increased fears, increased risk of abuse, injuries, and death. They also may internalize abusive behavior as a normal part of life and grow up to abuse their own or someone else's children. Domestic violence also creates problems at the societal level, such as increasing crime; legal, medical, and counseling costs; and reducing quality of life. Efforts are urgently needed to address and reduce the full spectrum of violence against women.

■■■■

Summary

Violence occurs in every country in the world, including the United States. Violence can be directed against the self, against another person, or against a community or group of people. Violence affects women when they are victims of crimes, and when they are the siblings, wives, girlfriends, mothers, daughters, and friends of victims. Because of violence, any women are left alone to raise children, girls are raised without fathers, and some women lose their sons. In addition to its direct physical consequences, violence often

■■■■

Topics for Discussion

1. How do interpersonal, collective, and self-directed violence affect women?

2. How do traditional attitudes about women's roles in society and place in society influence violence and its effects?

3. What are some of the major consequences of violence, in addition to the physical effects of the acts themselves?

4. Globally, how does violence in the developed world (the United States, Canada, Western Europe, and Japan) compare to the developing world?

Profiles of Remarkable Women

Lara Logan (1971–)

© ZUMA Press, Inc./Alamy Images

Lara Logan is a South African war correspondent and foreign affairs journalist. She has been the chief foreign correspondent for CBS News and for the television show *60 Minutes* since 2006. Logan has won many awards for her reporting. She reported from Baghdad as the U.S. military invaded the city; she has also reported on the Taliban's growth in Afghanistan, the Israeli-Palestinian conflict, violence in Northern Ireland, floods in Mozambique, and the U.S. embassy bombings in Kenya and Tanzania. She is married and has two children.

Logan was covering the Egyptian revolution in February 2011 when a mob of protesters separated Logan from her group and brutally beat and sexually assaulted her. Pulled in different directions and dragged along the ground, Logan later said she believed that she would die during the assault. Logan was rescued when a group of Egyptian women surrounded her, placing themselves between her and her attackers until a group of soldiers were able to fight off the crowd.

Logan revealed the details of her assault in a nationally televised interview after her return to the United States, saying that she wanted to break "the code of silence" that surrounds rape and sexual assault among female journalists, and to draw attention to the frequency of sexual harassment and assault of women in Egypt. Since then, she has chosen not to be defined by her assault, but to continue as a journalist, reporting from within the United States and nationally.

Profiles of Remarkable Women

Yvette Cade (1974–)

Yvette Cade is a survivor. In 2005, 3 weeks after a judge dismissed her protective order against her husband in a district court in Maryland, Cade's husband showed up at her place of employment, doused her with gasoline, and set her on fire. She suffered third-degree burns over 60% of her body. After undergoing multiple surgeries, Cade pulled through and has become an advocate for domestic violence victims. She has spoken out numerous times about her abusive relationship, including telling her story to a national audience on Montel Williams and Oprah.

Yvette and her family have used her personal tragedy to encourage other sufferers of domestic violence to leave their abusive partners and find freedom. She and her family speak about the importance of family support to get through a tragedy such as this. Yvette's situation resulted in significant changes in several states, including her home state of Maryland, regarding enforcement of protection orders and the court's responsibility to treat domestic violence as a serious crime.

Yvette was honored in 2007 by the U.S. Congressional Victim's Rights Caucus for being a survivor and offering hope to victims of domestic violence. She and her family started the Yvette Cade Fund to help fund Yvette's continued need for medical treatment and further surgeries, as well as raise money for domestic violence awareness activities.

5. What can a woman do to reduce her risk of assault?

6. What would you do if you think that a friend is in an abusive relationship? What would you do if a friend is being stalked?

7. What similarities exist between child abuse and elder abuse?

8. What steps may be involved during a rape exam? What evidence may be collected to help in making a case against a rapist?

■■■■
Key Terms

Battering: Repeatedly subjecting a person to forceful and coercive physical, social, and/or psychological behavior.

Child abuse and neglect: Physical or mental injury, sexual abuse or exploitation, negligent treatment, or maltreatment of a child by a person who is responsible for the child's welfare under circumstances that indicate that the child's health or welfare is harmed or threatened.

Cyberstalking: Threatening behavior or unwanted advances directed as another person using the Internet and other forms of online communications.

Date rape: Rape in which the victim and the rapist were previously known to each other and may have interacted in some socially appropriate manner. Also know as "acquaintance rape."

Domestic violence: Subjecting a spouse, partner, or family member to any forceful physical, social and psychological behavior so as to coerce that person without regard to his or her rights. Also known as battering.

Elder abuse: The injury, maltreatment, or neglect of an older person from a physical, psychological, or material perspective.

Family and intimate violence: The injury, maltreatment, or neglect of an older person from a physical, psychological, or material perspective.

Self-mutilation: Any self-directed repetitive behavior that causes physical injury. Self-mutilation acts are not usually suicide attempts but rather behaviors meant to express or release emotional turmoil. Examples include skin cutting with razors or knives (the most common pattern); burning or biting oneself; picking ones skin or hair; and extreme injuries such as auto-enucleation (self-removal of the eye), castration, or amputation.

Sexual harassment: Behavior that may include unwanted sexual attention or advance an/or the use of threats or bribery to obtain sexual favors. The offensive conduct often interferes with a person's ability to perform regular duties at work and creates an intimidating or hostile work environment.

Stalking: Behaviors directed toward a specific person that involve repeated visual or physical proximity; nonconsensual communication; verbal, written, or implied threats; or a combination of these behaviors that would cause fear in a reasonable person.

■■■■
Websites

Children's Defense Fund: http://www.childrensdefense.org

Futures Without Violence: http://www.futureswithoutviolence.org

National Center for Missing and Exploited Children: http://www.missingkids.com

National Center on Elder Abuse: http://www.ncea.aoa.gov

National Committee for the Prevention of Elder Abuse: http://www.preventelderabuse.org

NYC Gay and Lesbian Antiviolence Project: http://www.avp.org

Rape, Abuse, and Incest National Network (RAINN): http://www.rainn.org

Self-Abuse Finally Ends (SAFE): http://www.selfinjury.com

U.S. Department of Justice, Office on Violence Against Women: http://www.ovw.usdoj.gov

■■■■
References

1. World Health Organization. (2002). *World report on violence and health: Summary*. Geneva: WHO.

2. United Nations Department of Public Information. (2008). Unite to end violence against women fact sheet. DPI/2498. Geneva: UN.

3. United Nations Population Fund. (2010). Ending widespread violence against women. Available at: http://www.unfpa.org/gender/violence.htm

4. Tjaden, P., & Thoennes, N. (2000). Extent, nature, and consequences of intimate partner violence: Findings from the National Violence Against Women Survey. Washington, DC: National Institute of Justice, Office of Justice Programs, U.S. Department of Justice.

5. D'Emilio, J., & Freedman, E. B. (1998). *Intimate matters*. New York, NY: Harper and Row.

6. Davis, A. Y. (1983). *Women, race, and class*. New York, NY: Vintage Books.

7. Centers for Disease Control and Prevention. (2005). Behavioral risk factor surveillance system survey data. Atlanta, GA: U.S. Department of Health and Human Services, CDC.

8. Greenfeld, L. A., & Henneberg, M. A. (2001). Victim and offender self-reports of alcohol involvement in crime. *Journal of the National Institute on Alcohol Abuse and Alcoholism* 25(1): 20–31.

9. Bureau of Justice Statistics. (2004). American Indians and crime, 1992–2002. Washington, DC: Bureau of Justice Statistics, U.S. Department of Justice.

10. Sparks, G. (2012). *Media effects research: A basic overview*. New York: Cengage Learning.

11. Centers for Disease Control and Prevention. (2003). *Costs of intimate partner violence against women in the United States*. Atlanta, GA: U.S. Department of Health and Human Services.

12. Kyckelhahn, T. (2011). *Justice expenditures and employment, 1982–2007*. Bureau of Justice Statistics. Washington, DC: U.S. Department of Justice.

13. Campbell, J., Jones, A. S., Dienemann, J., et al. (2002). Intimate partner violence and physical health consequences. *Archives of Internal Medicine* 162: 1157–1163.

14. García-Moreno, C., Jansen, H. A. F. M., Watts, C., et al. (2005). *WHO multicountry study on women's health and eomestic violence against women. Initial results on prevalence, health outcomes and women's responses*. Geneva, Switzerland: WHO.

15. National Center on Domestic and Sexual Violence. (2008). *Darfur: Gendered violence and rape as a weapon of genocide*. Available at: http://www.ncdsv.org/images/darfurgenderedviolencerapeweapon.pdf

16. National Institute of Justice. (2007). *Stalking*. Available at: http://www.nij.gov/topics/crime/stalking/welcome.htm

17. National Center for Victims of Crime. (2003). *Stalking technology outpaces state laws*. Available at: http://www.ncvc.org/src/main.aspx?dbName=DocumentViewer&DocumentID=37137

18. Greenfeld, L. A., Rand, M. R., Craven, P., et al. (1998). *Violence by intimates: Analysis of data on crimes by current or former spouses, boyfriends and girlfriends*.

Bureau of Justice Statistics Factbook. Washington, DC: U.S. Department of Justice.

19. McDonald, R., Jouriles, E. N., Ramisetty-Mikler, S., et al. (2006). Estimating the number of American children living in partner-violent families. *Journal of Family Psychology* 20(1): 137–142.

20. Family Violence Prevention Fund. (2003). The effects of domestic violence on children. Available at: http://www.endabuse.org.

21. Voices for Change: Immigrant Women and State Policy Center for Women in Government and Civil Society. (2004). *Building bridges to stop violence against immigrant women: Effective strategies and promising models for reaching and serving immigrant women.* Albany, NY: University at Albany.

22. Raj, A., & Silverman, J. (2002). Violence against immigrant women: The roles of culture, context, and legal immigrant status on intimate partner violence. *Violence Against Women* 8(3): 17–20.

23. Greenfield, L. (2005). *Criminal victimization in the United States, 2003 statistical tables.* National Crime Victimization Survey (NCJ 207811). Washington, DC: U.S. Department of Justice.

24. National Institute of Justice. (2010). *Measuring intimate partner (domestic) violence.* Available at: http://www.nij.gov/topics/crime/intimate-partner-violence/measuring.htm

25. Wijma, B. (2003). Gynecologists could help identify sexual, physical, and emotional abuse. *Lancet* 361: 2107–2113.

26. National Coalition of Anti-Violence Programs. (2012). *Lesbian, gay, bisexual, transgender, queer and HIV-affected intimate partner violence 2010.* Available at: http://avp.org/documents/IPVReportfull-web_000.pdf

27. Peterson, R., Saltzman, L., Goodwin, M., et al. (2004). *Key scientific issues for research on violence occurring around the time of pregnancy.* National Center for Chronic Disease Prevention and Heath Promotion, and the National Center for Injury Prevention and Control, Centers for Disease Control and Prevention. Atlanta, GA: CDC.

28. Lipsky, S., Holt, V., Easterling, T., et al. (2003). Impact of police-reported intimate partner violence during pregnancy on birth outcomes. *Obstetrics and Gynecology* 102: 557–564.

29. Liebschutz, J., Frayne, S., Saxe, G., et al. (2003). Violence against women: A physician's guide to identification and management. Philadelphia, PA: American College of Physicians/American Society of Internal Medicine.

30. Nosek, M. A., Hughes, R. B., Taylor, H. B., et al. (2004). Violence against women with disabilities: the role of physicians in filling the treatment gap. In: S. L. Welner & F. Haseltine (eds.), *Welner's Guide to care of women with disabilities* (pp. 333–345). Philadelphia, PA: Lippincott, Williams and Wilkins.

31. U.S. Department of Health and Human Services, Administration on Children, Youth and Families. (2012). *Child maltreatment 2010.* Washington, DC: U.S. Government Printing Office.

32. National Center on Child Abuse Prevention Research. (2001). *Current trends in child abuse prevention, reporting, and fatalities: The 1999 fifty state survey.* Chicago, IL: Prevent Child Abuse America.

33. U.S. Department of Health and Human Services, National Center on Child Abuse and Neglect. (1996). *Third national incidence study of child abuse and neglect: Final report (NIS-3).* Washington, DC: U.S. Government Printing Office.

34. Heyman, R. E., & Slep, A. M. S. (2002). Do child abuse and interparental violence lead to adulthood family violence? *Journal of Marriage and Family* 64: 864–870.

35. OWL. (2009). *Elder abuse: A women's issue.* Available at: http://www.owl-national.org/Mothers_Day_Reports_files/OWL_MothersDay_Report_09_Final_2.pdf

36. National Center on Elder Abuse. (2005). *Elder abuse prevalence and encidence.* Available at: http://www.ncea.aoa.gov/Main_Site/pdf/publication/Final Statistics050331.pdf

37. Truman, J. (2011). *Criminal victimization, 2010.* Washington, DC: U.S. Department of Justice.

38. Bureau of Justice Statistics. (2012). *National Crime Victimization Survey (NCVS), 1973–2010.* Available at: http://bjs.ojp.usdoj.gov/index.cfm?ty=dcdetail&iid=245

39. National Institute of Justice. (2003). *Youth victimization: Prevalence and implications.* Washington, DC: U.S. Department of Justice.

40. Kilpatrick, D. G., Amstadter, A. B., Resnick, H. S., et al. (2007). Rape-related PTSD: Issues and interventions. *Psychiatric Times* 24(7): 315–318.

41. Langton, L. and Planty, M. (2011). *Hate crime, 2003–2009*. Washington, DC: U.S. Department of Justice.

42. U.S. Equal Employment Opportunity Commission. (2012). *Sexual harassment charges EEOC & FEPAs combined: FY1997–FY2011*. Available at: http://www.eeoc.gov/eeoc/statistics/enforcement/sexual_harassment.cfm

43. American Association of University Women. (2006). *Drawing the line: Sexual harassment on campus*. Washington, DC: AAUW.

Chapter Fifteen

Women in the Workforce

Chapter Objectives

On completion of this chapter, the student should be able to discuss:

1. Historical trends related to women in the workforce.

2. How the recession of 2008–2009 has affected employment opportunities.

3. Work-related barriers specific to low-income women and women on welfare.

4. The wage gap between the two genders and the concepts of the "glass ceiling" and the "sticky floor."

5. Connections between work, family, and personal life.

6. The importance of benefits and family-friendly work policies, and how the lack of these policies hurts women.

7. How housework, child care, elder care, and the work environment influence women's well-being.

8. How work-related stress effects women's mental health.

9. Common types of injuries and hazards in the workplace, and ways to protect against them.

10. Global dimensions of women in the workforce.

11. Ways for employers and employees to increase productivity and satisfaction.

womenshealth.jbpub.com

Women's Health Online is a great source for supplementary women's health information for both students and instructors. Visit

http://womenshealth.jbpub.com

to find a variety of useful tools for learning, thinking, and teaching.

Introduction

Over the past century, women have gone from being a workplace rarity to an essential part of the workforce. In 1900, women made up roughly one-fifth (18%) of the labor force. By 1950, these numbers had risen to 30%, and today women make up just under half of the labor force (47% in 2011).[1,2] Today, women become doctors, accountants, astronauts, politicians, or members of any other occupation with greater ease than any previous generation. It is difficult to overstate the importance of these changes. Throughout the 19th century and through a good deal of the 20th century, women were banned, either explicitly or in practice, from entering a number of vocations. Women who did have jobs systematically received less pay than men working those same positions and were more likely to be working in low-paid, low-status positions. Discrimination also existed in universities and colleges that offered the necessary training for many jobs. Major universities like Princeton and Yale did not admit women until the 1960s, and a few public military colleges did not admit women until the 1990s. Women's participation in the workforce and enrollment in colleges and universities grew throughout the 20th century. In addition, the amount of money they earned steadily increased (**Figure 15.1**).

Despite this progress, sexism and discrimination against women in the workplace continue to exist in many forms. On average, women only make less money than men working in comparable jobs. The average gender gap has remained at about 81% over the past decade, with wider income gaps in many industries. In addition, women are still not reaching the highest echelons of the work world in great numbers. In 2010, just 18 of *Fortune* magazine's top 500 companies had female CEOs (roughly 4%); only 14% had women holding at least one-fourth of their officer positions.

The greater presence of women in the workforce has highlighted many new issues, including pay differentials between genders, the balancing of work and family, health and safety in the workplace, and the struggle for many women between choosing a career and choosing to stay home. Women typically shoulder more of the burden of family and household responsibilities than men, often working at their paying jobs and then taking on a "second shift" of responsibilities when

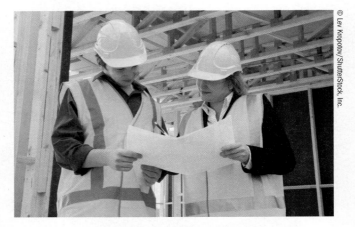

■ While women make up half of the workforce, they continue to earn less than their male counterparts for the same responsibilities.

they return home. Some women who choose to stay home feel conflicted by their choice, as do some women who choose to pursue a career and leave their child with a surrogate provider.

Health and safety issues also affect women in the workplace. Workstations, tools, and protective equipment have traditionally been designed for men and therefore may compromise the health and safety of women. Health hazards from biological, chemical, and disease-causing agents exist in many predominantly female occupations, including

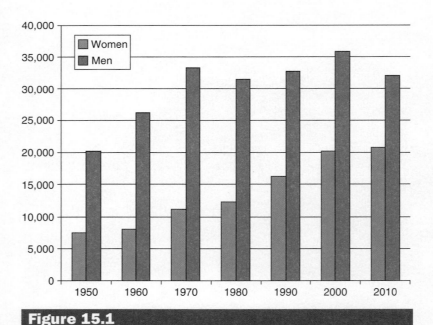

Figure 15.1

Median U.S. Incomes by Sex, 1950–2010*

Source: Data from U.S. Census. (2011). Historical Income Tables: People. Available at: http://www.census.gov/hhes/www/income/data/historical/people/

the textile, laundry, and meat industries; health care; and food preparation. Additionally, physically intense activities or exposure to certain substances while on the job can harm working women who are pregnant.

In addition, women currently in their 20s and late teens face the toughest job market in decades. Today, there are millions more qualified people looking for work than there are positions. Most women graduating college 10 or 20 years ago could count on their degrees and hard work to provide them with full-time employment, but today's college graduates have no such guarantees. National and global economic crises, followed by slow economic growth, have caused millions of people to lose their jobs and many companies and organizations to delay or stop creating new positions. Although employment levels have started to recover, today the average unemployment rate is more than 50% more than what it was before the recession of 2008–2009. For men and women

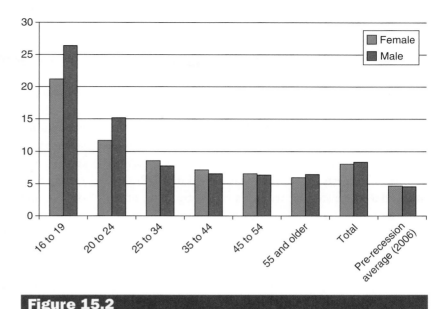

Figure 15.2

Unemployment rates by age and sex, July 2012

Source: Data from Bureau of Labor Statistics. (2012). Labor Force Statistics.

25 and under, the unemployment rate has more than doubled (**Figure 15.2**).

This chapter discusses gender differences in the workplace, the balancing of work and family, and occupational safety issues. In addition, the chapter presents strategies for reducing job stress and increasing workplace satisfaction.

Trends and Issues

Historical Issues

In colonial times, all members of the family worked together as an economic unit. Most of women's jobs outside the home appeared to be extensions of their household duties—making clothing, cleaning house, teaching, or cooking—but some women worked as blacksmiths, silversmiths, and shopkeepers. When their husbands were off at sea or at war, some women operated family businesses; other women accompanied troops to war and served as nurses and cooks.

The Industrial Revolution brought women into the factories, providing many with new skills, educational opportunities, and social outlets. Many European women immigrated to the United States to work as indentured servants, with hopes of a more promising future. Workplace violence, sexual harassment, and unfair pay were a fact of life, and many women were physically and sexually

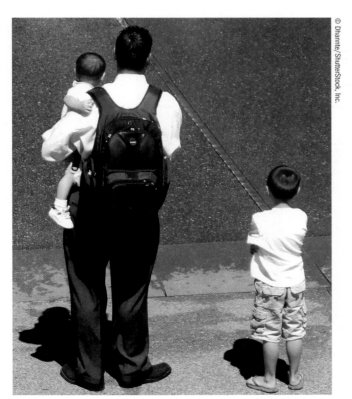

■ Men and women are redefining traditional roles and responsibilities for their families.

abused on the job, or deprived of personal freedom and financial compensation. Because many women's positions were viewed as temporary, many working women earned enough wages to help make ends meet, but not enough to make a comfortable living.

In the mid-1800s, women's rights advocates like Charlotte Woodward campaigned to allow women rights to their earnings (under existing laws, husbands had full ownership of their wives' money). The New York Married Women's Property Act, which was passed in 1848, represented a major step for women's rights; by 1860, other states had passed similar laws. It was not until 1974, however, that Congress passed the Equal Credit Opportunity Act, which barred creditors from discriminating against women on the basis of sex or marital status.

Throughout the 19th and early 20th centuries, many women found opportunities to earn wages, often working as nurses, governesses, cooks, domestic servants, and teachers. In 1869, Wyoming became the first state to provide equal pay for female teachers; California followed soon thereafter.[5] Although exceptions did arise, most women continued to work in positions where men defined their authority and control.

When the United States entered World War II in 1941, jobs available to women increased dramatically. "Rosie the Riveter," the factory worker appearing on posters underneath the slogan "We can do it!" became the symbol for women workers in the U.S. defense industries. More than 6 million women, from all backgrounds and from all over the country, worked at industrial jobs that challenged traditional notions of women's capabilities and ensured U.S. productivity that helped win the war. During the war years, women became streetcar conductors, taxicab drivers, machine operators, business managers, and railroad workers. They unloaded freight, worked in lumber mills and steel mills, and made munitions. This trend led to a rise in salaries and an overall commitment by women to their jobs; however, most of these women lost their positions when the war ended in 1945.

Women became more likely to enter the workforce grew throughout the 20th century. As women became more likely to work and began earning more money,

their contributions to family incomes increased. In 1970, women contributed 27% of the average family income; by 2009 that number had risen to 37%.[2] Women also started becoming more educated. Today, women are more likely than men to attend college, a major change from 30 years ago. The desegregation of college majors has led more women into fields such as architecture, business, and the sciences.[3] Many women are postponing childbearing and marriage, having smaller families, or focusing on their careers and personal development before taking on the roles of wife and mother. Women have opened up numerous opportunities for themselves by attending college, fighting for equal rights in the workplace, and breaking barriers in many occupations traditionally associated with men. Despite all of the advances, however, gender discrimination in jobs persists.

Occupation Trends of Women

Of the 120 million women in the United States, 59% are either working or looking for work.[2] Women between the ages 35 to 44 are more likely to be working than women in other age groups (**Figure 15.3**). This may be partly due to the fact that mothers are more likely to participate in the

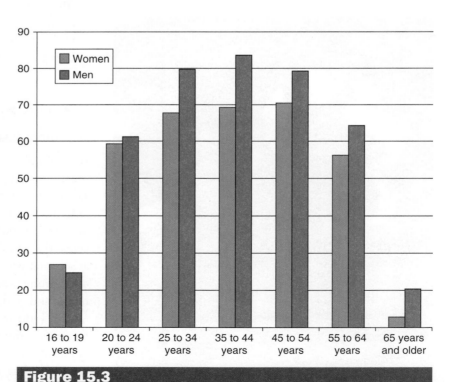

Figure 15.3

Percentage of Working Men and Women by Age, 2010*

Source: Data from U.S. Bureau of Statistics. (2011). Women in the Labor Force.

Table 15.1	Employment Rates and Average Weekly Income of Women, Ages 25–64, by Educational Attainment, 2010

	Average Weekly Income ($)	Employment Rate
Total	704	66.4
Less than high school	388	41.4
High school graduate, no college	543	61.3
Some college or associate's degree	638	69.0
College graduates, total	986	76.3
Bachelor's degree	909	74.7
Master's degree	1,127	78.5
Professional degree	1,362	79.6
Doctoral degree	1,352	86.1

Source: Modified from U.S. Department of Labor. (2011). *Women in the workforce: A databook.*

Table 15.2	Selected Occupations with Strong Gender Divisions, 2010

Occupation	Women's Percentage of the Workforce
Preschool and kindergarten teachers	97.0%
Registered nurses	91.1%
Elementary and middle school teachers	81.8%
Librarians	82.8%
Medical and health service managers	72.5%
Psychologists	66.7%
Tax examiners, collectors, and revenue agents	66.1%
Writers and authors	63.5%
Accountants and auditors	60.1%
Public relations managers	60.0%
Janitors and building cleaners	33.2%
Environmental scientists	26.2%
Dentists	25.5%
Chefs and head cooks	19.0%
Clergy members	17.5%
Broadcast and sound engineering technicians	9.9%
Civil engineers	9.7%
Television and video camera operators	7.2%
Fire fighters	3.6%
Electricians	1.5%

Source: Data from U.S. Bureau of Labor Statistics. (2011). *Employment and earnings.*

workforce as their children get older. The stronger an education a woman has, the more likely she is to be working, and the more money she is likely to make (**Table 15.1**). More than three-fourths of women age 25 years or older who are employed are college graduates.

Although women work in all industries and contribute in multiple ways to the economy, their participation is often concentrated in certain sectors. Women make up a strong majority of many positions in health care, education, communications, for example, but continue to be underrepresented in the fields of engineering, computer science, and construction work (**Table 15.2**) Nearly one of every five employed women works as a teacher (excluding postsecondary positions), secretary, manager or administrator, or cashier.[3]

According to the U.S. Census Bureau, women own just under one-third (29%) of all nonfarm businesses, totaling nearly 6.5 million businesses.[4] More than half of such firms are in the services industry, particularly business services and personal services. Women cite a variety of reasons for starting their own businesses:

- Flexibility
- Independence
- Outlet for creativity
- Relief from sexual harassment in the workplace
- An exit from poverty[4]

Over the past generation, the number of women in the workforce who have young children has increased. Today, 64% of mothers with children under the age of 6, and 77% of mothers with children ages 6 to 17, are in

■ By breaking the barriers of traditionally male-dominated fields, women have created greater opportunities for themselves in the workplace.

the workforce.[2] The number of dual-earner families also has increased. Before World War II, less than 10% of the workforce was from a dual-earner family. Today, more than 57% are dual-earner families. In nearly 75% of dual-earner families, both partners work full time.[3] Despite this change, many two-parent families with young children are having difficulty making ends meet. Fifty percent of young children are members of families with incomes less than $40,000; 25% are in families making less than $20,000.[5]

Special Populations

Women with Disabilities in the Workplace

Just over 14 million women with disabilities live in the United States; one in five of these women are either working or looking for work.[2] Women with disabilities confront many barriers in the workplace:

- Lack of job opportunities or appropriate jobs
- Inaccessible work environments
- Discouragement by family and friends
- Fear of losing health insurance or Medicaid
- Little or no accessible parking or public transportation nearby

Women who are able to get a job may still need to spend time and energy obtaining functional assistance, flexible work arrangements or hours, handrails or ramps, or other equipment. The severity of a woman's disability has the greatest influence on her employment status. Women with mild disabilities are about four-fifths as likely as women without disabilities to have jobs, but women with severe disabilities are only one-third as likely.[2] Women with disabilities also earn, on average, less than women with no disabilities. Women with disabilities that directly affect their work are more likely to live below the poverty level than those people without work disabilities. Approximately 40% of women with a severe work disability are living in poverty.[15]

Older Women

Women have increasingly been participating in the part-time labor force during the traditional years of retirement. This trend is partly attributable to the recession of 2008–2009 disproportionately affecting younger workers, and partly because individuals are living longer and healthier lives, thus finding their retirement

savings insufficient to make ends meet. Older women may have special health needs as members of the workforce, including the need for easy or disabled access to a work site, close proximity to restrooms, and seats with supportive backs or armrests to assist in getting up and down. Employers should be aware of the special needs of older workers, as they provide a valuable and often highly educated supplement to the workforce.

Socioeconomic Issues

Low-income women—particularly those living in poverty—face many challenges when trying to find and keep a job. For these women, the consequences of not finding employment or the inability to maintain a job can have devastating consequences. Low-wage workers are disproportionately women and minorities with family responsibilities. Women heads of household represent a high percentage of this group. Welfare-to-work programs have helped some of these women move from welfare into paid employment. Most of these individuals work in service industries characterized by low hourly wages (averaging about $8–10 per hour), however, and are at significant risk for layoffs or workhour reduction in a weakened economy.

"I'm lucky enough to have a full-time house-husband. Rick stays at home and takes care of the boys, while I go in to work at the medical center. I'm able to earn enough to pay the bills, but with the long hours I work, there's no way I'd be able to clean up, cook, and take care of the kids. I don't know what I'd do without him."

33-year-old doctor and mother of two

■ Childcare remains a major challenge for working parents.

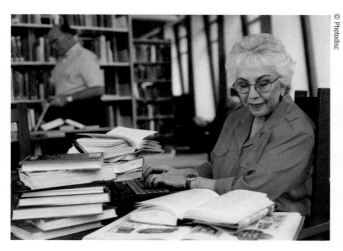

■ Older workers may have additional needs in their workplaces.

Work opportunities for low-income women or women on welfare are often limited because many persons in this situation lack education, training, transportation, or child care. Many jobs that are available either cover odd hours or have changing schedules. Both situations make transportation and finding childcare difficult. Low-income women who live in rural areas with little or no public transportation often have trouble getting to and from job training centers or jobs. Other women are caught between taking a job to put food on the table and leaving young children at home alone because of lack of child care. Even when women are able to find transportation and child care, the costs for these services may consume most of their incomes.

Low-wage jobs often provide few or no benefits, such as healthcare coverage, paid sick leave, or paid family leave. Furthermore, because the positions do not require advanced skills, employers are typically quick to replace a woman who may have to miss work because her child is sick.[7] Women who find work after receiving welfare are less likely than other working women to have jobs offering paid sick days, family leave, or flexible job schedules, even though they were more likely to have children with chronic health problems.[8]

Equal Pay for Equal Work

A great challenge for working women has been the battle of receiving equal pay for performing equal work. In almost every field, men in the same jobs earn more than women with the same education and years of experience. In 2010, women who worked full time, regardless of age, race, or educational attainment, earned an average weekly salary of $657 compared with $821 for men, or just over

Table 15.3	Women's Median Weekly Earnings Compared to Men's by Selected Characteristics, 2010	
Characteristic Age	**Women ($)**	**% of Men's Earnings**
Total, 16 years or older	657	80%
16 to 19	323	91%
20 to 24	445	93%
25 to 34	634	89%
35 to 44	709	78%
45 to 54	712	74%
55 to 64	727	75%
65 and older	602	76%
Race/Ethnicity		
White	684	81%
Black	592	94%
Hispanic or Latino	508	91%
Asian	773	83%
Marital Status		
Never Married	557	95%
Currently Married	708	76%
Divorced	680	85%
Separated	561	86%
Widowed	629	80%

Source: Data from Bureau of Labor Statistics. (2011). *Highlights of women's earnings in 2010*. U.S. Department of Labor.

four-fifths (81%) of what men make (**Table 15.3**).[2] Earning differences between genders varied by demographic features, with the greatest contrast arising between men and women aged 45 to 54, with women earning 74% as much as men in this age range. The narrowest gap between earnings was among workers 16 to 24 years old; in this demographic group, women earned 93% of what men earned (**Figure 15.4**). Wage gaps also exist by race, ethnicity, and other factors. There is less gender disparity among black and Hispanic/Latino workers than there is among workers who are white or of Asian descent. The wage gap narrows to 95% for women who have never been married, but rises to 73% among women who are currently married (Table 15.3). As a result of these differences, the average 25-year-old woman who works full time, year-round, until retiring at age 65 will earn more than half a million dollars less over her lifetime than the average working man.[9]

The pay gap is closing in some fields, but not in others and not quickly enough. In some professions, pay discrepancies are quite small, but in others they remain much

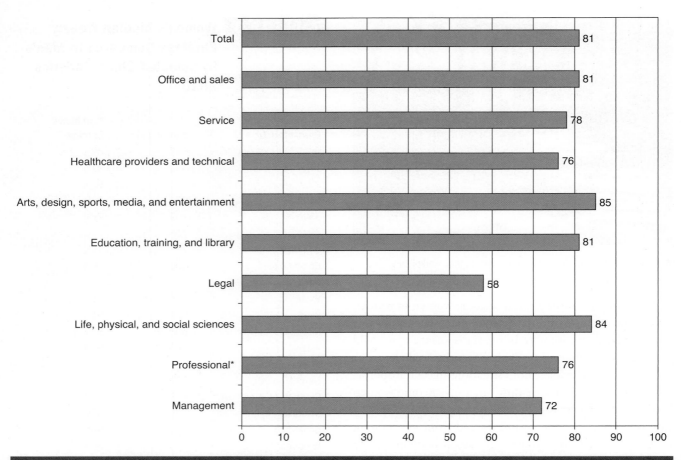

Figure 15.4

Women's Earnings as a Percent of Men's for Selected Occupations, 2010

Source: Data from Bureau of Labor Statistics. (2011) Women in the Workforce: A Databook.

larger (Figure 15.4). For example, in comparison to men in the same occupation, on a weekly average:

- Women lawyers make almost $500 less
- Women bartenders make about $70 less
- Women engineers make about $150 less
- Women doctors make nearly $500 less
- Women registered nurses make about $100 less
- Women professors make nearly $300 less[2]

Not only do women make less money than men in virtually every profession, but women are clustered in low-paying professions. Many women are worried about the "sticky floor"—employment practices that keep full-time, working women right at the poverty threshold level. One-fourth of women who work full time do not earn enough to move their families above the federal poverty threshold. Women also fight against the "glass ceiling"

phenomenon—employment practices that effectively keep working women out of top-ranking positions. Women remain strongly underrepresented in leadership positions in industry, politics, and other areas.

Besides lower wages, a grim reality for working women is the lack of paid sick or family leave; childcare benefits; flexibility of schedule associated with employment; and employer-provided health insurance, pension plans, or retirement benefits. According to an AFL-CIO survey:

- 97% of women are worried about healthcare costs
- 88% do not have retirement benefits
- 78% are concerned about a lack of job benefits
- 57% do not have equal pay for equal work
- 39% do not have affordable health insurance
- 29% do not have paid sick leave
- 24% do not have paid vacation time[10]

Pay gaps in women's earnings affect families as well as women. With more women in the workforce, more families depend on dual incomes. In addition, women are the head of households with no spouse present of one in eight (12%) of households. Women maintain 14% of White families, 47% of Black families, and 24% of Hispanic-origin families. Nearly one-third of all families maintained by women live below the poverty level.[11] Women occupy a greater proportion of low-paying jobs than men and generally receive fewer benefits and less flexibility in their working conditions. Minorities, especially minority women, are even more likely to be in these less desirable positions. The average weekly earnings for White women are 17% higher than Black women's and 32% higher than those of Hispanic women.[2] While women overall are more likely than men to be among the working poor, African American and Hispanic women are two to three times more likely than White women to be members of the working poor.[12]

Achieving Equal Pay

One key factor for women who are seeking to help themselves is education. Completing high school is the first step in increasing one's potential income. Women with high school diplomas earned an average of $540 per week in 2010—about 40% more than women without a diploma. Women's average earnings increases steadily with income: Women with bachelor's degrees earned an average of $910 a week, and women with doctoral degrees earned an average of $1,350—roughly 2.5 and 4 times as much as women without high school diplomas.[2]

To achieve fair compensation for their work, women should learn what fair and equitable pay is for their position and experience, be aware of the laws that prohibit pay discrimination against women, and support efforts to bring "pay equity" to their workplaces. Employees should encourage their employers to implement a pay equity policy, along with a way of creating a grading system to categorize jobs based on education, skills, and experience.

Balancing Work and Family Life

Women today face a growing challenge of combining family and work.[13] Women may juggle many tasks to perform well at work, run a household, provide a loving home for their children, spend quality time with their partners, and provide care for their elders. Having these roles can be a source of satisfaction, but can also contribute to strain and stress.

© Ryan McVay/Photodisc/Getty Images

■ Many women who have entered the workforce continue to work on household chores and child care when they return home from work.

One in five working parents is a member of the "sandwich generation," meaning that the individual is caring for both children and elderly relatives. More than one-third of those with elder responsibilities—men and women alike—reduced their work hours or took time off to provide the necessary care.[14] Fifty-four percent of Americans say they will probably be responsible for the care of an elderly parent or other relative in the next 10 years. Women account for 70% of the unpaid people caring for the elderly; they also constitute the majority of paid workers, including nurses, nurse's aides, and home healthcare workers.[11]

Child Care

Childcare facilities, relatives, and nannies have become a necessity for working families with children. The United States is one of only three countries in the world that does not offer paid time off for new mothers. More than three-fourths of preschool-age children with employed mothers are regularly cared for by someone other than their parents. Almost two-thirds of children from birth to age 6 spend some time in nonparental child care.[15] A babysitter or nanny regularly cares for 6% of children in the child's home. Families with children between the ages of 3 and 5 say that child care is their third greatest expense after housing and food.[11] The cost of full-day child care can range from $5,000 to $25,000 per year per child. In addition to the high costs, 9 out of 10 Americans describe finding quality child care as "difficult."[11,15] Only 12 states require childcare providers to have any early childhood training before minding children in their homes.[16]

Child care does not always ease the stress for working women. In fact, 52% of women say that childcare problems affect their ability to perform well at work.[13] Eighty percent of employers reported that childcare problems force employees to lose work time. In addition, only 9% of sampled workers with children in daycare facilities report feeling "very successful" in balancing work and family.[17]

The Current Situation

Working Mother magazine rates the 100 best companies for working mothers every year, based on various measures of flexibility within the workplace, such as flextime, telecommuting, and job sharing. The magazine also rates companies based on their propensity to listen to employees by surveying them on work–life topics and, in response

to the survey results, adding features such as lactation rooms.[18] However, when these benefits are present, they do not always extend to those in greatest need. In many organizations, workers in low-wage jobs are half as likely as managers and professionals to have flextime; low-wage workers are also more likely to lose a day's pay when they must stay home to care for a sick child.[19]

Within many companies, only 20% of employees have access to childcare information and referral services; 25% have access to eldercare information and referral services. Only 12% of employees with children younger than age 6 have childcare services on or near their work site that are operated or sponsored by their employers, and these facilities are usually located at headquarters, where managers and executives work.[5] Even those lower-paid employees who have access to nearby childcare facilities usually find the fees too high for their earnings. Many of the company-operated daycare centers are open only during regular business hours, such as 8 a.m. to 6 p.m.; however, close to one-third of employees with young children have unpredictable or erratic work schedules, and these are the employees who are most likely to earn less than $25,000 per year.[5,10]

Maintaining Balance

Many women suffer from job- and family-related stress, but do not feel they have any options that would relieve

---

Gender Dimensions: Health Differences Between Men and Women

Motherhood

Motherhood is often a woman's principal source of stress; she may enjoy this role and be committed to it, but nevertheless may feel strained by it. Her stress may be exacerbated by society's normative expectation of "good mothering," which does not usually encompass full-time employment.[26,27] Working may increase a woman's opportunities for obtaining resources, power, social identity, positive self-esteem, and involvement with others, but is often a major source of stress. The benefits of work depend on the woman's working conditions, her marital status, her stability in her job, and her ability to handle many roles at once. The more demanding and difficult the job and the less supportive the workplace, the greater the negative spillover from one's work life to one's personal life.

Working mothers often feel the stresses of work significantly more than working fathers. Mothers, for example, often must juggle the responsibilities of maintaining high job performance and being the primary caregiver for children. Single mothers frequently carry this double burden alone, resulting in even greater stress. Although men perform more household responsibilities than they did 20 years ago, women spend more time than men doing housework even as their workloads outside the home have increased. One study showed that women spend 31 hours per week doing paid work and 26 hours on

family care; by comparison, men spend 40 hours per week doing paid labor and 14 hours on family care or housework.[28] Housework and family care tend to be more unbalancing to a person's sense of well-being because the tasks are often more repetitive, dirtier, menial, unending, and inflexible. When men do housework, it is often work that can be scheduled, such as lawn maintenance or repairs. In contrast, women are often responsible for cleaning, cooking, and caring for children—duties that cannot be postponed.[26] Married men are more likely to have partners who are willing to take care of tasks at home, making men's lives more balanced. On the other hand, men in general do not adjust their time in response to their wives' employment status.[29]

Besides doing more housework, mothers spend more time on average with their children than fathers do. Mothers spend an average of 3.2 hours per workday with their children, whereas fathers spend an average of 2.3 hours with their offspring. Seventy percent of parents feel that they do not have enough time to spend with their children. In fact, both parents have less time for themselves than they did 20 years ago; fathers have 1.2 hours during the workday, whereas mothers have 0.9 hour.[13] Couples also have less time together. Nearly 46% of married women or women living with someone work different schedules than their partners do.[22]

that stress. Some women aspire to the "superwoman" ideal of having a high-paying, successful career, while keeping a clean house, preparing homecooked meals, spending quality time with her children, and being a loving and supportive wife. Women need to find their individual balance of work and family responsibilities and make changes if they are dissatisfied with their situation. For women with partners, open communication about the sharing of responsibilities can help couples to establish a good balance within their home. In situations where both partners work, sharing of chores is essential to minimize stress and maximize quality family time. Single women should also find balance between work and home responsibilities. This may mean reviewing policies at work that allow flextime or telecommuting, or advocating for these options if they are not available. Women who own businesses should set examples for pay equity, fair workplaces, supportive work environments, and family-friendly policies.

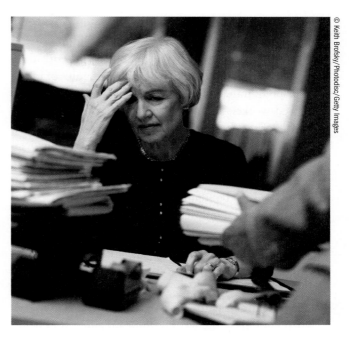

■ Long-term exposure to work-related stress can lead to higher levels of depression, anxiety, and other ilnesses.

Health and Safety in the Workplace

Work-related stress may come from unsupportive workplace policies, unfair pay, concerns for quality child care, inflexible scheduling, or lack of support and help at home. With the economy still recovering from national and economic recessions, concerns over downsizing and layoffs create added pressures. Other stressors revolve around lack of control at work, such as high workload demands, unreasonable deadlines, role ambiguity and conflict, repetitive and boring work, and strained relationships with coworkers or supervisors.[20] This kind of stress often produces little job satisfaction and a poor sense of well-being. The following jobs are associated with high stress because of the need to respond to others' demands and timetables with little control over events:

- Secretaries
- Waitresses
- Middle managers
- Police officers
- Editors
- Medical interns[21]

Long-term exposure to job stress can lead to higher levels of depression, anxiety, and other mental illnesses. As jobs become more demanding and less rewarding, employees often feel more stressed by the end of the workday and have less time and energy for their families. Twenty-five

percent of employees reported feeling stressed often or very often over the past 3 months, and 25% described feeling emotionally drained often or very often. More than one-fourth of employees are not in as good a mood as they would like for their families; 28% of people feel they have no energy for their families or other important people upon returning from work. This in turn creates a negative sense of well-being and results in negativity that affects a person's work performance.[21]

A person's work setting can create physical stress as well, because of noise, lack of privacy, poor lighting or ventilation, poor temperature control, or inadequate sanitary facilities. Physical stress on the body is a consequence of many different occupations. Jobs that require being on one's feet for long hours cause leg pain, swelling, and varicose veins; secretarial and desk-based jobs may cause neck and back aches and eye strain; and repetitive motions can cause musculoskeletal injuries to women on production lines. These difficulties are not restricted to gender, yet certain factors make women more susceptible to these types of injury. Equipment and workstations are often designed with men's larger body sizes in mind. Workstations and chairs that cannot be adjusted to the correct height for women promote poor posture; excessive reach; and strain on the neck, back, shoulders, and arms. Hand tools designed for larger hands may create unnecessary pain, stressed muscles, and calluses. Protective equipment and clothes that are too large are more likely to slip off, get caught in equipment, or create gaps for harmful chemicals to seep through.

Men are still more likely to be injured at work than women, in part because some jobs with high rates of injury are still predominately held by men. Almost two-thirds of injured workers are men, even though they work less than 60% of the total hours worked in the United States. However, in the fields of management, business, financial occupations, professional and related occupations, service occupations, and office and administrative support, women are more likely to be injured than men.[2]

Musculoskeletal injuries, also referred to as ergonomic injuries, disproportionately affect female workers. Although women account for only 33% of the people injured at work in the United States, they constitute 64% of repetitive motion injuries, which include the following conditions:

- **Carpal tunnel syndrome**—a condition that occurs when tendons in the wrist become inflamed after being aggravated
- **Tendonitis**—inflammation caused by friction from overuse of tendons
- Muscle strains from overexertion

Repetitive motions can injure the nerves, often those in the neck and hands. **Self-Assessment 15.1** discusses some of the common symptoms that nerve injuries can cause. Repetitive motion injuries account for more than half of all work time lost due to injuries and illness among women.[22]

Many women in low-wage occupations, or in occupations such as nursing aides, cashiers, maids, nurses, and assemblers that employ large numbers of women, are at significant risk of musculoskeletal disorders. Many of these jobs employ a large number of minorities, such as women who are Black, Hispanic, or of Southeast Asian descent. Back injuries are common among employees who need to lift large items or people. Correct lifting technique and using trolleys or coworkers to lift heavy objects greatly reduces the likelihood of injury.

Computer-related injuries have also become a significant concern in the workplace (**Self-Assessment 15.2**). Prolonged use of a keyboard or mouse, as well as sitting at a computer for long periods without stretching, can lead to

---

Self-Assessment 15.1

Symptoms of Repetitive Strain Injuries

- Do you have numbness and/or tingling in your hand that often feels worse when you lift your hand over your head?
- Do you often experience wrist weakness?
- Do you have numbness or tingling in the inside of your arm or into your fingers?
- Do you often feel numbness or tingling in multiple fingers and does your hand often "fall asleep" at night? Do you frequently drop objects?
- Do you have achiness, stiffness, tightness, or a burning sensation in your fingers, forearm, elbow, or shoulder?
- Do you experience muscle tightness at the side of your neck?

If you are experiencing one or more of these symptoms, you may have an overuse injury. Women should speak to their healthcare provider about preventing, reducing, and/or treating these types of disorders.

It's Your Health

Tips for Lifting Loads Safely

- Test the weight of the load before lifting. If too heavy or awkward, enlist a coworker to help or use a cart or dolly.
- Figure out where you need to move the load and how you are going to get to your destination before you lift.
- Lift with your legs shoulder-width apart and bend at your knees and hips, not your waist.
- Lift with tightened stomach muscles and using your leg muscles to reduce strain on your back.
- Hold the load close to your body at waist height.
- Avoid twisting during the lift; pivot your body or move your feet if necessary.
- Stretch and strengthen your back and stomach with exercises if lifting is part of your daily occupation.

It's Your Health

Tips for Preventing Injuries at Computer Workstations

- Reduce repetitive motions by alternating tasks throughout the day.
- Take frequent breaks, and stretch during the breaks if possible.
- Avoid bending or twisting your neck, or twisting your trunk.
- Keep shoulders relaxed and arms close by sides when working.
- Maintain good posture by keeping back and neck erect with shoulders relaxed.
- Keep your feet supported on the floor or on a footrest to reduce pressure on the lower back.
- Position your monitor so that it is centered directly in front of you and your neck is in a neutral or straight position when viewing it.
- Reduce glare on your screen by tilting the monitor, reducing overhead lights, and avoiding direct glare from windows.
- Every 30 minutes, look away from the screen and focus on something else.

Computer Workstation Evaluation Checklist

Posture

- Are your hands, wrists, and forearms straight, in-line, and roughly parallel to the floor?
- Is your head level or bent slightly forward and balanced?
- Is your head in line with your torso?
- Are your elbows close to your body and bent at 90 to 120 degrees?
- Are your feet fully supported by the floor or a footrest?
- Is your back fully supported when sitting vertical or leaning back slightly?
- Are your shoulders relaxed?
- Thighs and hips should be supported by a well-padded chair.
- Knees should be at the same height as the hips with the feet slightly forward.

Keyboard/Mouse

- Is your keyboard directly in front of you at a distance that allows your elbows to stay close to your body with your forearms approximately parallel with the floor?
- If you have limited desk room, do you use a keyboard tray to ensure adequate positioning?
- Is your keyboard in a position that lets you avoid reaching with the arms, leaning forward with the torso, and using extreme elbow angles?
- Can you reduce awkward wrist angles by lowering or raising the keyboard or chair to achieve a neutral wrist posture?

Seating

- Does your backrest support your lower back (lumbar area)?

- Does your seat width and depth accommodate your body?
- Does the seat front not press against the back of your knees and lower legs?
- Is the seat cushioning rounded and devoid of sharp edges?
- Do armrests support both forearms while you complete computer tasks?

Lighting

- Does your office have well-distributed diffuse lights that reduce glare on the computer screen?
- Does your office use light, matte colors and finishes on walls and ceilings to better reflect indirect lighting and reduce dark shadows and contrast?

Computer Screen

- Is your computer display screen at right angles to windows and light sources?
- Is the monitor clean and free of dust?
- Is the top of the screen at or below eye level?

Work Techniques

- Can you vary your computer tasks with other work activities or take short breaks and recovery pauses?

If you answered "No" to one or more of these questions, you are putting yourself at risk of injury. Use the checklist guidelines to improve your workplace health and avoid injuries.

Source: Adapted from the U.S. Department of Labor's Office of Safety and Health Administration's eTool, Computer Workstation Evaluation. (http://www.osha.gov/SLTC/etools/computerworkstations/checklist.html)

---

frequent muscle aches and nerve pain in the hands, arms, shoulders, neck, and back. Another common complaint of computer workers is visual discomfort, which is accompanied by eyestrain and headaches. Being aware of these risks and correcting improper posture and techniques can help prevent discomfort and injury.

Exposure to suspected carcinogens, allergens, or agents that cause respiratory illness are also serious concerns for many working women. Occupational exposures occur in many industries that employ large numbers of women and minorities:[23]

- Meat industry: exposure to suspected carcinogenic fumes
- Laundry/dry-cleaning industry: exposure to solvents that increase risk of kidney, cervical, bladder, skin, and liver cancer

- Textile industry: exposure to dust that causes a variety of lung diseases
- Metal-working industry: exposure to various chemicals that increase the risk of lung cancer
- Agriculture: exposure to pesticides and herbicides that may increase risk of non-Hodgkin's lymphoma and lung cancer
- Service industry: exposure to excessive cigarette smoke in bars or restaurants

Healthcare workers face additional hazards, including needlestick injuries, radiation, infectious diseases, and latex allergies. Approximately 600,000 to 800,000 needlestick injuries occur annually in healthcare settings, mostly involving nurses (more than 90% of whom are women). Needlestick injuries can cause serious infections from blood-borne pathogens, such as hepatitis C and HIV, creating both physical and emotional threats to workers.

In addition, 8% to 12% of healthcare workers who have frequent latex exposure develop sensitivity to this material. Symptoms can be as mild as contact dermatitis or as severe as **anaphylactic shock** (a severe and possibly fatal allergic response to a foreign substance, characterized by difficulty breathing and low blood pressure). The hazard from latex use is recognized in many different industries, including people in the latex-manufacturing industry, police, food handlers, and sanitation engineers. Pregnant women also appear to have a higher sensitivity to latex than the general population.[24]

The causes of most reproductive health problems are still unknown, but certain harmful substances can affect the health of pregnant women. Approximately 75% of all women of reproductive age are in the workforce, and more than half of all children born in the United States are born to working mothers. Women can be exposed to many different types of health hazards at work during pregnancy. Hazards from environmental pollutants in the workplace can cause multiple effects, depending on when the woman is exposed (see **Tables 15.6** and **15.7**). Substances may cause fetal damage, such as birth defects, low birthweight, developmental disorders, miscarriages, or stillbirths; infertility; menstrual cycle effects; and even childhood cancer. Other possible hazards to pregnant women include prolonged standing, lifting, and long work hours.

Other Health Concerns

Many women work in the informal work sector, employed in seasonal or domestic jobs that are not officially reported or recognized. Because these jobs often employ women who may not have official work permits or are "paid under the table" (meaning that the women do not receive benefits or declare taxes), women may face additional risks and insecurities. Injuries that occur during migrant crop picking, for example, often go untreated because the workers have few resources and are afraid of drawing the attention of authorities. Additionally, women who do odd jobs around the home, such as cleaning houses or painting, often do not have health coverage or disability coverage should an injury occur.

Hazardous work environments put many youths at risk of serious injuries. Young workers have been killed on construction sites, during robberies while tending retail establishments, and while working on farms.

Common nonfatal injuries incurred by young workers include sprains and strains, burns, cuts, and bruises. Homicide is the leading cause of death among youths in retail trade, accounting for nearly two-thirds of the youth fatalities in the industry. Most of these homicides are the result of robberies.[42]

Pregnant and lactating women may face additional stresses as they cope with sickness caused during pregnancy, co-workers' responses to pregnancy, and the time and privacy needs of nursing or pumping breast milk. Sexual harassment in the workplace is also a major form of stress (see Chapter 14).

© Photodisc

■ Needlestick injuries and latex allergies are two hazards faced by women working in health care.

I'm trying to get a permanent position in the United States as a research scientist so I don't have to go back to Russia. My boss makes me work long hours and always yells at me if I make a mistake. I was pregnant last year, and he still made me work with radiation in the lab. I was scared to complain for fear of losing my job. I didn't lose my job, but I ended up losing my baby.

32-year-old Russian scientist

Global Dimensions

Around the world, working women face many of the same challenges and opportunities that they do in the United States. Gender gaps in employment and pay persist, but have fallen in Europe and much of the developing world.[26,27] From 1990 to 2010, women's participation in the global labor market increased compared to men's. Progress in education has also occurred over the past generation. In the European Union, female students outnumber males in most universities.[27] Progress has been more uneven and slow in much of Asia, Latin America, and Africa, with large gender gaps in adult literacy and enrollment in primary schools, secondary schools, and universities.[26]

In spite of this progress, however, women continue to face discrimination, reduced pay, and fewer opportunities than men. These problems are strongest in the developing world. Women are less likely than men to be employed as politicians, managers, senior officials, and other powerful positions, and more likely to work as clerks, sales workers, and other lower-status, low-paying positions.[26] Women are working in greater numbers around the world, but still almost always have primary responsibilities for household chores, cooking, caregiving, and other housework. In all major areas of the world, women spend at least twice as much time as men doing unpaid household work.[26]

Women contribute to local, national and global economies through the informal sector. Informal work includes any position unrecognized or uncounted by government or other authorities; workers may grow food or make goods at home and sell them at an open market, or offer services such as manual labor, cleaning, or child care. Women make up the backbone of this growing movement. In some sub-Saharan African or Southeastern Asian countries, for example, nearly 90% of the female labor force is in the informal economy. Many economic experts believe that stimulating this informal sector may be an important way to promote long-term, healthy economic growth throughout the developing world. Examples of such efforts include microlending programs, where women receive small loans with reasonable interest rates to further their businesses without the need for collateral.

The rate of payback from these women-focused microlending programs has been higher than those observed with most other credit programs. Once women gain access to these loans, they can create sustainable and profitable business opportunities for themselves and their families, and protect themselves from the workplace health hazards that present themselves in many work environments. In addition, women typically reinvest the money they make in their local economies, and use it to improve the health of their families.

The United States, one of the richest countries in the world, is one of only three countries (the other two are Swaziland and Papua New Guinea, two developing countries with low incomes and poor infrastructure) that does

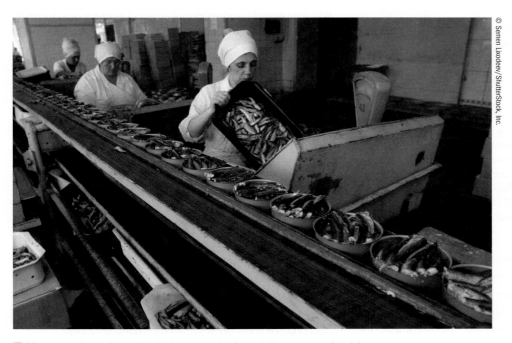

■ Women are becoming increasingly more active in workplaces across the globe.

not guarantee women any paid family leave.[28] Worldwide, 128 countries mandate some sort of paid family leave. For example:

- In Germany, a new mother receives 14 weeks of leave at full pay.

- In Canada, new mothers can take up to a full year off from work at 60% pay.

- In Norway, new mothers can take 1 year off from work at 100% pay.

- In Japan, new mothers can take up to 14 weeks at 60% of their pay.

- In South Africa, new mothers can take 4 months of paid leave, at up to 60% of their income.

- In Mexico, new mothers can take 12 weeks off from work at 75% pay.

Informed Decision Making

Sources of stress for women in the workplace may vary, depending on the profession they are in; their personality types; their age, race, or ethnicity; whether or not they have children; and other factors. All jobs, however, are likely to have some stress (being a homemaker has its own sources of stress, and for women looking for work, the search for a job can be a major source of stress). The key to improving one's mental health (and toward creating a more productive workplace) is to avoid stress when possible, and to deal with unavoidable stress in healthful ways. Supportive companies produce workers who are less stressed, feel more successful in the balancing of work and family, are more satisfied with both their work and home lives, and are more loyal and committed to their employers.[11]

I just had my second child, and I have 6 months off to care for him. My 2-year-old goes to day care at my firm's onsite childcare center. When I return to work, I'll work part time so I get to spend time with my children. The women of my firm have said that there's no problem with taking advantage of flextime and taking off 6 months to care for my newborn. I hope they're right! I feel very fortunate to be part of a firm that takes such good care of its employees.

30-year-old lawyer

Employers can help employees to better balance parenthood and work life by offering services related to family planning, preconception health care and counseling, and parenting classes. The Family and Medical Leave Act (FMLA) has been a valuable tool for many women. The

FMLA provides 12 weeks of unpaid, job-guaranteed leave for employees who need to care for newborns or a seriously ill relative, or to recover from a serious illness of their own. This benefit is available to employees who have worked at least 1,250 hours over the past year for employers with 50 or more employees. Currently, the act covers just over half of the country's private workforce. Workers in entry-level, low-paying jobs are less likely to be offered paid maternity leave than are managers and are less likely to get the time off after having a baby. More than half of the women who are covered by the FMLA do not know it. Although the FMLA was originally envisioned as dealing with a women's issue, almost half of those who have requested family and medical leave since its passage are men.

Employers can also ease new mothers' return to the workplace by providing breastfeeding support through lactation assistance programs and private breastfeeding rooms. Only 10% of working mothers continue nursing for 6 months following birth, compared with 24% of at-home mothers. Thirty-seven percent of employers currently provide opportunities for women who are nursing to continue to do so; this provision cuts down on absenteeism and healthcare costs for both mothers and infants.[5]

In addition, employers need to help employees find affordable, quality child care and elder care; develop childcare programs; or offer employee assistance for childcare facilities. Childcare assistance programs need to include more flexibility, by allowing for the needs of employees who work night and weekend shifts (**Figure 15.5**). Flexible work schedules, jobsharing programs, and prorated benefits for part-time and temporary employees also need to be enforced—two-thirds of part-time workers and three-fifths of temporary workers are women.[2] Some employers have established flexible work policies and are promoting the idea of a family-friendly workplace. Unfortunately, the people who need the extra support are the people who are often the least likely to receive it.

Women also need to be aware of their rights in the workplace. Women should not tolerate discrimination based on gender, race, religion, sexual orientation, disabilities, pregnancy, or other characteristics. Women who experience any of these forms of discrimination should promptly write down the details of the incident, and then report it to their supervisor or the company's human resources division. Women may also report a discrimination complaint with the Equal Employment Opportunity Commission (EEOC) or their state's fair employment agency.

Figure 15.5

Childcare Programs Need to be Developed with More Flexibility to allow for night and weekend shifts.

Profiles of Remarkable Women

Patricia Ireland (1945–)

Patricia Ireland began her career by working as a flight attendant for Pan American World Airlines from 1967 to 1975. Upon being told that her medical benefits didn't apply to her husband even though wives of male employees were covered, Ireland sued her employer and won—a victory that marked the beginning of her activism. Ireland received her law degree from the University of Miami Law School in 1975, then worked as a partner in a major Miami law firm. She served as legal counsel to Dade County and Florida National Organization for Women (NOW) for seven years. From 1987 to 1991, Ireland served as executive vice president and treasurer of the national NOW organization.

In 1991, Ireland became president of NOW, the largest, most visible, and most successful feminist organization in the United States. Her major contributions included organizing NOW activists to defend women's access to abortion, elect a record number of women to political office, work more closely in coalitions with other social justice and civil rights groups, and champion international feminist issues.

Ireland developed NOW's Project Stand Up for Women; in 1992, she led NOW in organizing a crowd of 750,000 for the organization's March for Women's Lives. In the same year, she initiated the "Elect Women for a Change" campaign. This campaign provided feminist candidates with experienced organizers who trained and deployed volunteers to staff phone banks, distribute leaflets and posters, organize fundraisers, and get people to the polls.

As part of NOW's work with the Up and Out of Poverty Now! coalition, Ireland delivered testimony and organized lobby days, news briefings, and protests on behalf of poor women. She served on the board of the Rainbow/PUSH Coalition and, in 1993, was a co-convener and keynote speaker for the 30th anniversary march on Washington commemorating the legacy of Dr. Martin Luther King, Jr. She has put forth significant efforts on behalf of lesbian and gay rights, including serving as a speaker and major organizer for the 1993 March on Washington for Gay, Lesbian, and Bi Civil Rights.

Ireland was the prime architect of NOW's Global Feminist Program. In 1992, she brought together women from more than 45 countries to participate in the Global Feminist Conference. Although no longer president of NOW, Ireland continues to champion many international feminist issues.

Profiles of Remarkable Women

Tina Fey (1970–)

© lev radin/ShutterStock, Inc.

Tina Fey is an actress, writer, producer, and comedian. For more than 15 years, she has worked and excelled in the field of comedy, a field traditionally and still largely dominated by men. Born and raised in Pennsylvania, Fey's interest in comedy began in the eighth grade, when she wrote an independent study project on the subject; during high school she joined the drama club and wrote comedy pieces for her school newspaper.[30] Fey studied drama and theater at the University of Virginia, where she was a self-described quiet, shy, and socially awkward student. After Fey graduated in 1992, she joined The Second City, an improv comedy group in Chicago that helped launch the careers of Dan Aykroyd, Gilda Radner, Steve Carell, and many other famous comedians.

In 1997, Fey accepted a writing position at *Saturday Night Live*. She wrote and performed on *Saturday Night Live* for 9 years, becoming the show's first female head writer in 1999, and becoming a recurring anchor on the show's Weekend Update sketches. Fey wrote about her experiences in the "boys' club" of the *Saturday Night Live* writing staff in her comedic memoir *Bossypants*. Fey enjoyed her work and appreciated the sense of humor of her male colleagues, even as she dealt with the challenge of writing and promoting sketches that did not come from an obviously male perspective. Fey wrote a sketch parodying feminine sanitary pads, but struggled for months to get the approval of her male cowriters, who were not familiar with the subject; when it aired, the sketch became one of the show's classic commercial parodies. As a performer, Fey also had to deal with the surface-obsessed entertainment industry in ways that her male colleagues did not: Fey only appeared in sketches after she lost a substantial amount of weight. While writing for *Saturday Night Live*, Fey wrote, produced and co-starred in *Mean Girls*, a teen comedy that explores high-school cliques.

Fey left *Saturday Night Live* to produce and star in *30 Rock*, a high-energy comedy series loosely based on her experiences on the show. As the show's protagonist Liz Lemon, Fey is both a role model and a comic figure: a capable and dedicated writer who regularly makes a mess out of her personal life; off the air, Fey married one of the show's composer, and gave birth to and raised two daughters while co-running the show. She also reappeared on *Saturday Night Live* to do a comedic take on vice-presidential candidate Sarah Palin during the 2008 election.

Fey has won seven Emmy Awards, two Golden Globes, and was the youngest winner of the Mark Twain Prize for American humor. Fey has dismissed male comedians who believe that women are not funny or less funny than men. In *Bossypants*, she wrote "It is an impressively arrogant move to conclude that just because you don't like something, it is empirically not good. I don't like Chinese food, but I don't write articles trying to prove it doesn't exist."

Summary

Women have become an integral part of the American workplace. The workplace can provide a social life, a support system, and opportunities for volunteering, and it affects people's moods and their values.

- Women are important parts of nearly every field and position, but inequities in pay and advancement persist.
- Women still shoulder the majority of the burden of children and home life, even when working.
- Millions of women have lost their jobs, received pay cuts, or been unable to find work as a result of the economic recession of 2008–2009.
- Women benefit greatly from quality, affordable, and accessible child care, enabling them to have choices about labor force participation.
- The stress of work and family, and the attempt to "do it all," creates stress and unhappiness for many women.

Employers must make an effort to create supportive and rewarding work environments. By promoting a healthy work–life balance, both employers and employees benefit. At the same time, women should strive to find such a balance in their lives, by setting priorities, discussing options with their employers and partners, and advocating for fairness and support in the workplace.

As both genders become accustomed to a more equitable sharing of responsibilities inside and outside the home, women will be afforded a more balanced existence between work and family. As Arlie Hochschild aptly states, "Up until now, the woman married to the 'new man' has been one of the lucky few. But as the government and society shape a new gender strategy, as the young learn from example, many more women and men will be able to enjoy the leisurely bodily rhythms and freer laughter that arise when family life is family life and not a second shift."[29]

Topics for Discussion

1. What questions should a woman ask before taking a job to ensure that she will receive all of the benefits that she may need?

2. Discuss how poverty creates additional barriers to employment opportunities for women.

3. What strategies could women use in the workplace to determine whether chemical, biological, or physical hazards are present?

4. How can women find balance in their professional, educational, and personal lives?

5. What are some strategies women can use when seeking greater equity opportunities in specific workplaces?

Key Terms

Anaphylactic shock: A severe and sometimes fatal allergic reaction to a foreign substance that causes symptoms such as weakness, shortness of breath, and falling blood pressure.

Carpal tunnel syndrome: A common, painful problem in the wrist and hand that occurs in the tendon and the carpal tunnel (a channel in the wrist for the nerve that serves the palm and thumb side of the hand). It is caused by pressure on the nerve that causes weakness; pain when the thumb is bent toward the palm; and burning, tingling, or aching that may spread to the forearm and shoulder.

Tendonitis: Inflammation caused by friction from overuse of tendons (connective tissues that attach muscle to bone).

Websites

American Federation of Labor—Congress of Industrial Organizations: http://www.aflcio.org

Business and Professional Women/USA: http://www.bpwusa.org

Institute for Women's Policy Research: http://www.iwpr.org

National Institute for Occupational Safety and Health—Women: http://www.cdc.gov/niosh/topics/women/

National Organization for Women: http://www.now.org

U.S. Department of Labor: http://www.dol.gov

U.S. Department of Labor—Bureau of Labor Statistics: http://www.bls.gov

References

1. U.S. Bureau of the Census. (1976). The Statistical History of the United States—From Colonial Times to the Present. Washington, DC: U.S. Department of Commerce.

2. U.S. Department of Labor. (2011). Women in the Labor Force: A Databook. Washington, DC: Bureau of Labor Statistics.

3. Parcel, T. L. (1999). Work and family in the 21st century: It's about time. *Work and Occupations* 26(2): 264–274.

4. Lowrey Y. (August 2006). Women in Business, 2006: A Demographic Review of Women's Business Ownership. Washington, DC: Office of Advocacy, U.S. Small Business Association.

5. Galinsky, E., Bond, J., & Sakai, K. (2008). *2008 National Study of Employers*. New York: Families and Work Institute.

6. Jans, L., & Stoddard, S. (1999). Chartbook on Women and Disability in the United States. An InfoUse Report. Washington, DC: U.S. National Institute on Disability and Rehabilitation Research, p. 18.

7. National Partnership for Women and Families. (2007). Where Families Matter: State Progress Toward Valuing America's Families. Washington, DC: National Partnership for Women and Families.

8. London, A., Scott, E., Edin, K., & Hunter, V. (2004). Welfare reform, work-family tradeoffs, and child well-being. *Family Relations* 53(2): 148–158.

9. Weichselbaumer, D., & Winter-Ebmer, R. (2005). A meta analysis of the international gender wage gap. *Journal of Economic Surveys* 19(3): 479–511.

10. AFL-CIO. (2006). Ask a Working Woman Survey. AFL-CIO Working Women's Department. Washington, DC: AFL-CIO.

11. DeNavas-Walt, C., Proctor, B. D., & Smith, J. C. (2008). Income, Poverty, and Health Insurance Coverage in the United States: 2007. U.S. Census Bureau, Current Population Reports, P60-235. Washington, DC: U.S. Government Printing Office.

12. AFL-CIO. (2003). Fact Sheet: Equal Pay for Women of Color. AFL-CIO Working Women's Department.

13. Goodwin, J. (2011). Multitasking stresses out working moms more than dads. *USA Today*. Available at: http://www.usatoday.com/news/health/wellness/story/2011-12-01/Multitasking-stresses-out-working-moms-more-than-dads/51545428/1

14. Lee, M., & Mather, M. (June 2008). U.S. Labor Force Trends. Washington, DC: Population Reference Bureau.

15. Federal Interagency Forum on Child and Family Statistics. (2006). America's Children: Key National Indicators of Well-Being, 2006. Washington, DC: U.S. Government Printing Office. Available at: http://childstats.gov/americaschildren/tables.asp

16. Wiggans, S., & Bergmann, B. (2003). America's Child Care Problem: The Way Out. New York: Macmillan.

17. Hochschild, A. R. (2001). *The Time Bind: When Work Becomes Home and Home Becomes Work*. New York: Holt Publishing.

18. Cartwright, C. (2007). 100 best companies for working mothers. *Working Mother*.

19. Holcomb, B. (2000). Friendly for whose family? *Ms.* 2(3): 40–45.

20. Wyn, R., & Soliz, B. (2004). Women's health issues across the lifespan. In Health Policy: Crisis and Reform in the U.S. Health Care Delivery System. Charlene Harrington, Carroll L. Estes, & Cassandra Crawford (Eds.), Sudbury, MA: Jones & Bartlett Publishers.

21. Judge, T. A., Jackson, C. L., Shaw, J. C., et al. (2007). Self-efficacy and work-related performance: the integral role of individual differences. *Journal of Applied Psychology* 92(1): 107–127.

22. U.S. Department of Labor. (2011). *Nonfatal occupational injuries and illnesses requiring days away from work, 2010*. Available at: http://www.bls.gov/news.release/osh2.nr0.htm

23. Centers for Disease Control and Prevention [CDC]. (2011). *Women's safety and health issues at work*. Available at: http://www.cdc.gov/niosh/topics/women/

24. Cheng, L., & Lee, D. (1999). Review of latex allergy. *Journal of the American Board of Family Practitioners* 12(4): 285–292.

25. U.S. Department of Labor Statistics, U.S. Department of Labor. (2012). *Census of fatal occupational injuries, 2010*. Available at: http://www.bls.gov/iif/oshcfoi1.htm

26. World Health Organization [WHO]. (2010). *The world's women, 2010*. Available at: http://unstats.un.org/unsd/demographic/products/Worldswomen/WW2010pub.htm

27. Blau, F. D., & Kahn, L. M. (2007). The gender pay gap. *The Economists' Voice* 4(4): 5–6.

28. European Union. (2009). *The EU and gender equality: Advancing women's full potential*. Available at: http://www.eurunion.org/News/eunewsletters/EUInsight/2009/EUInsight-GenderEqual-Apr-09.pdf

29. Yost, C. W. (2012). 3 reasons why card-carrying capitalists should support paid family leave. *Forbes*. Available at: http://www.forbes.com/sites/work-in-progress/2012/05/23/3-reasons-why-card-carrying-capitalists-should-support-paid-family-leave/3/

30. Hochschild, A. (1997). *The second shift*. New York, NY: Avon Books.

31. Murray, N. (2006). Interview with Tina Fey. *The AV Club*. Available at: http://www.avclub.com/articles/tina-fey,14025/